The Pregnancy Book
for
Today's Woman

D1401919

Also by
Howard I. Shapiro

The Birth Control Book

The Pregnancy Book for Today's Woman

Howard I. Shapiro, M.D.

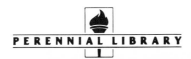

Harper & Row, Publishers
New York, Cambridge, Philadelphia, San Francisco
London, Mexico City, São Paulo, Singapore, Sydney

Permissions acknowledgments appear on page 463.

Designer: *Abigail Sturges*

Library of Congress Cataloging in Publication Data

Shapiro, Howard I.
    The pregnancy book for today's woman.

    Bibliography: p.
    Includes index.
    1. Pregnancy.   2. Childbirth.   3. Pregnant women—
Health and hygiene.   I. Title.
RG121.S495   1983   618.2   80–7916
ISBN 0–06–181766–X   84 85 86 87 10 9 8 7 6 5 4 3 2
ISBN 0–06–091059–3 (pbk.)   88 10 9 8 7

To
Jean Pike,
nurse extraordinaire and loyal friend,
and to
Bette, Suzanne, and Marjorie,
whose love inspired me to write this book

Contents

Tables

Boxes

Preface

Today's pregnant woman is far more fortunate than her sister of a decade ago. If her pregnancy is unwanted, she has the option of terminating it safely, thanks to the historic Supreme Court decision of 1973. If her pregnancy is welcome, the event of childbirth is now a time for happy anticipation, education, and participation rather than fear, ignorance, and isolation. Much credit for this healthy change of attitude must be given to the women's health movement in America. Feminists in particular and informed parents in general have helped force the medical establishment to make childbirth a more intimate and meaningful experience. If these consumers of obstetrical services had left it to their physicians to initiate change, they would probably still be waiting.

The patient-doctor relationship has also undergone a great upheaval during the past decade. The awe and docility with which women once approached their obstetricians has been replaced by a healthy skepticism and consumerism. As more information becomes available, fewer women are willing to accept a patronizing "doctor knows best" attitude. For some physicians, this change in female behavior has been intolerable. Others are yielding their power grudgingly, while a small number truly welcome and enjoy this new assertiveness and quest for education and participation on the part of their patients. Pertinent questions can no longer be answered in either a solicitous or a disdainful manner. If doctors expect to have obedient patients, they had better be prepared to provide intelligent reasons for the treatments they prescribe.

The questions asked by women of the eighties are different, more honest, and usually far more complex than their mothers or even their older sisters dared to ask.

"If I smoke marijuana, will it harm my baby?"

"How dangerous is pregnancy with an IUD?"

"Does LSD really cause chromosomes to break?"

"Can intercourse cause premature labor or miscarriage?"

"Is it true that a lovemaking technique has been responsible for the deaths of several pregnant women?"

"Is high-altitude air travel safe during pregnancy?"

"When traveling by car, is it all right to use a seat belt and, if so, how should it be worn?"

"Which vaccinations are safe to take before I travel abroad?"

"When I pass through a security system at an airport, does the radiation affect the fetus?"

"Is use of a microwave oven dangerous in pregnancy? How about radiation from my color television set?"

"Will one of the 'new' venereal diseases, such as herpes or chlamydia, harm my baby?"

This is not the usual pregnancy text dealing with heartburn, hemorrhoids, and how baby grows. There are already far too many books of that type. Instead, I have tried to pinpoint and discuss thoroughly the many different medical, social, and sexual problems that confront today's woman on each day of her pregnancy.

The book uses a question-and-answer format. Many of the problems covered here are those of the patients I saw as a practicing obstetrician over the past fifteen years. My greatest stimulus has been the questions these women asked. I am truly in their debt.

Acknowledgments

The author is indebted to Dawn Devaney for the hundreds of hours that she devoted to the typing and preparation of the manuscript. Her dedication and flawless effort is greatly appreciated. Thanks are also extended to Jo-Ann Friberg for her help in typing the earlier chapters. Joan Sjostrom and Jean Botts, the fine librarians at Norwalk (Connecticut) Hospital, helped me to locate the many references which were needed to successfully complete this project. I'm sure that they are as happy as I am that the book is finally completed.

Congratulations are extended to Carol Cohen, my editor and friend, for working so patiently with me over the past two years. Her knowledge of the subject and her enthusiasm and sensitivity have added immeasurably to the success of this book. I am also thankful to Russell Galen for instantly recognizing the importance of my work.

Finally, the encouragement I received from my beautiful wife Bette and my delightful daughters Suzanne and Marjorie will always be cherished.

The purpose of this book is to make you aware of the normal progress of pregnancy and the problems that may arise. You will need to consult your doctor to assess any problems or questions you may have; proper diagnosis and treatment of all symptoms connected with pregnancy call for careful attention to your concerns from your doctor.

1.
When Contraception Fails

Practical and serious problems can arise when pregnancy follows contraceptive failure. No method of birth control is 100 percent effective, and accidental pregnancies do occur even with the most reliable techniques. All methods, including the Pill, IUD, surgical sterilization, spermicides, and even rhythm, are associated with their own unique and potentially severe fetal and maternal risks. Sadly, few doctors take the time to inform couples of these risks when a contraceptive method is first prescribed. This chapter analyzes the various problems associated with pregnancy following contraceptive failure and the correct method of diagnosing and treating each specific complication.

Birth Control Pills

How do birth control pills prevent pregnancy?

Most birth control pills on the market today contain a synthetic estrogen combined with chemicals called progestogens or progestins and prevent pregnancy by stopping ovulation, the release each month of an egg from one of the two ovaries. The estrogen component of the pill inhibits the secretion of substances called releasing factors from an area of the brain, the hypothalamus. These hypothalamus releasing factors are vital for stimulating the hormones of the pituitary gland, which in turn act on the ovary to trigger ovulation. The estrogen and progestin contained in the Pill also prevent pregnancy by changing the endometrium, or lining of the uterus, in such a manner that even if ovulation did take place, implantation of a fertilized egg would be unsuccessful. Finally, the progestin produces a cervical mucus which is thick and hostile to sperm so that they are unable to penetrate and migrate through the cervical opening.

Pills which combine estrogen and progestin are taken each day for three weeks at a time, followed by one week of rest, during which time a menstrual period usually occurs. Commonly used brand names of combination pills are: Brevicon, Demulen, Lo/Ovral, Modicon, Norinyl, Norlestrin, Ortho-Novum, and Ovral.

Minipills are birth control pills which contain only progestin. They do not always prevent ovulation but exert their contraceptive effect by the dual action of thickening the cervical mucus and making the endometrium unreceptive to implantation of the fertilized egg. Unlike the combined pills, minipills are taken every day without interruption. Only three minipill brands are currently on the market: Micronor, Nor-Q.D., and Ovrette. A great advantage of the minipills is that they contain no estrogen and therefore are free of many of the serious complications found with the combination pills. However, they continue to remain unpopular because the high incidence of annoying bleeding is estimated to be almost 50 percent. In addition, the pregnancy rate among minipill users is significantly higher when compared to women using the more popular estrogen and progestin combinations.

If a pregnancy occurs while I am on the Pill, is it more likely to be in the tube rather than the uterus?

This depends on the type of birth control pill being used. A pregnancy located outside the uterus is called an ectopic pregnancy. By far the most common type of ectopic pregnancy is one in the fallopian tube, a tubal pregnancy. Rupture of the wall of the tube by an ectopic pregnancy may result in severe intra-abdominal hemorrhage and even death. Tubal pregnancies may also pass out the end of the tube. This condition is known as a tubal abortion. In extremely rare circumstances, the fetus will implant in the abdominal cavity and continue to grow after it is passed out of the tube. This type of pregnancy, known as an abdominal pregnancy, may go to term.

No reports suggest that users of combination-type oral contraceptives are more likely to suffer from an ectopic pregnancy if they accidentally conceive. However, data from at least eighteen separate studies strongly suggest a higher incidence of ectopic pregnancy among women who conceive while using the progestin-only minipill. One group of researchers suggested that the progestin norgestrel, the type found in Ovrette, was most likely to be the culprit; other studies have implicated norethindrone, which is found in both Nor-Q.D. and Micronor. In contrast, a progestin named lynestrenol, which is manufactured in Europe, has not been found to increase a woman's risk of ectopic pregnancy. The mechanism by which a minipill makes you more susceptible to an ectopic pregnancy is unknown. However, it is theorized that the progestin slows down the transport of the fertilized egg through the fallopian tube. As a result, it attaches itself within the tube rather than in its normal location within the endometrium of the uterus.

Your doctor should always consider the possibility of an ectopic pregnancy if you develop lower abdominal pain while on a progestin-only minipill.

Is it true that if I continue to take birth control pills without realizing I am pregnant, there is a chance that the genitals of my female fetus may be masculinized?

Yes. This has not been reported frequently, but it is a very real possibility. The reason for this is that the progestin in the Pill is a synthetic hormone more closely related to the male hormone testosterone than to the female hormone progesterone. The formation of a grossly enlarged clitoris, resembling a male penis, and a labia majora resembling a male scrotum is believed to be caused by the passage of progestins across the placenta at the time that these organs are being formed, between the seventh and twelfth weeks of pregnancy. If you stop the Pill before the seventh week, you can be assured that your female offspring will not be masculinized.

All birth control pills marketed in the United States today contain one of five progestins: norgestrel, ethynodiol diacetate, norethindrone acetate, norethindrone, and norethynodrel. By far the most potent and, theoretically, the one most likely to masculinize a female fetus is norgestrel, found in Ovral, Lo/Ovral, and Ovrette. Ethynodiol diacetate is next in potency and is found in Demulen and Ovulen. The least potent are norethynodrel and norethindrone.

Are birth defects more common among women who accidentally use birth control pills early in pregnancy or within two months before pregnancy begins?

The experts do not agree. Since 1973, there have been several reports noting an increased incidence of deformed babies born to women accidentally taking birth control pills early in pregnancy or given these and other hormones immediately before conception. In some cases the hormones were prescribed as pills or as an intramuscular injection to bring on a late period. In other cases the hormones were prescribed in an effort to maintain and support pregnancies threatening to end in miscarriage.

In 1973, Drs. James J. and Audrey H. Nora first described a characteristic pattern of anomalies in affected offspring to which they gave the acronym VACTERL (Vertebral, Anal, Cardiac, Tracheoesophageal, Renal, and Limb). They noted that when the hormone preparations were taken after a pregnancy had begun, the great majority of affected offspring were boys, but the distribution of affected males and females was equal if a woman stopped the Pill in the menstrual cycle just prior to conception. Several follow-up articles by the Noras, concluded that women who take hormones early in pregnancy are two to four times more likely than other women to bear children with one or several of these malformations. The validity of these findings has been questioned by scientists who rightfully claim that the number of patients studied over the four years was too small to be statistically reliable. In fact, the Noras did not uncover one case of the VACTERL syndrome associated with prenatal hormone exposure between July 1, 1973, and June 30, 1977. This is hardly convincing evidence of a major epidemic of such anomalies.

In 1974, epidemiologist Dr. Dwight T. Janerich of the New York State Department of Health in Albany studied 108 mothers of children with congenital limb-reduction defects and 108 mothers of normal children. Among the mothers of malformed children, 15, or 14 percent, were found to have been exposed to oral contraceptives or progestins during pregnancy. Only 4, or 4 percent, of the control mothers were similarly exposed. There was nothing unusual about the sex ratio among defective children who had not been exposed to hormones, but the 11 defective children who had been exposed to hormones were all males. Other researchers in 1974 noted increased chromosome breakage in cultures taken of women using oral contraceptives.

In 1980, doctors at the Hadassah-Hebrew University Medical Center in Jerusalem studied 108 infants conceived while their mothers were taking oral contraceptives. A significantly higher number of these infants died at birth than other newborns. In addition 10 were born with a variety of malformations, and as in the Janerich study, more male babies (8) than females were malformed.

In a much larger study published in the January 13, 1977, issue of the prestigious *New England Journal of Medicine,* researchers presented further evidence linking fetal exposure to female hormones with cardiac birth defects. Among the 1,042 women receiving female hormones during the first four months of pregnancy, the incidence of cardiac defects was 18.2 per 1,000 births, compared to 7.8 per 1,000 births in the control group. Of these 1,042 women, a subgroup of 278 specifically used birth control pills. There were 6 children born with cardiac birth defects in this group, equal to an incidence of 21.5 per 1,000 births.

Not all investigators agree that inadvertent use of birth control pills early in pregnancy predisposes a woman to fetal anomalies. In fact, several highly respected epidemiologists have pointed out the various shortcomings of these previous reports. A very large study conducted by the Royal College of General Practitioners in England in 1974 failed to show any relationship between pill ingestion and birth defects. Similarly, an American study in 1971 concluded there was no significant difference in the incidence of birth defects between 1,250 previous pill users and 1,250 non–pill users. Doctors at the University of Helsinki reported in 1981 that a study of the contraceptive usage of 3,002 mothers of children with malformations detected at birth failed to show any link between Pill use and birth defects. The most convincing study, refuting the relationship between hormone use and congenital anomalies, was published in the *New England Journal of Medicine* in 1978. Researchers at the Harvard School of Public Health studied the birth certificates of 7,723 infants whose mothers had taken birth control pills. When compared to a control group, the number of recorded malformations was found to be essentially equal in both groups.

These contradictory reports can only confuse a woman seeking sound advice about this very important question. But there are vital lessons here. First, the entire problem can be avoided if the absence of pregnancy is confirmed before oral contraceptives are started. This may sound like a simple suggestion, but it is violated repeatedly by women and their doctors. Second, hormones should no longer be used as pregnancy tests or as a method of bringing on periods and should rarely, if ever, be used to support a pregnancy in jeopardy. In the rare cases where the last is necessary, pure progesterone preparations given intramuscularly appear to be safest for the developing fetus.

If you miss one or more pills during a cycle, followed by no period after the last birth control pill is taken, get a pregnancy test before starting a new box of pills. The risk to the fetus is greatest if you restart the pills when you are pregnant, since VACTERL anomalies are most likely to occur between the fifteenth and the sixtieth day of embryo development.

Though most authorities continue to argue over whether or not birth control pills taken early in pregnancy are harmful, the vast majority now agree that hormones taken before conception will not adversely affect the fetus. Despite this, most doctors still suggest that if you stop using the Pill, you should continue with another form of contraception for three months before trying to become pregnant. The reason for this is not a fear of fetal anomalies but a desire on the part of the doctor to determine the exact date of conception, since periods tend to be irregular for the first three months after stopping the Pill. If pregnancy should inadvertently occur during this time, elective abortion because of fear of a fetal anomaly would appear to be ill-advised. In fact, pregnancy following use of oral contraceptives has been evaluated by several research groups, and some interesting positive results are described below.

Does prior use of the Pill have any good effects when a woman does have a baby?

Yes. Two large studies from England in 1976 and one from the United States in 1977 all agree that women who conceive following the use of birth control pills actually have slightly lower miscarriage and stillborn rates. In 1977, Dr. Kenneth J. Rothman of the Harvard School of Public Health reviewed the pregnancies of 8,616 women who used oral contraceptives prior to conception. He noted fewer spontaneous abortions and stillbirths. He reported that when pregnancy followed pill use of at least six months' duration and conception occurred within one month of stopping the Pill, the twin pregnancy rate was actually twice that of the general population. The twin increase was among fraternal (nonidentical) twins, resulting from ovulation and fertilization of two different eggs by two different sperm. In a similar study from Yale University in 1979, it was reported that of 4,428 women who conceived within two months of oral contraceptive use, there was a doubling in the rate of non-identical-twin pregnancies. Others have concluded that the incidence of multiple births actually decreases among former oral contraceptive users. This finding was also observed by Israeli researchers in a 1979 published report. The only exceptions to this trend were the higher twinning rates among former pill users who were underweight in relation to their height at the time of conception, those who inadvertently conceived while taking the Pill, and users of products containing higher doses of estrogen.

An interesting 1978 report from the Hadassah-Hebrew University Medical Center in Jerusalem showed that former pill users' babies experienced a death rate of 10.4 per 1,000 compared with 15.3 for nonusers. The rate of infants born with heart defects was 1.7 per 1,000 for users compared with 3.7 per 1,000 for nonusers. However, on the negative side, the researchers were surprised to find a higher rate of Down's syndrome, or mongolism, among former Pill users. This chromosomal abnormality occurred at a rate of 3.3 per 1,000, compared to 1.8 per 1,000 among women who did not use the Pill (see chapter 10).

Has anyone ever evaluated the IQ and personality of children born to mothers who used birth control pills?

Amazingly, very little research has been done on the mental capacity of children whose mothers were exposed to sex hormones prior to gestation. The largest study of this type was conducted at the University of Puerto Rico School of Medicine in

1974. The children studied ranged in age from five to eight, and their mothers had previously taken birth control pills of a dosage much greater than is currently used today. Despite this, their average IQ was exactly equal to a group whose mothers used methods of contraception other than the Pill.

In 1978, the children of thirty-four women, given either progestin alone or in combination with estrogen during the first three months of pregnancy, were studied by a Rutgers University researcher, Dr. June Machover Reinisch. She noted definite personality differences among the children exposed to prenatal hormones when compared to a similar group of children not exposed to these hormones and she noted significant differences between the progestin and estrogen treatment groups. Progestin group children were described as "significantly more independent, sensitive, individualistic, self-assured, and self-sufficient than the exposed offspring of the estrogen group; while the estrogen group subjects were more group-oriented and group-dependent." The IQs of both groups were similar. When both estrogen- and progestin-exposed subjects were compared to unexposed siblings within their families, similar results were obtained. It is obvious that more extensive studies involving many more women are needed before definite conclusions can be reached.

Is it true that a woman is more likely to give birth to a girl if conception occurs soon after birth control pills are discontinued?

No. In 1974, a medical journal from England, *Lancet,* reported a nearly 2-to-1 female-to-male birth ratio when conception occurred immediately following use of oral contraceptives, but the study involved less than 200 pregnancies. A large study in 1976 from the Harvard School of Public Health noted the female-to-male ratio to be 1-to-1 among 6,000 recorded births which followed oral contraceptive use.

Can birth control pills cause vitamin or mineral deficiencies which may be harmful to a pregnancy which occurs soon after the Pill is stopped?

Yes. Several studies have indicated that the estrogen in oral contraceptives prevents the body from absorbing certain important vitamins and minerals, such as folic acid, vitamin B6 (pyridoxine), vitamin B12, riboflavin, zinc, and possibly vitamin C.

The longer a woman is on the Pill, the more likely she is to experience a depletion of her stores of folic acid, a B vitamin essential for normal development of a fetus and necessary for the formation of hemoglobin. Folic acid deficiency, though, rarely reaches the point of overt anemia. Many authorities suggest that women on birth control pills for longer than a year eat foods which are rich in folic acid, such as liver, veal, kidney, lean meat, yeast, raw green leafy vegetables, and citrus fruit juices. Others recommend vitamin supplements equal to 400 micrograms a day, which is the Recommended Daily Allowance (RDA). During pregnancy, the RDA for folic acid actually doubles to 800 micrograms per day (see chapter 8). If a woman is lacking in folic acid as a result of using the Pill, the hormonal changes of pregnancy will often worsen the deficiency. This may create a potentially hazardous situation for a developing fetus during the first three months of pregnancy, since there is ample evidence that such a deficiency may be associated with very serious birth deformities. Though this problem is admittedly rare, many experts believe that it can be totally prevented if all long-term oral contraceptive users have their folic-acid blood level determined prior to a planned conception.

Vitamin B6, most investigators agree, diminishes in concentration among women using oral contraceptives. Despite the fact that it has been studied intensively, no one is really quite sure if low levels of vitamin B6 in the bloodstream will adversely affect a woman's pregnancy. A deficiency of vitamin B6 appears to interfere with the metabolism of glucose, a sugar. This has led several investigators to theorize that diabetic abnormalities which develop among some women on the Pill and during pregnancy may be related to a B6 deficiency. Though adverse psychological effects of the Pill, such as depression, have been associated with the progestins they contain, some authors have attributed this symptom to a deficiency of vitamin B6. Several workers in the field have suggested that all women using oral contraceptives receive a vitamin B6 supplement daily. The RDA is 2 milligrams for adult women not using birth control pills. A daily dose over ten times that, or 25 milligrams, is recommended for women who use birth control pills. This will prevent a B6 deficiency if pregnancy immediately follows oral contraceptive use. Foods rich in B6 are wheat germ, liver, meats, fish, kidney, whole grain cereals, milk, soybeans, bananas, peanuts, and corn. Though vitamin C (ascorbic acid) requirements for women using the Pill have not been thoroughly investigated, it would appear that they are increased slightly. There are many adequate sources of vitamin C even in the diet of indigent women, and to my knowledge there has never been a case of severe vitamin C deficiency resulting from pregnancy occurring immediately after the use of birth control pills.

The serum level of vitamin B12 decreases during oral contraceptive use, but this is probably of no clinical significance during a subsequent pregnancy. Pernicious anemia resulting from a severe vitamin B12 deficiency is practically unheard of among pregnant women.

Riboflavin levels also decrease with the use of oral contraceptives. The need for riboflavin is often closely related to that of vitamin B6, since both vitamins are used by the body in a similar fashion (see chapter 8).

A deficiency of zinc secondary to use of birth control pills has also been reported. However, no clinical significance of this alteration has been observed, and therapeutic doses of minerals are not recommended.

Are there certain medical problems which, if they occur while I am on the Pill, are more likely to happen again during pregnancy?

Yes. An alert physician is sometimes able to predict which women may encounter difficulties during pregnancy based on their reactions to the Pill. The development of diabetes is a perfect example. Most investigators agree that oral contraceptives have a detrimental effect on blood sugar and blood insulin in healthy, as well as diabetic, women. The estrogen and progestin components have both been held responsible for these changes. Among women with normal glucose (sugar) tolerance tests before using the Pill, it is estimated that at least 10 percent develop an abnormal test while taking the Pill. This "chemical diabetes" produces no symptoms and reverts to normal when the birth control pill is no longer used. But this abnormality may reappear when predisposed individuals are subjected to the hormonal stimulation and stress of pregnancy. It is a good idea for your doctor to test you for this condition one or more times during pregnancy, especially if you exhibited glucose intolerance when using birth control pills.

An abnormal elevation of blood pressure, or hypertension, develops in approximately 5 to 7 percent of all women who use the Pill and usually drops to normal within six months after the Pill is stopped. Similarly, an elevation of blood pressure during the last three months of pregnancy, termed preeclampsia, or toxemia, appears more likely among these susceptible women. If you have a history of hypertension while using the Pill, you should be carefully watched during your pregnancy.

Both the Pill and pregnancy are responsible for alterations in blood platelets and certain blood substances called clotting factors. This in turn may subject a very small percentage of susceptible women to inflammatory blood clots in the veins of the legs and pelvis, a condition called thrombophlebitis. Thrombophlebitis of the deep veins of the legs and pelvis often presents a real threat to a women's life because these clots can become dislodged and travel through the circulatory system to a vital organ such as the lung, causing instant death. If you have a history of previous deep-vein thrombophlebitis while on the Pill, your obstetrician may want to consider anticoagulation, or medical thinning of the blood, with a drug called heparin.

Approximately 3 women out of every 100,000 using the Pill each year develop a benign though potentially fatal liver tumor called hepatocellular adenoma, or hepatoma. The growth of these tumors appears to be linked to the estrogen in the Pill, and those oral contraceptives with the highest doses of estrogen are the most dangerous. Some investigators believe it is the combined effect of the progestin and the estrogen which is to blame for this problem. Women who are most susceptible are those over thirty who have used the Pill for more than four years. Rupture of a hepatoma results in massive intra-abdominal hemorrhage, and often the only symptoms preceding this catastrophe are the suggestion of a mass (enlargement) or fullness and slight pain under the right rib cage or on the right upper side of the abdomen. The diagnosis of hepatoma before rupture usually can be accomplished by an x-ray scan of the liver. After the birth control pills are discontinued, the tumor usually diminishes in size and remains dormant.

However, reactivation of hepatocellular adenoma is possible days or even years later if the Pill is restarted or if pregnancy occurs. Several deaths from ruptured adenomas have been reported during the pregnancy of women with a previous history of pill-induced hepatoma. If a woman with a history of hepatoma does conceive, it is vital that a doctor see her often and palpate her abdomen for enlargement or upper abdominal pain during each prenatal visit. Pregnancy must be terminated at the first indication that the tumor has recurred in order to avoid the risk of continued enlargement and a potentially fatal rupture. Some doctors recommend delivery by cesarean section for women with a history of pill-induced hepatoma, even if there are no clinical signs or symptoms that the tumor has recurred. The reason for this is their fear that the bearing-down maneuvers during the final stage of labor may create excessive tension on a small, undiagnosed hepatoma. Since rupture of a hepatoma requires replacement with large volumes of blood, observation in a well-equipped hospital with a modern blood bank is essential. It is not known if cutting out a hepatoma prior to pregnancy will guarantee a problem-free gestation, since smaller tumors may have the capacity to grow under the influence of the pregnancy hormones. Furthermore, surgery of this type even under the best of circumstances is extremely difficult and potentially very dangerous.

IUDs

What is an IUD?

An IUD, or intrauterine device, is a device inserted into the uterine cavity and left there for various periods of time for the purpose of contraception. There are approximately three million women in the United States currently using the IUD for contraception. Ever since 1909, gynecologists seeking immortality have had IUDs of various sizes and shapes named after them. Names such as Grafenberg, Hall, Stone, Birnberg, Marguiles, Lippes, and Majzlin are remembered fondly by some women and with disdain and hatred by a great number of others.

Modern IUDs are made of polyethylene plastic coated with barium which makes them visible on x-ray. IUDs are divided into two groups: nonmedicated devices, consisting only of plastic, and medicated devices which contain plastic combined with either copper (like the Cu-7) or progesterone (Progestasert). Most IUDs have a nylon tail, or strings, which protrude from the cervix into the vagina. By touching the tail or viewing it with a speculum, you and your doctor can usually be assured that the IUD is in place.

How does an IUD prevent pregnancy?

Several theories exist. For example, the presence of an IUD in the uterine cavity is known to stimulate an inflammatory reaction. As a result, large microscopic cells called macrophages are released. These are believed by some researchers to be capable of destroying sperm before they can get into the tube to fertilize the egg. Medicated IUDs containing copper and progesterone are believed to further enhance the hostility of the uterine lining, or endometrium. Others insist that macrophages destroy an already fertilized egg each month, thereby causing an early abortion. Evidence supporting the first theory comes from a 1977 study at the University of Southern California in which twenty-four women with IUDs had their blood analyzed daily for the presence of the pregnancy hormone, called human chorionic gonadotropin, or HCG, during the second half of the menstrual cycle. These researchers were unable to find any elevation of HCG. The absence of pregnancy hormone would lead one to conclude from this study that the IUD did not cause a miniabortion but, instead, prevented the sperm from fertilizing the egg. Another study in support of this theory involved artificial insemination of five women volunteers wearing IUDs within an hour before a scheduled hysterectomy. In the absence of an IUD, it is known that sperm rapidly passes from the cervix and into the uterine cavity. From there they enter the fallopian tubes within minutes. However, at the time of surgery, sperm were not found in the tubes. This led the authors to conclude that the IUD caused macrophages to intercept and destroy the sperm.

Equally convincing evidence is available to support the miniabortion theory. In 1976, investigators from Cornell University and the State University of New York, Downstate Medical Center, reported that the levels of HCG were elevated in the second part of the menstrual cycle among women wearing the IUD. The reasons for the discrepancy between this study and those from California remain unanswered at the present time.

Another very strong point in favor of the IUD's acting as an interceptor of a fertilized egg, rather than a preventer of fertilization, is the fact that it can be used effectively as a morning-after method of contraception. Several studies have confirmed that an IUD inserted the morning after unprotected intercourse at midcycle, and even as late as five days after intercourse, practically always prevents an unwanted pregnancy, probably by creating an unfavorable environment for the fertilized egg entering the uterine cavity from the tube.

Another theory of IUD action is that its presence in the uterus as a foreign object increases the motility of the fallopian tubes and thus stimulates the movement of the egg down the tube at a rate which is faster than would normally occur. As a result, an egg too immature to implant into the uterine lining reaches the endometrium prematurely. Copper in high concentrations is known to enhance this increase in tubal motility.

What should I do if I become pregnant while using an IUD?

Regardless of the type of IUD you have, if you decide to continue with the pregnancy, your doctor should remove the device as soon as possible. By doing this, your risk of miscarriage is reduced to approximately 30 percent, compared to 50 percent if the IUD is left in place. (The risk of miscarriage is normally around 10 percent.) If the IUD strings cannot be seen, the device may be easily located by ultrasound. This modern technique has the great advantage of not exposing the fetus to radiation (see chapter 10). If early miscarriage does not occur when the IUD is left in the uterus, a woman is still at four times greater danger of experiencing premature labor during this pregnancy.

If it is determined that the IUD is in the uterus but cannot be removed, it is the duty of your obstetrician to warn you that you may develop a severe and even life-threatening infection during the pregnancy. The option of therapeutic abortion with removal of the IUD should be presented to all women in this predicament.

How can an IUD cause infection during pregnancy, and what are the symptoms?

A great variety of bacteria normally inhabit the vagina and are often found on the IUD strings as well. When these strings are taken up into the enlarging uterus during pregnancy, the bacteria they contain will have the potential in a small percentage of women to cause a severe infection within the uterine cavity. Spread of such an infection may then take place through the muscle of the uterus and out into the lower pelvis. During the infectious process, the fallopian tubes and ovaries may become matted together in a ball of pus called a tubo-ovarian abscess. Patients in which such an abscess ruptures have a very high mortality rate. Bacteria may also enter the bloodstream and attack distant organs, producing an overwhelming reaction and a drop in blood pressure called septic shock which may also be fatal. When infection occurs in a woman wearing an IUD, this type of infection is most apt to happen during the first six months of pregnancy.

The severity of IUD-related infections during pregnancy was never appreciated until 1974 when the A. H. Robins Company, maker of the now-infamous Dalkon Shield, reported that 4 women with this device had died of sepsis during pregnancy. Later in 1974, the Food and Drug Administration (FDA) reported that a total of 14 deaths and 219 cases of septic or infected abortion had been attributed to the use of the Dalkon Shield. Based on this information, the Dalkon Shield was taken off the market. However, few women are aware of the fact that all IUDs are capable of causing infection and even death during pregnancy. In the FDA hearings on the Dalkon Shield, it was pointed out that 15 septic deaths were also traced to the Lippes Loop, while 3 were attributed to use of the Saf-T-Coil. And recent studies have confirmed that the Cu-7 may also be associated with severe infection during pregnancy.

Sadly, IUD infections during pregnancy are often extremely difficult to diagnose. In many of the reported cases, the women did not develop symptoms specific to the pelvis until late in the course of the disease. Instead, the initial symptoms often appeared only as a general feeling of tiredness, possibly some respiratory symptoms accompanied with generalized muscle aching, fever, chills, headache, and other flu-like symptoms. These symptoms often rapidly progressed within a matter of hours to irreversible septic shock. When symptoms are present in the pelvis, more than half the women with infection will experience tenderness over the uterus accompanied by a pus-filled vaginal discharge. Other common symptoms are bleeding and leakage of infected amniotic fluid from the vagina.

Some doctors have suggested that if suspicious symptoms develop but the diagnosis remains uncertain, an amniocentesis (see chapter 10) should be performed immediately and the sample of amniotic fluid examined for evidence of infection, such as the presence of white blood cells and bacteria.

Regardless of the length of the pregnancy, the diagnosis of sepsis resulting from an IUD requires immediate termination of the pregnancy and aggressive antibiotic therapy. Though this may appear to be harsh treatment in a pregnancy that has progressed to six months, if it is not done the infection will rapidly spread to a point where even hysterectomy will not be able to contain it.

Is ectopic pregnancy more common in women wearing an IUD?

Yes. Women who become pregnant while using an IUD are more likely than other women to have an abnormal pregnancy in the tube or the ovary. Both types of pregnancy are called ectopic pregnancies, and both may cause severe abdominal hemorrhage and even death. Among women not using the IUD, the incidence of tubal pregnancy is approximately 1 out of every 250 pregnancies. Among users of all IUDs except the Progestasert, the incidence of ectopic pregnancy is between 2 and 3 per 100 accidental pregnancies, with progressively higher rates reported the longer the IUD is used. Furthermore, there is adequate evidence to suggest that the previous use of an IUD increases a woman's chances of suffering from an ectopic pregnancy. The increased incidence of ectopic pregnancy among IUD users is believed to be related to the greater likelihood of tubal infection among this group of women. Such infections hinder the fertilized egg from passing down the tube to its normal location in the endometrium. As a result, it becomes trapped in the tube and grows there instead. Since the IUD prevents pregnancy in the uterus but not in the tube, even in the absence of infection a high percentage of women who conceive with the IUD will have a tubal pregnancy. One very disturbing report published in 1977 claimed that the Progestasert IUD was responsible for a five times greater number of ectopic pregnancies than any other device. The cause of this is obscure, but one of the authors of this paper, Dr. Howard Tatum, believes that it is due to the fact that the progesterone in the device may prevent the fertilized egg from moving down the tube as fast as it usually does. As a result, the pregnancy grows in the lining of the tube rather than into the endometrium of the uterus. At the present time, the FDA has requested that the manufacturers of this device reanalyze their statistics to determine the exact frequency of this very serious condition.

Certainly, if you conceive while using the Progestasert or any other IUD, your doctor should strongly consider the diagnosis of ectopic pregnancy. Symptoms of pregnancy accompanied by lower abdominal discomfort and a slight amount of dark vaginal bleeding can indicate an ectopic pregnancy. Movement of the cervix, either through intercourse or pelvic examination, usually elicits extreme pain in the lower abdomen. Occasionally it is possible for your doctor to detect an enlargement in the tube which contains the ectopic pregnancy.

Often women suffering from an ectopic pregnancy will not have the typical pregnancy symptoms, and the possibility of this diagnosis may be overlooked by the examining doctor. In one study of seventy women diagnosed as having an ectopic pregnancy associated with an IUD, the symptoms of bleeding and pelvic pain were often attributed to the mere presence of the IUD and not the pregnancy itself. Significantly, in over 50 percent of these patients, the IUD was removed between one and eight weeks before the definitive diagnosis of ectopic pregnancy at surgery, presumably in the hope that the removal or changing of the IUD would alleviate the symptoms. Therefore, it is vital to remember that if you continue to experience pain and bleeding after the IUD is removed, the diagnosis of ectopic pregnancy should be strongly considered and a pregnancy test obtained to confirm this possibility.

An ectopic pregnancy which occurs in the ovary rather than in the tube is called an ovarian pregnancy. The incidence of this extremely rare condition in the general population is reported to be 1 out of 100 to 200 tubal pregnancies. However, among IUD users, the incidence increases to 1 ovarian pregnancy for every 7 to 9 tubal pregnancies. Symptoms of a pregnancy in the ovary are identical to those which occur when the pregnancy is located in the tube.

If only a minimal amount of tissue along with the IUD is removed during an abortion of an IUD user with a positive pregnancy test, ectopic pregnancy should be strongly suspected. Diagnosis of this condition prior to rupture is easily achieved by means of a laparoscopy and ultrasound.

Can an IUD cause injury to the fetus?

It has been estimated that 20,000 to 30,000 infants are born each year to American women with "IUD pregnancies." It is only natural that these women express fears that the IUD may harm or cause deformity of the fetus by entangling a limb or other parts of the body. Fortunately, this does not happen, since the IUD always lies outside the gestational or pregnancy sac of the baby. Of greater concern is our inability to predict the potential dangers of chemicals such as progesterone and copper lying in close proximity to the developing fetus.

To date, there have been no malformations reported among infants following exposure to the Progestasert IUD in utero, though the number of infants born under such circumstances is still too small to draw definite conclusions. It is not totally accurate to compare the fetal effects of progesterone released from the Progestasert with the synthetic progestins contained in birth control pills. Most authorities agree that the latter have a far greater potential for causing anomalies than progesterone, a hormone which is present in abundance throughout all pregnancies. Experimental IUDs containing progestin rather than progesterone are now being evaluated. I am far more concerned about the close proximity of these devices to the developing fetus than I am about the progesterone which is found in the Progestasert device.

A 1975 report in the *British Medical Journal* described 2 women who conceived while using IUDs containing copper. Both gave birth to infants with similar limb defects in which some of the bones in the leg, arm, hand, and foot were missing. Contrary to this is a 1976 study from the Population Council of New York. This extremely large project involved 157 women carrying a pregnancy to completion in the presence of a copper-containing IUD. Only 1 minor congenital anomaly was noted among the offspring of these women, and this was a benign growth on the vocal cord of one of the babies. There were no limb deformities in any of the offspring. Other studies measuring copper levels of spontaneously aborted fetuses, exposed to the Cu-7 in utero, revealed no increase in copper in the fetal brain, liver, or kidney. Finally, and most importantly, was a study conducted by scientists from the Centers for Disease Control. Mothers of 96 infants born with shortened and deformed limbs over a six-year period were interviewed and compared with two control groups. The results, published in the January 1979 issue of *Fertility and Sterility,* indicated that there was no significant increase in the occurrence of limb reduction deformities among babies exposed to the IUD at the time of conception.

Spermicides

Can contraceptive gels, creams, or foam used by a woman harm her fetus?

Vaginal spermicides or sperm-killing preparations are available without prescription at all drugstores in the form of creams, gels, aerosol foam, tablets, and suppositories.

All spermicidal preparations consist of the spermicidal agent and an inert base which physically blocks the sperm, disperses the spermicide, and holds it against the cervix. Nonoxynol-9 and octoxynol-9 are the names of the spermicides found in practically all of these preparations. Spermicides in the past contained mercury and chemicals named hydroquinones. There was some concern that these compounds might affect the genetic material in the sperm, leading to conception with birth defects, or be absorbed into the bloodstream, causing toxicity in women using them. As a result, these agents were taken off the market several years ago.

Until recently, it was believed that currently used vaginal spermicides were completely innocuous. Within the past three years, however, at least four separate reports have questioned the validity of this assumption. Two separate independent studies have noted limb reduction deformities among newborns whose mothers used spermicidal contraception. In 1980, researchers studied spontaneous abortions and found a higher portion of two lethal chromosomal abnormalities in the pregnancies of women who were using a spermicide at the time of conception. They speculated that spermicides may occasionally damage, rather than kill, sperm cells, and this may allow an abnormal sperm to fertilize an egg. Others have theorized that spermicides may be absorbed into the bloodstream and produce direct damage to the egg before conception. Recent scientific evidence from Germany has demonstrated that 1.5 percent of a measured amount of nonoxynol-9 was found in the urine samples of women twenty minutes after it was applied vaginally. Longer exposures produced a urine concentration of 10 percent. Another possible mechanism of spermicide damage would be a direct effect on the embryo if these products are inadvertently used after conception has occurred.

The most distressing of the recent reports came from the Boston Collaborative Drug Surveillance Program. This 1981 report found that women who had used a vaginal spermicide in the ten months before conception were more likely than other women to give birth to a baby with a major congenital anomaly. Among 763 infants whose mothers had used spermicides, there was a 2.2 percent incidence of major congenital anomalies, compared to 1 percent in a nonexposed control group of 3,902 babies. Specific defects included limb-reduction deformities, chromosomal abnormalities such as Down's syndrome (see chapter 10), and a defect of the male genitalia known as hypospadias. Certain rare neoplasms were also more likely to occur among these offspring. In addition, it was reported that pregnancies following spermicide use were 1.8 times more likely to end in spontaneous abortion requiring hospitalization when compared to pregnancies in the control group.

Many scientists and epidemiologists have pointed out several deficiencies in the study. As expected, pharmaceutical firms have presented several company-sponsored animal studies attesting to the safety of nonoxynol-9 and octoxynol-9 and have quoted other clinical reports showing no association between a woman's use of spermicides and the presence of birth defects or spontaneous abortions following conception.

Several long-term epidemiological studies will have to be instituted before the final answer on this vital topic can be given. The findings, however, are quite disconcerting. For the woman who is understandably concerned because she conceives while using a spermicidal preparation, it is somewhat reassuring to note that the risk of a poor pregnancy outcome would still be extremely low. In fact, while the Boston Collaborative Drug Surveillance Program group noted a 2.2 percent incidence of major congenital anomalies among offspring of women who used spermicides, this number is still well within the expected rate of 1 to 3 percent found in the United States population. In my opinion, pregnancy termination would not be warranted if conception follows spermicide failure.

DES, The "Morning-After" Pill

What is the "morning-after" pill?

Diethylstilbestrol, or DES, is the "morning-after" pill, which, when taken within seventy-two hours of unprotected coitus at ovulation, is highly effective in preventing survival of the fertilized egg. The drug is classified as a nonsteroidal synthetic estrogen, which is another way of saying it is made in the laboratory, not in the body, and is of a chemical structure which is totally different from the steroidal shape of natural estrogens and those contained in birth control pills.

How does DES prevent continuation of pregnancy?

Dr. John Morris of Yale University defines the term "interception" as the process of preventing implantation of the egg after fertilization has occurred. It is theorized that DES may act as a pregnancy interceptor at several locations. One of its main effects appears to be on the corpus luteum, causing it to malfunction and produce inadequate amounts of the progesterone which is essential for support of an early pregnancy. A decline of progesterone is occasionally reflected by a premature drop in the basal body temperature during the second half of the menstrual cycle.

A second and also very likely site of DES action is the endometrium, where it causes a deficiency of an enzyme called carbonic anhydrase. Without this enzyme, the fertilized egg cannot dispose of its carbon dioxide waste products and therefore dies. Other studies of the endometrium have noted microscopic retardation of growth, in addition to a lack of another enzyme called alkaline phosphatase.

In the past it was theorized that DES was responsible for both slowing down and speeding up the passage of the fertilized egg down the fallopian tube. This "tube locking" effect was believed to be responsible for the higher incidence of ectopic pregnancy in women who conceived despite DES treatment. However, it is now generally believed that DES prevents intrauterine pregnancy, not tubal pregnancy. Therefore, if pregnancy does take place, the chances that it will be in the tube are greater, though the actual number of tubal pregnancies is no higher.

What is the effect on the developing fetus if DES fails to successfully intercept a pregnancy?

If DES fails to successfully intercept a pregnancy, its effects on the fetus at that early stage, though still unknown, may be similar to those produced by birth control pills (see page 3). Due to its nonsteroidal configuration, DES, when inadvertently taken after a pregnancy is already a few weeks along will increase the risk of vaginal and cervical abnormalities, as well as cancer, in any daughter born from that pregnancy. The characteristic DES abnormalities only occur when it is taken after the seventh week from the last menstrual period. Furthermore, abnormalities, though possible, are less likely to occur among women who first take DES after the nineteenth week of pregnancy.

How is DES, given to a mother, related to vaginal cancer in her daughter?

Practically all medication given to a mother is capable of crossing the placenta and reaching the fetus (see chapter 7). Between 1940 and 1971, DES was widely used to prevent miscarriage, especially for women with a poor obstetrical history, diabetics, and others who experienced vaginal bleeding early in pregnancy. It has been estimated that approximately two million pregnant women took DES or two other equally harmful nonsteroidal estrogens, dienestrol and hexestrol. In most instances, treatment with these substances began in the seventh week of pregnancy. Coincidentally, that is the time when vaginal and cervical development and demarcation becomes most active in the female fetus.

In 1972, three Boston physicians noted a sudden increase among young women in the number of previously rare cancers of the vagina and cervix, called clear-cell adenocarcinomas. Upon further investigation they discovered that the majority of the mothers of these young women had taken nonsteroidal estrogens during their pregnancies. In addition, benign though highly abnormal changes in the cervix and vagina of many of the daughters exposed to DES, dienestrol, and hexestrol were also noted. The Registry of Clear-Cell Adenocarcinoma of the Genital Tract of Young Females was formed in 1972 with the purpose of reporting all such tumors in women born in the United States and abroad after 1940. In 1977, the name of the registry was changed to the National Cooperative Diethylstilbestrol Adenosis Project, or DESAD.

To date at least 250 vaginal and 100 cervical adenocarcinomas have been reported. Of these, use of nonsteroidal estrogen by the mothers has been confirmed in approximately 65 percent. So far more than fifty women have died of adenocarcinoma, while several others have undergone radical and mutilating operations to prevent the spread of the disease. Fortunately, our worst fears of an epidemic of genital cancer have not been realized. The risk of development of clear-cell cancer is estimated to be no more than 1.4 per 1,000 and possibly as few as 1.4 per 10,000 exposed daughters. The peak incidence appears to occur at the age of nineteen, with a precipitous decline noted after the age of twenty-four.

What are the benign cervical and vaginal changes caused by DES?

Using sophisticated diagnostic techniques, skilled gynecologists have noted adenosis in anywhere from 80 to 97 percent of daughters exposed in utero to DES: adenosis refers to the presence of strawberry red, mucus-secreting glandular tissue on the outer part of the cervix and the vagina. These glands are normally located inside the cervix and are usually not readily seen with a speculum.

In addition to adenosis, the cervix in approximately 40 to 50 percent of these women often appears characteristically deformed, so that the diagnosis of maternal DES ingestion can be made simply by viewing its unusual shape during the routine vaginal examination. One of these distorted shapes, called a vaginal hood or collar, is seen as a circular fold in the upper vagina into which the cervix containing adenosis appears to merge. Another is the classic cock's comb, a small triangular protuberance seen at the upper pole of the cervix. In addition to abnormalities of the cervix and vagina, uterine abnormalities were described by doctors at Baylor College of Medicine in 1977, including underdevelopment of the uterus combined with a peculiar T-shaped configuration of the uterine cavity, and constricting bands were noted in the uterine cavity along the horizontal arm of the T.

Do these abnormalities of the cervix and uterus in DES daughters adversely affect their chances of a successful pregnancy?

There is no doubt that women who were exposed in utero to DES are more likely to experience several types of reproductive difficulties. However, it has not been conclusively shown that the anatomic abnormalities caused by DES are responsible for infertility. In a 1980 study, doctors compared the fertility of 618 women who had prenatal exposure to DES with 618 control subjects and noted no significant differences in their ability to conceive. In contrast, doctors at the University of Chicago, comparing 226 DES-exposed and 203 DES-unexposed women, observed that twice as many in the former group reported infertility. Researchers at the University of North Carolina reported infertility among 31 of 106 DES-exposed women and also noted that they were more likely to experience irregular menstrual cycles and longer and heavier periods.

While the question of infertility remains controversial, all experts agree that the pregnancy of a DES-exposed woman must be classified as high-risk. In July 1978, Dr. Donald Goldstein of Harvard Medical School reported on the pregnancies of 5 women exposed to DES in utero. All had typical abnormalities of the cervix and all experienced symptoms characteristic of an incompetent cervix—one that is weakened and unable to carry the weight of a growing pregnancy—usually resulting in a spontaneous and premature dilatation or opening of the cervix followed by miscarriage during the second and third trimesters of pregnancy. Dr. Goldstein attributed this to underdevelopment of the cervix (hypoplasia) of these young women and suggested that the chances of successful pregnancy could be enhanced by suturing the cervix just after the twelfth week of pregnancy before it would begin to dilate. In a 1980 study, Dr. Goldstein and Dr. Merle J. Berger reported a dismal 31 percent spontaneous abortion rate among DES-exposed women, a 5 percent incidence of ectopic pregnancy (see questions on ectopic pregnancy, pages 2, 11) during the first trimester, and an additional 18 percent miscarriage rate during the second trimester. Sadly, only 34 percent of their patients ultimately experienced a full-term delivery.

On the brighter side of the DES problem, a statistic that must be emphasized is that 80 percent of all the DES-exposed women in two recent studies eventually achieved a successful full-term pregnancy. It is this favorable and encouraging fact that should be conveyed to women who are unfortunate enough to have been exposed to DES in utero. Even if you fail to carry one or two pregnancies successfully, the odds are still in your favor that your persistent attempts will be rewarded. Another cause for optimism is a 1980 study from Boston's Beth Israel Hospital in which doctors found that some of the vaginal and cervical abnormalities attributed to DES may decrease spontaneously and even disappear in time.

Since the DES-exposed woman is an increased risk for an unfavorable reproductive outcome, she must be carefully monitored throughout her pregnancy. This should include frequent office visits, periodic pelvic examinations to detect premature cervical dilatation, and serial ultrasonic studies (see chapter 10).

Are there other postcoital estrogens which, in the event that they fail to prevent pregnancy, will be less likely to harm the fetus?

Yes! The presence of genital tract abnormalities is believed to be influenced by the nonsteroidal chemical structure of DES (see page 15). Estrogens with a steroidal configuration, such as ethinyl estradiol, conjugated estrogens, esterified estrogens, and estrone are not known to cause genital defects and have proven to be equally as effective as DES as a postcoital contraceptive.

If I take DES early in pregnancy and then give birth to a son, what problems may I anticipate?

Research conducted at the University of Chicago in 1981 on 308 DES-exposed men has revealed abnormalities of the genital tract in 31 percent. Of these, approximately half had cysts of the epididymis which is the tube carrying sperm from the testes. Other genital defects noted were abnormally small testes, undersized penises, and thickening of the capsule of the testicle. Moreover, 18 percent showed severe pathologic changes in sperm shape, concentration, and motility, compared to only 8 percent in a control group. Similar findings have been noted in a smaller study by doctors at New York's Beth Israel Medical Center. It is still too early to determine whether lesions comparable to vaginal and cervical adenocarcinoma will develop in these males, though it appears unlikely. However, it was noted that 65 percent of the DES-exposed men with abnormally small testes had a history of undescended testes and it has long been known that such men may be at an increased risk of developing cancer of the testes at a later date.

The suggestion of doctors at the University of Chicago and the Beth Israel Hospital is that all DES-exposed men undergo a complete urological examination. Though data is scarce, researchers have found no evidence of effects on a third generation of males following DES exposure.

A psychosexual study, conducted at Stanford University, on boys exposed to DES in utero, concluded that they were significantly "less masculine" than a comparative group not exposed to this drug. Psychiatrists rated six-year-olds and twenty-year-olds according to masculinity factors, such as athletic coordination, behavioral movements, heterosexual experience, masculine interests, and aggression-assertion attitudes. While the potential inaccuracies of such a study are readily apparent, it does suggest that hormones may be capable of influencing some aspects of postnatal psychosexual development in boys.

If I inadvertently take DES without realizing that I am pregnant, what are the chances of my daughter developing adenosis?

Table 1–1 demonstrates the likelihood of adenosis, based on when DES was first taken.

Table 1–1. Percentage of Women with Adenosis Based on Week DES Was Started

Week of Pregnancy DES Started	Percentage
1–6	close to 0
7–8	100
9–10	89
11–12	70
13–14	20
15–16	less than 15
16–19	less than 5
after week 19	none

Surprisingly, the amount of DES is less important than the week of pregnancy in which it is begun. There are instances of adenosis resulting from use of very small amounts of DES for only a few days during the critical seventh week of pregnancy.

The Rhythm Method

What is the rhythm method?

Rhythm, or natural family planning, is a method of birth control based on limiting intercourse to those times of the month thought to be free from the threat of pregnancy. Since it is the only contraceptive method sanctioned by the Catholic Church, it obviously has worldwide use. However, in the United States the use of the rhythm method among Catholics dropped from 31.8 percent in 1965 to 5.9 percent in 1975. Comparison figures for non-Catholics are 3.6 percent and 1.7 percent.

Calculation of the safe and unsafe times of the month can be achieved by one of three techniques: the calendar technique, daily basal body temperatures, and the sympto-thermal method. The calendar method, rarely used today, is based on the length of previous menstrual cycles. More accurate is the daily basal body temperature method, which is based on the fact that a woman's temperature will rise soon after ovulation and stay elevated until menstruation begins. This elevation of temperature is due to the release of progesterone by the ovary following ovulation. Since it is presumed that an egg is incapable of being fertilized twenty-four hours or longer after ovulation, the elevation of temperature for three consecutive days practically always means that pregnancy will not take place if a woman has intercourse after that time.

The sympto-thermal method is the most accurate and combines the use of daily basal body temperatures with changing bodily symptoms indicative of ovulation. The most important of these symptoms is the evaluation of the mucus secreted by the glands of the cervix. As ovulation approaches, the glands of the cervix under the influence of estrogen secrete a progressively more abundant amount of thin, watery, lubricative, and stretchable mucus. Spinnbarkeit is the name given to the ability of the mucus to stretch, while "peak symptom" describes the raw-egg consistency and appearance of the mucus at ovulation. Typically, ovulation occurs within a day or two before or after the peak symptom and maximum spinnbarkeit. When the mucus stretches to a length of approximately four inches, ovulation is imminent or has just occurred. Following ovulation, the mucus becomes thick, tacky, and opaque and lacks spinnbarkeit. This is owing to the effect of progesterone produced by the corpus luteum in the ovary. To avoid conception, abstinence is necessary from the time the thin mucus is first noted until four days after the peak symptom. This method of rhythm, based on analyzing changes in the cervical mucus, is also known as the Billings method, named after E. L. and J. J. Billings, two of its most ardent proponents.

If pregnancy occurs while using the rhythm method, are there any dangers to the fetus?

There is considerable evidence to suggest that a wide range of pregnancy problems, such as abortion and birth defects, may be related to the use of the rhythm method. It has been demonstrated that the best chance for normal pregnancy occurs when fertilization of the egg takes place just at the time of ovulation. Users of the rhythm method are more likely to abstain from intercourse at that time and for the few days prior to ovulation. Coitus twelve to twenty-four hours after ovulation is more likely to expose an overripe unhealthy egg to fertilization. Whereas fertilization normally takes place in the portion of the fallopian tube closest to the ovary, late fertilization does not occur until the egg has traveled some distance along the fallopian tube or has entered the uterine cavity. This has been termed "postovulatory," "tubal," or "intrauterine" overripeness. In the second type of overripeness, termed "preovulatory" or "follicular," the egg is retained in the ovary beyond the normal time. As a result, structural defects take place in the egg which may produce an abnormal fetus when ovulation and fertilization finally occur. Both types of overripeness have been held responsible for pregnancy problems.

Statistical data from three different studies conducted in New England have indicated a significantly higher rate of congenital fetal central nervous system defects in the Catholic population than in the Protestant population. In the September 16, 1978, issue of *Lancet,* two researchers noted an association between infrequent intercourse and an increased incidence of Down's syndrome, or mongolism. Down's syndrome most often occurs when a particular pair of chromosomes do not divide when the egg is being formed. As a result, a child born with this condition will have an extra chromosome. This article was followed by a letter from Marie T. Mulcahy, of the State Health Laboratory Services, Perth, Australia, published in the October 21, 1978, issue of *Lancet*. Ms. Mulcahy suggested that the findings could probably be attributed to the rhythm method of contraception and presented statistics from Australia to prove her point. She noted that, in an epidemiological study of Down's syndrome patients born in western Australia between 1966 and 1975, the incidence among Catholic women was more than double that found when compared to all other religious groups.

Ms. Mulcahy noted that this high incidence remained more or less constant throughout the ten-year-period, was apparent in all maternal age groups, and was not related to birth rank or to ethnic origin of either parent.

Dr. Richard Juberg and his colleagues of Louisiana State University, recently studying the effects of delayed fertilization among 33 parents having children with chromosomal abnormalities such as mongolism, found 24 instances in which there was definite evidence of delayed fertilization. Though other variables may certainly be responsible, it appears likely that the rhythm method plays a significant role in some of these chromosomal abnormalities.

Menstrual Extraction and Early Abortion

What is the difference between menstrual extraction and first-trimester abortion?

A first-trimester abortion, one which is performed during the first three months of pregnancy, is most effectively carried out with a small flexible plastic cannula or curette attached to a suction machine. Menstrual extraction, also known as a mini-abortion, is usually performed within three weeks beyond the missed period, on a woman with a slightly enlarged or normal-sized uterus. At this early stage, the cervix rarely has to be dilated, and cannulas with a very small diameter may be used to evacuate the uterine contents. A woman requesting menstrual extraction is usually one whose period is late and who is fearful of pregnancy but prefers not to know if she is pregnant. It must be emphasized that the criterion for calling a procedure a menstrual extraction rather than an abortion is not determined by whether the pregnancy test is positive or negative.

Does menstrual extraction always terminate a pregnancy?

A woman undergoing menstrual extraction should be aware of the fact that her present pregnancy may not be terminated in a significant percentage of cases. This may occur because the pregnancy sac is so small that it may be missed by the suction apparatus. In addition, the smaller cannulas used for menstrual extraction are less likely to create suction which will adequately dislodge the fetal sac from the uterine wall. It has been estimated that in approximately 3 percent of all women undergoing menstrual extraction, the pregnancy will remain intact and uninterrupted. When the small 4-millimeter cannula is used, the incidence of this complication will be approximately 5 percent. However, with the slightly more uncomfortable 6-

millimeter cannula, the continuing pregnancy rate is a very low 0.7 percent. Regardless of the cannula size used, both a pregnancy test and reexamination should be performed two weeks following all menstrual extractions in order to be certain that the pregnancy has been terminated.

Is the fetus that survives a menstrual extraction injured?

Fetuses surviving a failed menstrual extraction have an intact gestational or pregnancy sac, and you need not fear a deformity or injury. However, the insertion of instruments into the uterine cavity at the time of the attempted procedure can occasionally cause a severe infection of the pregnancy tissues. Symptoms of this complication practically always appear within a week and include a temperature over 38° C. (100.4° F.) a foul-smelling vaginal discharge which may be blood-tinged, and lower abdominal cramps. If not treated rapidly, the infection may spread to the lower pelvis, tubes, and ovaries, causing permanent damage, adhesions, and impaired future fertility. Bacteria may also enter the bloodstream and attack other organs and even cause death. These potentially dangerous complications can be avoided with immediate hospitalization, high doses of intravenous antibiotics, and termination of the pregnancy with a D and C. Attempts at salvaging a pregnancy in the presence of a uterine infection are foolhardy and doomed to failure.

All Rh-negative women should receive an intramuscular injection of immune globulin (RhoGAM) within seventy-two hours after a menstrual extraction in order to prevent the formation of antibodies against Rh-positive babies during future planned pregnancies (see chapter 10). The one exception to this would be if the father is known to be Rh-negative, in which case the medication need not be given. If you are Rh-negative and the menstrual extraction did not terminate your pregnancy, be assured that the injection of RhoGAM will not cause harm. In fact, it will probably help in preventing you from forming antibodies against your Rh-positive fetus.

What complications may be encountered during a pregnancy which follows a previous first-trimester abortion?

To avoid most complications, the ideal time to perform a first-trimester abortion is probably between the seventh and ninth week of pregnancy, as measured from the last menstrual period. After the tenth week, complications such as hemorrhage, retained placental fragments, and infection, increase significantly.

At the present time a great controversy exists among gynecologists over the important question as to whether or not dilatation of the cervix at the time of an abortion is responsible for an incompetent or weakened cervix during subsequent pregnancies. A woman with an incompetent cervix will suffer from repeated second-trimester spontaneous abortions and premature births because her cervix will be unable to support the weight of the enlarging uterus. Though the cause of cervical incompetence is usually unknown, trauma in the form of forceful dilatation may be responsible for the problem in some women, and many researchers believe that women who undergo repeated abortions are more likely to have an incompetent cervix.

Yet, studies throughout the world are totally contradictory in their results. For example, reports from Hungary, England, and Japan, where abortion has been legalized for several years, indicate that the incidence of spontaneous second-trimester pregnancy loss may be significantly higher among women who have experienced previously induced abortions. Other researchers, from Japan and Yugoslavia, have failed to demonstrate such a relationship.

Studies in the United States are conflicting. Though some imply that spontaneous abortion and premature labor may be associated with prior induced abortion, others demonstrate no such relationship. In an impressive study from the University of Washington in 1977, researchers compared the obstetrical records of more than 500 women who had previously had an induced abortion with a similar control group who had not experienced the procedure and concluded that there was no significant differences in pregnancy complications between the two groups. Futhermore, the incidence of spontaneous abortions and premature births was not affected by the number of previous abortions or by the week of pregnancy in which the previous abortion was performed. A 1980 report from Hawaii, involving over 2,000 women, reached similar conclusions, but noted, that the risk of miscarriage was far greater when pregnancy occurred within one year after either an induced abortion or a full-term birth.

In contrast to these studies, doctors at the Boston Hospital for Women concluded that those who had two or more previously induced abortions were two to three times as likely to miscarry during subsequent pregnancies. Interestingly, the technique used during the prior abortion did not appear to be an important contributing factor. This last conclusion is in complete conflict with several other studies which stressed the importance of the abortion method in determining the success or failure of future pregnancies. Data from the World Health Organization, encompassing the statistics of seven European nations, showed that the use of a sharp curette, rather than the more gentle and modern suction apparatus, increased the likelihood of a subsequent midtrimester spontaneous abortion.

Though I have heard it said that an ectopic pregnancy is more likely to occur among women who have undergone a previous abortion, there are not studies available which conclusively demonstrate such a relationship. However, if an abortion is complicated by a severe postoperative pelvic infection involving the fallopian tubes, it is more likely that a tubal pregnancy may occur. Immediate reporting of postabortal fever, abdominal pain, or foul-smelling discharge followed by appropriate antibiotic treatment by your doctor should prevent this complication.

What should a pregnant woman who has undergone a previous first-trimester abortion be aware of?

If you have had a previous pregnancy termination, it is important for your obstetrician to know the specific details. You can request this information from an abortion clinic, a hospital record room, or the files of the doctor who performed the procedure. As unbelievable as it seems, there are a number of doctors in this country who still perform first-trimester abortions with a sharp curette rather than with the more modern and efficient suction device. In addition, if you underwent an abortion before 1973, it is a certainty that a sharp curette was used. The record of your previous abortion will also reveal the size of the dilators and curettes which were used. During the first eight weeks of pregnancy, as measured from the first day of your last menstrual period, an abortion may be easily accomplished with a 6-millimeter plastic cannula. After the eighth week, it is customary to use a cannula with an outside diameter in millimeters equal to, or 2 millimeters less than, the duration of the pregnancy in weeks, counting from the first day of your last period. During the first trimester, the suction curette size should never be greater than the uterine size in weeks, and should not exceed 12 millimeters. If you have undergone two or more induced abortions, if a sharp curette was used, and if your cervix was dilated to 12 or more millimeters, your doctor may want to examine your cervix at frequent intervals throughout pregnancy in order to be sure that it is not dilating prematurely. A cerclage operation, or placement of a cervical-tightening suture around the cervix, at the earliest evidence of cervical incompetence, often helps to prevent midtrimester abortion and premature labor.

Abortion After Twelve Weeks

What problems may be encountered by a pregnant woman who has had a previous second-trimester abortion, and how can they be remedied?

To terminate pregnancies beyond twelve weeks, many doctors inject hypertonic saline (salt) or substances called prostaglandins into the amniotic sac and then await the onset of labor and expulsion of the fetus and placenta. Prostaglandin vaginal suppositories are also effective in terminating midtrimester pregnancies.

A cervical fistula, an abnormal opening in the cervix, can result from a rupture or a laceration occurring at the time of a midtrimester abortion. This complication, estimated as occurring in 0.1 percent to 5 percent of midtrimester abortions, most often happens to those women who have never carried a previous full-term pregnancy. Prostaglandins, administered either as suppositories or as an intraamniotic injection, are more likely to cause this problem than intraamniotic saline because the uterine muscle contractions produced by these substances are more forceful and frequent and adequate time is not allowed for the cervix to gradually efface and dilate.

Fistulas are often difficult to suture, and even when the surgical repair appears perfect, a woman may still be left with a permanently weakened and incompetent cervix. If you have experienced a cervical fistula from a previous abortion, your doctor may want to place a cerclage suture around your cervix. Ideally, this operation is best performed during the fourteenth week of pregnancy since the risk of early miscarriage is passed and the weight of the uterus is still not great enough to cause excessive pressure on the cervix.

Opinion varies as to the best method of delivery following a successful cerclage operation. Many doctors will prefer to leave the suture in place throughout pregnancy and accomplish delivery via cesarean section. If you request vaginal delivery, the cerclage suture may be cut during the last days of pregnancy and labor allowed to take place under close supervision. One disadvantage of allowing vaginal delivery is that the pressure of the baby's head during labor may reopen the fistula. A second drawback is that the cerclage operation has to be repeated during each subsequent pregnancy.

Until recently, it was universally believed that pregnancy termination after twelve weeks with the suction device and other instruments was extremely hazardous, because of the greater risk of hemorrhage, uterine perforation, retained pregnancy tissue, and infection. Though some gynecologists still share this opinion, as of 1982 the majority of American doctors now favor D and E, or dilatation and evacuation, of the uterine contents. Some have even performed this procedure beyond twenty weeks of pregnancy. Since dilatation of the cervix is performed with instruments which have a diameter greater than 12 millimeters, many authorities are fearful that D and E will prove to be responsible for significantly greater numbers of women with cervical incompetence. Even the most ardent supporters of this method admit that this is a real possibility. If you have had a previous D and E, your doctor may want to examine you frequently in order to detect the earliest signs of premature dilatation and effacement of your cervix.

To reduce the incidence of cervical injury following midtrimester abortions, many gynecologists are now inserting laminaria digitata, or dried sea weed, into the cervix prior to the procedure. Due to its hydroscopic (water-absorbing) ability, a sterile piece of laminaria, when inserted into the cervix, absorbs the secretions and increases its diameter by three to five times over a period of six to eight hours. This slowly and painlessly dilates the cervix without excessive force prior to suction curettage, D and E, saline, or prostaglandin abortions. Though laminaria may greatly reduce the incidence of cervical injury and problems during subsequent pregnancies, one disadvantage is that it may be associated with a slightly higher incidence of uterine infection. This is especially true if it is inserted more than twenty-four hours prior to the abortion.

Tubal Sterilization

What is tubal sterilization?

Tubal sterilization refers to any operative procedure on the fallopian tubes which prevents fertilization of the egg by sperm within the tube. Traditional methods have usually involved tying (ligating), combined with cutting out a portion of the tube. Newer techniques have utilized coagulation or burning, as well as the placement of elastic bands and clips around a segment of the tube. This is accomplished through a viewing instrument called a laparoscope which is placed in the abdominal cavity through the navel. The abdominal cavity may also be entered and the tubes tied through the vagina if a vaginal incision is made behind the cervix.

The highly touted "minilap," or minilaparotomy, is a new method of abdominal tubal ligation which is gaining popularity in many countries throughout the world. In this procedure, an instrument is inserted through the cervix into the uterine cavity in order to push the uterus up against the lower abdominal wall. A one-inch skin incision is then made directly over the top of the elevated uterus. The tubes are then brought up into the operative field and are either tied or cut.

Is pregnancy possible following a tubal ligation?

Yes. Regardless of the method used, pregnancy occurring weeks or even years later is a definite possibility and may occur between 0.1 and 3 percent of all sterilization procedures.

What effect does tubal ligation have on pregnancy?

If pregnancy does occur, there is a significant risk of it being an ectopic gestation (see chapter 2). The techniques that destroy relatively more tube, such as coagulation or burning, lead to higher ectopic pregnancy rates, since these procedures leave fistulas or openings from the uterus to the abdominal cavity through which sperm can find their way to the end of the tube and fertilize an egg. In general, most mechanical methods of sterilization, such as tying of the tubes, elastic rings, and plastic spring clips, are associated with remarkably low ectopic rates but higher numbers of intrauterine pregnancies. Statistics suggest that if pregnancy does occur following the standard tying or ligation of the tubes it is seven times more likely to be an ectopic pregnancy if the procedure is performed abdominally rather than through the vagina.

**Has pregnancy ever occurred after a hysterectomy,
and if so, how can the fetus survive?**

There have been about twenty reports in the literature of ectopic pregnancies occurring following the surgical removal of the uterus, in which the tubes and ovaries were not also removed. This circumstance occurs when determined and powerful sperm actually find their way through a small opening in the surgically sealed fallopian tube.

The most bizarre case of all was reported from Aukland, New Zealand, in 1979. A healthy five-pound baby girl was born four weeks prematurely after her mother underwent hysterectomy eight months earlier. The amazed physicians concluded that the woman was two days pregnant when her uterus was removed. The fertilized egg, which fell from the fallopian tube or was dislodged during the operation, attached itself to the bowel and was nourished by its blood supply. The baby was removed through an abdominal incision.

Vasectomy   **Is a pregnancy which occurs following unsuccessful
vasectomy more apt to be abnormal?**

No. Offspring conceived following unsuccessful vasectomy, the cutting of a man's sperm tubes (vas deferens), are at no greater risk of congenital abnormalities. Vaso-vasotomy is an operation used to reverse the sterility resulting from a previous vasectomy. Use of newer and sophisticated microsurgical techniques have allowed some specialists to achieve pregnancy rates of over 75 percent without any evidence of abnormal offspring.

2.
Conception and
Early Pregnancy

A woman usually reacts to the discovery that she is pregnant with unequalled joy. Next comes the torrent of questions about pregnancy, and usually the first concern is how to select a competent obstetrician. Since questions relating to distressing pregnancy symptoms, such as "morning sickness," and potentially more ominous problems, such as vaginal bleeding, require accurate answers and immediate attention, this choice should not be made haphazardly. In this chapter I discuss the criteria you should use in choosing an obstetrician and answer some of the more commonly asked questions about conception and early pregnancy. Simple methods by which you can assess your uterine size and the growth and development of your baby during each pregnancy month are also presented.

Pregnancy
Tests

What does a pregnancy test measure?

Though there are a variety of pregnancy tests, they all measure the presence of the pregnancy hormone, called human chorionic gonadotropin (HCG). HCG is produced by cells in the placenta and is detectable in the serum or urine of a pregnant woman eight to nine days after ovulation. It reaches peak levels between the second and third month of pregnancy. Levels of this hormone are measured in International Units (IU) per milliliter. At ten days following fertilization, the average HCG concentration in the blood and urine is approximately 0.2 IU per milliliter. This rises rapidly to 3 IU/ml at thirty days of pregnancy and 50 to 100 IU/ml by fifty days.

How accurate are the standard laboratory pregnancy tests and the newer home pregnancy tests?

Contrary to popular belief, the various urine tests using rabbits, rats, mice, and frogs are rarely used today. The usual sensitivity to HCG of these biological tests ranges from 0.5 to 5 IU/per milliliter, and they are therefore not totally accurate until fourteen to twenty-eight days following the missed period. Another drawback is that some of these tests require several days before the results are available.

The so-called immunological pregnancy tests, first introduced in 1960, are the most commonly used in this country today. Though there is a wide variety of these tests, they all measure the reaction which occurs when previously prepared antibodies to HCG come in contact with a pregnant woman's urine containing the HCG antigen. Immunological tests can be performed either in test tubes or on glass slides, and there are advantages and disadvantages to both methods. Tube tests are usually more sensitive than slide tests and can detect urinary HCG levels of 0.25 to 1 IU/ml. They are most reliable beginning the second week after a missed period. Slide tests vary in sensitivity from 1 to 5 IU/ml and are not accurate until at least two weeks after a missed period. They are valuable if time is important in obtaining a diagnosis, since the slides can provide results in from one to two minutes while test tube results take thirty minutes to two hours.

The new self-administered home urine pregnancy tests, such as the e.p.t., Acu-Test, and Predictor, are variations of the standard immunological pregnancy test and may be purchased without prescription at most retail pharmacies for about $10.00. These tests are sensitive to 1 IU of HCG/ml of urine and may easily be performed within minutes by anyone who is able to read and follow simple instructions. If the home pregnancy test is positive ten days or more after the missed period, the chances are that it is correct 97 percent of the time, but if the first test is negative, the accuracy drops to only 75 to 79 percent. These results improve to between 86 and 91 percent when the test is repeated one week later. It is important to remember that a negative e.p.t. does not necessarily mean that you are not pregnant. Under no circumstances should you take hormones to bring on a late period when the e.p.t. is negative since all female hormones have been associated with abnormalities of the developing fetus (see chapter 1). Instead I would strongly recommend that you follow such a negative test with the more accurate Biocept-G pregnancy test (see p. 29). It should be noted, however, that regardless of which immunological pregnancy test is used, its ability to detect the low levels of HCG from an ectopic pregnancy or threatened abortion will be only 33 percent.

Although few doctors or patients realize it, false positive immunological pregnancy tests have been reported in the presence of protein in the urine from kidney disease or infection, an overactive thyroid gland, or high doses of aspirin, tranquilizers, antidepressants, or anticonvulsant medications. False positive results have also been obtained in 20 percent of patients with macroglobulins in their blood and urine. (Macroglobulins are antibodies found in people suffering from a group of rare illnesses called immunological diseases.) HCG is immunologically undetectable from the pituitary hormone called luteinizing hormone (LH). Therefore, it is possible for extremely high levels of LH (between 0.7 and 1 IU) to give a false positive immunological pregnancy test. LH levels are highest immediately before ovulation and during the menopause.

What do the newest pregnancy tests tell a doctor besides the fact that a woman is or is not pregnant?

The most sensitive pregnancy test available, and the only one that can differentiate between HCG and LH, is the radioimmunoassay (RIA). This incredibly sensitive blood test measures the small part of the HCG hormone called the beta-subunit (B-subunit). It is capable of detecting as little as 0.003 to 0.015 IU of HCG B-subunit per milliliter of serum, and it can accurately detect the presence of pregnancy tissue as early as eight to nine days following ovulation. By repeating the RIA at frequent intervals, doctors can now follow the progress of an early pregnancy which is in jeopardy. Under normal circumstances, the HCG levels will show a sharp linear rise during the first four weeks after conception, with a doubling of its concentration every two days. When a woman's HCG values do not follow this expected curve, impending abortion or ectopic pregnancy should be strongly suspected. Use of this technique has achieved an almost 90 percent accuracy in predicting a healthy pregnancy and a 76 percent accuracy in forecasting an eventual first-trimester abortion. Though the RIA will rarely miss the HCG of an ectopic pregnancy or a threatened abortion, it can take as long as 36 hours to perform and therefore is of no value during an acute emergency. Another disadvantage is that some laboratories lack the sophisticated equipment and skill to perform this test. Finally, the cost of the beta-subunit test may be as high as $25 or $30. Less expensive beta-subunit RIA kits are now commercially available to laboratories for both the qualitative and quantitative determination of HCG in serum and plasma. These tests detect first-week pregnancy with almost 100 percent accuracy in one to three hours. The lowest levels of detectable HCG are in the astounding range of 0.015 to as little as 0.003 IU/ml. These tests have been simplified to the point where they can be performed by most laboratories at a reasonable cost.

The radioreceptor blood test, more commonly known as the RRA or Biocept-G, has the ability to diagnose pregnancy with an accuracy of 98 to 100 percent at the time of the first missed period, or the fourteenth day after ovulation and conception. Amounts as little as 0.2 IU of HCG per milliliter of serum give a positive Biocept-G test. This sensitivity helps doctors to diagnose abnormal pregnancies, such as an ectopic or threatened abortion, at an early stage. It is less expensive than the beta-subunit test and has the added advantage of giving accurate results in less than one hour. Since the Biocept-G does not distingush between LH and HCG, a rare false positive test may occur in the menopausal woman and among some women during the preovulatory peak of LH secretion. A quantitative radioreceptor blood test, able to detect levels of HCG similar to the most sensitive RIA for the beta-subunit of HCG, is expected to be marketed soon.

A simple, accurate, and rapid urine pregnancy test which many doctors are now using in their office is the Sensitex, manufactured by Hoffman-LaRoche, Incorporated. This test is simple to use, easy to interpret, requires no complicated equipment, and can accurately detect 0.25 IU/ml of HCG. In addition, it may be performed in ninety minutes and has the advantage of having very little interfering reaction with LH. In a 1981 report published in the *Journal of Reproductive Medicine,* doctors were able to predict an eventual spontaneous abortion among 63 percent of women with low HCG levels noted on repeated Sensitex determinations. Furthermore, rising levels forecasted a successful pregnancy 92 percent of the time. Equally sensitive results have been obtained with the Neocept and UCG-Beta Stat urine pregnancy tests.

Choosing a Doctor

How can I select a competent obstetrician?

Ideally, your search for a competent obstetrician should begin before conception, when you will be less apt to make a hasty decision. For the woman living in a rural area served by a small number of doctors, the selection may be limited. Most women, fortunately, can choose from a wide variety of physicians. Despite the options open to her, however, all too often a woman will select a doctor solely on the recommendation of a neighbor or casual acquaintance. Yet "shopping around" to find the best doctor is the right of every pregnant woman—a right that should be exercised more frequently.

Of primary importance in the selection process are the doctor's qualifications. Though many general practitioners practice obstetrics, you will usually be in far better hands if you choose someone who has completed a three-to-four-year residency program in obstetrics and gynecology. It is also wise to find out if your doctor has been certified by the American Board of Obstetrics and Gynecology. While Board certification is no guarantee of excellence, it does mean that the doctor has taken an approved residency program and has studied for and passed a rigorous exam. Moreover, medical specialty boards are now moving toward mandatory recertification, requiring study of the latest obstetrical procedures and techniques. Thus, recertification, though optional at the present time, is an indication that these doctors have the desire and the ability to keep up to date in their specialty.

Another indication of a doctor's skill is hospital affiliation. You should be skeptical if the hospital in which the doctor works is not accredited by the Joint Commission on Accreditation of Hospitals. If a hospital has an approved residency program and is affiliated with a medical school, it is more likely to attract highly competent physicians. In fact, many university-affiliated hospitals will not allow general practitioners to do obstetrics.

The *Directory of Medical Specialists* published by Marquis Who's Who (200 East Ohio Street, Chicago, Illinois 60611) is an excellent book, updated every two years, that lists the training, qualifications, and hospital affiliations of all doctors certified by specialty boards in the United States. I have found it to be most helpful when referring patients of mine to new obstetricians in distant cities. The *American Medical Directory,* usually available at large public libraries, is another good source of this information.

One simple and effective way of finding a competent obstetrician is to speak to a resident in obstetrics and gynecology at a local hospital. Residents are notoriously critical of their attending physicians, and an enthusiastic endorsement of a particular doctor is a reliable guarantee of competence. If the resident is reluctant to recommend one particular doctor, ask for a list of two or three favorites from which you can make your own choice. Finding out which doctors are most frequently the personal physicians of nurses who work in the obstetrical unit can also be valuable. If you cannot get this information from a resident or an obstetrical nurse, try telephoning a childbirth education group, a local childbirth education instructor, or a branch of the La Leche League. All can provide you with lists of highly regarded obstetricians.

Unfortunately, the choice of a competent obstetrician is no assurance that your personal relationship will be harmonious. For this reason, you would be wise to arrange an initial meeting with the doctor, preferably with your husband or partner present. At this meeting you should ask the questions about childbirth which most concern you, whether they be about nutrition, childbirth preparation classes, "gentle birth," family-centered care, or other pertinent subjects (see chapter 11). Beware of the doctor who appears to be adamant and unyielding over minor points, such as avoiding the enema or "full perineal prep" on admission to the delivery room. In the event that you require anesthesia, it is nice to know which types are preferred and why. If the doctor appears annoyed by your questions, or avoids them with a "leave everything to me" attitude, consider whether you wish to make a commitment to that physician. I would also be suspicious of the doctor who calls you by your first name, unless of course you are allowed the same privilege. As Dr. Oliver Jelly, a retired British surgeon, said, "I regularly found in consultation practice that the practitioners who seemed to know their patients best had the least idea of what was wrong with them, and Christian-name familiarity was a total bar to correct clinical diagnosis."

Observing the activity in a doctor's waiting room is often a good indication of efficiency. The busiest doctor in town is not necessarily the best. An obstetrician who habitually keeps women waiting for an hour or more is one who has the least concern for patients, is undoubtedly inefficient and disorganized, and is best avoided.

The first prenatal examination should include a complete history and physical. An examination limited to the breasts and pelvis is inadequate. The doctor must examine your heart, lungs, and abdomen early in pregnancy in order to detect any possible abnormality. The pelvic examination should be gentle and considerate; there is no excuse for a doctor's not using a warmed speculum, and if you have never given birth before, a small speculum should be used. The examination is incomplete without a vaginal, rectal, and recto-vaginal examination (index finger in the vagina, middle finger in the rectum), performed with a well-lubricated glove to minimize discomfort.

Following the examination, you should expect a full discussion of the doctor's findings and all aspects of prenatal care. This should be carried out in the consultation room after you are dressed and feel more comfortable. Having a written list of questions is a good idea for the first visit, as well as for all subsequent visits.

The majority of obstetricians in the United States are in group practices of varying sizes. Some groups have as few as two doctors, while others may have as many as ten. You should not hesitate to ask what the evening and weekend on-call schedule is; in some groups the senior physician no longer works at these times. It is essential that all members of the group have the same attitudes about childbirth so that promises and assurances given you by one obstetrician are not rejected by another. If you are being cared for by an obstetrical group, it is a good idea to arrange visits on a rotation basis among the doctors so that you familiarize yourself with all of them. You may find one member of a group to be not to your liking. If so, request that another group member be called should you go into labor when the doctor you don't care for is on call. If such an arrangement is not possible, consider finding another doctor or group of doctors. Remember, it is never too late to switch if you are unhappy!

The obstetrician in solo practice is an endangered species. Obviously, continuity of care and a more intimate patient-doctor relationship are of great advantage to a pregnant woman. There are disadvantages to having only one doctor, however, especially if the obstetrical practice is a busy one. The hours these doctors work are often grueling and require sleepless nights. Most women would prefer an alert physician to one struggling to stay awake throughout a complicated labor and delivery.

Efficiency experts have noted that solo practice is far more disorganized than group practice and canceled office hours and other patient inconveniences are more likely to occur. When a solo practitioner takes a vacation or even a weekend off, he or she may sign out to a doctor with whom you are totally unfamiliar. If you choose such an obstetrician, be sure to ask about vacation times, as well as the name of the doctor who will care for you during these absences.

There are too many doctors who induce labor in order to meet the demands of a busy office practice or vacation schedule. This is mentioned only to be deplored. Induction of labor is a serious undertaking which should be carried out only for very strict medical and obstetrical reasons (see chapter 11), never for convenience.

Discuss the obstetrical fee with your doctor and the office staff and get an accurate estimate of the total hospital costs. A good office staff can usually tell you which of the obstetrical costs will be covered by your particular insurance policy. Many doctors add an additional fee if it becomes necessary to perform a cesarean section. Ask about such extras beforehand. Finally, find out how your doctor wishes to be paid. Some doctors require a percentage, usually a third to a half of the total fee, before your due date. Others require full payment by the last month of pregnancy.

Boy or Girl?

Are there any simple methods to predetermine the sex of a child?

Over the centuries, thousands of formulas have been devised to help couples preselect the sex of offspring. Aristotle advised the Greeks to have intercourse in the north wind if males were desired, and in the south wind if females were preferred. Hippocrates, the father of medicine, believed that boys developed in the right side of the uterus and girls in the left. As a result, his followers suggested that to conceive a male, a woman should lie on her right side after intercourse.

The sex of a baby is determined by its father at conception, although women throughout history have been blamed for not giving birth to a child of the desired gender. The adult male has two different sex chromosomes in his body cells; one labeled X and the other Y. Each sperm carries only one of these chromosomes—an X or a Y. The adult woman possesses two X sex chromosomes in each of her body cells but no Y chromosomes; therefore, her egg always contributes an X to the future offspring. If a sperm carrying a Y chromosome fertilizes the X egg, the result will be an XY male. However, if a sperm cell carrying an X gets there first, the result is an XX female (see illustration).

Sex preselection received some attention in the 1960s when Dr. Landrum B.

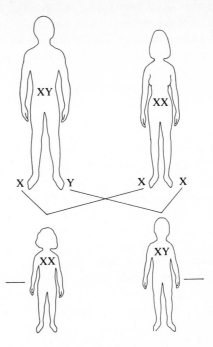

How sex is determined.

Shettles claimed that he was able to distinguish two types of sperm under a phase contrast microscope: a small, fast-swimming, round-headed, fragile sperm carrying the male-producing Y chromosome and a larger, stronger, slower-swimming, oval-shaped type carrying the female-producing X chromosome. Based on these differences, Dr. Shettles concluded that couples wanting to conceive a boy could improve their chances by timing intercourse as close to the moment of ovulation as possible, douching with baking soda and water immediately before intercourse, use of a rear entry coital position, and encouraging female orgasm. It was his theory that these measures would allow a greater number of weaker male-producing sperm to be deposited at the cervix. In contrast, to conceive a girl, Dr. Shettles attempted to create a less favorable vaginal environment in which the stronger female-producing sperm would be more likely to survive. To achieve this, he recommended that intercourse cease two or three days prior to ovulation, that it be preceded by an acid douche of vinegar and water, use of the face-to-face or "missionary position," avoidance of female orgasm, and shallow penetration by the male at the time of his orgasm.

Though the public was quick to test this theory, no one has been able to reproduce the 80 percent predictability rates claimed by Dr. Shettles. One investigator, using this method, artificially inseminated 85 patients and predicted the sex of the babies in only 40 cases.

There does seem to be some validity to Dr. Shettles' claim that the timing of intercourse may determine the gender of a baby. Records show that a preponderance of male offspring, estimated roughly at 130 males for every 100 females, are born to

Orthodox Jews who follow the practice of ritual separation between husband and wife in which intercourse is forbidden during menstruation as well as for an additional seven days. In a 1979 study from the Hadassah-Hebrew University Medical Center in Jerusalem, Dr. Susan Harlop noted the sex of 3,658 babies born to Jewish women practicing the ritual of sexual separation. Significantly, more male babies, specifically 65.5 percent, were born when intercourse was resumed two days after ovulation than when resumed one or two days before ovulation. Dr. Harlop correctly cautioned against advising couples desiring a male child to delay intercourse until after ovulation since a relationship may exist between congenital malformations and fertilization of an aged egg (see question on rhythm method page 20).

Studies in animals have suggested that what one eats before conception might have an effect on determining the sex of the fetus. In a 1980 report, published in the *International Journal of Gynecology and Obstetrics,* doctors in France instructed 260 couples to follow a specific diet starting at least four to six weeks before attempting conception. Those men and women desiring to conceive a girl followed a diet high in magnesium and calcium and low in salt. To conceive a boy, women followed a high potassium and salt diet. After pregnancy was confirmed, the couples resumed their normal eating habits. Amazingly, 212 of the 260 couples, or 82 percent, conceived an infant of the desired sex. Though these results are impressive, larger studies would be required before this method of sex preselection can be endorsed.

Are there any accurate methods to preselect sex?

Scientists have now been able to identify and separate X- and Y-bearing spermatozoa based on differences in their size, weight, speed of movement, and fluorescence patterns under ultraviolet light. Some have claimed success with centrifugation, or spinning, of semen specimens at high speeds, allowing the lighter Y-bearing sperm to stay suspended while the heavier X-bearing sperm settle to the bottom of the test tube. Others have used electrical separation techniques based on the fact that male sperm normally carry a slight negative charge on their surface while female sperm carry a positive charge. Some scientists have devised special filters and columns of concentrated albumin to achieve sperm cell separation. Supporters of the latter method claim that the final ejaculate used for artificial insemination may contain between 70 and 84 percent Y-bearing sperm. Unfortunately, most methods to date have had little success in isolating and preserving the X-bearing female sperm. At the present time, most authorities would agree that totally reliable and accessible sex preselection facilities will not be available for several years.

Is it possible to determine the sex of the fetus early in pregnancy?

At the present time, there are no reliable methods of determining fetal sex during the first trimester of pregnancy. During the second trimester, at approximately sixteen weeks of pregnancy, a sample of amniotic fluid may be obtained by placing a needle into the uterine cavity through the lower abdominal wall. This procedure, called amniocentesis, is simple and relatively painless. When the cells of the amniotic fluid are studied in the laboratory, the sex of the fetus may be predicted with an accuracy approaching 100 percent. The one important application of sex determination based on amniocentesis has been in the therapeutic termination of pregnancies in which there is a considerable risk of a woman giving birth to an infant with a sex-linked disorder (see chapter 10). Meanwhile, researchers throughout the world are attempting to develop reliable methods of determining fetal sex at an early stage of pregnancy, when a safe menstrual extraction or suction curettage can be performed.

In one very encouraging 1979 study Dr. Kurt Loewit and his Austrian colleagues were able to predict the fetal sex with 92 percent accuracy based on a measurement of the urinary excretion of the hormone testosterone. Male fetuses were noted to produce a significantly higher level of this hormone in their mothers' urine than did female fetuses. Though testosterone can be measured in the blood as well as the urine, its use in this manner to predict fetal sex has been unsuccessful. Doctors at Walter Reed Army Hospital, in a 1981 published report, measured levels of serum testosterone and concluded that there was no significant difference between women carrying a male fetus and those carrying a female fetus.

Researchers in Switzerland have successfully predicted fetal sex by use of a blood test. By isolating these fetal cells that pass into the maternal bloodstream and staining them, the Swiss scientists were correct in predicting fetal sex 86 percent of the time, but they were only able to accurately evaluate the cells after the fourteenth week of pregnancy. Investigators at Stanford University have discovered fetal cells in the maternal circulation as early as the twelfth week of pregnancy. They have actually calculated that there may be between two and twenty million fetal cells of various types which pass from the fetus to the mother. It is the aim of these scientists to develop a blood test which obstetricians could offer to all their patients early in pregnancy in order to detect both the fetal sex and a wide range of chromosomal and chemical abnormalities. Successful studies have been carried out in the People's Republic of China by sampling cells that are shed into the endocervical canal from the placenta. The cells are obtained in the same manner as a Pap smear, and the accuracy of sex prediction to date has been 94 percent. Similar encouraging reports on the use of endocervical cells for prediction of fetal sex have come from studies conducted at the University of Alabama School of Medicine; however, researchers at Southern Illinois University School of medicine were not able to duplicate these results.

Though the tests presently used to predict fetal sex during the first trimester of pregnancy are still considered experimental, eventual perfection of these techniques raises very important sociological and ethical issues. Some consider the early diagnosis of a disease and the ability to terminate a pregnancy a blessing, while others do not. Many people rightfully decry the use of modern technology to abort a potentially healthy fetus merely because a couple prefers a child of the opposite sex. The sociological implications of the perfection of these techniques are beyond the scope of this book, but they will certainly be important topics of discussion in the future.

**Length of
Pregnancy**

How can I accurately calculate my due date?

The chances are only eight out of one hundred that you will give birth on the exact date calculated for you by your obstetrician. The standard method of calculating the expected date of confinement (EDC) may be roughly determined by a formula called Naegele's rule: count back three months from the first day of your last period, and then add seven days. For example, if your last period began on June 10, subtracting three months gives you March, and adding seven days to the tenth gives you March 17 as your due date. This system works relatively well for women having the classic textbook menstrual cycle of twenty-eight days, who ovulate on day fourteen. However, women with longer cycles tend to ovulate later while those with shorter cycles will ovulate earlier (see question on p. 424). The most constant aspect of the menstrual cycle is the fact that ovulation will occur approximately fourteen days prior to the next period. Therefore, if your periods come every thirty-eight days, you will most probably ovulate on day twenty-four. Obviously, under such circumstances, Naegele's rule will be inaccurate unless you account for this delay by adding additional days. If you have periods every thirty-eight days, and your last period started on June 10, you have to add ten extra days over the standard twenty-eight. Therefore, your EDC would be March 27, or March 17 plus ten days.

Confusion in determining how far along you are in your pregnancy results from the fact that obstetricians traditionally determine your pregnancy length and your uterine size from the first day of your last menstrual period rather than from the actual onset of pregnancy, which begins with fertilization just after ovulation. Therefore, if your obstetrician says that your uterus is ten-weeks' size, he or she really means that you are 8 weeks from the day of conception. Pregnancy is said to last 40 weeks (280 days) from the last period, provided the start of your period is every 28 days. Actually, the length of pregnancy is closer to 266 days, or 38 weeks. Another source of confusion occurs because an obstetrician thinks of a pregnancy as lasting 10 lunar months, each having 28 days, while a patient views it over the usual 9-calendar-month span.

Dr. G. L. Park, an English physician, accurately noted the EDC of 2,100 pregnant women under his care and published his conclusions in 1969. Based on his findings, the long-accepted Naegele's rule may not be totally valid. The important point here is that 68 percent of the women studied went into labor after the fortieth week of pregnancy, with the peak period of births occurring between the end of the forty-first week and the beginning of the forty-second week. If the majority of normal births take place after the fortieth week, it would seem foolish for a doctor to induce labor at the forty-first week from the last menstrual period simply because of the fear that the baby may be postmature (see questions on induced labor and prolonged pregnancy, page 367). It is Dr. Park's practice to consider the forty-first, forty-second, and forty-third weeks of pregnancy as a period of nonintervention unless there is a good medical reason. His very low perinatal mortality figures of 4 per 1,000 attest to the wisdom of this policy. The logical suggestion following this study is that obstetricians should alter Naegele's rule and add 14 days instead of 7 to the first day of the last menstrual period. Most American obstetricians do not share Dr.

Park's optimism about pregnancies that have progressed beyond the forty-second week. Evaluation of fetal well-being in the form of electronic monitoring and sonography are often initiated at this time (see chapter 10).

What is the longest pregnancy on record?

There are numerous cases on record in which the duration of pregnancy is said to have exceeded 320 days from the onset of the last menstrual period. There is one well-documented case of a pregnancy lasting 334 days from the first day of the last menstrual period. The length of a prolonged pregnancy is of great medicolegal importance in cases where the husband has been away for ten months or more and the legitimacy of the child is in question. Pregnancies ruled legitimate in recent years have been of 331, 346, and 355 days, but the world's most liberal court decision took place in England in 1949. In this case, the husband's petition for divorce was dismissed despite the fact that the pregnancy was presumed to be 360 days!

Prolonged pregnancy is known to be associated with a fetal malformation called anencephaly. This condition is characterized by a complete or partial absence of the brain and overlying skull. One of the most unusual cases—and the longest documented pregnancy on record—was that of an anencephalic infant delivered by cesarean section one year and twenty-four days after the woman's last menstrual period.

Following the Progress of the Pregnancy

How can I follow the growth of the fetus?

The observant woman who has practiced previous self-examination can detect a pronounced softening of the cervix as early as a month after conception. This is one of the earliest signs of pregnancy. If you have a speculum, you may be able to observe a characteristic violet color of the cervix and vagina during the first few weeks of pregnancy. This is due to the increased blood supply, or vascularity, in these areas and when noted in the vagina it is called Chadwick's sign.

You can check your uterine growth as pregnancy progresses by following some very easy rules. Urinate to empty your bladder and then lie on your back on a flat, hard surface. You should be able to touch the top of the uterus starting at the twelfth week from the last menstrual period. At that time, the uterus is palpable just above the pubic bone. A second important landmark is your navel, or umbilicus. When the top of the uterus reaches the umbilicus, you should be approximately halfway or twenty weeks from your last period, with another twenty weeks to go until delivery. If the uterus is one finger's breadth below the navel, you are approximately eighteen weeks pregnant, while one finger's breadth above the navel means a pregnancy of about twenty-two weeks. In a pregnancy of sixteen weeks the distance is halfway between the symphysis bone and the umbilicus. The approximate uterine size with each month of pregnancy is presented in the illustration.

For greatest accuracy and enjoyment, have your husband or partner keep a record of these measurements throughout pregnancy. If you believe your uterine size is two weeks or more at variance with your dates, tell your doctor. A uterus that is growing at a faster than normal rate may indicate the presence of twins or a very

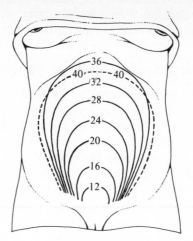

Height of uterus at various weeks of pregnancy.

large baby, while a uterus smaller than expected on the dates may mean that there are problems of fetal growth.

For greater accuracy in measuring your uterine height, you can use a tape measure having a centimeter marker. Between the fourteenth and twenty-seventh week of pregnancy you will find that the uterine height above the symphysis, as measured in centimeters, will be approximately equal to the number of weeks that you are pregnant based on the last menstrual period. A good point to remember during the last trimester is that uterine growth will usually progress at an average rate of 3 centimeters per month, with an ultimate height of 28 to 36 centimeters being reached. Don't panic during the last three or four weeks if the uterine height suddenly decreases by a few centimeters; probably your baby's head has dropped into the pelvis.

Can I detect fetal movement and heartbeat in monitoring the progress of my pregnancy?

The detection of fetal movement is an excellent guide for determining how far along in your pregnancy you are. Most women first become aware of a slight fluttering about the eighteenth to twentieth week after the last period. The first perception of this fetal movement has been termed "quickening." Among women who have carried previous pregnancies, "quickening" may be noted at the sixteenth or seventeenth week. Fetal movement will increase in intensity as pregnancy progresses, though the number of movements per day varies from one fetus to another. During the last trimester, it is very important to immediately report any sudden increase or decrease of fetal activity from the usual pattern.

If you have a stethoscope or are able to borrow one, you and your husband or partner can detect the fetal heartbeat at about the twentieth week of pregnancy. The rate varies between 120 and 160 beats per minute and should not be confused with the pulsations from your abdominal aorta, which usually are of a frequency of less than 100 beats per minute. The aorta rate is synchronous with the pulse in your wrist. The widespread belief that a fetal heart rate above 140 beats per minute means that you will have a girl, while one below 140 represents a boy, just isn't true. The fetal heartbeat varies from minute to minute throughout pregnancy, with wide variations between 120 and 160 being the usual and healthy pattern. A fetal heart rate below 120 or above 160 may represent a potential problem, and this too should be brought to the attention of your obstetrician.

One final helpful sign for following the progress of your pregnancy is the presence of frequent urination. This is caused by the enlarging uterus, which produces pressure on the urinary bladder, and often begins four to six weeks after the last period. More significantly, it disappears after the twelfth week when the uterus rises up into the abdomen from its position in the pelvis. Frequency reappears when the baby's head descends into the pelvis days or weeks before the onset of labor.

Is there any way to determine the height and weight of the fetus during each month of pregnancy?

Yes. Thanks to a man named Hasse, the approximate length of the fetus in centimeters can be determined during the first five months by squaring the number of lunar months from the last period; after the fifth lunar month of pregnancy, the fetal length will be equal to the lunar month multiplied by five (see table 2–1). It's a fantastic bit of information, and it really works. Table 2–1 also lists corresponding average weights at the end of each lunar month during pregnancy.

Morning Sickness

How can I safely combat nausea and vomiting during the first three months of pregnancy?

Though its cause is not definitely known, nausea of pregnancy is believed to be due to the elevated levels of human chorionic gonadotropin (HCG) in the blood. Studies

Table 2–1. Average Fetal Length and Corresponding Weight at End of Each Lunar Month of Pregnancy

End of Lunar Month	Length in Centimeters	Grams	Weight Pounds and Ounces
2	2 × 2 = 4	1.1	less than 1 oz
3	3 × 3 = 9	14.2	less than 1 oz
4	4 × 4 = 16	100.0	3 oz
5	5 × 5 = 25	300.0	10 oz
6	6 × 5 = 30	600.0	1 lb 5 oz
7	7 × 5 = 35	1,001.0	2 lbs 4 oz
8	8 × 5 = 40	1,675.0	3 lbs 11 oz
9	9 × 5 = 45	2,340.0	5 lbs 2 oz
10	10 × 5 = 50	3,250.0	7 lbs 3 oz

have shown that women who do not experience nausea during pregnancy are far more likely to have a pregnancy in jeopardy of miscarriage. Similarly, the sudden disappearance of nausea during the first two months of pregnancy may represent an impending miscarriage. If you experience nausea it usually first appears at the end of the first month and subsides by the end of the twelfth week, or third lunar month, following your last period.

Though "morning sickness" during the first three months of pregnancy is often a sign of a healthy pregnancy, it is nonetheless a distressing, unpleasant, and frustrating problem. Nausea and vomiting in varying degrees of severity are known to afflict almost half of all pregnant women, often beginning at the time of the first missed period and persisting until the twelfth week of pregnancy. Though the condition is often more likely to occur in the morning, for many women it may more accurately be described as "all-day sickness."

A woman who is suffering from morning sickness during her fifth week of pregnancy finds little consolation in the fact that her symptoms will eventually subside spontaneously. Most drugs that are capable of controlling nausea and vomiting have not been proven safe for the developing fetus, and the recent adverse publicity associated with the use of Bendectin (see chapter 7) has influenced both obstetricians and their patients to seek more conservative remedies.

Certain simple measures may greatly reduce the severity of morning sickness. For example, those beverages and soups which are either very hot or icy cold are least likely to elicit nausea. Bouillon, apple juice, grape juice, ginger ale, and cola beverages are usually the most easily tolerated. Liquids, including soups, are best handled when taken between meals. For this reason it is best to eat meals without soup or drink and then drink the liquid about one hour later. Eating as many as six or seven light snacks during the day is less likely to cause nausea than two or three large meals. Even if you aren't hungry it is best that you try to eat, since nausea may become more bothersome when your stomach is empty. Carbohydrate foods such as bread, crackers, unbuttered popcorn, and baked potatoes are usually well tolerated. Eating dry crackers every two hours during the day is an excellent way to combat nausea. Some women wisely carry dry crackers in their purse during the day and eat one whenever they begin to feel sick. Another good idea is to keep crackers or dry toast next to your bed as a snack immediately upon awakening in the morning. Many women report that hard-boiled eggs are easy to digest and cause little if any nausea.

If you discover that certain stimuli, such as particular foods or smells, make you sick, try to avoid them whenever possible. Also stay away from fried or highly seasoned foods until the nausea is no longer bothersome. Occasionally, aromas of coffee, fried fish, or cauliflower precipitate an attack, so these items are best avoided. To eliminate most kitchen odors, you should cook with the exhaust fan on and the kitchen windows open.

Most prenatal vitamins contain iron supplements which may irritate the stomach and intestinal lining. In the presence of severe morning sickness it is best to temporarily avoid all iron-containing preparations.

If all the above measures fail to bring relief, medications which are both helpful and safe for the developing fetus are available. Emetrol is a pleasant-tasting, mint-flavored liquid which may be purchased without prescription at any pharmacy. It contains balanced amounts of the sugars levulose and dextrose, combined with orthophosphoric acid. One or two tablespoons, taken at fifteen-minute intervals until nausea is relieved, is an extremely effective and absolutely safe course of action. Antacids, such as Maalox, Camalox, and Mylanta, may also prove helpful in neutralizing stomach acidity. Vitamin B6, or pyridoxine, taken orally in a dose of fifty milligrams twice daily, has been enthusiastically endorsed by some gynecologists as a safe and effective antinauseant. If vomiting prevents ingestion of oral pyridoxine, it may be given as an intramuscular injection.

A very small percentage of women vomit to the point of severe dehydration and weight loss. When this occurs, the use of stronger medication is imperative (see chapter 7). On rare occasions, hospitalization and intravenous feedings are necessary to control symptoms and restore mineral and chemical balance.

Early Pregnancy and Women over Thirty

What problems of early pregnancy may I expect if I am over thirty?

Ten years ago, the vast majority of women in the United States had their first child in their early or midtwenties. Today, many women are delaying motherhood in hopes of completing their education and establishing careers. This trend is confirmed by a recent study which showed that first births among women over thirty almost doubled between 1972 and 1978. In addition, statistics from the National Center for Health show that 5 percent of births in the United States are to women over thirty-five years of age. Estimates for the year 1982 from the U.S. Bureau of Census predict that the percentage of births to women thirty-five years or older will increase by 37 percent in the 1980s. The key reason for this is that women born during the so-called baby boom between the late 1940s and mid-1950s will reach their thirty-fifth birthday during the 1980s. According to one census projection, the total number of American women between the ages of thirty-five and forty-four will increase by an astounding 42 percent during this period, a rise from 13 million to 18.5 million women.

Statistically, women over thirty are at a slightly greater risk of experiencing first-trimester bleeding and spontaneous abortion. Despite this, the vast majority of women between the ages of thirty and forty easily breeze through pregnancy and childbirth with few if any complications. These women should be encouraged in their desire to achieve a successful birth. I am far less optimistic about childbirth for women over the age of forty-five. In a study conducted by Dr. David H. Kushner of Columbia Hospital for Women in Washington, D.C., for example, women over forty-five accounted for a significantly higher number of pregnancy complications, including an alarming 40 percent spontaneous abortion rate.

Chromosomal abnormalities have been detected in 50 to 60 percent of embryos and early fetuses that are aborted spontaneously. The likelihood of such abnormalities becomes progressively greater each year in women beyond the age of thirty and men after the age of fifty-five. The older woman is also at greater risk of carrying a chromosomally abnormal infant to term (see chapter 10). This, however, need not serve as a deterrent to childbearing since chromosome analysis of an amniotic fluid sample during the sixteenth week of pregnancy can easily and accurately diagnose these problems. Women carrying a chromosomally abnormal infant may be offered a therapeutic abortion.

Leiomyomas, also known as fibroids and myomas, are benign tumors of the uterus which are commonly found in women over the age of thirty. These tumors tend to grow much larger during pregnancy and then regress in size following delivery. Even if a woman has several large fibroids, they rarely cause abortion. It is the location of these tumors, rather than their size, which determines the risk of early pregnancy complications. Fibroids which lie just under the endometrium, or lining of the uterine cavity, are most likely to create problems. Fortunately, these tumors, known as submucous myomas, account for less than 5 out of every 100 fibroids.

On rare occasions, an enlarging fibroid outgrows its blood supply and degenerates during pregnancy. Symptoms of this complication are pain and tenderness to touch over the site of the fibroid and occasionally a low grade fever. Treatment should be conservative, consisting of analgesics and bed rest since most often the signs and symptoms abate within a few days.

Diseases, such as diabetes and hypertension, are more likely to complicate the pregnancy of the older woman. Problems caused by these conditions, however, usually arise toward the end of pregnancy (see chapter 11) rather than during the first few months.

On a more optimistic note, several epidemiological studies have confirmed that infants born of older women are much less likely to experience sudden infant death syndrome (SIDS) or "crib death." The reasons for this phenomenon remain obscure despite the fact that many theories have been offered.

Spontaneous Abortions

Is vaginal bleeding during the first three months of pregnancy a danger sign?

As many as 22 percent of all women carrying healthy pregnancies may have one or two incidents of bloody discharge early in pregnancy. This may be caused by the fertilized egg implanting in the lining of the uterus and is appropriately called "implantation bleeding." However, you should report any bleeding to your doctor. Often, the bleeding is due to an erosion or inflammation of the cervix and totally unrelated to the developing pregnancy. This bleeding is more apt to occur with penile contact during intercourse and is never a cause of miscarriage.

For unknown reasons, bleeding during the first three months of pregnancy appears to be three times more frequent among women with one or more children (multiparas) than among women having their first baby (primigravidas). There is a widespread belief that pregnancy bleeding may normally occur each month at the time of the expected period. Such stories are of questionable authenticity, and vaginal bleeding at any time during pregnancy should be regarded as abnormal and investigated by your obstetrician. It is comforting to know that if your bleeding is minimal in amount and soon subsides, your chances of giving birth to a healthy baby are excellent. When bleeding represents a potentially serious condition, the most likely cause is a threatened miscarriage.

If I experience bleeding early in pregnancy which then subsides, are my chances of a successful birth equal to those of a woman who has never bled?

Probably not. Several studies have demonstrated that women experiencing bleeding for several days early in pregnancy have a significantly higher incidence of babies born prematurely or with birth defects.

What are the symptoms of impending abortion?

Doctors use the term "threatened abortion" to describe any bloody vaginal discharge or vaginal bleeding which occurs during the first half of pregnancy. Obviously this is a fairly common diagnosis, since at least one out of five women experience some bleeding early in pregnancy. Among women who experience bleeding, approximately half actually abort. Doctors prefer to see bleeding of a dark brown rather than a bright red color, because the former usually indicates "old blood" from bleeding that has occurred several days before. A threatened abortion may be accompanied by mild cramps or low back pain resembling that of the menstrual period. It has been demonstrated that when bleeding persists for longer than a week, the prognosis for successful pregnancy greatly diminishes.

A threatened abortion becomes an inevitable abortion when uterine contractions become intense, the cervix dilates, bleeding becomes heavy, with the passage of clots, or the membranes of the pregnancy sac rupture. The fetus and placenta are usually passed soon thereafter. In early pregnancies of eight weeks' duration or less, the fetus and placenta are often expelled together. When this occurs, it is termed a "complete spontaneous abortion." If the placenta, in whole or in part, is retained in the uterus, it is termed an "incomplete abortion." Under such conditions it is necessary for your doctor to remove the placental fragments retained in the uterus. Despite the fear and disappointment which spontaneous abortion at home may provoke, it is vital that you collect all tissue which is passed in a glass jar and take it to your obstetrician. Any type of alcohol or formalin can be added to the jar to preserve the tissues. If your obstetrician sees that you have passed the entire pregnancy sac, a D and C (dilatation and curettage) or suction procedure to remove retained fragments may not be necessary. In addition, your doctor and the hospital pathologist will be able to examine the tissue for a possible cause of your miscarriage.

What is the treatment for threatened abortion during the first three months of pregnancy?

There is no convincing evidence that any treatment changes the course of an early threatened abortion. Therefore, it is cruel and unusual punishment for an obstetrician to prescribe bed rest. Orgasm may be responsible for uterine contractions and should be avoided for at least two weeks after the bleeding stops. Remember, it is orgasm, not the penile trauma caused by intercourse, that produces miscarriage, and orgasm achieved through clitoral stimulation may be equally harmful. (As a matter of fact, studies suggest that orgasm achieved through masturbation may produce more intense contractions than that produced through intercourse.)

Occasionally, slight bleeding without cramps may persist for weeks while a woman suffers the anguish of not knowing whether the outlook for her pregnancy is favorable or hopeless. Though weekly examinations by an obstetrician are helpful in determining if the pregnancy is healthy and the uterus is growing, the use of ultrasound is far more accurate (see chapter 10). This modern technique is capable of discovering if the gestational sac is well formed and intact. In the presence of an impending abortion, defects in the development of the sac may be accurately diagnosed. Occasionally the findings are in doubt, but a repeat ultrasound examination one week later will practically always give the correct answer.

One type of ultrasound, known as real-time (see chapter 10), is capable of detecting fetal movement as early as the seventh week of pregnancy. When fetal movement is absent at or after the seventh week, it is often a reliable prognostic sign that abortion is inevitable. In a 1980 report, published in *Obstetrics and Gynecology,* doctors at the Bowman Gray School of Medicine, in North Carolina, used real-time to evaluate women threatening to abort. Only two of sixty-five women who eventually aborted demonstrated fetal movement, while seventy-two of seventy-four pregnancies with fetal motion continued successfully to term.

If the diagnosis of an unhealthy gestation is confirmed by ultrasound, the pregnancy may be immediately terminated by curettage, thereby sparing many women the grief of carrying an unhealthy fetus week after week.

Serial beta-subunit HCG determinations are also helpful in predicting the outcome of a threatened abortion. Failure of HCG levels to rise significantly over a period of several days is usually predictive of an eventual miscarriage. However, a doctor should not act solely on this information but should seek confirmation with ultrasound before terminating the pregnancy.

The prognosis for successful pregnancy in the face of heavy vaginal bleeding and severe cramps is poor. Under such circumstances, termination of the pregnancy by curettage is indicated.

Women likely to abort naturally should not be treated with oral and intramuscular preparations of progesterone and progestins. This form of treatment is mentioned only to be condemned. It has no proven beneficial effects and may actually increase the incidence of birth defects (see chapter 1).

What are my chances of a miscarriage, and why does it occur?

The term "miscarriage" describes what doctors call a spontaneous abortion, a natural termination of pregnancy before the fetus is sufficiently developed to survive. Ten to 15 percent of all pregnancies end in spontaneous abortion, and about nine out of ten cases will occur during the first three months.

The most common cause of spontaneous abortion appears to be an abnormality in the development of the egg (ovum) which makes it incompatible with life. In studying the microscopic chromosomal structure of these so-called abortuses, researchers have noted gross chromosomal abnormalities 50 to 60 percent of the time. If the fetus is abnormal, it is best that it be allowed to spontaneously abort. Furthermore, at this early stage, abortion will occur even if a woman is lying in bed. The only activity that pregnant women with vaginal bleeding should avoid is orgasm. Among some women orgasm may cause uterine contractions and subsequent expulsion of a normal fetus (see chapter 4). Spontaneous abortions caused by a "blighted" ovum occur in the early weeks of pregnancy.

Anatomical abnormalities of the uterus existing at birth—two separate uteri connected by a bridge of tissue, for example, or the presence of a wall, or septum, within the uterus—may also be responsible for early miscarriage. Occasionally an abnormally small uterus will be unable to hold a developing pregnancy. Some daughters of women who took DES during pregnancy may have an abnormal T-shaped uterus which may be responsible for miscarriage after the first three months (see question on the "morning-after" pill, page 15).

Myomas, or fibroids, are commonly found benign tumors of the uterine wall which may be responsible for spontaneous abortion, although rarely. Infections and scarring of the endometrium may have a similar effect. Early spontaneous abortion is known to occur when the corpus luteum of the ovary does not produce amounts of progesterone adequate to support an early pregnancy. Such endocrine imbalances as thyroid dysfunction and diabetes, as well as a wide variety of systemic diseases, may also be responsible. In 1 percent of all spontaneous abortions, the fault lies with an abnormal chromosomal pattern in one of the two normal-appearing parents.

Spontaneous abortion beyond the first trimester is rarely the result of a blighted ovum or chromosomal abnormality of the fetus. Often the cause is unknown, though the anatomic factors described above may occasionally be responsible. A weakening of the cervix, termed an incompetent cervix, has been implicated in many second-trimester pregnancy losses.

Can emotional or physical trauma cause spontaneous abortion during the first three months of pregnancy?

No. Contrary to popular opinion, there is no evidence that emotional or physical trauma is responsible for early spontaneous abortion. In seeking to explain an early miscarriage, a particular accident might be associated with the abortion that follows soon after. However, in the medical literature there are many examples of severe trauma which failed to interrupt existing pregnancies. Furthermore, most spontaneous abortions occur sometime after the death of the fetus has taken place. If abortion were caused by trauma, it would not be a very recent event but one that had occurred some weeks earlier. Since the height of the uterus is below the pubic symphysis bone until the twelfth week of pregnancy, it would be nearly impossible for physical trauma to the lower abdomen to cause injury to the fetus before this time.

How soon after a spontaneous abortion is it safe to try for a baby again?

A couple can safely resume sexual relations two weeks after a spontaneous abortion, but most doctors advise waiting at least two regular menstrual cycles before attempting another pregnancy. It is important for your obstetrician to be able to accurately estimate your day of ovulation and conception. By knowing this, it is easier to determine if your uterus is growing at a rate compatible with your presumed date of conception. This is especially important if the symptoms of threatened abortion recur.

If I have one spontaneous abortion, am I more likely to have another during my next pregnancy?

Following one spontaneous abortion, your chances of successful pregnancy are almost equal to those of a woman who has never experienced an abortion. The risk of recurrent abortion is slightly higher if the abortus is chromosomally normal rather than abnormal. Moreover, the risk is highest, perhaps 35 to 50 percent, if the abortus is chromosomally normal *and* the mother has no liveborn offspring. Even if you experience two consecutive spontaneous abortions, it is comforting to know that your risk of its happening a third time is only 5 percent above that of the general population. Habitual abortion is defined as the consecutive occurrence of three or more spontaneous abortions. In the United States, 5 percent of all spontaneous abortions are of the habitual type. Following three consecutive such abortions, a woman's risk of a fourth will be about 32 percent, or 17 to 22 percent above the 10 to 15 percent rate expected in the general population. Though the causes of habitual abortion may be varied, they must all be investigated by your obstetrician. Referral to a geneticist is also mandatory, since approximately 7 percent of habitual aborters or their husbands demonstrate chromosomal abnormalities, some of which preclude successful pregnancy. Spina bifida is a congenital abnormality of the spinal cord in which the covering membrane is incomplete. It is often associated with hydrocephaly, an abnormal enlargement of the fetal head. One recent study from England, reported in the *British Medical Journal* in 1979, confirmed the findings of previous authors that this abnormality is significantly more common among women experiencing two or more previous spontaneous abortions.

Abnormal Pregnancies

How do I distinguish between an ectopic pregnancy and a threatened abortion?

An ectopic pregnancy is one which grows outside its normal location in the endometrium. Though ectopic pregnancies have been reported to occur in the abdominal cavity, ovary, and cervix, the fallopian tube is by far the most common site. (It is for this reason that the term ectopic pregnancy is often used synonymously with tubal pregnancy.) Cramping, pelvic pain, and vaginal bleeding are symptoms common to both ectopic pregnancy and threatened abortions. As a result, an ectopic pregnancy is often mistaken for the more common threatened abortion. Approximately 1 out of every 200 pregnancies is ectopic, and if your doctor does not have a strong suspicion for this diagnosis it will be missed.

The internal hemorrhage resulting either from rupture of an ectopic pregnancy through the tubal wall or from passage of the pregnancy out of the tube and into the abdominal cavity is a far more dangerous threat to a woman's life than the heavy vaginal bleeding which may occur with a spontaneous abortion.

Ideally, it would be nice to diagnose an ectopic pregnancy before rupture and internal hemorrhage, and this is possible if you and your doctor are alerted to certain differences in the symptoms of ectopic pregnancy and threatened abortion. Though both conditions are characterized by lower abdominal pain, the pain of a spontaneous uterine abortion is generally milder, likely to be rhythmic, and located lower in the midline of the abdomen. With a tubal pregnancy the pain may be on the side of the affected tube or it may be generalized, but it is usually far more severe. The external vaginal bleeding noted with an ectopic pregnancy is usually not heavy and is dark in color, while the bleeding associated with a threatened or incomplete abortion is usually heavier and accompanied by the passage of blood clots. A careful pelvic examination performed by your doctor will usually give further clues as to the correct diagnosis. Characteristically, a woman carrying an ectopic pregnancy will experience severe tenderness upon motion of her cervix. Though the uterus, under the influence of pregnancy hormones, may be slightly enlarged when a pregnancy is in the tube, it will tend to be larger and softer when it is intrauterine. Occasionally, your doctor may be able to feel the enlargement of the tube produced by the ectopic pregnancy, but in most cases this is unreliable. As mentioned in chapter 1, if you have an IUD, the above symptoms should be a red flag of warning to your obstetrician that an ectopic gestation is a distinct possibility.

Rupture of an ectopic pregnancy is a frightening, life-threatening emergency. It is characterized by sudden severe lower abdominal pain often described as sharp, stabbing, or tearing in character. Symptoms of impending shock such as nausea, dizziness, and fainting soon follow. Treatment at this point must include immediate abdominal surgery, with removal or excision of the pregnancy and control of bleeding from the site of rupture. Often this involves removal of the affected tube. Blood transfusions are usually required to replace the large amount of blood lost following tubal rupture. Modern technological advances have allowed doctors to diagnose most ectopic pregnancies prior to rupture. This includes use of the more sensitive pregnancy tests, such as the Biocept-G and beta-subunit, to determine the presence of a pregnancy, combined with ultrasound and laparoscopy to locate its site.

Are pregnancies more likely to be abnormal if they result from artificial insemination?

Offspring conceived following artificial insemination are at no greater risk of being born with congenital abnormalities than are offspring conceived naturally. In recent years, many men undergoing vasectomy have elected first to store several ejaculates in special sperm storage facilities called frozen-semen banks, or cryobanks. The sperm are preserved in glycerol and then frozen in liquid nitrogen at -197 °C. for months or years. If a couple desires children at a later date, the sperm may be thawed and used for artificial insemination at the time of ovulation.

Several researchers have confirmed that pregnancies resulting from thawed sperm may be healthier than those conceived naturally. The reason for this is that freezing may have the effect of killing off weak and unhealthy sperm. In a University of Arkansas study of 1,000 children conceived following insemination with previously frozen sperm, it was found that fewer than 1 percent had birth defects, compared to 2 to 3 percent in the general population. In addition, it was noted that the miscarriage rate was less than 6 percent in the inseminated group, compared with the standard 10 to 15 percent which is generally quoted.

Another major benefit of cryobanking is that it is now possible to store the sperm of men who must undergo a prostate operation or chemical and radiation treatment for cancer, procedures that may make a man permanently sterile. In the days between the diagnosis and treatment, a man can deposit his uncontaminated and healthy sperm for use at a later date. It generally takes from three to six ejaculates to provide sufficient semen for artificial insemination attempts for six cycles. This should provide a couple with a reasonable chance for conception to occur. The conception rate with frozen semen from donors whose semen tolerates freezing well is close to 90 percent, but only about 37 percent of all patients can have their semen frozen and thawed while still maintaining an adequate percentage of motile sperm.

Cryobanking Facilities in the United States

**Atlanta Center for
Reproductive Health**
1285 Peachtree St. N.E.
Atlanta, Georgia 30309
(404) 892–8608
Idant Division

Cryo Lab Facility
100 East Ohio St.
Chicago, Illinois 60611
(312) 751–2632

Cryogenic Laboratories, Inc.
1935 West County Rd. B–2
Roseville, Minnesota 55113
(612) 636–3792

Frozen Semen Bank
Department of Anatomy
University of Arkansas
for Medical Sciences
Little Rock, Arkansas 72201
(501) 661–5184

Frozen Semen Bank
University of Oregon
Medical School
3181 S.W. Sam Jackson Park Rd.
Portland, Oregon 97201
(503) 225–8261

Genetic Semen Bank
Human Genetics Dept.
University of Nebraska
Medical Center
Omaha, Nebraska 68105
(402) 541–4570

Idant Corporation
645 Madison Ave.
New York, New York 10022
(212) 935–1430

International Cryogenics, Inc.
189 Townsend St. Suite 203
Birmingham, Michigan 48011
(313) 644–5822

Dr. Z. H. Marcus
University of Cincinnati
Internal Medicine Dept.
Cincinnati, Ohio 45267
(513) 872–4701

Dr. Stephen Seager
Texas A. and M. University
College Station, Texas 77843
(713) 845–7254

So. Calif. Cryobank
2080 Century Park East
Los Angeles, California 90067
(213) 553–9828

Dr. Pierre Soupart
Department OB/GYN
Vanderbilt Medical Center
Nashville, Tennessee 37232
(615) 322–6585

Reproductive Genetic Center
8320 Old Courthouse Rd.
Vienna, Virginia 22180
(703) 821–3790

Tyler Clinic
921 Westwood Blvd.
Los Angeles, California 90024
(213) 477–6765

**Washington Fertility
Study Center**
2600 Virginia Ave. N.W.
Washington, D.C. 20037
(202) 333–3100

Xytex Corporation
1519 Laney-Walker Blvd.
Augusta, Georgia 30904
(404) 724–5615

Erie Medical Center
50 High St.
Buffalo, New York 14203
(716) 883–2213
Idant Division

Since there is a strong chance that a man's semen may not survive frozen storage adequately, cryobanks routinely have a specimen undergo freeze-thaw analysis prior to accepting it for storage. Another disadvantage of cryobanking is that it may be quite expensive, and this cost may be a deterrent for many couples. Cost will vary from $20 to $60 for an initial semen analysis and evaluation of its thaw and freeze survival. Preparing and freezing each ejaculate may cost from $50 to $60, and long-term storage may range from $30 to $35 per year for each specimen.

Is the incidence of congenital malformations higher among women who take "fertility drugs"?

There are many women today who in the past were unable to conceive because they do not ovulate. Over the past decade, newer drugs popularly referred to as "fertility drugs" have allowed these women to achieve successful pregnancy. There is a popular misconception that ovulation-inducing drugs are the cure-all for every infertility problem. In reality, they do not enhance the fertility of the women who ovulates regularly. If your gynecologist determines that your infertility is not due to a failure of ovulation, there is nothing to be gained by taking these drugs.

Of all medications used to induce ovulation, clomiphene (trade name Clomid) is the most popular and the safest. It is taken in pill form over a period of five or more days and is believed to exert its effect by stimulating the hypothalamus to secrete its releasing factors. One complication of this form of therapy is a higher incidence of fraternal twins, owing to the release of more than one egg. The normal frequency of twin pregnancies in the United States is approximately one out of eighty-eight pregnancies, but this increases to approximately 8 percent following use of clomiphene.

Though clomiphene has proven to be safe for the induction of ovulation, there is some evidence that it may adversely affect the developing fetus when it is inadvertently administered after pregnancy is established. For this reason, it is imperative that you are certain that you are not pregnant before you attempt to begin a course of ovulation induction.

A smaller group of women who are unable to ovulate with clomiphene, or who have a malfunction of their pituitary gland, may achieve ovulation and successful pregnancy with the use of human menopausal gonadotropin (trade name Pergonal). This very expensive drug consists of the pituitary hormones FSH and LH. It is manufactured from, of all things, the urine of menopausal women, which is known to be rich in these two hormones. When administered as a daily intramuscular injection over a period of one to two weeks, Pergonal causes the follicle in the ovary to ripen in preparation for ovulation. Ovulation is then triggered by injecting the pregnancy hormone HCG following the last Pergonal injection. Numerous studies have confirmed that pregnancies achieved through this regimen are at no greater risk of congenital abnormalities, though the spontaneous abortion rate may be increased slightly. Of greater concern is the risk of multiple pregnancy, which may be as high as 20 percent. Usually this will be a twin pregnancy, though multiple births of three or more children, as reported by the media in recent years, may result. If the dose of Pergonal and HCG is not carefully controlled, a woman taking these medications may encounter significant risks to herself caused by hyperstimulation of the ovaries. For this reason Pergonal should be administered only by gynecologists having extensive experience with this therapy and who have easy access to a laboratory which can perform sophisticated hormonal assays on a daily basis, so that the doses of Pergonal and HCG can be appropriately adjusted and complications avoided.

Bromocryptine (trade name Parlodel) has recently been approved by the FDA for treatment of amenorrhea (absence of menses) and galactorrhea (milk secretion from the nipples). These conditions are due to a malfunction involving the releasing factors of the hypothalamus which are necessary for initiating the process of ovulation. One releasing factor of the hypothalamus prevents the pituitary gland from releasing prolactin, the hormone which causes galactorrhea. Bromocryptine lowers prolactin levels and allows the normal ovulatory mechanism to reestablish itself. The FDA has recently also approved this drug as a treatment for infertility, and several women have conceived while using it. In addition, it has been successfully used to treat postpartum lactation and breast engorgement. The safety of bromocryptine when inadvertently taken early in pregnancy has not been definitely determined. However, evaluation of more than 500 infants conceived while their mothers were taking bromocryptine has not demonstrated a higher incidence of spontaneous abortion or congenital abnormalities, nor has extensive research on rats and rabbits shown a relationship between birth defects and the use of this medication.

Interesting Pregnancy Statistics

Until what age is pregnancy a real possibility?

Successful pregnancy is extremely rare in women past the age of fifty. Though one-fourth of all women over fifty have regular menses and microscopic evidence of ovulation, pregnancy rarely succeeds because the corpus luteum of the ovary is incapable of providing adequate amounts of progesterone to support it. In one study in New York City, there was only 1 mother over the age of fifty for every 50,000 births reported. In another review of the literature covering birth statistics for over 100 years, only 26 women with normal pregnancies over the age of fifty were recorded. The oldest mother among these was a sixty-three-year-old woman! (The youngest mother on record is Lina Medina of Lima, Peru, who on May 15, 1939, age five years and eight months, was delivered by cesarean section of a 6½-pound boy.)

What is the size of the largest and smallest babies ever delivered?

The smallest surviving newborn on record was a girl delivered on August 2, 1979, at Albert Einstein Medical College, in New York City, who weighed slightly less than 15 ounces. Fantastic technological developments have enabled pediatricians to save many infants of similar weight who until recently were doomed to die.

The largest baby ever delivered was a stillborn female in 1916 who weighed 25 pounds, but delivery of a baby weighing more than 13 pounds is extremely rare. I recently delivered a 12-pound-3-ounce baby boy. Amazingly, his mother weighed a mere 105 pounds before her pregnancy.

3.
Sports and Physical Fitness

Until recently, the enjoyment of sports and physical fitness was considered the private domain of men; even women with natural ability and a love of sports often avoided participating in athletics for fear of being considered unfeminine.

Times have changed! During the past decade tremendous numbers of women have taken up a great variety of physical activities. One reason for this is an increased awareness of the importance of physical fitness, but of far greater significance is the influence of the feminist movement in this country. Women who previously assumed they were physically inferior to men now find themselves chuckling with glee while sprinting past a man during a marathon run. The feminine incursion into the sports world has occurred so rapidly that there is little unbiased research on measuring and predicting a woman's potential for athletic accomplishment.

Sports-related aspects of women's health have been overlooked or ignored by many obstetricians. Many of the old myths about the harmful effects of physical activity on pregnancy still persist. Other equally misinformed individuals believe that *no* limitations should be set on physical activity during pregnancy. This advice is far more dangerous. This chapter provides practical information and advice about the effects of sports and physical activity on the pregnant woman.

Safe Limits

How can I determine the safe limits for exertion during pregnancy?

Unfortunately, there are not enough data available to draw definite conclusions. However, most authorities agree that the way to determine the amount of training appropriate for any particular pregnant woman is to consider her prepregnancy fitness and activity level. While the physically fit woman can continue most activities at or slightly below her levels, prior to pregnancy, it is probably not wise for her to strive to exceed these limits. Extremely sedentary women will probably benefit from mild and gradual exercises such as walking, water exercises, and kinetics (see pages 63–69). These are safe and excellent methods of increasing strength and flexibility for all women.

Before you embark on an exercise program during pregnancy, it is vital for you to have a complete physical examination and medical clearance by your obstetrician. Ideally, you should start a physical fitness program prior to pregnancy. However, if

you have not done this, you can undergo a modified stress test on a bicycle ergometer or a treadmill during pregnancy to determine your exercise tolerance. These
studies are performed in the physical therapy or cardiology departments of most
hospitals by an exercise physiologist, and the results are often valuable in tailoring
an exercise program to your particular abilities. To benefit the cardiovascular and
circulatory systems, exercise must produce an increase in the heart rate to at least
150 beats per minute over a period of at least thirty minutes, excluding warm-up
and cool-down exercises. You should exercise at least three times a week, or every
other day, but not more than sixty minutes or six days per week. By using a complex
formula of your resting heart rate and maximum rate during vigorous activity, the
exercise physiologist is able to determine a target or ideal heart rate for you to hold
during each exercise session.

How do I determine my exercise tolerance
if I don't have an exercise therapist to guide me?

If, like most women, you do not have the luxury of an exercise therapist, you can
easily determine your safe exertional limits by understanding and applying some
very basic definitions. The pulse rate is simply the rate per minute that your heart
beats in transporting oxygen and nutrients throughout your body. Taking your pulse
is a simple task which may be accomplished by placing the index and middle fingers
on the underneath surface of the wrist just above the thumb. It can also be taken on
the outside of the neck, just below the junction of the jaw on one side. (Be careful
not to press too hard in this location, because you may impede the blood flow and
cause dizziness.) By counting the pulsations for 10 seconds and then multiplying by
6 you will know your number of heartbeats per minute. The resting heart rate is best
determined before getting out of bed in the morning. This is an important measurement of fitness because it tells you how hard your heart is working to keep you alive.
While the average resting heart rate for women is between 78 and 84 beats per
minute, it is not uncommon for runners and other well-conditioned athletes to have a
resting pulse of less than 50 beats per minute. You should be aware of the fact that
the resting pulse rate increases by 10 to 15 beats per minute throughout pregnancy.
It may also be higher following a meal, and especially after you drink tea or coffee.
Strong emotional responses, fever, and recent intercourse also elevates the pulse rate.

The pulse rate which is taken immediately upon stopping an exercise is appropriately known as your exercise rate. Maximum heart rate, or MHR, is defined as
the highest attainable heart rate recorded during an exercise. (The MHR is directly
affected by age, and the older one becomes, the lower the MHR should be.) It is
dangerous and foolish to exert yourself to the point of exhaustion during pregnancy
in order to determine your MHR. Instead, this information can be obtained by a
special formula:

220 beats per minute minus number of years of age equals estimated MHR

It should not be your goal to achieve your MHR during exercise. Instead, strive
for the *target heart rate,* that rate which, when attained, will provide a sufficient

level of exercise to efficiently stimulate your cardiac and respiratory system. Depending on your previous physical condition, this would be between 60 and 85 percent of your MHR. It is ill-advised for a woman in poor physical condition to even attempt to approach a target heart rate above 70 percent. Regardless of your physical condition, if maximum benefit to your cardiovascular system is to be achieved, you must maintain this target rate for at least thirty minutes per exercise session. Table 3–1 lists the target heart rate that you should try to achieve based on your physical condition.

Table 3–1. Target Heart Rate for Women Based on Physical Condition

Target heart rate (% of MHR)

60%—New participants in the program who have not been exercising
70%—Those who have been participating in a cardiovascular program for more than five weeks, twice weekly
80%—Those who have been participating in a cardiovascular program on a regular basis
85%—Those who are well-conditioned athletes

In Table 3–2 I list the approximate MHR according to age, as well as the corresponding target heart rate for the well-conditioned and poorly conditioned woman.

The ability to exercise usually decreases significantly during the first three months of pregnancy. This is due to nausea, vomiting, and general discomfort which is so common during the first trimester. Do not be disillusioned, because activity levels usually increase to near prepregnancy capacity after your third month. Regardless of your physical condition, it is a good idea to reduce your efforts slightly during the first three months.

Table 3–2. Maximum Heart Rate and Estimated Target Heart Rate for Women Based on Physical Fitness

| | | | Target Heart Rate | |
| | | | Unconditioned (60% MHR for 10 sec.) | Good Condition (85% MHR for 10 sec.) |
Age	*MHR/min.*	*MHR/10 sec.*		
20–25	200	33	20	28
26–30	190	32	19	27
31–35	185	31	18	26
36–40	180	30	18	25
41–45	175	29	17	25
46–50	170	28	17	24

**Effects of
Exercise on
Pregnancy**

**Is it true that physically fit women experience easier pregnancies
and labor than women who do not exercise?**

Though there is a general feeling that women with good physical fitness do better in
labor than those who do not exercise, this has never been proven scientifically. The
few studies that have been reported are contradictory. In 1974, the *American Journal of Obstetrics and Gynecology* reported the work of researchers at the University
of California, San Diego, who tested fifty-four women on a bicycle ergometer between the thirty-fifth and thirty-seventh week of pregnancy. Surprisingly, women
with the worst fitness scores fared equally well with their physically fit sisters later
when comparing length of pregnancy, complications, and health and weight of their
newborn babies. Nor was the length of labor among women having their first baby
significantly different in the two groups. However, among women who had previously given birth, the more physically fit individuals had significantly shorter labors.

Can too much exercise early in pregnancy cause a miscarriage?

No. Following an early miscarriage, women are often left with feelings of guilt for
having played too much tennis or jogged too many miles—or even stood or walked
for prolonged periods of time. These are myths. Research on aborted fetuses clearly
demonstrates that a very high percentage are abnormally developed or have gross
chromosomal defects.

Can too much exercise have any adverse effects on pregnancy?

It has been found that excessive exercise diverts oxygen-carrying blood away from
the uterus to the muscles and skin. Though there are no studies to show how strenu-
ously a woman can safely exercise before compromising the blood supply to her
uterus, it is known that women who experience prolonged inadequate blood flow to
the uterus tend to give birth to smaller babies. It would seem foolish, therefore, for a
woman to exercise beyond her capabilities.

Increased body temperature, or hyperthermia, is also a problem that can be
caused by excessive exercise (see question on increased body temperature from exercise, hot showers, or saunas, page 55).

Fortunately, the trend in obstetrics appears to be away from treating pregnancy
as a pathological condition. The implantation of a healthy egg into the uterine lining
(endometrium) is very strong; the egg cannot easily be dislodged. This fact can be
attested to by the millions of women who, prior to legalization of abortion by the
Supreme Court, spent hours jumping up and down in attempts to dislodge their
unwanted pregnancies.

Can a blow to the abdomen or a fall cause a miscarriage?

The uterus does not ascend to a level above the pubic symphysis bone until the
twelfth week of pregnancy, counting from the last menstrual period (see page 45).

Until that time it cannot be injured by a blow to the lower abdomen, and vigorous sports, such as gymnastics, competitive skiing, and football, can be played without fear. After the twelfth week of pregnancy, the uterus rises enough to be seen and to be palpated abdominally. At this point, the chance of injury to the uterus by a direct blow increases but is still highly unlikely. Injury to the fetus is even more unlikely, since the amniotic fluid acts as a protective cushion. Nevertheless, it is probably best to avoid contact sports or sports which might involve a direct blow to the abdomen. Many women find training physically uncomfortable after the fifth month because of the increasing size of the uterus and the bouncing inside which occurs while running. This type of movement, however, is not harmful to the baby.

Your risk of injury during athletic endeavors is likely to increase as pregnancy progresses. No matter how agile you are, you will become progressively less nimble with each month, and any activity in which there is a danger of falling should be curtailed.

Can the stress of athletic competition adversely affect my pregnancy?

Though the "thrill of victory and the agony of defeat" have been glorified on *Wide World of Sports,* the stress produced by intense athletic competition may be detrimental to the developing fetus. Under emotional stress due to any cause, body chemicals called catecholamines are secreted in greater amounts. Increased catecholamine levels produce a decrease in the uterine blood flow, which in turn lowers the amount of oxygen passing to the fetus. In one 1970 study of 150 healthy pregnant women having their first baby, the more anxiety-prone mothers gave birth to infants of lower birth weights. British doctors, in a 1979 report, found that 67 percent of women delivering between four and seven weeks prior to their due dates had experienced major psychological stresses which may have precipitated labor. Among women giving birth earlier than this, 84 percent reported experiencing major psychological traumas before the onset of labor. In comparison, only 43 percent of women delivering full-term infants had experienced major mental stress before labor. Other investigators have found a positive correlation between anxiety scores and prematurity in stillbirth rates. In a sense, some of these studies tend to support the folklore that a pregnant woman who is frightened or subjected to great anxiety may "lose her baby." Based on these reports, the best advice for the pregnant athlete is to enjoy sports but don't try too hard to win.

Can increased body temperature from exercise, from hot showers, or from saunas cause birth defects?

Though definite proof is lacking, several worrisome articles have been published recently suggesting that women who exercise so hard during the first trimester of pregnancy that they become overheated risk giving birth to offspring with central nervous system defects. Prolonged maternal hyperthermia, or increased body temperature, may be associated with a wide variety of spinal cord abnormalities and faulty development of the brain and skull of the fetus. The most critical time for this to occur would appear to be the third, fourth, and fifth weeks of pregnancy, though anomalies have been reported following an episode of hyperthermia as late as the fourteenth week. While a person's normal body temperature is 37°C. (98.6°F), elevations above 38.9°C. (102°F) appear to be associated with fetal abnormalities. Intermittent high fevers are not as threatening to the fetus as a sustained temperature rise.

Some competitive marathon runners sustain increases of temperature into the "high fever" range, though an objective study of the offspring of women marathon runners has not been conducted.

Hyperthermia itself, regardless of its cause, may be associated with the same abnormalities. In one study, seven out of sixty-three women giving birth to offspring with anencephaly (a severe defect of the brain and skull) had a history of high fever early in pregnancy. In most of these women the fever was caused by viral or bacterial infections, though two women had possibly experienced periods of increased body temperature while sauna bathing. Doctors from Dartmouth and the University of Washington medical schools, in a 1981 article, observed that fetuses affected by hyperthermia displayed similar patterns of facial deformities and central nervous system dysfunction. Mental deficiency, loss of muscle tone, abnormally small skull bones surrounding the eye, nose, and ear, cleft palate, and cleft lip were observed. In a study from Australia of 602 babies born with central nervous system defects, researchers found that the rate was 26 percent higher for infants born in the spring, compared with a control group of babies born at other times of the year, and 28 percent lower for infants born in the fall. Dr. Gordon Parker hypothesized that this seasonal variation was caused by maternal hyperthermia, which is more likely to occur when the first three months of pregnancy occur during the summer, and advised his patients to avoid excessive exercise during hot weather, to stay out of saunas during the first three months of pregnancy, and to keep temperatures down during illnesses in which there is a tendency toward a high fever. It is interesting that aspirin has recently been blamed as being the culprit in some birth defects (see chapter 7), but Dr. Parker notes that fever, not aspirin, might be the cause of these disorders.

Safe limits of exposure in a hot tub or sauna during pregnancy have not been established. However, one group of doctors has recently determined that a woman can stay in a 39°C. bath for fifteen minutes or a 41°C. (106°F) bath for ten minutes without risk of her body temperature rising above the critical abnormality-causing level of 38.9°C. Sauna bathing, because it allows for evaporation and convection, requires longer exposure. This may explain the lack of any apparent excess of hyperthermia-associated malformation problems in Finland, where maternal sauna bathing is usually limited to six to twelve minutes.

Until more evidence is available, I would urge pregnant women not to take very hot baths or showers and to avoid the sauna during the critical period of central nervous system development. The temperature in the sauna is on the average 40°C. (104°F) to 55°C. (131°F) (wet bulb) during use, and the average time in the sauna is five to twenty minutes. According to several investigators, a person's rectal temperature rises during a sauna from the normal of 37°C. (98.6°F) to between 37.6°C.

(99.7°F) and 40°C. (104°F) depending on the temperature and humidity of the sauna and the time spent within the sauna room. In one reported instance of a fetal central nervous system deformity resulting from a sauna, a woman had used it for forty-five minutes on four occasions during the fifth week after conception. On one of these occasions the temperature of the sauna rose to 43°C. (109.5°F).

What effect does exercising have on laboratory tests?

Several important laboratory blood tests may be temporarily altered following vigorous exercise. These abnormal values will usually return to normal within forty-eight hours. Elevation of three important enzymes in the blood, known as LDH, SGOT, and CPK, are extremely helpful in the diagnosis of a wide variety of diseases. All are abnormally high immediately following vigorous exercise. Measurements of uric acid in the blood aid in the diagnosis and management of preeclampsia during the last trimester of pregnancy. However, intense physical activity can cause uric acid levels to rise. Another exercise-associated change is a lowering of the hemoglobin, or red blood cell mass. This occurs because there is an increase in the plasma volume in relation to the number of red blood cells. As a result, a doctor may be given a false impression that a pregnant runner is anemic even though her actual number of red blood cells has not decreased.

Nonpregnant women who exercise vigorously and have amenorrhea or absence of periods, are known to have low blood estrogen levels. FSH and LH are the two pituitary hormones responsible for ovulation. The former is low and the latter is abnormally high among runners. Testosterone, cortisone, and prolactin are three important hormones which, when measured immediately after running, have been found to be high. When measured after a rest period of twelve hours, however, their levels all return to normal limits. TSH is released by the pituitary gland and stimulates the thyroid gland to secrete its hormones. TSH has been found to be reduced in amenorrheic runners, though this has not been associated with decreased thyroid function.

What is carpal tunnel syndrome?

The carpal tunnel is an anatomical site on the front of the wrist through which passes the major nerve supply to the hand, called the median nerve. Carpal tunnel syndrome refers to the burning, pain, stiffness, numbness, and tingling in the hands which may occur when the median nerve is compressed by the surrounding ligaments in the wrist. It may result from a variety of disease conditions, but it is also common during pregnancy, when fluid retention in the wrists and hands causes compression of the median nerve. As many as 10 percent of all pregnant woman may have symptoms of carpal tunnel syndrome, and it is often sports-related, being precipitated by activities involving strenuous or repetitive use of the wrists. Many pregnant women who fish and play tennis and golf will notice that the symptoms are intensified at the end of the day. Others will wake up in the middle of the night to shake their hands in order to "wake them up." Occasionally, the pain may spread to the elbow or even up to the shoulders.

Since carpal tunnel syndrome during pregnancy is benign and will abate after delivery, treatment in the form of corrective surgery is rarely if ever indicated. Of all the many so-called cures for this condition, the best advice is to drastically reduce activities which use repetitive hand motion. A removable splint applied and fitted to the wrist by an orthopedic surgeon will bring significant relief. If only one hand is involved, it is best to sleep on the opposite side. A low salt diet is helpful in relieving hand edema, as are mild diuretics, or "water pills." Though diuretics are rarely if ever indicated during pregnancy, this is one of the few conditions in which their advantages greatly outweigh the disadvantages.

What is hematuria, and how does it relate to physical exertion?

Hematuria is an abnormal condition in which red blood cells are present in the urine. With many blood cells the urine will turn red. If only a few cells are present it will remain a clear yellow color, but the red blood cells can still be detected by simple microscopic urinalysis. In addition, rapid urinary screening tests for protein will be positive in the presence of red blood cells. Though doctors are taught in medical school that the presence of red blood cells in the urine often indicates serious diseases of the urinary tract such as stones, infection, or even malignancy, exercise-related hematuria is a frequent and benign condition. If you are a jogger and your urine test is positive for red blood cells or protein shortly after running, tell your obstetrician to relax and retest your urine forty-eight or more hours later.

Limitations and Precautions

To what types of bone and joint injury is the pregnant athlete most susceptible?

The pregnant athlete experiences the same types of bone and joint injuries as the nonpregnant woman. However, the likelihood of injury is greater because the progesterone produced during pregnancy increases joint flexibility.

The most common of all athletic injuries are sprains and strains. A sprain is a rupture or tear of a ligament, the band of tissue that connects one bone to another. A strain is a rupture of the muscle-tendon-bone unit. Women seem to be particularly susceptible to sprains of the ankles and fingers, and knee sprains are far more common among female skiers than male skiers. The most common joints involved in partial dislocation among women athletes are the ankle, knee, elbow, and wrist.

The pubic symphysis bone is actually composed of two separate bones joined together in the midline of the pubic area by a strong ligament. This ligament, under the influence of progesterone during pregnancy, becomes so relaxed that the two bones actually separate considerably. A woman with a marked degree of this so-called symphyseal separation can actually feel the movement of the bones when walking or during any exercise involving movement of the legs. Occasionally a tight girdle will limit movement of the symphysis and relieve the discomfort felt, but frequently the movement causes extreme pain and limits all activity as pregnancy progresses.

How do the bodily changes of pregnancy limit a woman's ability to participate in exercises?

Though physical fitness fanatics are quick to point out that Evonne Goolagong Cawley played tennis professionally through her fourth month, that skier Andrea Mead Lawrence won two gold medals in alpine racing at the 1952 winter Olympics while three months pregnant, and that May Jones successfully ran thirteen miles in her ninth month of pregnancy, these events are certainly unusual phenomena that need not be emulated by even the most enthusiastic or skilled pregnant athletes. Physical activity should be a part of every pregnancy, but it is important to understand the natural bodily changes which limit optimal performance. Knowing these physiological changes and adjusting for them in your daily exercise is far more rational than denying their presence while trying to achieve unrealistic and potentially harmful goals.

The most important changes during pregnancy involve the heart and circulation. The cardiac output, or amount of work performed by the heart, increases during the first trimester. This will be reflected in your resting pulse rate, which typically increases about 10 to 15 beats per minute during pregnancy. Take this fact into account when measuring your pulse rate in response to vigorous exercise. Ninety percent of all women will develop a slight heart murmur during pregnancy due to the greater circulatory load. This is harmless and subsides soon after delivery but may confuse an examining doctor if he or she is unaware that you are pregnant. During pregnancy, there is a greater tendency for circulating blood to pool or stagnate in small, peripheral blood vessels. As a result, sudden shifts in head position may not allow adequate time for oxygen-carrying blood to reach the brain, and you may experience sudden lightheadedness and dizziness.

It is now firmly established that when a pregnant woman lies on her back during the last four months of pregnancy, the enlarging uterus will flop back and compress the veins that return blood from the lower half of the body. This hindrance of blood return to the heart may result in a dangerous lowering of the blood pressure, referred to as the supine hypotensive syndrome. Therefore, during the last four months of pregnancy, you should not rest, perform exercises, or labor for long periods of time on your back. It is much better to lie on your left side. This position takes the weight from the enlarged uterus off the vena cava, the major vein carrying blood to the heart from the pelvis and lower extremities.

The pressure in the veins of the legs increases at least threefold during pregnancy. The tendency toward stagnation of blood in the lower extremities throughout the latter part of pregnancy is due entirely to the pressure of the enlarged uterus on the pelvic veins. This is of great importance since it contributes to the ankle edema, or swelling, frequently experienced by a woman as she approaches the end of her pregnancy. It is also responsible for the development of varicose veins in the legs and vulva, as well as enlargement of the hemorrhoidal veins during gestation. Obviously, women vary a great deal in their susceptibility to these problems.

Respiratory changes occur early in pregnancy and are often felt as a shortness of breath or increased awareness of a desire to breathe. This increased respiratory effort is believed to be due to the stimulation of the respiratory center in the brain by progesterone hormone. The slight increase in respiratory rate is associated with a greater amount of work performed by the respiratory muscles. During the last two months of pregnancy, breathing may be more difficult because the enlarging uterus, which elevates the diaphragm, limits lung expansion.

Gastrointestinal changes may seriously inhibit a pregnant woman's ability to engage in physical exercise. Nausea and vomiting are usually worse during the morning but may continue throughout the day. Fortunately, this symptom usually subsides by the end of the third month of pregnancy. Heartburn, one of the most common complaints of pregnant women, is usually caused by reflux, the backing up of acidic gastric contents into the lower esophagus from the stomach. Heartburn may persist throughout pregnancy. Profuse salivation (ptyalism) is another source of distress to some pregnant women. The cause of this excess stimulation of the salivary glands is unknown, though some women may obtain relief by reducing their intake of starch-containing foods.

Most women feel unusually tired and feel the need for more sleep early in pregnancy. Headaches early in pregnancy are also a frequent complaint. All these symptoms have an unknown cause but fortunately will usually subside after the third month. You are not neurotic if you have these complaints, and you should never feel guilty for resting instead of exercising during the time that these symptoms are present.

The pressure of the enlarging uterus on the urinary bladder may cause involuntary and frequent urination during pregnancy. This is most common during the first twelve weeks of pregnancy. The problem disappears after the third month, but then reappears when the fetal head descends into the maternal pelvis during the last month of pregnancy. It is unfortunate that many books dealing with physical fitness and with pregnancy rarely mention this embarrassing physiological condition which may deter active sports participation.

There are very important skeletal and muscular changes which a pregnant woman must adjust to while participating in sports. The major change is that her center of gravity becomes lower due to the increased weight gain and enlarging abdominal girth. As a result, dexterity in sports requiring balance such as gymnastics, skiing, and diving may be affected. Backache occurs to some extent in most pregnant women. Minor degrees follow excessive strain or fatigue and excessive bending, lifting, or walking. Lordosis, a forward curvature of the spine, tends to increase as the uterus enlarges in size. Lordosis often puts excessive strain on the back muscles of some women, so that it occasionally becomes necessary to reduce all activities requiring sudden forward movement. This strain on posture usually begins at about the fifth month and is always noticeable by the seventh month. In some women there is a relaxation of the ligaments which connect the two halves of the pubic symphysis bone. This condition, previously mentioned, may result in excruciating pain on walking. Relaxation of the lumbosacral joints of the back and general relaxation of the pelvic ligaments occurs in all pregnant women and is believed to be due to an excess of circulating progesterone. This is most marked after the seventh month, and athletic injury from laxity of ligaments is most likely to occur after this time. For this reason, most gynecologists wisely recommend that women curtail strenuous exercise after the seventh month.

Breast tissue is markedly altered by hormonal changes. Though the pregnant athlete should take particular care to protect her breasts, the fear of breast trauma far exceeds the actual incidence of serious injury. (The only exception to this was noted by the team physician for the Fillies, a New York women's football team, who noted a high incidence of breast hematomas, or collections of blood in the breasts, in his players.) A pregnant woman's breasts are heavy, more glandular, and require a greater degree of support even during minimal amounts of exercise. Specially designed bras provide the extra support that the expectant athlete needs. Irritation of the nipples commonly occurs in both male and female runners due to the friction created by a shirt against the nipple. Though nipple abrasion may become a real problem as the nipples enlarge during pregnancy, it may be alleviated by wearing adhesive strip bandages or nursing pads while running. Pregnant women should be encouraged to exercise and maintain physical fitness, but all benefits of such activity will be lost if proper precautions are not taken.

Backache resulting from lordosis of pregnancy may be relieved by sleeping on a firm to hard mattress or by putting a bedboard under your mattress. Psychoprophylactic exercises are also beneficial in relieving back pain. Edema, or swelling of the ankles and feet, is a normal physiological occurrence of pregnancy created by pressure on the veins of the lower extremities by the enlarging uterus and is more likely to occur during warm weather. Diuretics should rarely be used as treatment for ankle edema during pregnancy and are mentioned only to be discouraged and deplored. A guaranteed decrease of ankle edema can be accomplished by lying in bed for twenty-four hours on the left side with your legs elevated. This will have the effect of displacing the uterus from the pelvic veins which carry blood from the legs. This treatment may have to be repeated every few days, but it is far better than taking diuretics.

Exercising under extremely hot and humid conditions may create severe discomfort and result in dizziness because the body is unable to adequately cool itself. Sports scientists say your body will not indicate its need for fluid until it has lost two to four pounds of water, so don't wait to feel thirsty before drinking. During exercise in hot weather, the formula for safeguarding against dehydration is to drink eight to twelve ounces of fluid every ten to fifteen minutes. Ice cold drinks are best because they are absorbed more quickly than liquids at body temperatures. Contrary to popular belief, sucking ice cubes won't bring on cramps and may actually help to rapidly absorb fluids. Commercial drinks and fruit juices should be diluted with half or even two-thirds the amount of water because the sugar they contain may cause cramps and slow the absorption of water into your body. You must never use salt tablets when exercising because they can increase your chances of becoming dehydrated.

The combination of excessive perspiration and intense humidity will predispose the pregnant woman to annoying Monilia vaginal infections. This condition is easily treated during pregnancy, but may be a source of great discomfort. "Jock itch" is a rash in the genital area caused by a superficial skin fungus. It is most likely to be present under conditions favoring an increase in moisture and was formerly believed to occur only in the male athlete. However, gynecologists often see this condition in their physically active patients. The incidence of "jock itch" can be reduced by wearing cotton undergarments and loose-fitting jogging shorts and avoiding exercising under extremely humid conditions. Taking prolonged hot baths also increases moisture in the genital area and should be avoided. Though there are no known detrimental effects of cold weather on exercise during pregnancy, high-altitude sports participation may be associated with decreased oxygenation to the fetus and result in the birth of a smaller baby. (A complete list of potentially dangerous high altitude areas in the United States is found in chapter 6). A black woman with sickle-cell trait may be most in jeopardy at these higher altitudes.

Which medical conditions keep the pregnant woman from active sports participation?

As mentioned previously, consult your obstetrician before undertaking or continuing any sport or training program during pregnancy. The decision on how active a woman with a particular medical problem, such as diabetes or heart disease, should be is a difficult one and may require consultation with one or more specialists. For example, exercise in moderation is often beneficial for the diabetic woman, but too much physical activity may result in severe metabolic imbalance. Insulin requirements usually increase significantly during pregnancy, and this, as well as many other factors, must be taken into consideration. Similarly, the treatment of a woman who has a history of heart disease requires frequent consultation with a cardiologist. Though a full discussion of the multitude of medical problems is beyond the scope of this book, it is important to remember that many diseases are altered in their severity by the hormonal changes of pregnancy. Diseases which have been inactive for many years may suddenly recur with greater severity, while other conditions such as arthritis may dramatically improve, thereby allowing a greater degree of physical activity.

Obstetrical complications may also dictate that physical activity be limited. Vaginal bleeding during the second half of pregnancy may indicate the presence of a low-lying placenta (placenta previa) or a premature separation of the placenta (abruptio placenta). Under these circumstances, physical activity should be severely restricted. Women with hypertension, or elevation of blood pressure, should also curtail activity. Occasionally, the medications used to treat hypertension may be associated with dizziness and loss of balance. Hypertension which specifically occurs during pregnancy is called pre-eclampsia. Pre-eclamptic women do best on bed rest and careful medical supervision. Though exercise in the presence of a threatened abortion during the first three months of pregnancy is unlikely to precipitate a spontaneous abortion, this may not be the case after the third month if a woman has an incompetent cervix. Exercise of any type must be avoided both before and after corrective surgery is performed on the cervix. Weakening of the ligaments which support the uterus may occasionally cause it to prolapse, or drop. This situation is more likely to occur among women who have carried previous pregnancies. The cervix may actually protrude through the vaginal opening and require a pessary device to reposition it and support the uterus. Women with a significant degree of uterine prolapse should not engage in physical activity during pregnancy.

What precautions should I take while exercising?

Total awareness and acceptance of your body's cardiovascular and respiratory alterations, postural changes, relaxation of ligaments, and weight gain will allow you to safely enjoy exercise and sports throughout your pregnancy. You can continue any activity or sport you practiced before pregnancy at or near the same level of exertion (for exceptions, see questions on specific sports, pages 63–69).

Exercises involving sudden shifts in head position should be avoided because of the dizziness which may result from the cardiovascular changes of pregnancy described above. Similarly, you must remember not to exercise on your back for prolonged periods of time during the second half of your pregnancy. This position may not only lower your blood pressure but may also be harmful to your baby. While it is beneficial to stress the cardiovascular system to some degree, it is unwise to push yourself to a point beyond your predesignated target heart rate. Movement of the legs in any sport during pregnancy is helpful to the circulation and increases the flow of blood from the veins in the lower extremities. Support stockings and pantyhose are often beneficial in improving the blood circulation if you are predisposed to varicose veins.

Regardless of the type of exercise you may perform during pregnancy, the risk of injury to ligaments, muscles, and tendons can be diminished if the activity is preceded by proper warm-up and flexibility exercises (pages 76–82). In addition, maximum physical activity must not be stopped abruptly, but should taper off slowly. This slowing down phase is usually called the cool-down period.

Exercises and Sports for the Pregnant Woman

How do specific sports affect a pregnancy?

Cross-country skiing can be an invigorating form of aerobic exercise for the pregnant woman. If you are an accomplished downhill skier, participate on a slope which is one step below your normal level; in other words, if you are an expert skier you should ski at an intermediate level or lower. Many accidents occur on icy terrain, so it is best to ski only under conditions which are optimal. Many skiing accidents result from collisions; try to do most of your skiing on weekdays when the mountain is likely to be less populated. Avoid rapid changes in head position, which may cause dizziness. Because skiing at high altitudes may decrease the oxygen supply to the fetus (see chapter 6), stay below 7,000 feet above sea level.

Ice skating should present no problems if you are an accomplished skater, though changes in your body's center of gravity can hinder your balance. It is a good idea to wear heavy clothing as a buffer against falls. Ankle and foot edema combined with the greater ligament relaxation of pregnancy will make you more susceptible to injuring your ankle or knee. For this reason, it is best not to learn to ice skate during pregnancy.

Bowling is a sport which offers little in the way of aerobic benefits. Nevertheless, it is a popular and safe activity for the pregnant woman.

Though the walking involved in golf is excellent exercise, don't expect to improve your golf swing during pregnancy. Many pregnant golfers actually have to drastically flatten their swing after the fifth month in order to compensate for their increasing abdominal enlargement. It is important to play golf in loose comfortable clothing and to avoid playing on very hot and humid days.

The racket sports of squash and racquetball provide excellent aerobic activity for the pregnant woman. If singles competition is too exhausting, you may want to play squash doubles, paddle tennis, or regular tennis doubles. Singles tennis provides far greater exercise than doubles, but it also requires first-rate physical conditioning. After the fifth month of pregnancy, I advise my patients to limit their tennis to doubles.

Regardless of the sport you choose, remember to do it for fun and never with the unhealthy competitive attitude of winning at all costs. Such an attitude may actually be harmful to your fetus (see page 55).

What sports provide the best exercise for the pregnant woman?

There is ample evidence to show that the circulatory system is best served by participation in aerobic exercises. Aerobics literally means "with oxygen," and aerobic exercises are those which are most likely to bring in oxygen and deliver it to the tissue cells, where it is combined with foodstuffs to produce energy. Aerobic exercises benefit your cardiorespiratory system because you are able to take in more air with less effort, and your heart becomes stronger because it is able to pump more blood with fewer strokes. Aerobic exercises include walking, jogging, cycling, swimming, and cross-country skiing. All these sports utilize the whole body in rhythmic and continuous movement. Swimming and cycling are the best because they are weight-independent, meaning that by performing the exercise you do not have to support your body weight. On the other hand, weight-dependent exercises, such as walking and jogging, require that the body weight be supported and therefore require greater effort to do the same amount of work as pregnancy progresses.

Participant sports such as golf, tennis, volleyball, and bowling are not as aerobically beneficial as the above-mentioned activities. Isometrics, weight lifting, and most calisthenics improve strength and flexibility but are aerobically the least beneficial. Few people look on dancing as an aerobic exercise, but many excellent aerobic dancing programs have been developed throughout the country. Aerobic dancing is an attractive alternative to the drudgery and boredom of a rigid exercise class incorporating the graceful movements of dance with the beneficial bodily effects of aerobics. Aerobic slimnastics is derived from aerobic dancing and combines the basics of dancing with calisthenics, muscle stretching, and strengthening maneuvers.

What sports should be avoided during pregnancy?

Definite hazards are associated with water skiing, and this sport is best avoided. There are several reports in the medical literature of severe vulvar and vaginal lacerations and hematomas (collections of blood) caused by a direct blow from a water ski. In addition, falling into the water at high speeds while skiing has resulted, on rare occasions, in water rapidly entering through the vagina and cervix and into the uterus and fallopian tubes. Spillage of this water into the pelvis has caused peritonitis or abdominal infection. Furthermore, there is a documented case in the medical literature of an early miscarriage occurring shortly after an involuntary vaginal douche while water skiing. Inadvertent water enemas resulting from a fall while water skiing are fairly common, though it rarely causes more than moderate discomfort. However, perforation of the bowel from this type of accident has been described. The standard swimsuits worn by the majority of water skiers allow water at high pressure to reach the vulva and enter the rectum and vagina. If you plan to water ski despite advice to the contrary, it would be much safer to wear a rubber wet suit or rubber pants rather than a standard swimsuit.

Scuba diving has gained great popularity, and many women today are engaged in sport, military, commercial, and scientific diving. However, most experts in the field of diving medicine agree that pregnancy is not the time to learn how to scuba dive. The question as to whether or not it is safe to continue to scuba dive during pregnancy is unanswered at the present time, but one 1979 animal study suggests that scuba diving may be potentially hazardous to the fetus. Researchers monitored the umbilical arteries of fetal sheep in utero during dives of varying depths and time spent underwater followed by decompression. At the greater depths, the fetal sheep died from massive intravascular air bubbling, although the mothers had no bubbles in their bloodstream. The human placenta is similar in structure to that of the sheep, and since humans are generally more susceptible to decompression sickness than are sheep, the authors concluded that the human fetus would also be susceptible. On the basis of this study, experts conclude that diving during pregnancy should be avoided. If you insist on diving, avoid depths greater than 60 feet and spend only a short amount of time on the bottom. One interesting and unexplained observation, reported in 1982, is that women married to male divers are twice as likely to give birth to a female than a male.

Horseback riding is another sport that should probably be avoided throughout pregnancy. There are no objective studies to prove that the bouncing movement of a horse is detrimental to the well-protected fetus, but aside from the obvious dangers of a fall, the pregnant equestrienne may be more prone to tenosynovitis (inflammation of the tendon and joint attachment) of a muscle in the thigh called the adductor longus. This muscle is attached to the pubic symphysis bone, and symptoms of inflammation are vulvar pain and tenderness. This condition is the most common pelvic complaint among nonpregnant riders. It hurts more during pregnancy because of the increased softening of the ligaments, which causes greater movement of the two halves of the pubic symphysis bone.

Data collected from the athletic departments of several colleges indicate that of the many sports in which women participate, the greatest number and variety of injuries occur in basketball. This is followed closely by volleyball and gymnastics. The sports which produce the most serious injuries, including major fractures, head injuries, and dislocations, are basketball, field hockey, softball, and gymnastics. Participation in these sports with any degree of intensity would appear to be a foolish endeavor during pregnancy.

Is kinetics a good form of exercise for a pregnant woman?

Yes. Kinetics is a form of exercise which combines the disciplines of calisthenics, yoga, and isometrics to help the body develop strength and stamina. According to its creator, Ms. Gail Pudaloff, kinetics is ideal for the pregnant woman who wants to keep in shape but is unable to participate in the more strenuous and exhausting forms of exercise of better-conditioned women. Movements in kinetics are never vigorous, and the goal is to build stronger and firmer muscles with a minimum amount of exertion. Students concentrate on specific muscle groups, working on them section by section in slow, small, controlled movements. Ms. Pudaloff emphasizes that correct breathing is important to the success of kinetics exercises. She advises that women take a deep breath when they reach the maximum stretch in a movement and hold that breath for two to three counts for the goal of five counts.

Is walking a beneficial exercise during pregnancy?

Yes. Though we usually don't think of walking as an exercise, it is an excellent way of promoting physical fitness without risking the injuries which may occur with jogging. Walking is especially suitable for pregnant women who are not athletic, are overweight, or are accustomed to a sedentary life-style. When practiced at regular intervals, it can prevent the gaining of excessive amounts of weight during pregnancy. On the average, a three-mile walk in an hour's time by a 160-pound woman will use up about 285 calories. The same activity by a 120-pound woman will use about 215 calories (see chapter 8). In a 1980 report, doctors at Tel Aviv University Medical School observed a significant improvement in physical fitness within three to four weeks when their patients walked half an hour a day, five days a week, at a pace of three miles an hour while carrying a 6½-pound load.

If you are in less than ideal physical condition and are considering walking as an exercise during pregnancy, be sure to start slowly. You can begin with a two-mile-an-hour pace for twenty minutes and gradually work your way up to a pace of three or four miles an hour for at least half an hour at a time. To achieve maximum benefits, you must walk purposefully, rather than stroll, and you should exert yourself enough to increase your heart rate to at least 130 beats per minute. Fitness can also be enhanced if you carry a backpack, shopping bag, or briefcase weighing six to thirteen pounds.

Walking is an ideal exercise—anyone can participate, it can be done at your convenience, it is free, and requires no special equipment other than a good pair of shoes.

How does jogging affect the mother and the fetus?

In one carefully controlled study from the University of Hawaii in 1978, Dr. Rudolph H. Dressendorfer noted the effects of a strenuous jogging program on a woman whom he followed through two pregnancies over a period of four years. He observed no disturbance to mother or fetus when the maternal heart rate reached as high as 95 percent of her maximum heart rate. He also noted that his subject was able to increase her maximum oxygen intake and endurance to levels above normal through a carefully planned exercise training program during pregnancy. Though her exercise schedule called for long-distance runs of six to eighteen miles, she remained healthy throughout the four years that the test was conducted and both pregnancies resulted in the delivery of healthy infants weighing over seven pounds. Women should not draw premature conclusions from this limited study since it involves only one closely monitored individual.

Most women, unlike Dr. Dressendorfer's subject, run in moderate amounts of one to two miles several days per week. The safety of this degree of activity has recently been evaluated in an article published in the *American Journal of Obstetrics and Gynecology* in March, 1982. Doctors evaluated the fetal status of seven pregnant women who jogged approximately one and a half miles three times a week. Electronic monitoring of the fetal heart rate was performed before and immediately after jogging on several occasions during the last three months of pregnancy. Normally, the fetal heart rate ranges between 120 and 160 beats per minute, and all seven joggers were within this range prior to exercise. Postjogging fetal heart rates accelerated to between 180 and 204 beats per minute, and it took an average of twenty-two minutes for the heart rate to return to the prejogging level. Nonstress testing (NST), indicating the possibility of fetal distress (see chapter 11), was also performed before and immediately after jogging. Of thirty NSTs performed, all indicated a healthy fetus and this diagnosis was confirmed at delivery. The authors concluded that moderate amounts of maternal jogging were probably safe, but they also noted that an alternative and contradictory conclusion would be that the consistent postexercise fetal rapid heart rate represented a fetal compensatory state, perhaps in response to undetected fetal distress.

There is little scientific evidence to support the view that jogging benefits pregnancy. Most sports medicine experts agree that exercise to the point of hyperthermia, or greatly elevated body temperatures, during the first trimester may cause birth defects (see question on hyperthermia, page 55). Also, strenuous running programs late in pregnancy may lead to a significant shifting of blood flow from the uterus to the leg muscles. This in turn may decrease the amount of oxygen carried to the placenta. Though such changes are unlikely to affect a healthy baby, they may cause significant distress for the compromised infant.

What are some of the physical problems that pregnant joggers may experience?

The greater amount of relaxation of the joints of the knee and ankle during pregnancy, believed to be caused by the rise in progesterone hormone levels at this time, makes the pregnant jogger more susceptible to joint injuries than the nonpregnant woman. Even a slight increase in weight may produce enough added stress on the lower body during jogging to cause joint damage. The continual bouncing of the jogging motion may also strain abdominal muscles and pelvic ligaments. Though support hose is of some benefit, it is more important that jogging be done correctly and efficiently to prevent muscle and ligament injury. Novices at jogging should ask more accomplished runners to observe and make corrections in their style where indicated.

Edema, or swelling of the ankles, is a normal occurrence of late pregnancy created by pressure on the veins of the lower extremities by the enlarging uterus. Since edema limits ankle movement there is a greater likelihood of injury. When a pregnant woman with foot and ankle edema does injure a ligament or sprain an ankle, healing is slower than if edema was not present. In such cases a sprain can take several months to heal.

To reduce the risk of ankle and knee injuries wear proper jogging shoes and avoid extensive running on a hard surface. Do correct warm-up and flexibility exercises (see exercises, pages 76–80) before jogging and follow jogging with a cool-down period.

Gradually increasing lordosis, or forward curvature of the spine, is a major problem for the pregnant jogger. As the uterus enlarges, the muscles of the back are increasingly strained in their attempts at maintaining normal posture. This condition is especially noticeable after the fifth month of pregnancy. Backache resulting from lordosis of pregnancy can be relieved by sleeping on a firm to hard mattress or by putting a bedboard under your mattress. Psychoprophylactic exercises (see page 79) are also beneficial in relieving back pain.

Irritation of the nipples commonly occurs in both male and female runners due to the friction created by a shirt against the nipple. This condition, known as "jogger's nipples," may produce redness and bleeding and create a real problem as the nipples enlarge during pregnancy. It may be alleviated by wearing a specially designed runners bra and adhesive strip bandages or nursing pads while running. Coating the nipples with petrolatum or applying protective dressing and wearing shirts with satin-like finish, such as those made of synthetic fabrics, should alleviate the irritation.

There is no scientific validity to the claims that jogging during pregnancy contributes significantly to permanent sagging of the breasts and the weakening of the pelvic muscles and tissues which support the uterus and bladder. Nevertheless, it is recommended that all women wear a good supportive bra while jogging to prevent breast pain and contusions caused by the force of the breasts striking against the chest wall.

Despite the claim that jogging is responsible for weakening of pelvic support and prolapse or droppage of the uterus and urinary bladder, American gynecologists have not observed an epidemic of prolapse among their nonpregnant joggers. In fact it has been reported that 25 percent of women with symptoms suggestive of urinary bladder prolapse actually improved when they started a running program. To quote gynecologist Dr. Robert Hedequist, "If female organs are going to drop down during jogging, think what male organs will do."

The loss of urine with weight-bearing exercises, such as jogging, may increase during pregnancy due to the pressure of the enlarging uterus on the urinary bladder. Pregnant joggers should wear a pad when they run. Urine loss during pregnancy may also occur when you laugh and sneeze—but this is no reason to give up these activities.

If you experience uterine or urinary bladder prolapse following childbirth, be assured that it was caused by your beautiful child and not by your activity levels. Whether or not you will develop prolapse is determined by the inherent strength of your connective tissues and muscles which support your uterus and bladder. There are many women with five or more children who have better pelvic support than others who have had only one child. Inheritance is an important aspect of this condition—if your mother experienced prolapse associated with childbirth, there is a good chance that you will too.

Is it safe to swim or dive while pregnant?

Women often express fear that water may enter the vagina while swimming and cause infection, especially during the last months of pregnancy. Such fears are groundless. You can prove this to yourself by inserting a tampon and seeing if it gets wet while swimming. Though the outer portion may become slightly dampened, you will find that most of the tampon will remain dry. Water and air can be thrust upward into the vagina following a high feet-first dive, and higher dives should be avoided, but diving head first into the water should be safe for at least the first three months of pregnancy, when the uterus is well protected by the pubic symphysis bone. Diving after this time should be avoided even though it is probably safe. If you accidentally land on your abdomen, injury to you or your baby will be highly unlikely since the amniotic fluid surrounding the baby will easily cushion the impact.

In an attempt to evaluate the effect of scuba diving on human pregnancy, a 1980 report surveyed 208 female divers. The number of fetal anomalies for those who dove during pregnancy did not exceed the range for the general population. However, the data suggested that women who dove during pregnancy, especially if they made deep and decompression dives, tended to have more fetal anomalies than women who did not dive when pregnant. On the basis of these studies, most experts conclude that diving during pregnancy should be avoided. However, if you insist on diving, you should avoid depths of 60 fsw (feet of sea water) and the duration of time spent on the bottom should be one-half the limits established by the United States Navy no-decompression tables.

What to Wear While Exercising

What should I wear in order to be most comfortable and avoid injury while exercising?

Since foot and ankle injuries are more likely to occur while running during pregnancy, it is very important to select well-cushioned, properly fitting shoes. Instead of running in an old pair of tennis shoes, buy shoes specifically designed for running. One popular brand is Nike Lady Roadrunner, which has a long-lasting rubber sole, making it suitable for long-distance running. Lady Waffle Trainer, another shoe from Nike, has a waffle sole for extra cushioning. New Balance W320 is a narrower shoe giving a snugger fit. When purchasing shoes, always try them on over cotton athletic socks and wear these thicker socks while running in order to prevent blisters from forming.

Despite good running shoes, many joggers still injure their ankles, knees, hips, bones, and muscles because they inadvertently pronate—roll their feet inward—as they move forward. Often misdiagnosed as "flat feet," excessive pronation can easily be corrected by adding special inserts called orthotics to shoes. Orthotics are also helpful in preventing stress fractures of the leg and knee, as well as hip problems in people with high arches. They can be purchased in a surgical supply store or custom made through a podiatrist or orthopedic physician.

Properly fitting support stockings and pantyhose are helpful in reducing edema of the feet and ankles and in preventing pooling of blood in the varicose veins of the legs. Hanes and Slenderalls Support Stockings are functional and also fashionable; they may be purchased in most department stores. Parke Davis, a drug company, sells a variety of good maternity support pantyhose and stockings for approximately twice the cost of the above brands. They may be purchased either at pharmacies or surgical supply stores and are well worth the added expense. The Truform Elastic Legotard costs approximately $35 but is of excellent quality. Legotards may be purchased at most pharmacies or surgical supply companies. Kendrick Stockings are also expensive but worth the investment. They come in a variety of sizes and require some fitting. The Kendrick knee-length stocking sells for about $30 a pair, while the thigh-length stocking costs a little more per pair. Jobst stockings are the Rolls-Royce of maternity support stockings. They must be fitted to the exact contour of your leg and in my opinion give better support than any other stocking. A knee-length Jobst stocking costs about $20; the thigh-length stocking sells for slightly more, and the pantyhose costs approximately $60.

To help prevent "jock itch" caused by a superficial fungus, and vaginitis and vulvitis caused by monilia (see chapter 5), the physically active woman should wear cotton panties or panties having cotton inserts.

The Flexnit High Back Maternity Girdle gives added support to the pregnant woman's enlarging abdomen while she is exercising. Vassarette and Olga also offer a wide variety of panty girdles and panty briefs. The Vassarette sports brief is excellent for exercise early in pregnancy, but not after the fifth month.

Because of the hormonal changes which take place in the breasts during pregnancy, a bra with good support is essential. Studies have demonstrated that standard bras are inadequate for the needs of women athletes, especially those who are pregnant. American manufacturers have recently introduced several brands of extrasupport "sport bras." Select one that is fairly rigid so that it limits breast motion but does not bind. Dr. Christine Haycock, a physician who has done research on this subject, suggest that you jump up and down while trying on a bra. A properly fitting bra will allow a very slight bounce to the breasts without producing pain. It is important to be sure that all metal fasteners are covered in order to prevent chafing, and seams should be padded. Dr. Haycock suggests nonelastic bra straps to prevent stretching. In addition, the straps over the shoulders should be wide so they do not slip. The strap across the back must be wide and fit low if it is to provide adequate support. "Cut and sew" rather than one-piece bras are recommended. All-cotton bra cups are preferred because they allow maximum absorption of perspiration and are less abrasive than nylon. Some women with large breasts prefer under-wire bras. However, they are not recommended because they tend to cut into the breasts.

Bras recommended by Dr. Haycock include the Tryform Serious Runner's Bra, Lily of France, Lovable Sport Bra, Splendorform, and Lady Duke. Two excellent maternity bras providing excellent support are Bali and Smoothie. Warner and Smoothie produce bras which may be used for sports participation during pregnancy, though they are not specifically sold as maternity bras. The Running Free bra from Vassarette is a 100 percent cotton knit "cut and sew" bra which gives excellent support. Playtogs, manufactured by Playtex, is the latest of the specially designed sports bras.

Water Exercises

What advice do you have for participation in water sports during pregnancy?

Regardless of your level of ability, you will derive great benefit from the positive aerobic effects of swimming during pregnancy. In doing laps in a pool, it is important to pace yourself and do them slowly without exertion to the point of exhaustion. Even if you are a nonswimmer or very poor swimmer, you can still participate in the prenatal water exercise classes offered by many Ys. All these exercises are simple and cause no undue stress to muscles, tendons, or ligaments. Below is an outline of the prenatal swimming exercise program offered at the Westport, Connecticut, YMCA.

Prenatal Water Exercises
1. Warm-ups.
   a. Jog in chest-deep water in a big circle with both hands on shoulders; jog back against current.
   b. Stand in chest-deep water. With feet apart, arms stretched out, push water from side to side with both hands. Push water from side to side and reach up into the air.

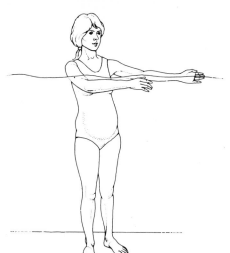

Warm-ups.

c. Stretch arms out to the sides and make circles, first with your fingers, then with your hands, lower arms, and whole arms. Reverse. Finish by pushing water from side to side again.

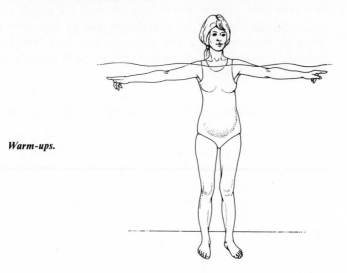

Warm-ups.

d. Jog to pool wall.
2. Waistline. Stand with feet apart, hold onto pool wall with one hand. Reach other hand over your head and make ten side bends. Repeat on the other side.

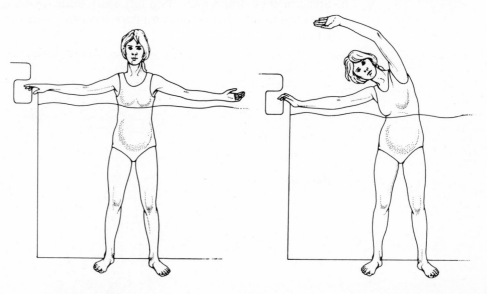

Waistline exercise.

3. Pelvis and thighs. Hold onto wall with right hand and underarm, stretch left foot out in front of you so it touches the wall, bring it out to the side, back, down, and up to the wall again ten times. Place same foot on the wall and reach your toes ten times. Turn and repeat exercise with the other foot.

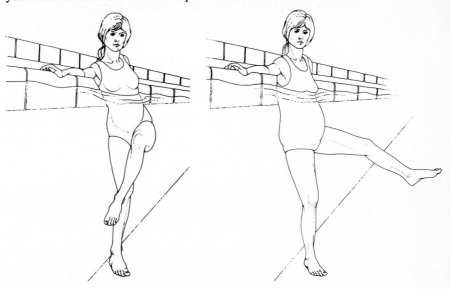

Pelvis and thigh exercise.

4. General stamina. Walk around in a big circle with arms moving in crawl strokes. Walk back against the current.
5. Leg muscles and pelvis.
   a. Hang onto wall and bicycle forward. Bicycle with knees outward. Bicycle backward. To prevent cramps, do not point toes.

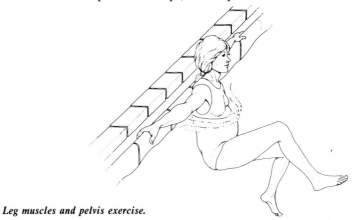

Leg muscles and pelvis exercise.

b. Walk around in a big circle with arms moving in breast strokes; walk back against the current.

6. Stomach.

a. Hang onto wall, back tight against it, then lift up both legs in front of you. Swing your legs apart, together, and down. With back still tight against wall, lift legs up, bend knees, stretch legs out, and lower slowly. Repeat both five times.

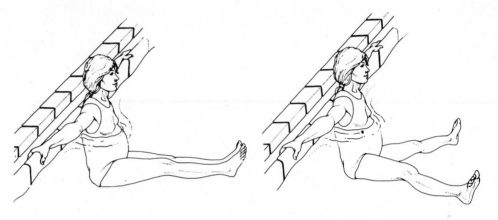

Stomach exercise.

b. Walk around in a big circle with your arms moving in butterfly stroke. Walk back against current.

7. Legs and waistline. Hang onto wall and do crossover bicycling.

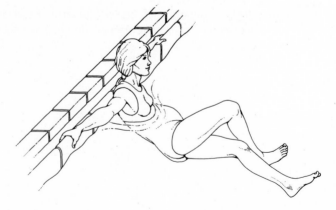

Legs and waistline exercise.

8. Pelvis and inner thighs. Face the wall, hang on with both hands, and walk up the wall with your feet outside your arms; "frog walk."

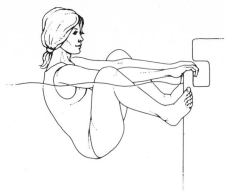

Pelvis and inner thigh exercise.

9. Varicose veins.
   a. Life one leg, make small circles with foot out in front, sideways to the wall. Repeat with other foot.

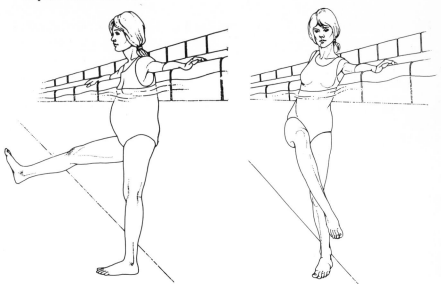

Varicose vein exercise.

   b. Walk around in a big circle, grabbing the air, really stretching. Walk back against current.
   c. Finish with two or three laps of swimming with two kickboards, one under each arm. If you have any back problem, or if it is late in your pregnancy, swim on your back.

10. Knee-to-nose kick for legs and thighs: Hold wall with both hands and bring knee up toward face. Don't point toe. Bring leg down and back up to surface of water. Do this four times with each leg before changing to the other.

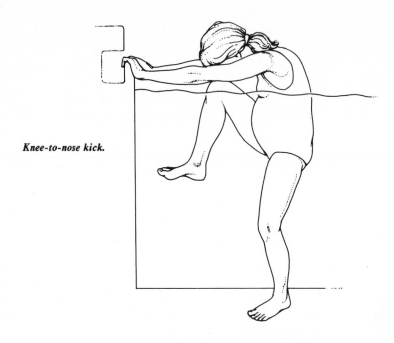

Knee-to-nose kick.

An Exercise Program for a Healthier Pregnancy

What exercises are recommended for a healthier pregnancy which will also help avoid injury when participating in sports?

Women who exercise regularly and thoughtfully during pregnancy often note a greater sense of emotional and physical well-being. Properly performed flexibility exercises loosen the muscles, strengthen the legs, and enhance the strength and resilience of the shoulders and elbows. The muscles and tendons of the legs, back, and shoulders are most vulnerable to strains, and a regular exercise program, emphasizing careful stretching of these muscles, can prevent most sports-related injuries. Vigorous jerking movements, which can only have the reverse effect of contracting the muscles should be avoided. Instead, the stretching exercises should be done slowly and carefully, holding the body for several seconds in the stretch position. Many of these exercises are used by women studying the Lamaze method of childbirth. In addition to their obvious physical benefits, they also provide an efficient method of psychological relaxation and satisfaction.

Leg and Thigh Exercises

To prevent what can be a crippling injury to the calf muscles and the Achilles tendon, wall push-ups are extremely helpful. Stand 12 to 15 inches from the wall, facing it. Place your palms on the wall while keeping your heels on the floor, your knees back, and your arms and body straight. Next, bend your elbows and move the upper part of your body toward the wall until your chest presses against it. You should feel a pull in your calf muscles. Hold this position for 10 seconds, slowly push away from the wall, and then return repeating 10 times. This exercise should be performed every morning and night until you no longer feel the pull in your calf muscles. As your muscles become more flexible you can move back to a distance of 2 feet from the wall.

Wall push-up.

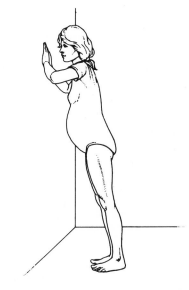

Injury to the thigh muscles and tendons can be quite painful and incapacitating. One simple exercise for increasing flexibility of the thigh muscles is to bend from a standing position and touch the floor with your fingers while keeping your knees straight. Hold this position for 10 seconds, and repeat the exercise 4 more times per day. If you can't touch the floor with your feet close together, it is permissible to spread your feet apart, provided you don't bend your knees. This is called a split stretch.

Split stretch.

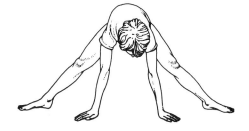

If even the split stretch is too difficult, particularly after the fifth month of pregnancy, place the heel of one foot on a low table or desk, making sure to hold the knee straight with your hands. Then bend the other knee until the leg on the table is resting evenly on the tabletop with the foot pointing up and backward toward your face. Repeat this 5 times, once a day, on each leg until the tightness in the thighs is relieved. After you are experienced at this maneuver, you can try leaning over toward your raised foot and holding that position for a count of 10.

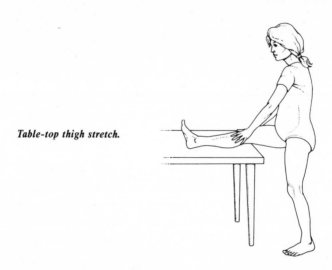

Table-top thigh stretch.

The hurdlers stretch also helps stretch the muscles along the backs of your legs. This is done by sitting on the floor with one leg outstretched and the other at your side. Lean forward to grasp the foot of your outstretched leg. Hold this position for a count of 10 and then release. Do this a total of 5 times with each leg once a day.

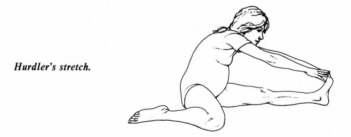

Hurdler's stretch.

Another exercise benefits the front of the thigh: stand with one hand resting on a wall or table while grasping your ankle with your other hand. Pull your foot back until either your heel touches your buttock or you feel a pull in the thigh. This exercise should be repeated 5 times with each foot, holding each time for a count of 10, once a day, until the pull in the thighs disappears.

Back and Abdominal Exercises

There are several exercises which are specifically designed to strengthen and relax your abdominal muscles and lower back and which help prevent the accentuated forward curvature of the spine during pregnancy. If these exercises are performed diligently, the low back pain which often accompanies the lordosis of pregnancy may be significantly reduced. The pelvic tilt is performed by lying on your back with your feet on the floor and knees bent. In this position, tighten your buttocks and abdominal muscles, then rotate your pelvis backward, then upward, lifting your hips off the ground. Hold this position for a count of 10, then release and rest for a count of 5. This can be repeated 20 times a day.

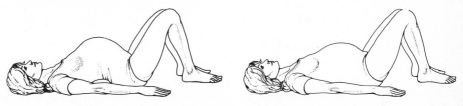

Pelvis tilt.

Bent-leg sit-ups are done in the position shown, never with the knees straight. Start with 10 per day and gradually work up to 30. Before rising from the supine position touch your chin to your chest, then let a deep breath out as you begin to sit up. Easier sit-ups may be done with your hands reaching toward your knees. When you have mastered this technique, try sitting up with your arms folded across your chest, placing one hand on each shoulder.

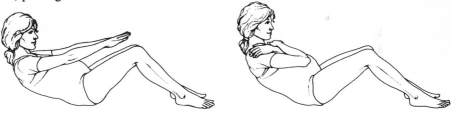

Bent-leg sit-up.

A good muscle-relaxing exercise to perform after sit-ups is the hip twister. Lie on your back with your knees bent and slowly move your knees from side to side while turning your head in the opposite direction. Continue this for a period of 30 seconds, gradually increasing to 1 minute.

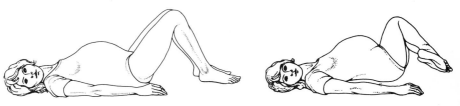

Hip twister.

Some of the best exercises for preventing and relieving low back pain during pregnancy are the knee presser and curl exercises. To perform the knee presser exercise, lie flat on your back and pull one knee up to your chest, holding it in this position with your hand. Hold this stretch position for a count of 5; each leg a total of 5 times. After this, bring both legs up together for 5 times. Do these exercises slowly, without jerking.

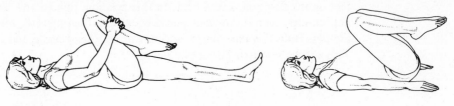

Knee presser.

Lying on your back, the curl position is assumed by bringing the knees to the chest and the head to the knees. Breathe out during the curl and hold the position for a count of 6. Relax and then repeat the exercise 4 more times.

Curl.

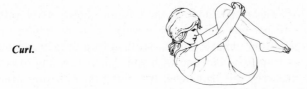

Shoulder Exercises

A simple apparatus can be used at home to strengthen your shoulder muscles. Hang a pulley on a clothes hook on the wall and run a 6-foot length of rope on a firm cord through the pulley. With hands held together and raised in front of you, grasp an end of cord in each hand, pulling one end toward you while the other arm rises as high as comfort permits. Hold your elbows straight. Pull up and down 20 consecutive times a day.

Shoulder exercise with pulley.

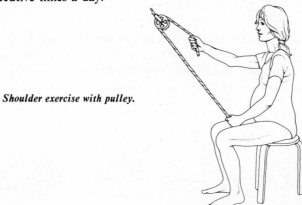

Exercises with Weights

The orthopedic surgeon Dr. James A Nicholas recommends the use of weights for women who are interested in significantly strengthening their legs. If these exercises are performed carefully, I see no reason why a pregnant woman cannot benefit from them. They are also helpful in strengthening one leg if it is weaker than the other as a result of a previous injury. Expensive equipment is not needed; all that is required is a group of weights, such as whole or half bricks in sizes of 1½ to 5 pounds. Traction weights and metal weights through which a belt can be passed also serve well. Dr. Nicholas recommends an old handbag, a pail, a flour sack, or other receptacle for holding the weights, as well as a belt or strap for attaching the weights to the foot.

To strengthen the thighs, sit on a high desk or table with your legs hanging down. Place a folded towel under the thigh at the edge of the table. Suspend a comfortable amount of weight from one foot. This should probably be no more than 10 pounds at first. Raise your thigh about 8 inches above the table and hold it there for 1 second; then return to the starting position. Do not persist if you experience pain. If you do not experience pain, do the exercise a total of 10 lifts with each leg. This can be increased gradually to 20 lifts for each leg, and weights may be added gradually. I would not advise lifting more than 15 pounds during pregnancy.

To strengthen the legs, assume the same position. Start with no more than a 10-pound weight. Straighten your leg and hold the extended position for 1 second. Then, return to the starting position for 1 second, and hold for 1 second. It is important not to swing the weight up and down. Repeat the exercise 6 to 10 times, depending on your strength, and repeat this group of exercises 2 more times while taking a 2-minute rest period between each 6 to 10 lifts.

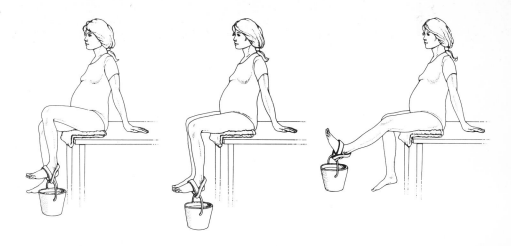

Thigh exercise with weight.   *Leg exercise with weight.*

Side lifts serve the purpose of strengthening the legs and hips but should be done with a weight of 5 pounds or less.

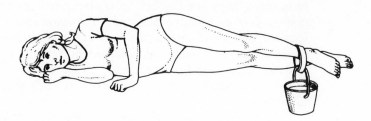

Side lift with weight.

Lift your leg about 12 inches from the top of a bench or low table. Hold it there for 1 second and then return to the starting position. This should be done 10 times with each leg followed by a 2-minute rest period. Gradually increase to a maximum of 30 side lifts with each leg.

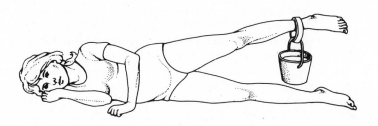

Side lift with weight.

Has the value of intercourse as a form of exercise ever been studied?

Recent studies suggest that intercourse is an excellent form of exercise. Scientists have determined that a woman will lose approximately 100 calories during one act of coitus, though this will vary depending on your enthusiasm and vigor as well as the endurance and skill of your partner. On the average, the amount of energy used is equivalent to a brisk walk around a city block, and intercourse also has an advantage over other activities in that it requires no special equipment and does not need a large playing field.

No subject of pregnancy has aroused more curiosity or misunderstanding than sexuality. In the next chapter I will try to dispel some old misconceptions on this important subject.

4.
Sexuality During Pregnancy

Since the days of Hippocrates, who was the first to suggest that sexual intercourse might bring about a miscarriage, very little has been learned about the medical aspects of sexuality during pregnancy. Even the most up-to-date obstetrical textbooks devote just a few lines to this vital subject, with the result that the majority of obstetricians practicing today know less about sexuality than the women they treat. Few doctors mention anything to their pregnant patients about sexual behavior or alternative coital positions during pregnancy and rarely are sexual techniques other than intercourse discussed.

The medical profession owes a great debt to William H. Masters and Virginia E. Johnson for their pioneering work in the field of human sexuality. As a direct result of their innovative and brilliant research, many taboos and misunderstandings about sexuality in pregnant and nonpregnant women have been dispelled and replaced by a greater open-mindedness between women and their doctors. Educational seminars based on the teachings of Masters and Johnson are regularly scheduled throughout the United States, while most medical schools now require a human sexuality course as a prerequisite to graduation. Let's hope that young obstetricians in the 1980s will be able to share with their patients a greater awareness and knowledge of the physical and emotional aspects of sexuality during pregnancy and the postpartum period.

Unlike other medical topics presented in this book, many questions about sexuality have no absolute answers. My discussion of what we do know about this important subject is based on the available literature.

The Female Orgasm

What are the components of the female orgasm and how do they differ for pregnant and nonpregnant women?

Our knowledge of the female orgasm is derived from the extensive research conducted by Masters and Johnson. They were able to divide the female orgasm of both nonpregnant and pregnant women into four distinct and sequential phases: excitement, plateau, orgasm, and resolution. Each phase is characterized by distinct changes in the breasts, external genitals, internal genitals, and vagina.

The Excitement Phase

During the initial stage of sexual response the breasts increase in size because of engorgement, or vasocongestion of the veins within each breast. The nipples become erect. In the genital area, the clitoris increases in length and width while the labia, or inner lips, increase in size and extend outward.

At the same time as these external changes are taking place, the vagina begins to lubricate as well as lengthen and distend. The uterus and cervix actually elevate higher in the pelvis to make room for the penis.

Vaginal lubrication usually occurs within ten to thirty seconds after sexual stimulation is initiated. For years, doctors were taught that this lubrication came from the glands of the cervix and the two Bartholin glands at the vaginal opening. Masters and Johnson demonstrated that vaginal lubrication results from the passage of droplets of fluid from congested and dilated veins surrounding the vaginal walls.

Masters and Johnson studied the excitement phase in six pregnant women, three of whom were having their first baby, who had also been evaluated before they became pregnant. They found that during the excitement phase, the vasocongestive reaction of the breasts and genitals to sexual stimulation is superimposed on the hormonal changes resulting from pregnancy. As a result, the rush of blood to the enlarged breasts can cause tenderness and pain. This was particularly evident in the first trimester, and especially among the women having their first baby (nulliparas, or primigravidas). During the second and third trimesters of pregnancy there was usually a marked reduction in these women's complaints of breast tenderness.

The genitals of the nulliparous woman undergo little change in the excitement phase of sexual arousal during pregnancy. However, for women having a second (primiparas) or later baby (multiparas) there is excessive engorgement and swelling of the labia majora and labia minora. By the third trimester, the external genitals are so swollen by pregnancy that further swelling due to sexual excitation is difficult to detect.

All six women reported a significant increase in the production of vaginal lubrication, beginning at the end of the first trimester and persisting throughout pregnancy. Additional vaginal lubrication in response to sexual excitement also developed more rapidly and extensively during pregnancy.

The Plateau Phase

The bodily changes of the plateau phase in the nonpregnant woman are a continuation and intensification of the excitement phase. The breasts continue to swell. The areola, or pigmented area around the nipple, also enlarges significantly, giving the impression that the nipples are retracted and smaller than they are during the excitement phase. The characteristic change in this phase is that the blood vessels surrounding the outer third of the vagina become markedly congested with blood. This vasocongestion is so pronounced that the outer vaginal opening is reduced in diameter by at least one-third from that noted during the excitation phase. Masters and Johnson named this outer area of congestion the "orgasmic platform."

Another important change occurring during the plateau phase is the retracting of the clitoris under the hood created by the two labia minora. At this point, the clitoris is often difficult to locate and is so tender that efforts to touch it directly may cause discomfort.

At the end of the plateau phase, other muscles in the body begin to tense, the pupils dilate, and a feeling of lightheadedness frequently occurs as orgasm approaches.

The main difference between the plateau phase in pregnant and nonpregnant women is that the vasocongestion of the outer portion of the vagina is far more pronounced during pregnancy. Among the nulliparous women studied, the vaginal opening was noted to be reduced in size by 75 percent. The effect was even more pronounced among multiparous women, where it was noted that vasocongestion occurred to the point that the two lateral or side walls of the vagina were actually touching each other. This condition tended to become more pronounced as pregnancy progressed and explains why some couples complain that "there is no room" or that the vagina is "too tight" when intercourse is attempted.

The Orgasmic Phase

The basic characteristics of the female orgasm are identical in all women and are triggered by direct or indirect stimulation of the clitoris. During orgasm, the congested outer part of the vagina contracts strongly at regular 0.8-second intervals. With each orgasmic experience, the total number of contractions ranges from three to fifteen, while the interval between contractions lengthens after the first three to six. The number of orgasmic platform contractions varies from woman to woman and within the same individual from one orgasmic experience to the next. Usually a mild orgasm consists of three to five contractions, while there may be eight to fifteen strong contractions in a more intense orgasm.

In addition to the contractions of the orgasmic platform, the uterus also contracts at regular intervals every few seconds. Uterine contractions, unlike orgasmic platform contractions, are less frequent, usually begin two to four seconds after a woman is aware of the onset of an orgasm, and may last for several minutes following orgasm. Masters and Johnson made the interesting observation that the uterine contractions initiated in response to masturbation were of greater intensity and duration than those induced through orgasm via intercourse.

Other changes which occur during orgasm are a further retraction of the clitoris, a tightening of the anal sphincter, a curling of the toes, and an increase in the heart and respiratory rates. Orgasm rarely lasts longer than ten to fifteen seconds.

Masters and Johnson observed one very important difference between orgasm in the pregnant woman when compared to the nonpregnant woman. During the last trimester of pregnancy, and especially during the last four weeks, instead of normal orgasmic contractions, the uterine muscle may go into a spastic and continuous contraction without relaxing. During the last month of pregnancy, some of these contractions have been noted to last as long as one minute and to recur as late as a half-hour after orgasm. Masters and Johnson observed that the fetal heart rate slowed during such contractions, but they noted no further evidence of fetal distress. Other investigators have not shared their optimism.

The Resolution Phase

Following orgasm, there is a period of calm and relaxation. In the nonpregnant woman, the blood filling the veins of the breasts and pelvis slowly flows to the other areas of the body, while anatomy and physiology return to normal.

The resolution phase is an uncomfortable experience for the pregnant woman because the intense vasocongestion in the pelvis subsides very slowly following orgasm. According to Masters and Johnson, this condition gets progressively worse as pregnancy advances. During the second trimester, it took ten to fifteen minutes for vasocongestion to subside in the women having their first baby and approximately thirty to forty-five minutes for this to occur in the others. During the third trimester, vasocongestion may not be relieved at all following orgasm, and this may result in an increase in sexual stimulation, sexual tension, and frustration for some pregnant women. All six pregnant women who were intensively studied by Masters and Johnson reported no relief of their sexual tension levels during this period despite the fact that three of the women were suddenly able to experience multiple orgasm for the first time.

What is the G spot and how is it related to the female orgasm?

The G spot or Grafenberg spot is an erotically sensitive area located just beneath the urethra on the anterior vaginal wall at a point approximately 2 centimeters deeper into the vagina than the inner border of the pubic bone. It was first described in 1950 by a man of the same name, but it was not until 1982 that its presence was documented in hundreds of women. Most women and their gynecologists have never seen the Grafenberg spot because it is only apparent upon sexual stimulation when it swells and forms a small nodular area just below the urethra. In some women, further stimulation will actually result in simultaneous orgasm and ejaculation of a small amount of fluid from the urethra. Analysis of this fluid has shown that it is chemically similar to prostate fluid ejaculated with the male orgasm. Electronic measurements of orgasmic uterine contractions following Grafenberg spot stimulation have been found to be of far greater intensity than those resulting from clitoral orgasm.

The rediscovery of the Grafenberg spot has revitalized the prejudiced Freudian view of the vaginal orgasm. Freud claimed that this was a more mature and true orgasm than that emanating from the clitoris, which he labeled immature and neurotic. This idea is in direct conflict with the findings of contemporary sex researchers, such as Masters and Johnson, who regard the vaginal orgasm as a myth, believing that all female orgasms involve clitoral stimulation.

Declining Sexuality During Pregnancy

Does a woman's interest in sex decline during pregnancy?

Usually, yes. Many men erroneously believe that a woman's increased hormonal levels during the first trimester, as manifested by enlarged breasts and a new voluptuous body contour, produce a heightened sexual desire at this time. Nothing could be further from the truth. Unpleasant physical factors in early pregnancy such as nausea, vomiting, and fatigue tend to significantly reduce coital and noncoital sexual interest for many women. Masters and Johnson interviewed 111 pregnant women in an attempt to learn more about a woman's pattern of sexual interest and response throughout each trimester of pregnancy. They concluded that women having their first baby were most likely to experience a significant reduction in sexual interest and in effectiveness of sexual performance during these early months than women having a second or later baby.

During the second trimester, most women in both groups reported a significant increase in eroticism and effectiveness of sexual performance. Of 101 women studied at this time, 82 noted this positive effect.

Masters and Johnson had difficulty evaluating the sexuality of women during the last trimester of pregnancy, since intercourse was discouraged by their obstetricians during this time. Despite the limitations of this inquiry, the majority of the women studied reported that they gradually lost interest in sexual activity during the last three months.

Thus, the sexuality of the pregnant women studied by Masters and Johnson demonstrated a roller coaster effect: low in the first trimester, greatly accentuated during the second three months, and diminished again during the last trimester.

Other researchers studying patterns of sexuality during pregnancy do not agree with Masters and Johnson. The vast majority of reports demonstrate that most women experience a steady and consistent decline in sexual activity, libido, and satisfaction throughout pregnancy. While some investigators have noted a slight improvement of sexual performance during the second trimester when compared to the first trimester, the level of sexual interest for most women remains far below their prepregnancy levels.

One of the most intensive studies of all aspects of sexuality during pregnancy was performed in 1974 by Drs. Nathaniel N. Wagner and Don A. Solberg of the University of Washington, who interviewed a total of 260 middle-class women. Though coital rates for these women declined progressively throughout pregnancy, the most dramatic changes were noted during the seventh, eighth, and ninth months. Unlike Masters and Johnson, Wagner and Solberg noted no relationship between coital frequency and the number of times a woman had been pregnant. When asked to rate the intensity of their orgasms during pregnancy in comparison to those preceding conception, the majority reported less intense orgasms as their pregnancy continued, particularly in the seventh, eighth, and ninth months.

Wagner and Solberg also studied noncoital methods of achieving orgasm. Although 50 to 60 percent of those women who masturbated to orgasm prior to pregnancy abstained from this practice while pregnant, the rate of the remaining group was the same as before pregnancy. Similarly, fewer women reported manual stimulation by their partners as a method of attaining orgasm during pregnancy. Of those who continued to use this method, the incidence of achieving orgasm did not vary from their prepregnancy rates. However, in contrast to masturbation and manual stimulation, orgasmic rates achieved by oral-genital stimulation declined significantly during pregnancy. During the prepregnancy period, 16 percent of the women reported no or only rare orgasms from oral-genital stimulation. This number rose to about 60 percent in the ninth month of pregnancy.

What factors are most responsible for a woman's declining sexuality during pregnancy?

Many interrelated physical and psychological changes may adversely alter a woman's sexual response throughout pregnancy. Women asked by Wagner and Solberg to list the factors which were most responsible for their changing sexual behavior during pregnancy mentioned physical discomfort most frequently (46 percent), followed by fear of injuring the baby (27 percent), and physical awkwardness (17 percent). (More than one reason was accepted and recorded.) Approximately one-third of the women interviewed had been told by their physicians to abstain from intercourse at times ranging from two to eight weeks prior to their expected date of confinement. Despite this, only 8 percent of the women cited their doctors' recommendations as a reason for altering their sexual behavior, and only 4 percent cited loss of attractiveness in the eyes of their partners as a reason for diminished sexual intensity.

As previously mentioned, the extensive vascular congestion within the breasts during pregnancy may cause great sensitivity and pain, especially in the nipple and areola. The fact that this previously sensual area is now off limits is often a source of frustration to a couple.

The congestion of the genital tissues during pregnancy may cause a feeling of vaginal discomfort and "tightness" for a woman during coitus. Another rarely discussed deterrent to sexual enjoyment is the greater quantity of vaginal discharge during pregnancy. Many women report a much stronger aroma to their vaginal secretions, which they often characterize as unpleasant and embarrassing during oral stimulation of the vulva and the vagina, so that they are less likely to enjoy this lovemaking technique. Moniliasis, or "yeast" infection, is a common cause of vaginal and vulvar irritation and discharge during pregnancy. Though this is not a serious condition and is easily treated (see chapter 5), it can be a source of annoyance for a woman and diminish her sexual interest and participation.

The uterine contractions which follow orgasm during pregnancy may last for half an hour or more in some women. Sometimes these contractions of the so-called postorgasmic syndrome are so painful that a pregnant woman may prefer to avoid sexual intimacy entirely.

Hormonal changes of pregnancy often cause marked alterations in the blood supply to the cervix. Spotting of blood from the cervix following coitus with deep penetration is harmless but can be very frightening to the couple who has not been forewarned by their doctor that this may occur.

What other factors might inhibit a woman's sexuality during pregnancy?

Psychologically, most pregnant women experience a heightened body preoccupation, feelings of insecurity, and a strongly increased need for affectionate rather than sexual touching. Pregnancy seems to have the effect of lowering the erotic component of a woman's sexual functioning while increasing her desire for affection.

The greatest dependency period and time of maximum vulnerability appears to occur during the ten weeks before birth. It is at this time that affection and emotional support are essential to the psychological well-being of most pregnant women. It is sad that many men fail to understand this basic and powerful need.

Many women express resentment against sexually demanding husbands who are unable to understand, appreciate, or accept their decreased inclination for coitus and orgasm. Several surveys have demonstrated that as pregnant women become less interested in sexual contact, they tend to masturbate their husbands more frequently. For some couples this is an acceptable form of lovemaking, but many women object to repeatedly "servicing" their "selfish" husbands.

Ten of the nineteen women interviewed by Dr. Celia J. Falicov of the University of Chicago experienced fear, frequently recognized as unrealistic, of harming of the fetus or producing miscarriage as a result of coitus. Several reported a "subconscious holding back" from orgasm because of fear of fetal injury. The survey of Wagner and Solberg as well as many others, confirmed that this fear is quite prevalent and persists throughout the entire pregnancy.

What happens to a man's sexuality during his partner's pregnancy?

Pregnancy is a stressful period for most men. Feelings about their own dependency, masculinity, childhood attachments, and identification with their mothers may surface at this time. For many it represents sudden changes in a previously organized life-style, combined with the need to plan for new economic responsibilities and pressures.

The overwhelming number of surveys clearly demonstrate that most men experience a decreased desire to be sexually intimate with their wives, particularly as pregnancy progresses and she appears more visibly pregnant. A man's sexual response is influenced by a variety of factors, the most obvious of which is his wife's sexuality. If she is plagued by discomforting symptoms or is totally preoccupied with her unborn baby, it will adversely affect his enthusiasm and response. Even a mature man may feel somewhat threatened and jealous of this new entity who has suddenly disturbed a previously happy relationship. Under such circumstances, he may prefer not to make demands on his wife. Other men, whose wives stimulate them to orgasm without themselves experiencing sexual gratification, often report feelings of guilt for not being less demanding. While some men note a greater sexual attraction to their wives' larger breasts and more rounded body contours, this interest is usually not reciprocated. Repeated spurning of his sexual advances may be frustrating and rather than risk repeated rejections a man may simply stop trying. The opposite may also occur: a woman's larger breasts, swollen vaginal tissues, increased vaginal lubrication, and stronger scent during pregnancy may overwhelm some men to the point of creating loss of erection and sexual dysfunction.

The fear of injury to the fetus is often cited as a common reason for a man's declining interest in coitus during pregnancy. This becomes most pronounced after "quickening," the woman's first detection of fetal movement, which occurs at approximately the twentieth week of pregnancy. For many men it is only at this point that the baby as a living human being first becomes a reality. For some immature men, this stated fear of injury may merely reflect an underlying ambivalence about the pregnancy and feelings of hostility toward both woman and unborn child.

As strange as it seems, there are reports of men who have avoided coitus because of an irrational fear that the fetus may be watching them or is attempting to grasp or even bite their penis. These fears, though realized as being ridiculous, are for some men impossible to abandon.

Many expectant fathers report that they are frustrated by their wives' extreme breast tenderness, which prohibits manual and oral stimulation. Others state that they avoid oral contact with their wives' genitals (cunnilingus) because of the greater amount of vaginal lubrication and discharge, which most men agree has neither a pleasing flavor or aroma. In addition, as previously mentioned, a couple may note a slight amount of bleeding from the cervix following intercourse. Though this is rarely if ever serious, it may further contribute to a man's anxiety and sexual alienation.

Psychiatrists have attributed the sexual dysfunction of some men during pregnancy to what is termed the "madonna image" or the "mother-mistress conflict." It is theorized that early teachings cause these men to associate all pregnant women with the purity of the Madonna. Subconsciously, having sex with someone who is so obviously a mother seems akin to incest.

There is some evidence that 10 percent of expectant fathers actually experience physical symptoms during their wives' pregnancies. Most commonly observed is a loss of appetite, nausea, and heartburn. These symptoms seem to reflect a man's desire to be part of an experience that he was very much involved in initiating.

What can a couple do to avoid a sexual crisis during pregnancy?

Problems of sexual adjustment during pregnancy can threaten the stability of the most comfortable and secure relationship. A couple alerted beforehand to the possibility of a woman's diminished libido and sexuality during pregnancy will not be frustrated and disappointed by unrealistic expectations about sexual performance.

Dr. Elizabeth Wales, in her excellent article published in the journal *The Female Patient* of September 1979, emphasized the fact that most men do not understand a woman's need for affection in preference to erotic stimulation during pregnancy. A typical sequence of events that often leads to conflict and misunderstanding begins when a woman initiates physical contact merely because she is seeking affection. Her mate may interpret this as a request for intercourse and seek to establish sexual contact leading to orgasm. She in turn may interpret his aggressive behavior as demanding and selfish and may respond by rejecting his advances, leaving him hurt, confused, and angry. A man must be helped to understand that the words "Not tonight, honey" doesn't mean "I don't love you."

Masters and Johnson introduced the beautiful term "pleasuring" to describe the way a man and woman can think and feel sensuously about each other without any pressure to proceed to orgasm. The end result of all intimate contact, especially during pregnancy, is not necessarily orgasm. There are many ways that a man can communicate his love, and often a hug, a kiss on the cheek, a backrub, or a body massage can be far more meaningful and gratifying to a pregnant woman than an intense orgasm.

The key to averting a sexual crisis during pregnancy is good communication between a couple. If a woman does not desire to have intercourse, she should be able to say so. He, in turn, should be encouraged to ventilate his feelings and frustrations rather than let them build, to surface angrily at a later date. A couple should experiment with various positions which facilitate comfortable intercourse during the second half of pregnancy. Positions which avoid deep penetration not only add to a woman's comfort, but also help to avoid disturbing bleeding from the superficial capillaries of the cervix. The knowledge that orgasm may bring uncomfortable uterine contractions helps to allay anxieties for most women when this occurs. Noncoital lovemaking techniques should also be freely discussed. If a man is suddenly turned off by cunnilingus because of his wife's excessive lubrication, he should be comforted in knowing that these feelings are not uncommon and are experienced by most expectant fathers. Some men report that they can still enjoy oral sex by limiting it to the drier clitoral area while using their fingers to stimulate the labia and vagina. A woman who is self-conscious about her increased lubrication and odor can shower or wash the vulva immediately before lovemaking. Another helpful tip is to apply a natural oil, such as coconut or sesame, to the vulva prior to lovemaking. A couple should also realize that self- and mutual masturbation may also increase in frequency as coital interests decline and that there is no reason for the guilt feelings many individuals experience about the natural and harmless act of masturbation.

If your obstetrician instructs you to avoid intercourse at any stage during pregnancy, ask for the reasons for this decision, the length of time that the restrictions are in effect, and whether or not noncoital alternatives leading to orgasm can be safely substituted.

How can unpleasant odors originating in the genital area be avoided?

No society has a greater preoccupation with body odor, and genital odor in particular, than ours. In recent years a variety of perfumes, feminine hygiene sprays, creams and jellies have appeared on the market, many with a musk, civet, or ambergris base—all of which have their origin in animal scent-producing sex glands. (The word "musk" is Persian, taken from the Sanskrit for testicle.)

Despite the propaganda of Madison Avenue, soap and water are more effective in promoting genital hygiene and male sexual interest than any of these potentially irritating products. Pregnant and nonpregnant women should be meticulous about personal hygiene, washing the labia and perineum no more than once a day with a mild, nonperfumed, nondeodorant soap. This should be followed by a thorough rinsing and drying. Cleansing the perineum following urination should be performed by wiping the labial area first and then continuing the wipe toward the anal region.

Excessive perspiration and odor of the genital area may result from wearing tight-fitting panty girdles, jeans, or slacks. Synthetic fabrics for underwear, panty hose, and panty girdles lack absorbency and therefore retain the moisture of the vaginal excretions, as well as perspiration. This moisture acts as an irritant to the vulva and perineum, causing chafing and burning. The pregnant woman is extremely susceptible to monilial infections resulting from excessive wetness in the genital area (see page 61).

Are some women and men allergic to these new feminine hygiene sprays?

Yes. Allergic contact reactions to feminine hygiene sprays or "gynacosmetics" as well as new "erogenital cosmetics" for both sexes are now being seen with great frequency by both dermatologists and gynecologists. Both the propellants and the ingredients of these sprays are capable of causing vulvar, vaginal, and penile irritation. A severe cellulitis, or spreading bacterial infection, of the pubic area has also been reported among women using these preparations. On rare occasions an allergic contact dermatitis can be caused by exposure to the propylene glycol found in K-Y Lubricating Jelly. Women often apply this popular product to their inner labia before intercourse in order to decrease friction and enhance the coital experience. Men may experience the identical allergic reaction following application of the jelly to the penis or contact with it during intercourse.

Why do some women experience greater sexual drive throughout pregnancy?

Women undergo a complicated series of physical, hormonal, and psychological changes during pregnancy, and as a result it is extremely difficult to categorize women in this regard. However, researchers have found that most women who enjoy high levels of eroticism, sexual performance, and orgasm during pregnancy are likely to have very high levels of sexual interest when they are not pregnant. These women are not only more likely than other women to masturbate when they are not pregnant, but they do so at a far greater frequency than women whose sexual interest decreases during pregnancy. Women with more liberal attitudes toward sexual behavior and those who are more comfortable with their own sexuality are far more likely to engage in a variety of noncoital sexual behavior and to experiment with a variety of coital positions during pregnancy. However, there are many extremely sensual women who react negatively during pregnancy.

Is it true that some sexually frigid women become surprisingly sexual during pregnancy?

No. This is a myth. Several studies have demonstrated that women who rarely or never achieve orgasm have coitus and orgasm significantly less often when they are pregnant.

Are men more likely to engage in extramarital affairs when their wives are pregnant?

Although the evidence is certainly not conclusive, several researchers have noted that a man is more likely to engage in an extramarital affair for the first time during his wife's pregnancy, especially if significant sexual incompatibility existed earlier.

The two most common excuses given by men for their infidelity are an inadequate sex life both before and during pregnancy and forced sexual abstinence as ordered by their wives' obstetrician. A significant number of men say they sought extramarital encounters because they felt rejected by wives too immersed in their pregnancies to devote any time to the emotional needs of their husbands.

In 1966, Masters and Johnson interviewed 79 men and found that 12 reported sexual release outside their marriage during pregnancy, while an additional 6 did so right after the delivery. In another survey, 8 out of 110 men had taken lovers, although a considerably larger number reported that they were spending more time thinking about an extramarital relationship and fantasizing about covert and exotic sexual encounters.

Most psychologists conclude that if a couple is not encountering marital difficulties, the odds are well over 90 percent that a husband will not take a mistress during his wife's pregnancy. To relieve sexual tensions, many men will masturbate more frequently during pregnancy. In one survey it was noted that men tended to masturbate significantly more often during the first and third trimesters when intercourse rates are much lower. It is unfortunate that many men experience guilt feelings about masturbation, since it is a healthy and acceptable method of releasing sexual energy.

Coital Positions

Which coital positions are most satisfying during pregnancy?

While the traditional male-superior (or face-to-face missionary) position is the most commonly used before pregnancy and during the first two trimesters, a woman's increasing abdominal girth in late pregnancy markedly limits the use of this position. The women surveyed by Drs. Wagner and Solberg listed the side-by-side position as most popular. Rear-entry and female-superior positions also increased in popularity during the last three months but remained less popular than the male-superior position.

The missionary position can be successfully employed if a man lies partly sideways so that most of his weight is off the pregnant uterus. Many couples find that a more comfortable variation of this position is for the man to kneel at the foot or the side of the bed while the woman rests on her back with her buttocks at the edge of the bed and both feet touching the ground. Depending on the height of the bed and the size of the man, adjustments can easily be made by placing one or more pillows under her buttocks or his knees. This variation takes all his weight off her enlarged abdomen and allows him greater freedom to stimulate her breasts and clitoris than does the standard missionary position.

Variations of the side-by-side position are very popular in late pregnancy because they allow for shallow penile penetration. This is especially important during the last month when the baby's head may be engaged or deep in the pelvis and deep penetration becomes painful.

Many women favor the female-superior (woman-on-top) position in late pregnancy because it puts no weight on the abdomen and allows the woman to control the depth of penile penetration.

Men often find the many variations of the rear-entry position extremely exciting and sexually gratifying. However, during pregnancy several of my patients have stated that they prefer the intimacy of face-to-face contact (which the rear-entry position does not provide). The most common variation of the rear entry position is the "spoon" position, in which the couple curls side by side. In this position the male is unable to thrust deeply because he is behind the woman and has little leverage. Another advantage is that it is comfortable while still allowing the woman to enjoy breast and clitoral stimulation during intercourse. For added comfort and a smoother penile entry, the woman may prefer to raise her upper leg with the help of a pillow or two.

Rear entry may also be performed with a woman resting on her knees and elbows. While this position is possible and even satisfying for some women late in pregnancy, most find it uncomfortable and difficult to maintain for more than a couple of minutes. Rear entry from a sitting position, with the woman on the man's lap, is far more comfortable and pleasurable. Be sure that the chair, table seat, or table that you select to sit on is strong enough to hold the weight of both of you.

The rear-entry standing position has several disadvantages. One major problem is that the man is often taller than the woman and must crouch in order to enter her. The angle of entry of the penis is most comfortable if a woman bends forward as far as possible, but her ability to do this is severely limited during the second half of pregnancy. For maximum comfort in this position it helps if the woman can rest her head on a pillow placed on a sturdy table or desk under her.

Possible Hazards of Sex During Pregnancy

Can male sperm cause miscarriage?

Many body cells, including sperm, contain substances called prostaglandins, which have been synthesized in the laboratory and are used medically to induce abortion by causing intense uterine contractions leading to expulsion of the fetus. It has been suggested that sperm prostaglandins, absorbed through the vaginal wall, may be responsible for recurrent miscarriage and premature labor. It has also been theorized that this may be prevented if a man wears a condom while having intercourse during pregnancy.

The great majority of researchers refute this theory. Some have actually calculated that in order to deposit enough prostaglandin in the vagina to cause miscarriage and premature labor it would take fifteen simultaneous ejaculations of equal volume and potency. Swallowed prostaglandin in an ejaculate are also believed incapable of being absorbed and causing laborlike contractions.

As previously mentioned, orgasm itself is much more likely to cause involuntary uterine contractions than is the presence of prostaglandins from an ejaculate, and Masters and Johnson demonstrated that the uterine contractions which accompany orgasm with masturbation are far more intense than those resulting from coital orgasm.

Can orgasmic contractions of the uterus cause miscarriage during the first three months of pregnancy?

There are practically no scientific studies to substantiate the claim that orgasm during the first three months of pregnancy increases the risk of spontaneous abortion. In his book, *Spontaneous and Habitual Abortion* (1957), Dr. C. T. Javert stresses the importance—for women who had had three or more consecutive spontaneous abortions—of eliminating any factor which would stimulate even a mild amount of sexual arousal leading to a uterine contraction.

Current opinion is that coital and noncoital orgasm as a primary cause of spontaneous abortion is extremely rare. However, if a woman has a history of repeated miscarriage, or notes intense and painful uterine contractions following orgasm, abstinence is the best policy for at least the first twelve weeks of pregnancy. If bleeding follows orgasm, and your doctor can demonstrate with a vaginal speculum examination that the blood flow is from the uterus, rather than the capillaries of your cervix, which is harmless, it would be advisable to avoid further orgasm during the first trimester.

Are orgasmic uterine contractions ever responsible for premature labor?

Yes. Each year, 200,000 infants are born prematurely, and their prematurity is associated with a significantly higher incidence of severe physical and mental disability. The criteria for prematurity, as defined by most medical researchers, are a gestational age of less than thirty-seven weeks and/or a birth weight of 2,500 grams (5½ pounds) or less.

Dr. Robert C. Goodlin of Stanford University Medical Center, in a letter published in *Lancet* in September 1969, was one of the first physicians to alert the medical profession to the possibility that orgasm during the second and third trimester might make premature labor more likely. Among twenty-five women surveyed, twenty-one reported painful uterine contractions and pains and pressure in the back or pelvis following orgasmic coitus. Of six women who delivered four or more weeks prematurely, four believed that their premature labors probably began with orgasmic experience, as did three out of five who prematurely ruptured their amniotic membranes prior to the onset of labor. (When this membrane ruptures, an abundant amount of amniotic fluid is released vaginally. Labor often will begin within twenty-four hours of this event, but if it doesn't, medical induction is sometimes necessary to prevent fetal and maternal infection.)

In 1971, Dr. Goodlin and his associates expanded their research by interviewing 200 women. Among this group, a total of 155 (77 percent) were orgasmic during the second and third trimesters of pregnancy. Of these 155 orgasmic women, a surprisingly high number of 127 complained of postorgasmic discomfort in the form of uterine contractions, pelvic pain or pressure, backache, and thigh pain. Whereas the incidence of premature labor prior to the thirty-seventh week of pregnancy is estimated at 10 percent of the general population, it was found to be 21 percent among women who achieved orgasm after the thirty-second week of pregnancy.

As part of this same study he noted that coitus in the absence of orgasm had no relationship to premature labor. As part of another study, Dr. Goodlin and his associates asked five women who were seen on vaginal examination to be "ripe" for labor to initiate an orgasm at a specific time. Of the five women, two were admitted to the hospital in labor within three hours and the third within nine hours after orgasm. A fourth woman experienced false labor contractions which soon stopped.

Though Masters and Johnson were unable to document a higher incidence of prematurity among orgasmic women, they did note that four women who were uninvolved in their study had an experience which was almost identical to that of the five women studied by Goodlin. All four women were within eighteen days of their due date, and three began labor immediately after orgasmic intercourse. The fourth woman initiated labor within minutes of a multiorgasmic masturbation.

Support for Dr. Goodlin's orgasm-prematurity relationship was reported in *Fertility and Sterility* of August 1976, by Drs. Nathaniel N. Wagner and Julius C. Butler, who obtained complete sexual histories from nineteen mothers of premature infants and compared them to a control group of nineteen women who gave birth to full-term infants. During the first trimester, fourteen of the nineteen mothers of premature babies, or 74 percent, reported experiencing orgasm from three-fourths of the coital times to "always," while only seven, or 37 percent, of the controls noted orgasm this frequently. Though the incidence of orgasm decreased as pregnancy progressed, it remained higher for the mothers of premature infants.

In 1979, Dr. Richard P. Perkins of the University of New Mexico School of Medicine reported detailed sexual and obstetrical data from 155 women who had recently given birth. Based on the responses to his questionnaire, Dr. Perkins concluded that sexual activity, regardless of technique, appeared to have no adverse effects on the incidence of premature rupture of the amniotic membranes, premature labor, and infants of low birth weight. One surprising finding was that orgasmic women, especially those who masturbated to orgasm, had a *lower* incidence of premature infants than women who did not achieve orgasm. This relationship appeared to be true throughout all stages of pregnancy. Furthermore, more women who had sex within twenty-four hours of labor were admitted with ruptured amniotic membranes if their most recent sexual stimulation was not accompanied by orgasm. These findings led Dr. Perkins to theorize that the sexually unfulfilled individual may be more prone to premature labor than those engaged in regular satisfying sexual relationships. In other words, Dr. Perkins believes that if you're going to be sexual in the third trimester, do it with feeling or don't do it at all. Unlike other researchers, such as Masters and Johnson, Dr. Perkins did not note as strong a relationship between a woman's attainment of orgasm and her perception of uterine contractions. Though women perceived more contractions after coitus with orgasm than with any other type of sexual behavior and response, coitus itself seemed to be as strong a stimulus to uterine contractions as was orgasm.

Support for Dr. Perkins' findings may be found in an article published in *Lancet* in July 1981. In this review of almost 11,000 pregnancies, doctors concluded that coitus during the third trimester did not increase the incidence of premature labor, infants of low birthweight, or perinatal deaths.

In the presence of these contradictory findings, it is difficult to offer specific advice to women about the relationship between intercourse, orgasm, and premature labor. However, there does appear to be a small number of susceptible individuals who will, as a result of their sexual activity, deliver prematurely. If you have previously given birth to a premature infant, avoidance of orgasm during the last three months of pregnancy would appear to be a sound suggestion.

Can orgasmic uterine contractions affect the fetus?

It has been demonstrated that the uterine contractions associated with orgasm may be related to a slight temporary decrease in the amount of oxygen carried to the fetus. This in turn may result in a slowing of the fetal heart rate. However, the opinion of most experts is that this is of little consequence. The safety of orgasm late in pregnancy was illustrated in one study in which a woman in her ninth month was attached to an ultrasonic recorder in a hospital for 106 minutes. During this time, her husband manually stimulated her to orgasm five times. With each orgasm there was a decrease in the fetal heart rate and a progressive increase in the intensity of the uterine contractions. She delivered a healthy and intelligent 8-pound 5-ounce infant a few days later. When last seen, mother, father, baby, and ultrasonic recorder were all reported to be doing well.

In the past there have been scattered unscientific and speculative reports claiming that the lack of oxygen to the fetus during orgasm was responsible for lower IQs in the newborn, as well as severe mental retardation and some couples reported an increase in fetal activity associated with coital and noncoital orgasm. Few doctors took these claims seriously, until a 1979 letter from St. Bartholomew's Hospital Medical College of England was published in *Lancet* under the heading "Does Sexual Intercourse Cause Fetal Distress?" Of seventy women delivered of their first baby, thirty engaged in coitus during the four weeks before delivery while forty abstained. The researchers noted that the women who had intercourse showed a higher incidence of fetal distress as measured by the Apgar score (see page 328) and by the presence of meconium staining of the amniotic fluid. Though this research involved only a small number of women, I would agree with the authors that there is a clear need for further investigation.

Can the act of intercourse increase a woman's risk of infection during pregnancy?

No obstetrical condition has received more attention in the news than the research on this subject by Dr. Richard L. Naeye of the Pennsylvania State University College of Medicine. Dr. Naeye analyzed 26,886 pregnancies which took place between 1959 and 1966 to determine the relationship between coitus during the second half of pregnancy and the incidence of infection of the amniotic fluid surrounding the baby. Dr. Naeye noted a frequency of 156 infections per 1,000 births when mothers reported intercourse once or more per week during the month before delivery, compared with 117 per 1,000 when no coitus was reported. More significantly, of those infants who contracted infections, 11 percent died when there was a history of coitus, as compared to 2.4 percent of infants whose mothers abstained. Dr. Naeye also found that babies born of mothers who had coitus during the month prior to labor were twice as likely to experience the consequences of prematurity, such as lower Apgar scores, respiratory distress, and jaundice.

It is known that there are powerful antibacterial substances in the amniotic fluid which are capable of destroying a wide variety of bacteria. These substances first appear at the end of the third month, and their strength in combating infection increases progressively until the end of pregnancy. It has been theorized that infection occurs when sperm or enzymes in the sperm facilitate the passage of bacteria through the protective mucus of the cervix and into the amniotic fluid membrane. If too many bacteria enter the amniotic fluid, the protective bacterial-fighting mechanism may be overwhelmed and an infection will spread. Since the concentration of these bacterial-fighting substances increases as pregnancy progresses, their ability to combat greater numbers of bacteria should also increase. Confirmation of this theory was demonstrated microscopically among the women studied by Dr. Naeye. At twenty to twenty-four weeks of pregnancy, 82 percent of the women with acute inflammation had microscopic evidence of spread. This rate decreased to 78 percent at twenty-five to twenty-eight weeks and 63 percent at twenty-nine to thirty-eight weeks.

Dr. Naeye also observed a second intercourse-associated increase in the frequency of amniotic fluid infections after the thirty-eighth week of pregnancy. Women engaged in coitus at least once a week were noted to have a 50 percent greater risk of contracting a serious amniotic fluid infection than women who abstained from intercourse at this time. He theorized that this was probably due to the dilatation and effacement (shortening) of the cervix which normally occurs in the last weeks before the start of labor. These changes of cervix increase the exposure of the amniotic membrane to semen and bacteria from the vagina and cervix.

From a practical point of view, what decision regarding intercourse should a pregnant woman make during the second half of pregnancy?

Even the most knowledgeable authorities on this subject do not really know what advice to give to their patients. Dr. Naeye is currently conducting research to determine if the use of condoms during pregnancy can reduce the frequency of amniotic membrane infections and improve the outcome for babies who become infected. However, one of his concerns is that other complications which these babies experience, such as respiratory distress and jaundice, are not always associated with infection and would not be significantly reduced simply by use of a condom. Following publication of his article, Dr. Naeye said he was not prepared to recommend prolonged abstinence in pregnancy, simply because of the marital discord that it might cause. Whereas many obstetricians recommend abstinence at some point during the last few weeks of pregnancy, Dr. Naeye suggested that it made more sense to abstain in the fifth through seventh months, when the bacterial-fighting substances in the amniotic fluid were at their lowest concentration.

Some of Dr. Naeye's research techniques and conclusions have been challenged by several researchers. For example, his criteria for diagnosing an infection was based on finding a small number of white blood cells in the amniotic fluid. This finding, however, is not necessarily indicative of a clinical infection in either a woman or her baby, and some pathologists will not diagnose an amniotic fluid infection unless there is a significant number of white blood cells present. The only definite proof of an infection is a positive bacterial culture, and even Dr. Naeye admits that his diagnosis of infection was not based on this absolute evidence. Another criticism of his widely publicized paper is that there is no mention of the length of labor of the women studied, the presence of complications in labor, or the time elapsed between rupture of the membranes and delivery of the baby. This is unfortunate, since the last of these factors is the most important in determining if an infection will occur. Another challenge to Dr. Naeye's conclusions is a 1981 analysis of 10,477 births in which doctors demonstrated no deleterious effects between coitus in late pregnancy and the development of an amniotic fluid infection.

These conflicting findings have created uncertainty and anxiety for couples seeking sound advice about sexual activity during pregnancy. They have also posed vital questions to researchers involved in prenatal health care and human sexuality. Studies by psychologists have confirmed that serious emotional turmoil and tension may result when abstinence is prescribed for prolonged periods of time. On the other hand, a couple who attributes their newborn's infection to their coital activity may face far greater and longer-lasting feelings of guilt.

Though further studies are necessary before definite advice can be given, there are sensible guidelines that women should follow. Those women who have a history of previous reproductive failure and premature labor and those women who, when examined by their obstetricians, are noted to have premature dilatation or effacement of their cervix should avoid orgasm, as well as intercourse, during the last three months of pregnancy. In addition, abstinence is also advised for women whose amniotic membranes have ruptured prematurely. If a woman has previously given birth to one or more healthy full-term infants despite having experienced both coital and noncoital orgasms throughout her pregnancy, it would appear foolish for a doctor to insist on abstinence for prolonged periods of time during a subsequent pregnancy. In all probability, her current pregnancy will remain normal in either case, and she would be unlikely to heed medical advice which appears contrary to her own personal experience.

How common is anal intercourse, and what are its dangers to the pregnant woman?

In a 1975 survey, the incidence of heterosexual anal intercourse was reported at 3 percent. However, in a more recent study of 528 married women under the age of thirty-five, it was found that approximately 25 percent had engaged in this activity one or more times, although only 8 percent considered anal intercourse to be a regular, frequently used, and pleasurable part of their sex lives. Not too many years ago, this form of sexual activity was regarded as a perversion, but today many people engage in anal intercourse periodically, and many more try it as an experiment. Couples also report using this method as an alternative to vaginal intercourse, especially during the mid-cycle fertile period of the menstrual cycle.

The most common injury resulting from anal intercourse is a split or crack in the skin and the mucous membrane of the anal canal. This condition can usually be prevented by liberal use of a lubricant, such as K-Y Jelly, for both the penis and the anus prior to entry. Rough and forceful insertion and vigorous thrusting of the penis are much more likely to cause injury than is a disproportion in size between anus and penis. The muscle surrounding the anus, called the anal sphincter, can be gently and gradually dilated to easily encompass the diameter of the average or even the largest penis.

Many proctologists believe that repeated anal intercourse may be responsible for aggravating previously existing conditions of the rectum such as colitis and hemorrhoids, though it is an unlikely cause of these disorders. Certainly the gross enlargement, bleeding, and discomfort of hemorrhoids, which occurs in practically all women during pregnancy, is likely to become far worse if anal intercourse is attempted during this time. While stretching of the anal sphincter is uncomfortable and unpleasant to many women, this same sensation is erotic to others. With repeated episodes of anal coitus, the sphincter may become dilated and lose its tone, causing hemorrhoids to protrude more and a small percentage of women to experience involuntary passage of gas, rectal mucus, and fecal soiling of their underwear.

A common myth is that the rectum, like the vagina, lubricates in anticipation of intercourse. Actually, the lubrication of the anal canal is very scanty, and any discharge noted is usually the result of an excessive secretion of rectal mucus in response to a low-grade inflammatory reaction caused by the trauma of previous anal coitus. Some leakage of rectal mucus also occurs when weakened sphincter muscles are unable to hold the mucus within the anus.

The rectum and anus normally harbor a wide variety of bacteria which are capable of entering a man's urethra during anal intercourse. In addition, any skin abrasion, cut, or sore on the penis may be a potential site for multiplication of these bacteria. If rectal intercourse immediately precedes vaginal intercourse, bacterial contamination of the vagina, or vaginitis, may occur. Symptoms of this condition are a watery, usually malodorous, and irritating discharge. In the nonpregnant woman this form of vaginitis, though usually not dangerous, requires antibiotic therapy. During pregnancy this type of infection is potentially more serious since it can spread to the cervix and amniotic membranes. Merely washing the penis with soap and water between vaginal and anal entry is hardly sufficient to remove all bacteria, but it is far better than not washing at all.

When bacteria multiply within a man's urethra they may cause an inflammation, or urethritis, even if he vigorously washes his penis with soap and water. A scant yellowish urethral discharge, frequency of urination, burning on urination, and passage of cloudy urine are signs of this type of urethritis. Occasionally, these symptoms may be accompanied by an elevated temperature and chills. Obviously, passage of the infection to the vagina is more likely to occur with future vaginal intercourse once a man has contracted urethritis. The only adequate precaution to prevent infection requires that a man either wear a condom for the anal portion of coitus or restrict each intercourse to the vagina or to the anus. It is important to remember that similar hygienic precautions must be taken to avoid contamination of the vagina following insertion of a finger into the rectum. At the very least, the finger should be thoroughly washed with soap and water and the nail cleaned with a brush before inserting it into the vagina. Anilingus is the licking of the anus as a means of erotic stimulation. If cunnilingus immediately follows anilingus, bacteria may be transferred to the vagina.

As with vaginal intercourse, anal intercourse should not occur during pregnancy when a woman experiences vaginal bleeding of unknown cause, when ultrasound examination reveals that the placenta is low-lying or even completely covering the cervix (placenta previa), if the membranes have ruptured and fluid is leaking and if obstetrical history and vaginal examination suggest that the cervix may be effacing and dilating prematurely.

Can a doctor tell if I practice anal coitus, and why should a doctor need to know?

If the anal sphincter is stretched excessively, it usually means frequent anal intercourse. When it is not, some doctors perform the so-called sphincter relaxation test, gently placing an index finger against the anus to see if relaxation of the anal sphincter muscle and marked dilatation of the anus takes place, almost by reflex. (While the physician who first described this test claimed that it was nearly infallible, it seems to me to be more an indication of the patient's ability to relax during an examination, and of the doctor's gentleness, than of her preference for anal coitus.)

Rather than speculate as to whether or not a patient practices anal coitus, the easiest way is simply to ask. It is unfortunate that many physicians consider this question off limits, because by obtaining this information a doctor is able to advise patients about the various hygienic precautions that should be taken if infection and injuries are to be prevented.

Can erotic stimulation from an enema cause premature labor?

A klismaphiliac is an individual who derives intense erotic pleasure from receiving an enema. Some individuals introduce this practice to their partners and both derive sexual pleasure through mutual enema-giving. Contrary to popular belief, enemas administered during pregnancy will not cause premature onset of labor, and other than aggravating and causing bleeding from enlarged hemorrhoids, they are usually harmless. However, in the presence of obstetrical conditions such as undiagnosed uterine bleeding, a prematurely dilated and effaced cervix, a low-lying placenta, or a placenta previa (placenta covering the cervix), enemas should not be used.

Are there any hazards associated with oral-genital contact during pregnancy?

There are no medical reasons to stop oral-gential contact during pregnancy provided that one bizarre maneuver is avoided. Many deaths have occurred among pregnant women whose lovers have forcibly blown air into their vaginas. When exhaled air is held under pressure by the tight application of the mouth to the vaginal opening of a pregnant woman, the air may enter the circulation via the enlarged and dilated veins of the vagina and cervix, travel to the heart, lungs, and brain, and cause instant death. When air moves through the circulatory system in this fashion it is called an air embolus.

As far as I know, there have been no reported deaths from air embolism in nonpregnant women engaged in this form of sexual behavior. Women who have engaged in this type of sexual stimulation report that the pleasure derived comes from the release from the vagina of the air under pressure. My own feeling is that the sex life of both pregnant and nonpregnant women can remain quite satisfactory without this maneuver.

Can air be accidentally introduced in a similar fashion if a woman douches or uses a bidet during pregnancy?

Maternal deaths due to air embolism have been recorded in numerous cases where the cause was a douche administered with a bulb syringe. Usually the douche was administered in an attempt to induce an abortion. However, in at least four cases there seems to be clear evidence that the douche was used for hygienic purposes. For this reason, I prohibit douching during pregnancy and explain to my patients that their increase in vaginal discharge is a normal physiological reaction which requires no treatment. If a discharge causes a severe itch and irritation or is malodorous, it is abnormal and does require treatment. However, regardless of the cause, all discharges can be treated adequately during pregnancy without resorting to use of a douche (see question on treatment of vaginitis on page 144).

A bidet is a basin about the size and height of a toilet bowl, usually equipped with fixtures for running water and a built-in spray. With this method of cleansing, the spray of water irrigates only the vulva. Since no air enters the vagina under pressure, use of a bidet is perfectly safe during pregnancy.

Can a woman be allergic to a man's semen?

Though it is not a common occurrence, instances of allergy to seminal fluid have been reported regularly, and several of these women have had this condition start during pregnancy. Allergic reactions never occur with a woman's first exposure to an ejaculate; it takes several contacts before she becomes sensitized. Seminal fluid allergy may be mild and localized to the vulva and vagina, or severe and generalized throughout the body.

Until recently, treatment of seminal fluid allergy consisted of a man wearing a condom during all coital episodes. If a pregnancy was contemplated and a woman's previous sensitivity had been a severe generalized one, coitus without a condom on the day of ovulation was probably best performed with an intravenous running and injectable epinephrine ready at the bedside! A more practical solution to this problem has recently been suggested by researchers at the University of California at San Francisco, who were able to significantly reduce the severity of one woman's generalized allergic reaction with biweekly skin injections of dilute samples of her husband's seminal fluid over a period of several months. This form of immunothera-py shows great promise for women with this unfortunate and unusual problem.

Is it safe to use a vibrator as a method of sexual gratification during pregnancy?

There are a wide assortment of battery-powered mechanical devices classified as vibrators. External vibrators are used specifically to stimulate the labia and clitoris. If used too vigorously, they may cause abrasions, or a hematoma, which is a collec-tion of blood below the skin. However, if care is taken, they can safely be used during pregnancy. It is important for a woman to remember that a vibrator-induced orgasm may bring about uterine contractions of greater intensity than those associ-ated with coitus. If these contractions cause great discomfort, or if a woman has a history of premature labor, she should probably abstain from using the vibrator.

Women using intravaginal vibrators are strongly advised to abstain from this practice during pregnancy. If a couple insists on using these devices, it is important that penetration take place slowly and with great care, since the vaginal tissues are more vascular and engorged at this time. If a woman is on top when using an intra-vaginal vibrator, she will be able to more carefully regulate the pressure and pene-tration speed and thus avoid abrasions, lacerations, and hematomas of the vaginal wall. Abundant lubrication with K-Y Jelly is also helpful in reducing the risk of these injuries.

Can breast stimulation induce labor?

There have been several interesting studies confirming that labor can be successfully induced by breast stimulation. Ancient people would actually put a suckling baby to the breast of a woman in labor in order to stimulate contractions and hasten deliv-ery. Women who nurse their babies readily detect simultaneous uterine contractions, or "after pains," and when nursing is initiated immediately after delivery it dimin-ishes postpartum blood loss by keeping the uterus in a contracted state. The mecha-nism behind this phenomenon is the fact that breast stimulation causes impulses to be sent back to a part of the brain called the posterior pituitary gland. This gland then releases oxytocin, a hormone which stimulates uterine muscle contractions. Oxytocin is the same hormone which, under the trade name Pitocin, is used by doctors to induce labor.

Probably the most complete investigation of the induction of labor by breast stimulation was reported in 1973 by Drs. A. Jhirad and T. Vago, of the Barzilai Medical Centre, Ashkelon, Israel, who attempted breast stimulation with electric breast pumps as a method of inducing labor in 204 patients at the time of their expected delivery date. Labor was successfully induced in 142 women, or 69.6 per-cent, and the interval from the onset of breast stimulation to the time of delivery averaged eight and a half hours, with 52 women giving birth in six hours or less. Those women with the greatest number of children had the highest success rates and the shortest labors; with women who had given birth to five or more full-term infants, breast stimulation achieved a successful labor induction rate of 73 percent. This finding has great practical significance because standard medical methods of labor induction are potentially dangerous for such a woman since her uterus, weakened by previous childbirth, is at greater risk of rupturing.

One additional advantage of breast stimulation noted by Drs. Jhirad and Vago was the absence of breast engorgement and a plentiful secretion of milk in all these women during the postpartum period. Several of my patients have had labor successfully initiated by their husband's use of gentle manual nipple stimulation. To prevent irritation, a lubricated jelly such as K-Y should be applied to the nipple and areola. If your pregnancy is uncomplicated and you are at or beyond your expected date of confinement, it can't hurt to try this safe technique. Doctors have recently used nipple stimulation during the last trimester as a test of fetal well-being (see chapter 10).

Postpartum Sexuality

Is it true that some women experience orgasm at the moment of birth?

Some imaginative authors have described the final agonizing effort of labor as a sensual and even an orgasmic experience. My observations and careful questioning of hundreds of women over the past few years does not in any way confirm this impression. The sensation most often reported is that of intense pain followed by a feeling of exhaustion and relief.

How soon after delivery can sexual contact be resumed?

Contrary to what most doctors recommend, there is no scientific evidence to show that a couple must wait a standard six weeks before resuming intercourse. Following an uncomplicated vaginal delivery, in which there are no vaginal lacerations and no episiotomy is performed, coitus should be perfectly safe at two weeks postpartum. One good indication of when to resume intercourse is the quantity and character of the postpartum vaginal discharge, or lochia. For the first few days following delivery, it consists of a bloodstained fluid called lochia rubra. This soon changes to a paler fluid called lochia serosa. Finally, after ten to fourteen days, it becomes lochia alba, which is white in color and minimal in amount. At this point, the cervix is usually closed, infection is not present, and intercourse may be attempted without fear of introducing infection. However, if the lochia is foul-smelling, infection of the endometrium, the lining of the uterus, may be present. A persistence of a reddish color for more than two weeks often signals the retention of small portions of the placenta or failure of the uterus to contract adequately over the site where the placenta was located. Both conditions may require a dilatation and curettage (D and C). It is best to avoid coitus until these symptoms are evaluated by your obstetrician.

If you have an episiotomy or a sutured laceration, the stitches will usually be completely dissolved three weeks later. At that time intercourse can be attempted gingerly, and if you do not experience discomfort there is no need to abstain.

Following a cesarean section, the abdominal incision usually takes two weeks to heal and, barring unusual medical complications, intercourse should be safe at this time.

As far as noncoital lovemaking techniques are concerned, I instruct my patients who have delivered vaginally not to engage in cunnilingus too soon postpartum. The mouth contains a variety of potentially harmful bacteria which, when introduced into a periurethral, vaginal, or vulvar laceration resulting from childbirth, are capable of causing an infection. If you are contemplating oral-genital sex less than three weeks after delivery, first carefully inspect your vulva and vagina with a hand mirror for evidence of a laceration that has not healed. If you are unable to do this, consult your obstetrician.

Some obstetricians believe that bacteria from a man's mouth can be introduced into the nipple of a nursing mother during lovemaking. When these bacteria multiply, breast inflammation may result. In contrast to this, babies and mothers usually share the same bacterial flora, and therefore the risk of introducing new and different bacteria during nursing is minimal.

How does the response to sexual arousal during the postpartum period compare to the prepregnancy response?

The six women previously referred to who were studied intensively during their pregnancies by Masters and Johnson were also evaluated for sexual response between the fourth and sixth postpartum week, between the sixth and eighth postpartum week, and at the end of the third postpartum month.

Although four of the six women reported a return of erotic interest during the first postpartum evaluation, Masters and Johnson found that the sexual target organs responded more slowly and with less intensity when compared to prepregnancy levels. Vasocongestive reactions of the labia, which usually begin in the excitement phase of sexual stimulation, were found to be delayed in development well into the plateau phase. Vaginal lubrication developed slowly, and the quantity was significantly less during the postpartum period. Distention of the inner two-thirds of the vagina was also noted to be reduced in rapidity of development, as well as in the amount of enlargement that took place during sexual excitation. Though all six women were noted to have a thinning atrophic appearance of their vaginal walls, this was most pronounced among the three women who were nursing. (The reason why the vagina of a nursing mother resembles that of a postmenopausal woman is because the usual pathway for hormonal stimulation between the hypothalamus and pituitary gland becomes disrupted when a woman is nursing. Prolactin hormone, produced by the pituitary gland, is responsible for milk secretion but also prevents the release of other hormones which are helpful in stimulating estrogen synthesis by the ovary. It is estrogen which thickens the vaginal tissues and gives them a healthy appearance.)

Masters and Johnson also noted a reduction in development of the orgasmic platform during the plateau phase, as well as a marked reduction in the intensity and duration of uterine contractions with orgasm among patients questioned between the fourth and sixth postpartum week.

At the six-to-eight week postpartum evaluation, the six women studied showed essentially the same physiological responses that they did at four to six weeks. However, at the end of the third postpartum month, the picture changed completely, with all six women showing evidence of full return of estrogen hormone production and prepregnancy sexuality. These beneficial effects included thickening of the vaginal walls, quick vasocongestive response of both labia to sexual stimuli, abundant and rapid development of vaginal lubrication, and full expansion of the vaginal canal. With orgasm, all six women were noted to have a normal intensity and frequency of their orgasmic platform contractions.

Do the breasts undergo physiological changes in response to sexual stimulation during the early postpartum period?

Unlike the vasocongestion of the breasts which is intensified by sexual stimulation during pregnancy, little if any physiological change is detected during the postpartum period. If milk production has been suppressed by use of hormones, it may be six months after delivery before any definite vasocongestive reaction can be observed in the breasts in response to sexual stimulation. Similarly, the breasts of nursing women do not demonstrate a consistent increase in size during the excitement phase or during increased levels of sexual tension. For some there is an uncontrollable spurt of milk from both nipples as soon as they are sexually aroused; for others, this occurs only with orgasm.

How do these postpartum changes influence a woman's subjective evaluation of her sexuality during the postpartum period?

Needless to say, women will demonstrate a variety of sexual responses during the postpartum period. Many will experience return of erotic interest within four weeks, despite the fact that physiologic testing tells us she should not be enjoying herself that much. The meaning and affection involved in a relationship can increase a woman's subjective rating of the strength or goodness of her orgasm despite the decrease in strength and rapidity of the measured physiologic response. For this reason, postpartum women initially resuming intercourse often experience full satisfaction despite the fact that they have not yet returned to prepregnancy levels of functioning.

What factors are most responsible for an early return to prepregnancy sexual enjoyment?

Based on interviews of 101 women in the third month after delivery, Masters and Johnson concluded that female eroticism was not significantly associated with a woman's age or number of children but could be related to whether or not she was breast-feeding. The highest levels of postpartum sexual interest were reported by a group of twenty-four nursing mothers. Furthermore, the nursing women who had the longest delay in the the return of ovarian function and menstruation reported the highest levels of eroticism. While the group of twenty-four nursing women stated that suckling by their infants was sexually stimulating, six said they were anxious to resume normal marital relationships with their husbands as quickly as possible in order to relieve guilt feelings about perverted sexual interests. Patients of mine have voiced similar concerns. It should be reassuring to know that it is perfectly normal to experience erotic sensations with nursing, and there is certainly no reason to feel guilty about them.

An interesting finding by Dr. Celia Falicov, of the University of Chicago, was that most women, though having intercourse less frequently, were enjoying it more. Similar conclusions have been reached by Masters and Johnson. The reasons for this are varied, but the majority of those interviewed commented that pregnancy, labor, and delivery helped them to shed traces of their timidity in relation to bodily functions and they found that they were less inhibited following childbirth.

How common is sexual dysfunction during the early postpartum period, and why does it occur?

Sexual dysfunction during the early postpartum period is a far greater problem than is generally realized. For example, of the 101 women interviewed by Masters and Johnson in the beginning of the third month following delivery, 47 described low or essentially negligible levels of sexuality. The reasons given were excessive tension and fatigue in caring for the new baby, pain with attempted intercourse, discomfort related to breast engorgement, persistent vaginal discharge, and fear of pregnancy. Falicov reached similar conclusions in her study of eighteen postpartum women.

One should not underestimate the trepidation that most women feel in anticipation of their resumption of intercourse during the postpartum period.

If a woman is afraid that her episiotomy is not completely healed, or even if she may know that all her stitches are dissolved, she may still experience a fear, often realized as irrational, that coitus will be painful. This may lead to vaginismus, or painful spasms of the vagina resulting from contractions of the vaginal walls. If this psychological reaction occurs to a significant degree, the vaginal walls may close completely when intercourse is attempted and penetration may become extremely difficult, if not impossible. Other women express concern that their vaginal tissues have become "too loose" as a result of being stretched while accommodating the birth of the baby.

Few doctors tell their patients that the vaginal tissues of the nursing woman most often resemble those of a postmenopausal woman, because they are thin, atrophic, and lacking in estrogen. The reason for this is the disruption of the usual pathway for hormonal stimulation. Without estrogen the vaginal walls do not thicken, and intercourse may be uncomfortable and even painful.

For many women, breast-feeding is an extremely sensual experience which carries over to their sexual relationship. However, others report marked sensitivity of the breasts and nipples, and a partner's usual caresses may be unwelcome. In addition, as noted earlier, it is not uncommon for nursing women to experience uncontrollable spurts of milk from their nipples during orgasm or as soon as they are

sexually aroused. Regardless of when it occurs, the abundant amount of milk released may both literally and figuratively dampen a man's sexual response.

Occasionally, the fear and dysfunction associated with coitus may originate
with the man, who, having witnessed his partner's labor, episiotomy, and birth, becomes fearful of inflicting further trauma. Under such conditions, it is not uncommon for him to lose his erection during early coital attempts.

What can be done to relieve some of the problems and reduce postpartum sexual dysfunction?

Good communication is a couple's best asset in dealing with the problems of postpartum sexual dysfunction. It is important to talk about these feelings and frustrations,
and for men to understand and respect the fact that many women are just not interested in resuming sexual contact during the first eight weeks following delivery. Sex
for many postpartum women is more than intercourse; it is touching, pleasuring,
massaging, sharing responsibilities, and understanding the reasons why the person
you love feels a certain way at a certain time. While fatigue in caring for a new baby
often saps a woman's sex drive, some researchers believe that the lack of estrogen
and progesterone hormones may also contribute to the postpartum decline in libido
experienced by some women. I recommended to all my patients that they set aside a
few hours every week to go out alone with their spouse so that they have the opportunity to focus on each other in a quiet, anxiety-free environment.

Some women delay resumption of sex or fail to reach orgasm because they are
afraid of becoming pregnant again. Postpartum contraception should be discussed by
the obstetrician before a woman leaves the hospital so that adequate precautions are
taken and fears allayed.

The most common fear of the postpartum woman is that coitus will cause severe
pain in the area of the episiotomy. For this reason a man must be extremely gentle
during the first few attempts at intercourse. Occasionally, the stitches may actually
be too tight, and a doctor can show a woman how to carefully stretch the vaginal
opening at home with plastic dilators or a speculum. When apprehension about coital injury is so intense that it causes muscular spasms (vaginismus), an obstetrician
should be able to demonstrate to a woman and her partner how to gently overcome
this problem, first with fingers, then with increasingly larger dilators.

To minimize discomfort related to the episiotomy, try varying your positions for
intercourse. Women with a mediolateral episiotomy, one that goes off to one side,
say that it is helpful if their partner leans to the opposite side. Most episiotomies are
median (in the midline). This type of incision is far more comfortable and usually
heals faster and with less of a scar. Nevertheless, try to choose a position in which
the penis presses against the front part of the vagina and clitoris, rather than the
tender area in back. Couples should try those positions in which the woman can
control the depth of penetration as well as the point of maximum penile pressure.
The best in this regard are the side-by-side, woman-on-top, and "spoon" positions.

The lack of vaginal lubrication, caused by a postpartum estrogen deficiency and
most pronounced in nursing women, can be easily overcome with liberal use of K-Y

Jelly or natural oils such as sesame and coconut. Some doctors have advocated the use of estrogen vaginal cream. However, this preparation is absorbed through the vaginal walls and into the circulation. Since this could not only diminish milk production but also pass into the breast milk and be ingested by the baby, I never prescribe vaginal estrogen preparations for a nursing woman.

To alleviate the problem of spurting milk from the nipples during sexual arousal, try wearing a bra or nursing pads that provide enough pressure to stop the flow of milk or at least absorb it. One excellent suggestion is to nurse the baby immediately before lovemaking; this will have the dual advantage of decreasing the amount of milk which leaks and reducing the chances of an interruption from a hungry baby. But though all these suggestions are helpful, the best medication for curing postpartum sexual dysfunction is time. Patience, love, understanding, and communication will usually overcome even the most difficult problems.

Do you have any suggestions for couples who continue to experience sexual dysfunction beyond the immediate postpartum period?

It has been my experience that the overwhelming majority of couples who have a good sex life prior to pregnancy will return to their level of enjoyment within a reasonable amount of time. Most sex therapists believe that pregnancy and the immediate six-week postpartum period is not the time to seek help, especially if a couple has had an adequate prepregnancy sexual relationship. Pregnancy introduces many temporary emotional and physical variables which often subside spontaneously, thereby making therapy unnecessary. During pregnancy and postpartum, minor sexual problems may be magnified and appear much more serious than they actually are.

However, a significant number of couples have deep-rooted sexual difficulties which have antedated the pregnancy. Problems among men, such as premature ejaculation, impotence, and inability to maintain an erection, and dysfunction among women in the form of inability to experience sexual interest or orgasm, all require treatment. While pregnancy is not the time to seek this type of therapy, there is no reason to delay evaluation later than eight weeks postpartum. Without help, these problems will not suddenly subside spontaneously but will only worsen.

Couples seeking sexual counseling should realize that most family doctors and obstetricians lack the training and expertise needed to deal with these serious problems. Furthermore, few doctors have the time in a busy office practice to personally treat their patients' serious sexual dysfunctions on an intensive basis. As a result of the new openness in discussing and treating problems of sexuality, many sexual dysfunction clinics have opened throughout the United States. Dr. William H. Masters has referred to the vast majority of these clinics as "institutions operated for money by pure charlatans" and states that only 1 out of 100 can be considered legitimate. Most reputable sex therapists are accredited by the American Association of Sex Educators, Counselors, and Therapists (AASECT), 600 Maryland Ave. S.W., Washington, D.C. 20021, and the American Society for Sex Therapy and Research (ASSTAR), c/o Oliver Bjorkater, M.D., 171 Ashly Ave., Charleston, S.C. 29403.

Each of these organizations can provide a listing of approved sex therapists in a particular area.

Effects on Pregnancy of Drugs Taken to Enhance or Heighten Sex

What effects do aphrodisiacs have on a pregnant woman?

Aphrodisiacs are drugs, medications, or concoctions which are used to enhance erotic desire and sexual performance. Lovers throughout history have sought the perfect aphrodisiac without success. All too often, women inadvertently take one of these drugs before they are aware that they are pregnant. Others try these preparations with the foolish intention of enhancing a waning sex drive during pregnancy.

Amyl nitrite and isobutyl nitrite

Amyl nitrite is probably one of the most popular aphrodisiacs used in this country. It comes in small glass ampules, and it is used as an aphrodisiac by breaking the glass and inhaling the contents just before orgasm. Isobutyl nitrite, also used as an aphrodisiac, is packaged in a small bottle with a screw cap. For this use, the cap is removed and the contents inhaled. Both are classified as vasodilators, which means they open the blood vessels, and amyl nitrite is used medically to relieve the pain of angina. In addition to dilating blood vessels, both drugs lower the blood pressure and speed the heart rate. Sexual sensations are enhanced: orgasm feels more intense and prolonged and the drugs are effective in relaxing the vaginal and anal openings, thereby permitting easier penetration. Sexual activities which may have seemed repugnant or were rejected because of inhibitions often become desirable.

Because amyl nitrite is used in the treatment of heart disease, it has been studied more extensively than isobutyl nitrite. Surprisingly, there are few if any harmful side effects of this drug, and in the medical literature there are no documented deaths or permanent injuries resulting from its recreational use. However, the sudden drop in blood pressure which it is capable of causing could be theoretically dangerous for women with either high or low blood pressure, as well as for individuals with certain heart conditions.

Though there are no reports that I know of which link use of amyl or isobutyl nitrite to congenital anomalies, neither should be used for sexual enhancement during pregnancy. Even a transient drop in blood pressure at any time during pregnancy may be associated with a decrease in the blood flow to the uterus. When this occurs, less oxygen is carried to the fetus, which has the potential to cause permanent fetal damage. Recreational use of these drugs is especially dangerous among women with hypertension or pregnancy-induced hypertension (preeclampsia). Among these individuals, the drop in blood pressure is often more dramatic and more likely to compromise the oxygen supply to the fetus.

Cocaine

Cocaine, a very popular and expensive aphrodisiac, is, unlike amyl nitrite, an illegal drug having no approved medical use. It achieves its effect by constricting the blood vessels, the exact opposite action of that of amyl nitrite. It acts as an aphrodisiac by stimulating the central nervous system to produce enormous energy, referred to as a "rush." The response to cocaine varies widely from one user to another, and though there are no scientific studies to prove its effectiveness, the majority of men and women who use this drug report a heightened sexuality. Some men have claimed that while snorting (inhaling) cocaine powder they are capable of multiple orgasm without loss of erection, a phenomenon which most men rarely, if ever, experience. Cocaine has also been used as a surface anesthetic which, when applied to the tip of the penis or clitoris, decreases sensation and permits longer and more varied sexual activity.

Cocaine users in increasing numbers are smoking the drug rather than snorting it. This is very dangerous because a far greater amount of cocaine is rapidly absorbed into the circulatory system. Cocaine smokers have been noted to experience intense anxiety, paranoia, auditory and visual hallucinations, and psychoses.

Though there are no known reports of birth defects resulting from a woman's use of cocaine during pregnancy, in recent laboratory studies deformities were produced in mice given low doses of cocaine early in pregnancy. Defects included those to the eye, brain and bone. There is also a very real possibility that cocaine's vasoconstricting effect on blood vessels may decrease the blood flow to the fetus later in pregnancy. It is known that women who suffer from certain diseases in which there is vasoconstriction of the uterine arteries are far more likely to give birth to premature and growth-retarded infants. For this reason, cocaine should not be used at any time during pregnancy.

Marijuana

Marijuana, also known as pot or grass, is probably the most popular drug used in this country to enhance sexuality. The potency of a particular sample of marijuana depends on its concentration of THC (9-tetrahydrocannabinol), the drug's chief active ingredient. While some users feel more sensuous, erotic, and aroused after smoking marijuana, the majority of studies have concluded that this drug either hinders or has little influence on sex drive or frequency of intercourse. Those who report that marijuana has a positive effect on sexuality claim that it makes the act feel as though it lasts longer, though it probably does not. Users also claim a heightened concentration on the details of the sexual act, to the exclusion of all other distractions.

Several studies show that men who smoke marijuana on a daily basis are more likely to experience a significant decline in their blood levels of testosterone, the male sex hormone. This in turn may lead to impotence or infertility. Although complete reversibility of these changes was not observed after marijuana use was stopped, sperm motility was significantly improved two weeks later.

Researchers have concluded that infertility and other reproductive and endocrine problems are more common among women who smoke marijuana. Though there is no convincing proof that marijuana causes chromosome damage to the egg or sperm, research on both rodents and monkeys suggests that maternal exposure to marijuana and pure THC may be toxic to the fetus in utero and also cause deaths of the newborn. Though experience with women who smoke pot during pregnancy is quite limited, a Canadian investigator recently noted that those who smoke five or more joints a week during any one trimester of pregnancy were more likely to give birth to an infant with tremors, unusual startle reactions, a high-pitched cry, and abnormal visual and auditory responses. It was also noted that the severity of symptoms in the newborn was directly related to the amount of marijuana smoked by its mother. Of great concern was the fact that the tremors and abnormal startle reactions were still evident at nine days of age, while the visual disturbances persisted for longer than thirty days. Marijuana use was not found to adversely affect the course of pregnancy or delivery, the baby's Apgar score (see page 328), birth weight, length, or head circumference. In a 1982 study from the University of California in Los Angeles, doctors studied the effect of marijuana use in thirty-five pregnancies. They found that infants born to marijuana users were more likely to pass greenish fecal material, or meconium, into their amniotic fluid. This condition is occasionally associated with fetal distress. Users of marijuana also experienced a higher incidence of prolonged and difficult labors than nonusers. Most recently, investigators at Boston University School of Medicine noted that women who smoked marijuana were more likely to give birth to smaller infants and infants with anomalies similar to those described with fetal alcohol syndrome (see page 118).

It has been clearly demonstrated that THC crosses the placenta from mother to fetus and is also found in maternal milk. Suckling male offspring of rodents treated with marijuana for six days postpartum were observed to have both endocrine and behavioral changes. In humans, there are a few unconfirmed reports of drowsiness reported in nursing infants after their mothers smoked marijuana.

The anatomic and physiologic response of monkeys is very similar to that of humans. Therefore, the results of experimental research on these animals are of greater significance than those attained from studies of lower forms of animal life. In a 1979 report from the University of California, THC was administered to monkeys at a dose equivalent to that obtained by a person smoking two marijuana cigarettes per day. Forty percent of these animals experienced reproductive failures which included fetal death, stillbirth, and early infant death. Monkeys not exposed to THC experienced these problems only 11 percent of the time. Though all fetuses and infants of the THC-treated monkeys appeared normal, closer examination of the internal organs revealed developmental abnormalities in the nervous, cardiovascular, or urinary systems. These defects were often accompanied by abnormalities of the placenta.

These data seem sufficiently ominous to discourage women from even occasional marijuana use during pregnancy. The pot-smoking couple contemplating pregnancy should abstain at least two weeks, and preferably one month, before attempting conception.

Amphetamines

Amphetamines, also known as "speed," "uppers," and "bennies," are addictive drugs which stimulate the central nervous system and produce a feeling of excitation and euphoria. Amphetamines, such as benzedrine, dexedrine, and preludin, are often initially prescribed as diet pills by doctors who are either too ignorant or too lazy to seek safer alternatives for their overweight patients.

Claims about the sexual benefits of amphetamines vary greatly. However, most researchers believe that while these drugs may enhance the libido of the occasional user, they diminish the sex drive of the chronically addicted individual.

Amphetamines should rarely if ever be taken by the nonpregnant woman and never by the pregnant woman. Laboratory studies on animals suggest that amphetamines may damage and produce abnormalities of the developing fetus (see chapter 7). Amphetamines are particularly dangerous because they are capable of causing a marked elevation of the blood pressure, which is especially hazardous for women with a borderline elevation of blood pressure as a result of preeclampsia.

Barbiturates

Barbiturates, also known as "downers," "goofers," and "dolls," act on the central nervous system to produce sedation and sleep. Common trade names are Tuinal, Seconal, Nembutal, and Amytal. Their prolonged use results in both physical and psychological dependence, and withdrawal is more serious and dangerous than from narcotics. Though barbiturates have some very important medical applications (see chapter 7), it is amazing how many unnecessary prescriptions for barbiturate capsules are written by doctors in this country each year. If sexuality is at all improved with barbiturates, it is because the sedation which results from these drugs tends to lower inhibitions. This effect may last for one to eight hours.

In both animal experimentation and studies of pregnant women, there is strong evidence to suggest that barbiturate use during the first three months of pregnancy increases the likelihood of fetal abnormalities (see chapter 7). If barbiturates are taken within eight hours of delivery, the drug can pass through the placenta and cause sleepiness and respiratory depression in the newborn. This type of medical problem is one of the most difficult for neonatologists to treat. Though barbiturates are known to pass into the breast milk, there is only one report in the medical literature of questionable drowsiness of a nursing infant.

Methaqualone, another type of "downer," creates bodily reactions similar to barbiturates, despite being chemically unrelated. It is sold under the trade name of Quaalude, and though it is referred to by devotees as the "love drug," there is no substantial evidence to show that it enhances sexuality. Because of its potency, it should never be taken during pregnancy.

Anxiety-reducing Drugs

When used in small doses, and for a short term, certain anxiety-reducing drugs, or tranquilizers, are capable of stimulating erotic desire and in lifting certain inhibitions. When used for prolonged periods of time, these drugs depress eroticism. Prolonged use, however, leads to both physical and psychological dependence. The most popular drugs in this group are meprobamate (trade names Miltown and Equanil), chlordiazepoxide (trade name Librium), and diazepam (trade name Valium). Diazepam has the dubious distinction of being one of the most commonly prescribed drugs in the United States.

None of these drugs should be used during the first trimester of pregnancy because of the risk of congenital malformations in the fetus. Also, these drugs, administered to a woman in labor, can be transferred to the fetus via the placenta, causing drowsiness, abnormally low body temperature, poor muscle tone, and respiratory depression in the newborn.

It is very important that a breast-feeding woman be aware that the concentration of Miltown or Equanil will be two to four times greater in her breast milk than in her bloodstream. While Librium and Valium are transmitted to breast milk in lower concentrations, research studies do show that infants metabolize Valium more slowly than adults, possibly resulting in accumulations of the drug in a baby's body. Breast-feeding mothers who take diazepam may thus produce drowsiness in their infants.

Hallucinogens

Hallucinogens are a group of dangerous drugs which, though not associated with addiction, physical dependence, or physical withdrawal, may cause permanent emotional damage and psychological dependence. The most notorious drugs in this group include LSD (D-lysergic acid diethylamide), peyote (a mescaline-containing cactus), and PCP (phencyclidine hydrochloride).

LSD is the most potent and potentially the most hazardous. An LSD trip may last eight to twelve hours, during which time total contact with reality may be lost. The effects of LSD on the fetus have been studied with more intensity than most other medications, and several investigators have demonstrated significant breaks in the chromosomes of LSD users and their offspring. In one study of forty-four women known to have taken LSD before and during pregnancy, six (13.5 percent) gave birth to infants with serious deformities of both the lower and upper extremities. In addition, five of twenty-one aborted fetuses of LSD users had similar deformities. The usual incidence of these defects in the normal population is only 0.1 percent. It is frightening to note that the damage caused by LSD is random; one cannot predict which infants will be immune from injury and which ones will be deformed. The dose of LSD taken by the mother apparently is not a determining factor.

If a woman has taken LSD at or after the time of conception, therapeutic abortion is recommended. If pregnancy has progressed beyond the fourteenth week, analysis of fetal chromosomes may be performed by amniocentesis (see chapter 10). The chromosomes in the fluid may then be studied for abnormalities but this is far from foolproof, since not all LSD-deformed infants have broken chromosomes.

Peyote does not cause the chromosomal damage associated with the use of LSD. Members of the Huichol Indian tribe of northern Mexico have a lifelong history and a 1,600-year cultural tradition of peyote ingestion. Researchers from the University of California, in studying these Indians, were unable to detect chromosomal abnormalities among peyote users or their offspring.

Phencyclidine hydrochloride, or PCP, also known as "angel dust" is a hallucinogenic drug that has been responsible for an alarming increase in the number of people treated in hospital emergency rooms for fatal or near-fatal coma and respiratory depression following its use. One recent case in the medical literature describes the appearance of an infant born of a woman who used PCP daily throughout her pregnancy. At birth, the baby experienced respiratory depression, lethargy, coarse tremors, poor feeding, and abnormal eye movements. In addition, its face had an unusual triangular shape with a pointed chin and abnormal angle to the jaw. While there are no other studies concerning similar infant abnormalities, such effects must be considered a possibility in light of this report. Recent laboratory studies have demonstrated that PCP concentration in breast milk may be 10 times greater than those found in the maternal bloodstream.

Narcotics

Narcotics are effective in relieving pain, but they also elevate mood, counteract depression, and induce euphoria, sedation, and sleep. Prolonged use produces severe physical and psychological dependence. Drugs in this group are heroin, morphine, methadone (trade name Dolophine), opium, codeine, and meperidine (best known by its trade name Demerol).

Heroin is the most deadly of these drugs. Though it is impossible to obtain exact figures, there are probably about 700,000 heroin addicts in the United States. Approximately one-fourth are women, and of these about 140,000 are of childbearing age. Heroin users report that, in the beginning, sexual encounters are intensely gratifying. However, with prolonged addiction, both sexes experience a loss of erotic desire and sexual function.

Some investigators have attributed chromosomal abnormalities to narcotic addiction. In one of the largest studies of 99 methadone- and heroin-addicted pregnant women and their babies, both mothers and offspring were found to have a far greater percentage of chromosomally damaged cells than is usually noted in the general population. Interestingly, the chromosomal changes were unrelated to the dosage or duration of drug use. Similar studies on laboratory animals have confirmed these findings.

It has been estimated that only 10 to 20 percent of all addicted pregnant women bother to seek prenatal care. Of this group, one-third register late in the third trimester. Women who do not have a secret supply of heroin stashed away in their possessions brought to the hospital show evidence of withdrawal symptoms—nausea, tremors, abdominal pains, and cramps—within twenty-four hours of delivery. To prevent this from happening, most addicts sign out of the hospital immediately after delivery unless placed on methadone. Though methadone is probably more addicting than heroin, it has the ability to block the "high" produced by heroin without causing physical withdrawal. In addition, it can be given as a medically supervised daily dose. For this reason, it is important to substitute methadone maintenance for heroin as soon as possible during pregnancy.

The incidence of obstetrical problems is significantly greater in the pregnant addict. Included among these complications are ectopic pregnancy, low birth weight, premature rupture of the membranes, toxemia, abruptio placenta or premature separation of the placenta caused by a blood clot which forms behind it, and multiple births.

One of the most tragic medical conditions is narcotic addiction of the newborn resulting from transmission of drugs via the placenta. Approximately 70 percent of all babies born of addicted mothers will show some evidence of a withdrawal reaction within a few hours after birth: irritability, tremors, vomiting, high-pitched cry, sneezing, hyperactivity, respiratory distress, and diarrhea. These babies must be treated with the greatest care and skill by medical personnel who are experienced in dealing with this very difficult problem. Even with the best of care, the newborn mortality rate will be approximately 3 to 5 percent.

Many female addicts resort to prostitution in order to maintain their drug habit. As a result, they are much more likely to contract venereal diseases, such as syphilis, gonorrhea, and herpes, which can be transmitted to their infants during pregnancy or at the time of birth. One study found that 20 percent of pregnant addicts had a blood test which was positive for syphilis.

Though all narcotics are capable of passing from mother to child in the breast milk, the highest and most unpredictable concentrations occur with heroin. There are cases in the medical literature of infants of heroin-addicted mothers showing withdrawal symptoms when breast-feeding was delayed or discontinued. Nursing mothers on maintenance doses of methadone do not need to discontinue breast-feeding, since the average daily dose received by the infant is minimal. The limited reports available on morphine and codeine also indicate that little if any of these narcotics are present in the breast milk.

Is it true that Spanish fly is the ultimate aphrodisiac?

Every teenage boy has heard the legend of the frigid woman turned into a sex-starved nymphomaniac following the use of Spanish fly; in my youth, there was always some neighborhood madman who claimed to be in possession of a secret supply. Even today, there are many street drugs being sold under this name.

Spanish fly does exist; its scientific name is *cantharides*. However, it is not an aphrodisiac but an irritating and poisonous powder derived from dried insects. When applied to the genitals it causes intense irritation and inflammation of the vulva, vagina, urinary bladder, and urethra which may result in permanent damage to the genitals and kidneys. Deaths have even been reported following use of Spanish fly.

Does vitamin E increase libido and sexual potency?

No. Ever since the discovery of vitamin E in 1923, people have claimed that it can cure everything from hiccups to hemorrhoids. None of these claims have ever been scientifically substantiated, though the myths persist. In actuality, vitamin E is anything but a glamorous vitamin. It is found in just about all foods, having its highest concentration in vegetable oils such as safflower oil, wheat germ oil, and peanut oil. A vitamin E deficiency is practically unheard of in this country.

There is absolutely no truth to the widespread belief that vitamin E heightens sexual potency; in fact, there is some evidence suggesting that massive doses may actually reduce the functioning of the reproductive organs.

Does alcohol have an aphrodisiac effect?

Alcohol in small amounts has the effect of stimulating sexual desire in both men and women. This occurs because it depresses centers in the brain which are responsible for creating fear, anxiety, and socially inhibited behavior. Unfortunately, there is a fine line between the amount of alcohol which will create this positive sexual effect and that which will bring sedation, sleep, intoxication, and lack of sexual interest.

How much alcohol can be drunk safely during pregnancy?

The ancient Romans believed that intoxication at the moment of conception resulted in the birth of a damaged child. The Carthaginians forbade the drinking of wine by bride and groom on their wedding night for fear that a defective child might result. This sound advice was neglected for thousands of years, and until very recently intravenous alcohol was extensively used with some success in preventing or stopping premature labor. In 1968, the association between maternal ingestion of alcohol and a variety of developmental abnormalities in the newborn was firmly established. The term "fetal alcohol syndrome" was coined in 1973 to describe the gross malformations, prenatal and postpartum growth retardation, and permanent intellectual and psychomotor defects of some infants born of alcoholic mothers. The classic facial appearance noted in fetal alcohol syndrome is that of a small head circumference (microcephaly), underdevelopment of the jawbone (micrognathia), low-set ears, abnormalities of the eyelids, and underdevelopment of the bridge of the nose (hypoplasia). In addition to these distinctive features, bone and joint abnormalities, abnormal creases in the palm, cardiac defects, and female genital anomalies have been found in over 50 percent of these children. In addition to the fetal alcohol syndrome, researchers have found that women who drink may also be at significantly greater risks of spontaneous abortion, stillbirths, prematurity, and the birth of babies with low birth weights and retarded growth.

While most reports have focused on the chronic alcoholic woman, in whom the risk of fetal abnormality is estimated at 40 percent or more, it has also been found that sporadic but excessive intake of alcohol at critical stages of pregnancy may lead to a poor pregnancy outcome. Even moderate amounts of alcohol consumption may be dangerous. Doctors at Columbia University in New York City recently noted a significantly higher rate of spontaneous abortions among women who consumed as little as one drink twice a week. When drinks were broken down according to type of liquor, the investigators found that women who drank wine and spirits ran a greater risk of miscarriage than those who preferred beer. The reason for this is believed to be the greater concentration of alcohol contained in each ounce of wine and spirits. In a 1980 study from the National Institute of Child Health and Human Development, doctors concluded that pregnancy loss between the fifteenth and twenty-seventh weeks of pregnancy was higher for women taking one or two drinks per day than those who averaged less than one drink daily.

Furthermore, the widely held belief that alcohol is harmless if one has an adequate diet is just not true. There are several reports in the literature of alcoholic women delivering babies with characteristics of fetal alcohol syndrome despite the fact that they maintained excellent nutrition throughout pregnancy. For this reason, when patients ask me how much they can safely drink during pregnancy, I tell them that abstinence is certainly the safest policy. I am in full agreement with the Surgeon General's 1981 advisory that pregnant women avoid all alcoholic beverages and food and drugs which contain alcohol. While no safe level of maternal alcohol intake during pregnancy has been established, the U.S. Food and Drug Administration has concluded that six drinks per day is sufficient to establish a major risk to the developing fetus, while two drinks daily may carry an increased risk for growth and developmental abnormalities.

Fetal alcohol syndrome has also been noted on rare occasions among babies born of previously alcoholic mothers who abstained throughout pregnancy. However, in most cases abstinence or marked reduction of alcohol consumption during pregnancy, including the third trimester, will significantly lower the risk to the fetus.

Until 1979, no hypothesis could be offered to explain why many women who are heavy drinkers deliver normal babies, while others who drink minimally give birth to abnormal offspring. Researchers now theorize that the reason for this lies not with the alcohol itself but with one of its breakdown products, called acetaldehyde. It is known that high blood levels of this chemical are capable of causing cell damage and fetal abnormalities. In most individuals, these high levels are never reached following alcohol consumption because acetaldehyde is rapidly eliminated from the circulation. However, some people have either an inherited or an acquired defect in their ability to rapidly lower the blood levels of acetaldehyde even after modest alcoholic intake.

In the future it may be possible to detect those women who can safely drink during pregnancy and those who must abstain simply by measuring how quickly they break down the alcohol they consume.

Based on an evaluation of recent reports, it has been estimated that variations of fetal alcohol syndrome may occur with an astonishing frequency of 4 to 7 cases per 1,000 live births. If these calculations are correct, it would make this syndrome the most common cause of mental deficiency in the United States.

Alcohol is excreted in breast milk in small amounts, and alcoholic beverages taken in moderation by a nursing mother appear to have little effect on the infant, although in one report an infant developed symptoms of drunkenness with a high alcohol blood level after the mother drank one and a half pints of port wine. In another dramatic case, a well-meaning mother said she drank seven beers a day plus other alcoholic beverages in order to increase her milk supply. Her four-month-old daughter became obese, lethargic, and experienced stunted growth. The child improved dramatically when her mother's alcoholic intake was curtailed.

5.
Sexually Transmitted Diseases

The sexual freedom of the past decade has unfortunately been accompanied by an overwhelming increase in the incidence of sexually transmitted diseases. In the past, venereal disease, or VD, meant either syphilis or gonorrhea, which still threaten our population. Other diseases such as herpes, mycoplasma, and chlamydia have only recently become a source of great concern to health professionals. According to the most up-to-date estimates, approximately twenty different diseases are now known to be transmitted sexually. Susceptibility to precancerous and cancerous disease of the cervix also correlates strongly with a woman's sexual history, so these diseases, too, may be classified as venereally transmitted.

By definition, venereal disease refers to diseases spread by sexual intercourse. Considering the sexual preferences of today's society, however, the term "sexually transmitted disease" more accurately reflects the many conditions that may be passed to others, not only by vaginal intercourse but also by anal intercourse, oral-genital contact, and anilingus.

Many women are totally uninformed about the sexually transmitted diseases which may afflict them and their babies. Even more discouraging is the fact that a great many doctors, too, are unfamiliar with the changing patterns of disease transmission. Medical textbooks published as late as 1975 take little if any notice of diseases such as penicillin-resistant gonorrhea and nongonococcal urethritis. Treatments considered correct for a variety of sexually transmitted diseases in 1970 are in many cases not adequate today. And many doctors waste more time in moralizing than in understanding and effectively treating their patients. The woman who fears she may have VD is not particularly interested in a lecture on the evils of promiscuity. And a physician's shyness in obtaining a complete sexual history from a married upper-middle-class patient may only delay the prompt and accurate diagnosis of her disease.

While some sexually transmitted conditions pose little if any threat to the developing fetus or to the baby at the time of birth, others are potentially lethal and require instant detection and therapy. Several of these diseases are totally without symptoms, thereby making the diagnosis particularly difficult. This chapter discusses current methods of diagnosing and treating those sexually transmitted diseases that may affect the pregnant woman and her baby.

Syphilis

What causes syphilis, and what are its symptoms?

Syphilis is caused by a spiral-shaped microscopic bacterium called a spirochete and known by the scientific name of *Treponema pallidum*. The U.S. Public Heath Service estimates that there are at least 80,000 new cases each year in this country.

For syphilis to be transmitted, the skin or mucous membranes of a susceptible individual must come in contact with the skin or mucous membranes of an infected person. The incubation period (the time between exposure to the infection and development of the first symptoms) may vary from ten to ninety days. The usual time, however, is two to four weeks.

The initial infection may be single or multiple and usually begins as a flat sore on the skin which soon erodes to form a hard, firm-edged, painless ulcer called a chancre (pronounced *shanker*). A chancre is teeming with millions of highly contagious bacteria. Since it is a painless sore, it often goes unnoticed, though the spirochetes are easily spread during coital or noncoital contact. While most chancres appear on the genitalia, they may also be found on the lips, tongue, fingers, nipples, or anus if these areas come in direct contact with areas harboring spirochetes. The lymph nodes in the area surrounding a chancre are usually enlarged but are not painful to touch.

An untreated primary chancre usually heals slowly over a period of three to eight weeks, leaving a thin scar. Its disappearance ends the primary stage of the disease and is often falsely considered as a sign that all is well. However, the secondary stage usually appears within three months after the first stage has healed although it may be delayed for many months or even years. Its appearance means that the spirochete is now disseminated throughout the body.

Symptoms of secondary-stage syphilis vary, though some form of skin rash is usually noted on the trunk, palms, and soles, and often with a scaly appearance. Occasionally it is most prominent on the moist skin surfaces such as the underarms, the genitals, and the anus. The hair on the head may fall out in patches. The inside of the mouth may show secondary syphilis lesions, known as mucous patches, which have a grayish-white necrotic area surrounded by a dull red border and cause a severe sore throat. All these skin and mucous membrane lesions are extremely infectious. Whereas only the local lymph nodes are enlarged during the primary stage of syphilis, 50 percent of individuals with secondary syphilis experience a generalized lymph node enlargement throughout their bodies: in the groin, under the arms, in the neck, and under the jaw. Since the disease is widespread throughout the body during the secondary stage, it is often accompanied by generalized symptoms, such as headache, weakness, loss of appetite, and aching in the long bones, muscles, and joints.

Amazingly, if left untreated, the lesions of secondary-stage syphilis also will heal without scarring within two to six weeks. A latent period follows in which there are no signs or symptoms of the disease. During the first two years of this period, known as early latent syphilis, the individual is usually not contagious unless a relapse occurs. After the second year, the disease enters the late latent period, during which time it is not contagious either.

Three to ten years after the primary stage, the earliest lesions of the final stage, called tertiary syphilis, appear. Tertiary syphilis is a devastating disease, capable of causing permanent damage to practically every organ in the body.

One characteristic lesion at this stage is a gumma, or localized destructive ulcer, which may vary in size from one millimeter to several centimeters in diameter, or from the size of a pinhead to the size of a silver dollar. Gummas usually occur in groups on any part of the skin or on mucous membranes such as those of the mouth, throat, palate, pharynx, larynx, and nasal septum. However, they may also occur in the outer lining of the bones, in muscles, in the stomach, intestines, liver, spleen, lungs, and kidneys, and even in the genitals. When gummas involve structures, such as the hard palate and nasal septum, they destroy the supporting bone and cartilage and cause permanent deformities.

About 10 percent of all patients with tertiary syphilis will experience permanent damage to the muscles and valves of the heart, as well as the aorta, pulmonary arteries, and vena cava, which are the three major blood vessels carrying blood to and from the heart. *Treponema pallidum* can also invade the brain and spinal cord, resulting in a wide variety of crippling neurological disturbances and cytological abnormalities.

What are the effects of syphilis on pregnancy?

A fetus is usually well protected from the ravages of syphilis at the beginning by a layer of cells, the Langhans' layer, which is present in the placenta until the eighteenth week of pregnancy. After this point, the Langhans' layer is absorbed, and the infection may then be transmitted from the mother to the fetal bloodstream by the passage of spirochetes across the placenta. (One recent microscopic finding suggests that the Langhans' layer may not offer as much protection as previously believed, since *Treponema pallidum* was detected in the bodies of fetuses aborted during the first trimester of pregnancy.)

The presence of an overwhelming syphilitic infection in the fetus may result in a stillbirth. This is most likely to occur when the mother is in the primary or early secondary stages of infection.

Infection in the newborn is termed congenital syphilis. Congenital syphilis may be difficult to detect at birth, since physical signs and symptoms do not usually appear for several weeks and they may not develop until later in childhood, when the manifestations are different from those in infancy. If syphilis is obvious at birth, the infection is usually severe.

"Early congenital syphilis" is the term used to describe untreated syphilis before the age of two. One of the most frequent signs of this stage is a skin rash similar to that of the adult with the disease. Equally as frequent is the presence of "snuffles," a heavy mucuslike discharge from the nose and throat, which makes breathing and sucking difficult and irritates the skin that comes in contact with the discharge. There may also be anemia, inflammation of the long bones of the body, and enlargement of the liver and spleen.

Late congenital syphilis is syphilis which has persisted beyond two years of age.

While the disease is not contagious at this stage, the effects may be devastating: inflammation of the cornea of the eye, unusual configurations of the teeth, deafness, bone and joint deformities, skin fissures, involvement of the central nervous system, and damage to the valves of the heart.

How is syphilis diagnosed?

A sore or ulcer in the genital area, anus, mouth, or tongue, or the presence of a generalized rash, lymph node enlargement, or sore throat should alert your doctor to order appropriate laboratory tests for syphilis. The simplest method of screening patients for syphilis is with one of several nonspecific preliminary blood tests called nontreponemal tests. The more popular nontreponemal tests are Wassermann, Kolmer, Kline, RPR, and VDRL. Positive results appear for practically all patients within seven days after the ulcer first appears. In a very small percentage of cases it may take as long as twenty-one days for these tests to become positive. It is well to remember that a false positive diagnosis of syphilis based solely on this preliminary testing is possible. Conditions such as infectious mononucleosis, acute infections, upper respiratory diseases, malaria, so-called collagen diseases, such as systemic lupus erythematosis and arthritis, and even pregnancy, may all give false positive results for syphilis. Similarly, certain vaccinations and immunizations, as well as heroin addiction, may cause a false positive reaction.

So more sensitive tests, called treponemal antibody tests must be performed to confirm the positive diagnosis of the preliminary test. A positive reaction to these tests confirms the diagnosis of syphilis, while a negative test means the nontreponemal test was incorrect and syphilis is not present. The most popular of these treponemal antibody tests are the FTA-ABS (fluorescent treponemal antibody absorption tests), the TPI (treponemal pallidum immobilization), and the MHA-TP (microhemagglutination treponemal pallidum).

The diagnosis of syphilis may also be made by obtaining a sample from an ulcer with a cotton swab and a glass slide. Viewed under an ordinary microscope, using a special technique called a dark-field examination, the organism appears white against a dark background.

What should be done to ensure the early diagnosis of syphilis during pregnancy and prevent congenital syphilis?

All pregnant women should have a nontreponemal blood test for syphilis, such as the VDRL or Wassermann, at the time of their first prenatal visit. Since syphilis may be contracted later in pregnancy, when it is most likely to damage the fetus, many authorities now recommend a second nontreponemal blood test for all women during the third trimester. If either of these tests is positive, a more specific evaluation such as the FTA-ABS test should be done immediately to confirm or refute the diagnosis. If the FTA-ABS is also positive, antibiotic treatment must be begun for both the pregnant woman and her sexual partner or partners. (If the man has engaged in intercourse with others his contacts should be located and treated, too.)

If a woman has had syphilis in the past, tests such as the VDRL and FTA-ABS often remain positive for years following successful treatment. In such situations, it may be difficult to interpret the usual tests. This problem can usually be resolved by a quantitative nontreponemal test in which the strength, or titre, of the syphilis reaction is measured. If a woman has contracted syphilis anew, there will be at least a fourfold rise in titre within three to four weeks. However, if syphilis is not active, the titre will remain unchanged. After treatment of syphilis with antibiotics during pregnancy, a woman should be followed closely with monthly quantitative nontreponemal blood tests throughout the remainder of her pregnancy. If a fourfold-or-more rise in titre is noted, it usually means that she has been reinfected and requires treatment again.

The risk of congenital syphilis in the baby will be minimal if maternal syphilis is adequately treated before delivery. Even in the absence of infection, most healthy newborns will still inherit their mother's nontreponemal antibodies, which are passed across the placenta. These so-called 7-S antibodies are responsible for an elevated titre, which will become negative within the first year of life.

If the newborn's titre rises above that of the mother, it is a good bet that the baby has active congenital syphilis requiring immediate treatment. Infected infants are frequently without symptoms at birth, and this blood test may be negative if the maternal infection occurred late in pregnancy. A far more accurate blood test for detecting syphilis in the newborn is a fluorescent antibody procedure which detects the presence of large antibodies, called 19-S or IgM (immunoglobin M) antibodies. Since these antibodies are too large to cross the placenta, their presence in the newborn indicates an active infection. Infants must also be treated with antibiotics if signs or symptoms of the disease are present or recur, if the mother's treatment is inadequate or unknown, if the nontreponemal test either increases or fails to show a significant decrease, or if adequate follow-up of the infant cannot be guaranteed.

What is the correct treatment for syphilis?

Penicillin remains the treatment of choice for all stages of syphilis; fortunately. *Treponema pallidum* has never developed resistance to this antibiotic. However, too many people falsely believe that a "shot of penicillin" provides an instant cure. It is not this easy; all penicillins are not the same and doctors must adhere to the specific treatment recommendations established by the U.S. Public Health Service if a cure is to be guaranteed. If you, your partner, or your baby have been diagnosed as having syphilis, be sure your doctor follows the current treatment recommendations of the U.S. Public Health Service. Fortunately, all forms of penicillin are safe to take during pregnancy.

How is syphilis treated if a person is allergic to penicillin?

From 0.3 to 1 percent of the population is allergic to penicillin, with life-threatening reactions occurring 1 to 3 times per 1,000 individuals treated. Tetracycline and erythromycin offer effective alternative treatment for men and nonpregnant women, but tetracycline should never be prescribed for pregnant women or infants because it may cause damage to the bones of the fetus and bluish discoloration of the permanent teeth. Erythromycin, however, is safe for mother and fetus, although its efficacy in the fetus is not well established. It may be taken as erythromycin stearate, erythromycin ethylsuccinate, or erythromycin base; erythromycin estolate should not be prescribed because it may be potentially harmful to the pregnant woman and her fetus.

Gonorrhea

What causes gonorrhea and what are its symptoms in a woman?

Gonorrhea is caused by a bacterium called a gonococcus with the scientific name *Neisseria gonorrhoeae*. While syphilis is caused by a spiral-shaped bacterium, the organism responsible for gonorrhea is described as a diplococcus because it is present in pairs (diplo) and is round in shape (coccus) when viewed under the microscope. Rapid microscopic identification is made possible with use of a special dye-staining technique called a Gram stain.

In the United States, gonorrhea remains the most frequently reported of all contagious diseases, over one million new cases each year. Despite the availability of a variety of antibiotics, the disease has reached epidemic proportions over the last twenty years.

One of the problems in controlling the spread of gonorrhea is the fact that an estimated 30 to 70 percent of men harboring the disease are totally without symptoms, yet these so-called asymptomatic carriers are capable of transmitting the infection to a susceptible woman, and in one study of a group of men with gonorrhea it was found that the one-third with signs of the disease nevertheless denied the symptoms and continued to transmit their infection. The problem of the asymptomatic carrier is even greater among women: perhaps 80 percent of all those who have contracted the disease. The initial site of infection is practically always the inner lining of the cervix, with the urethra often involved as well. (Interestingly, the vaginal walls are totally resistant to gonorrheal infection.) Symptoms include a purulent discharge from the cervix combined with frequency and discomfort in urination. A yellowish discharge and inflammation may occur in the glands near the urethral opening and those located on either side of the vaginal opening. From its primary location within the cervix, the gonococcus will move along the surface of the endometrium and pass into the fallopian tubes. Here it is capable of causing severe infection and permanent damage and distortion. If the infection remains untreated, pus will pass out through the ends of the fallopian tubes and into the abdominal cavity, causing acute pelvic inflammatory disease (PID). Symptoms of PID are fever and severe lower abdominal pain. The presence of upper abdominal pain usually indicates further spread of the infection. Often, the tube and ovary will become matted together in an inflammatory mass called a tubo-ovarian abscess. Spontaneous intra-abdominal rupture of a tubo-ovarian abscess is a life-threatening medical emergency which usually requires immediate surgical removal.

Following the acute phase of gonorrhea, chronic flare-ups of infection may occur from time to time over a period of years. This stage is called chronic PID. The bacteria involved in these infections are usually not the gonococcus which initiated the problem; instead, they are organisms which thrive in tissues damaged by previous infection. Women suffering from chronic PID are often in pain caused by the presence of adhesions, or abnormal attachments of scar tissue, between the intestines and the pelvic organs. Hysterectomy with removal of the fallopian tubes and ovaries usually offers the only permanent cure.

In healthy women, fertilization normally occurs in the outer third of the fallopian tube. The fertilized egg then passes downward into the endometrium (lining of the uterus) where it attaches and grows. But scarring from gonorrheal infections may completely block the fallopian tubes and prevent fertilization of the egg by the sperm. If the tube is only partially blocked, the sperm may be able to reach the egg but the tubal scarring may then prevent the rapid passage of the fertilized egg in its destination to the endometrium. This results in a significantly greater danger of an ectopic pregnancy within the fallopian tube among women with a previous history of gonorrhea.

The gonococcus may also enter the bloodstream and be transported to distant locations. The large joints of the body, such as the knees, ankles, and wrists, are the most common sites for so-called gonococcal arthritis to occur. Symptoms of this condition are tenderness, swelling, and redness of the joint accompanied by fever. In addition, a nonspecific skin rash may develop in any location on the body. Though extremely rare, gonorrhea has been known to cause myocarditis (inflammation of the heart muscle), pericarditis (inflammation of the membrane enclosing the heart), and endocarditis (inflammation of the tissue lining the inner surface of the heart). In addition, uveitis (inflammation of the iris of the eye), meningitis (inflammation of the membrane surrounding the spinal cord and brain), perihepatitis (inflammation around the liver), liver abscesses, glomerulonephritis (kidney inflammation), myositis (muscle inflammation), pneumonia, and osteomyelitis (inflammation of the bone) have all been reported.

An increasingly recognized form of gonorrhea is pharyngitis, or sore throat, which occurs two to three days following fellatio with an infected male. The area in the back of the throat, especially around the tonsils, is extremely likely to harbor the gonococcus. In addition to the sore throat, redness of the tonsillar area and enlargement of the lymph nodes under the jaw may be noted. Gonorrheal proctitis is an inflammation of the anus and rectum which may occur following anal intercourse with an infected male.

What are the effects of gonorrhea during pregnancy?

A plug of mucus which forms within the inner lining of the cervix, called the endocervix, prevents the ascent of *Neisseria gonorrhoeae* into the uterine cavity and tubes of pregnant women. For this reason, acute pelvic inflammatory disease caused by gonorrhea is practically unheard of during pregnancy. Instead, the bacteria stay quietly within the endocervix until the time of delivery, when the protective mucous plug is lost. They can then pass through the cervix to infect the tubes. If symptoms of pelvic pain, fever, and a purulent discharge from the vagina occur one week to ten days following delivery, the diagnosis of pelvic infection caused by gonorrhea is a strong possibility.

Two different bacteriological studies have demonstrated that women with positive cervical cultures for gonorrhea during pregnancy have a higher incidence of prematurely ruptured amniotic membranes with inflammation and the onset of premature labor.

How is gonorrhea diagnosed in the pregnant woman?

Women usually have many harmless bacteria in the vagina, cervix, and urethra. Therefore, the Gram stain diagnosis is likely to be inaccurate, and treatment should not be initiated solely on the results of this test. The only definite proof of gonorrhea in a woman is a positive Thayer-Martin culture and sugar fermentation test.

Gonorrhea in the pregnant woman may be diagnosed by taking an endocervical culture without fear of harming the pregnancy. Many doctors and obstetrical clinics perform routine endocervical cultures on all women during their first prenatal visit and again in the weeks before delivery. A negative culture at the end of pregnancy is a reassuring sign that the baby will not be infected with gonorrhea as it passes through the birth canal. When gonorrheal pharyngitis or proctitis is suggested, the diagnosis can be confirmed by cultures taken from the involved areas.

What is the Gonosticon Dri-Dot test and what are its limitations?

The Gonosticon Dri-Dot is the first blood test to be developed which is capable of detecting gonococcal antibodies. Manufactured by Organon, Incorporated, it was released for nationwide distribution in 1980.

The Dri-Dot is a useful and rapid screening test for alerting a doctor that a possible gonorrhea infection may be present in a patient who does not have a history of the disease. It is easily performed in a doctor's office and is of great help in determining which patients should then undergo cultures to confirm the presence or absence of active gonorrhea. However, the test has definite limitations. While it identifies individuals with antibodies, it does not prove the presence or absence of current gonococcal infection, and individuals with a positive test may have developed these antibodies as a result of an infection years earlier. For this reason, the Dri-Dot must never be used as a substitute for a culture since the latter is the only accurate method of detecting an active infection. In addition, a false negative blood test may occur in patients who have had gonorrhea too recently for detectable antibody levels to develop.

What is the recommended treatment for gonorrhea during pregnancy?

While penicillin remains the drug of choice for most patients with gonorrhea, infectious disease experts have expressed great concern about the growing resistance of certain strains of *Neisseria gonorrhoeae* to this antibiotic. These resistant strains, which originated in the Far East but are now found throughout the United States, produce enzymes which have the ability to destroy penicillin, as well as ampicillin,

Table 5–1. Gonorrhea Treatment Schedule

Gonorrhea in Pregnancy	Probenecid: 1 gm orally followed with APPG: 4.8 million units intramuscularly divided into 2 doses and injected in each buttock at one visit.	Ampicillin: 3.5 gm or amoxicillin: 3.0 gm orally, either given with 1 gm probenecid by mouth.	For women allergic to penicillin or probenecid: Spectinomycin hydrochloride; 2 gm intramuscularly in one injection. Safety for the fetus has not been established with this drug. or Erythromycin: succinate stearate or base: 0.5 gm orally four times daily for 5 days. Erythromycin is only about 70 to 75 percent effective, but is at least considered safe for use in pregnancy by the FDA.	The tetracyclines are not recommended in pregnancy or in nursing mothers because of potential adverse effects to the fetus, the newborn, and the pregnant woman.

amoxicillin, and tetracycline. For this reason, the U.S. Public Health Service is constantly changing and updating its recommended treatment schedules for this disease. The amount of penicillin needed to cure an uncomplicated case of gonorrhea is approximately eight times greater now than it was fifteen years ago. Obviously, if your doctor is following an old treatment protocol, the dosage you receive may be less than adequate (see table 5–1).

The use of penicillin, ampicillin, and amoxicillin combined with probenecid has proven to be safe for both mother and fetus. The dose is identical for pregnant and nonpregnant women. Tetracyclines should not be used during pregnancy. If a woman is allergic to penicillin, intramuscular spectinomycin is safe and effective. While some doctors have used oral erythromycin instead of spectinomycin for the penicillin-allergic pregnant woman, it is not recommended because investigators have noted a treatment failure rate as high as 25 percent.

If laboratory tests confirm the presence of strains of gonorrhea resistant to penicillin, ampicillin and amoxicillin, spectinomycin is considered the treatment of choice. A new antibiotic named cefoxitin (trade name Mefoxin) combined with probenecid has been found to be equally as effective against these mutant bacteria. Fortunately, both of these antibiotics can be safely used during pregnancy.

How should gonorrheal pharyngitis be treated?

Gonococcal infections of the pharynx will usually respond to the same dose of antibiotic that is used for uncomplicated gonococcal infections. If ampicillin is used, however, it is best to take an additional 500 milligrams orally, four times daily for two days. A pregnant woman who is allergic to penicillin and ampicillin may safely take oral erythromycin in a dose of 500 milligrams four times daily over a period of five days.

What are the effects of maternal gonorrhea on the newborn?

If gonorrhea is present within the mother's endocervix at the time of delivery, the eyes of the newborn will be exposed to the organism while the baby is passing through the birth canal. This may result in severe inflammation and scarring of the cornea, called ophthalmia neonatorum. If not treated promptly, permanent blindness may result. The early symptoms of a gonorrheal eye infection usually appear two to three days following delivery and consist of swelling and inflammation of the eyelids a cloudy appearance of the cornea, and a yellowish discharge from both eyes.

A syndrome recently noted among these newborns is an infection of the upper respiratory tract and throat. This is caused by the infant's swallowing infected cervical secretions in its passage through the birth canal during labor. Treatment with penicillin cures this condition.

Is the routine procedure of giving eye drops to newborns to prevent gonorrheal eye infections recommended?

The most popular form of eye drops given to prevent gonorrheal eye infections is 1 percent silver nitrate drops applied to the eyes just after birth. Many respected physicians question the benefits of routine eye prophylaxis, arguing that silver nitrate too often causes a chemical irritation on the inner membrane of the eyelid, called chemical conjunctivitis. Another argument is that drops can mask a serious eye infection caused by chlamydia which may be present. Under such conditions, the onset of the infection will be delayed until several weeks after the baby has left the hospital and is no longer under the close supervision of the pediatrician. Finally, the method is not infallible since 1 percent of infected babies still develop gonorrheal eye infections even if the drops are given.

Only ten states presently have legislation requiring that prophylactic eye treatment be given to all newborns in order to prevent gonorrheal eye infections. Despite this, all newborns are treated with a 1 percent silver nitrate solution, as a routine procedure in almost 100 percent of hospitals in this country. Alternative treatment is erythromycin or tetracycline eye drops; the once popular use of penicillin is rare now since its use may sensitize a newborn and eventually cause an allergy to the drug at a later date.

If an infant is born to a mother with gonorrhea, that baby is at high risk of infection and requires immediate treatment with a single intravenous or intramuscular injection of aqueous crystalline penicillin G. Eye drops should be used, but never as the sole treatment for these infants.

If a newborn contracts gonorrheal eye infection, immediate isolation is indicated since these infections are highly contagious. Aqueous crystalline penicillin G should be given and eyes should be irrigated with a dilute saline, or salt, solution.

Silver nitrate, penicillin, or erythromycin eye drops are of no benefit at this stage of the disease.

PGU and NGU

What is PGU?

PGU stands for postgonococcal urethritis, the presence of a urethral discharge in a man following successful treatment of his gonorrhea with antibiotics. Cultures taken of this discharge are negative for *Neisseria gonorrhoeae.*

Until recently, doctors could not understand why some men developed PGU while others did not, though it was known that it could be cured with tetracycline. Bacteriologists now believe that men treated for gonorrhea who later develop PGU actually harbor other bacteria in the urethra in addition to gonorrhea. These bacteria are resistant to penicillin treatment and have the potential to cause urethritis in the absence of gonorrhea. Researchers have determined that the organisms which cause PGU are also responsible for the worldwide epidemic of NGU.

What is NGU?

NGU stands for nongonococcal urethritis, or urethral inflammation in a man caused by organisms other than *Neisseria gonorrhoeae.* Although many bacteria have been suggested as possible causes of NGU, at the present time only one, *Chlamydia* (pronounced *clam-ID-ia*) *trachomatis,* has been definitely incriminated. Organisms called mycoplasmas have been implicated as another cause of NGU, though the relationship is not as firmly established.

Can a man with NGU transmit the infection to his sexual partner?

Yes. NGU is the most common sexually transmitted condition affecting males; probably more than 3 million cases occurred in the United States in 1981. Chlamydia is easily transmitted from the urethra of a man to the cervix and vagina of a woman during coitus. Most women harboring the organism in the vagina and cervix are completely without symptoms and enjoy good health. However, more than half the women excreting *Chlamydia trachomatis* in the urethra experience symptoms such as burning on urination and urinary frequency. In recent years, epidemiologists have become concerned that some female contacts of men with chlamydial NGU can develop an inflammation of the Bartholin glands at the vaginal opening, cervicitis (inflammation of the cervix), salpingitis (inflammation of the fallopian tubes), and pelvic inflammatory disease. Chlamydia may also increase a woman's risk of amniotic fluid infections, premature labor, and stillbirths.

How does chlamydia affect newborn babies?

It has been estimated that 4 percent of women attending prenatal clinics will have cultures which are positive for *Chlamydia trachomatis.* Infants born to women infected with this organism may acquire chlamydia while passing through the birth canal during labor. The symptom most commonly apparent is a characteristic eye infection called congenital inclusion conjunctivitis. While the exact risk of an infant's contracting inclusion conjunctivitis from its mother has never been accurately determined, most authorities believe it is somewhere between 40 and 70 percent. If this is so, over 50,000 babies get this disease each year in the United States.

Symptoms of conjunctivitis, such as eye redness and discharge, usually do not appear until the second or third week of life. (This is unlike the eye infection caused by gonorrhea, which is far more destructive and produces symptoms during the week following delivery.) Chlamydial inclusion conjunctivitis responds to treatment with sulfa or tetracycline eye ointment over a period of two to three weeks, though some authorities consider oral erythromycin preferable. Silver nitrate drops, so useful in the prevention of gonorrheal eye infections, are of no help in preventing chlamydial inclusion conjunctivitis. Unlike gonorrhea conjunctivitis, it usually heals without producing residual scarring or blindness.

In addition to conjunctivitis, *Chlamydia trachomatis* may also cause pneumonia and infections of the middle ear, nose, and throat of the newborn. Authorities estimate that approximately half of all babies with conjunctivitis, or at least 25,000 infants per year, will develop chlamydial pneumonia. Other reported problems include poor weight gain and stomach and intestinal infections.

How do mycoplasmas affect pregnancy?

Though the mycoplasmas have been blamed for a variety of complications in pregnancy, there are no large, carefully controlled studies which support such a relationship. It is known that the organisms may cause endometritis, or inflammation of the lining of the uterus, and from this site may even enter the bloodstream. In addition, mycoplasmas have been isolated from the bloodstream, amniotic fluid, and placenta of patients with fever following abortion and full-term delivery, but the association between genital mycoplasma infections and habitual spontaneous abortion has not been adequately demonstrated.

What is the correct treatment for chlamydia and mycoplasma infections?

Tetracycline is the drug of choice for NGU caused by chlamydia or mycoplasmas, although the ideal dose and duration of therapy has never been established. Since tetracyclines should not be used during pregnancy, erythromycin may be substituted for fourteen days as treatment for chlamydia and infections caused by the mycoplasma named *Ureaplasma urealyticum.* The other mycoplasma, named *Mycoplasma hominis,* is resistant to erythromycin, and in these cases the antibiotics kanamycin, gentamicin, and spectinomycin may be used. Infected partners must also be treated at the same time in order to prevent reinfection.

Herpes

What is herpes?

Genital herpes was the most common sexually transmitted condition diagnosed by American physicians in private practice in 1982; probably 5 million to 20 million

Americans have it. Amazingly, textbooks of gynecology published ten years ago rarely if ever mention this disease, which now claims an estimated 500,000 new victims each year.

Herpes is one of a group of viruses, called DNA viruses, which can be transmitted from person to person through sexual and nonsexual contact. Members of this group include the herpes simplex virus Type I (also known as HSV-I); herpes simplex virus Type II (also known as HSV-II); cytomegalovirus, or CMV; the EB or Epstein-Barr virus, which causes infectious mononucleosis, or mono; varicella-herpes zoster, which causes chicken pox; and a nonvenereal disease called herpes zoster.

HSV-I is officially named *Herpesvirus hominis,* Type I, and is known to cause so-called oral herpes, fever blisters and canker sores of the mouth and lips. Until recently, researchers believed that HSV-I could only be found "above the waist" and was not sexually transmitted because it most commonly occurs in young children. However, ample evidence now suggests that a significant number of sexually active men and women contract HSV-I in the genital and rectal area through oral-genital and oral-anal contact.

HSV-II, or *Herpesvirus hominis,* Type II, is usually transmitted to the genital area through sexual intercourse, but it has frequently been cultured from the mouth and lips of individuals engaged in oral-genital contact with an infected partner.

The DNA viruses as a group have been called "the viruses of love." A perfect example of this is the Epstein-Barr virus, the cause of infectious mononucleosis, known also as the "kissing disease," since kissing is believed to be its most usual mode of transmission. Cytomegalovirus is known to be transmitted via sexual intercourse.

Though chicken pox and herpes zoster are not transmitted through sexual intercourse, close contact with an infected individual is still necessary for transmission of the virus.

What symptoms does a woman experience during her first genital attack of HSV-II virus?

Following intercourse with an infected male, there is usually an incubation period of three to seven days, though there are reports that this period may be as short as twenty-four hours and as long as twelve days. The virus first forms a small, almost undetectable blister on the skin of the external genitals. One of these small blisters may contain millions of viruses which multiply and produce new blisters. Early in the course of this primary infection, symptoms are often very mild and a woman may notice only a slight itch or mild irritation. At this stage, it is not uncommon to misdiagnose the condition as moniliasis, or yeast infection.

The external genitals soon become covered with extremely painful blistering sores, often accompanied by swelling of the entire genital area. Often, these individual sores coalesce, or come together, to form larger sores which, after about twenty-four to forty-eight hours, break down into open, shallow, painful, grayish ulcers. The disease is now at its most highly contagious stage. Within five days after the ulcers begin to form, the pain finally starts to lessen.

In addition to its attack on the external genitals, HSV-II often invades the vagina and cervix, where it may produce a profuse, irritating, watery discharge. The urinary duct leading to the bladder is particularly vulnerable. The virus produces blisters and ulcers in the urethral lining which cause intense burning on urination. This pain is intensified when urine comes in contact with the sores on the outer vaginal area. Occasionally, the pain on urination is so severe that a woman will retain urine rather than void, requiring insertion of a urinary catheter in order to relieve her discomfort.

The acute stage of the disease may be accompanied by chills, low-grade fever, headache, painful enlargement of the lymph nodes in the groin called inguinal nodes, and a dull aching pain in both legs, accompanied by a general feeling of fatigue.

Spontaneous healing of the skin ulcers usually begins about ten days after the first appearance of the disease and is usually complete without evidence of scarring in three to six weeks. On rare occasions, a secondary bacterial infection at the site of the ulcers not only delays the healing process but may cause permanent scarring.

For the more fortunate, the primary attack represents their one and only episode of herpes. However, approximately one-third to two-thirds experience reappearance of the disease at a later time. It is theorized that in these unlucky individuals the virus travels from the infected areas on the skin to several of the nerves just below the skin surface and from this location migrates up the nerves to the central nerve cells located near the lower part of the spinal cord, where it remains in a latent state for variable periods of time. When the virus becomes reactivated, it begins to multiply within the nerve cells and retraces its path down the nerve to the genital skin area supplied by that particular nerve. This causes a recurrence of the herpes blisters on the skin surface. Unlike the first infection, which may involve the entire genital area, recurrences usually appear as single blisters or a small group of blisters, and usually in the same location they appeared before, since the virus migrates up and down the same nerve each time.

The first recurrence will usually take place within eight weeks after the primary infection has completely healed, but there have been several reports of the first recurrence taking place as late as two years or more after the primary infection. The frequency of recurrences varies, ranging from as often as every two weeks to as infrequently as every few years. The most usual pattern of recurrences is four to five during the first year, two or three the following year, and spontaneous disappearance of all recurrences during or after the third year, although there are many individuals who suffer from recurrences throughout their lifetime. Unlike the primary infection, the blisters of the recurrent attacks heal completely within ten days of their onset.

What causes herpes to reoccur?

It is not known what triggers the sudden reactivation of the virus, but it is unrelated to sexual activity. Factors reported capable of triggering recurrences in a susceptible individual include other illnesses, fatigue, lack of sleep, emotional trauma, fever, change of climate, excessive exposure to sunlight, menstruation, and premenstrual tension. When recurrences do follow sexual intercourse, they are usually due to direct trauma and irritation to the genital area, as might occur with a penis, douche, or vibrator, rather than to the reintroduction of the virus to the skin via one's infected sexual partner.

How is herpesvirus diagnosed?

There are several available laboratory tests for diagnosing a herpesvirus infection with certainty. The Tsanck test is a simple procedure which any doctor can perform. It consists of scraping the material from an ulcer or blister, placing it on a glass slide, staining it and viewing it under the microscope. Though the herpes virus is too small to view under the ordinary microscope, it does produce a characteristic reaction in the infected cells which is easily seen microscopically. This reaction consists of minute substances in the nucleus or center of the infected cells, appropriately named intranuclear inclusions. In addition, the presence of large inflammatory cells, named multinucleated giant cells, helps to confirm the diagnosis of herpes. Though viruses may be viewed under electron microscope, this expensive instrument is available in very few laboratories.

If a glass slide containing material from a herpes blister is treated with a fluorescent antibody specific against herpes, a detectable reaction can be noted and the diagnosis thereby confirmed. However, the most reliable diagnostic test for HSV-I or HSV-II is a culture of the lesion. Growth of HSV-I and HSV-II on the culture medium is detected by the presence of characteristic pockmarks within forty-eight hours. HSV-I can occasionally be differentiated from HSV-II because it produces a smaller pockmark. For maximum yield of positive cultures, it is best to obtain them within forty-eight hours after the lesions appear.

If a doctor has nothing else available, the Pap smear may be used to detect the characteristic intranuclear inclusions and multinucleated giant cells. While the Pap smear has the advantage of being readily available and inexpensive, it has a very high rate of false negative results compared to the culture technique and in situations such as the last month of pregnancy, the diagnosis of herpes is critical.

There are several blood tests available which measure the presence of antibodies to herpesvirus. Unfortunately, the test is performed by very few laboratories, and difficulties are often encountered in detecting HSV-II antibodies among individuals with prior HSV-I infections. It usually takes from one to four weeks following an infection for a person to develop herpes antibodies. Therefore, if an antibody blood test is to be used for the diagnosis, it is important to do the initial test at the first sign of infection. If antibodies are present at this time, it means that the person being tested has had previous herpes exposure. However, when the initial blood test is negative for herpes antibodies, but a convalescent serum obtained two to four weeks later is positive, it is considered proof that a primary herpes infection has occurred.

What is the recommended treatment for herpes?

There is no known cure for a genital herpes infection. Topical solutions applied to blisters are incapable of permanently curing the disease, since the virus lives in its inactivated form in the nerves deep below the skin surface. However, several agents have been tried with some success in bringing symptomatic relief and, in some cases, shortening the time that the lesions remain on the skin, among them alcohol and ether applications, Betadine, idoxuridine, adenine arabinoside, zinc, 2-deoxy-d-glucose, nonoxynol-9, and adenosine monophosphate. Other purported remedies include the amino acid lysine taken orally and a variety of intramuscular vaccines. When all local remedies for recurrent herpes fail, some doctors recommend surgical removal of the blisters under local anesthesia. Laser treatment also has its enthusiastic supporters.

To date, the most promising therapy for genital herpes has been an antiviral agent named acyclovir (trade name Zovirax). Available as an ointment, it is applied to the affected areas every three hours six times per day for seven days. Best results are obtained if treatment is started within eight hours after the blisters first appear.

Acyclovir works by mimicking another substance that the herpesvirus needs to reproduce. Once the virus is fooled in taking it in, however, acyclovir provides the wrong compound for growth and reproduction of the cells. As a result, the virus is unable to reproduce.

In clinical trials, acyclovir has been shown to decrease the healing time and the duration of viral shedding among a significant number of women suffering from primary herpes. In contrast, there is no convincing evidence that it will benefit a woman with recurrent disease. With continued use, the herpesvirus tends to develop resistance to acyclovir treatment.

The safety of acyclovir during pregnancy is unknown at the present time, though moderate doses given to rats, mice, and rabbits have produced no harmful effects. When exceedingly high doses are given, however, the drug appears to hinder the fertilized egg from attaching to the uterine lining at the onset of pregnancy. It is not yet known whether acyclovir is excreted in breast milk.

What can a woman do to relieve the intense pain of primary herpes?

Knowing that the acute attack is self-limited is of little consolation to the individual suffering from genital herpes. Mild analgesics, such as aspirin and Tylenol, are worthless, and if relief of pain is to be achieved, it is best to use narcotic preparations such as codeine or Demerol. Compresses of cool Burow's solution will relieve discomfort. Cold applications of potassium permanganate in a dilution of 1 to 8,000 or 1 to 12,000 is an old and effective remedy for relieving symptoms. Several applications a day may be used. The one drawback of this treatment is that it permanently soils linens and undergarments. The intense pain on urination can be alleviated if cold water is gently poured on the perineum during urination. Urinating from a standing position is helpful in directing the flow away from the ulcers on the labia. Though many doctors suggest that patients urinate while taking a hot tub bath, I discourage my patients from doing this during the acute stage of genital herpes. Prolonged and frequent soaking tends to cause maceration of the normal skin. In the presence of herpes, it has been demonstrated that new lesions may develop on the macerated area along with local spread of the infection.

Ice cubes wrapped in a pack or towel will afford relief when applied continuously to the perineum for ninety minutes at a time. This is an easy home remedy which will relieve symptoms of both primary and recurrent herpes. Some research even suggests that this form of cryo or cold therapy will also hasten the healing of the blisters.

It is important to keep the sores as clean and as dry as possible in order to prevent a secondary bacterial infection. This can be accomplished by taking a hot sitz bath no more often than twice a day. The sores can be gently washed with a germicidal soap such as Betadine. It is best to dab dry the vulva rather than rub a towel along the skin surface. Use of a hair dryer is a great way to keep the lesions dry without irritating the skin or spreading the infection. Women should wear only clean cotton underwear and avoid nylon underwear or pantyhose since these tend to trap moisture and prevent air circulation.

Healing of the blisters has been shown to be prolonged if they are covered with creams or ointments. However, if the sores around the urethral opening are irritated by urination, application of a thin layer of xylocaine anesthetic ointment may be helpful in relieving symptoms.

Are pregnant women more susceptible to genital herpes infections that nonpregnant women?

Yes. Epidemiologists believe that the pregnant woman is at least three times more susceptible to genital herpes infections than her nonpregnant sister. Though one out of three pregnant women infected with herpes have no visible external sores, when symptoms are present during pregnancy they tend to be more severe and persist for longer periods of time.

What effect does genital herpes have on early pregnancy?

If a woman experiences a recurrence of an old genital herpes infection during the first half of her pregnancy, she can be assured that the fetus is not at risk of developing an infection or a congenital birth defect at that time. Mothers with a previous history of herpes usually have the antibody IgG in their bloodstream, which is small enough to be transferred across the placenta to the fetus during pregnancy. The levels of IgG in the fetus are equal to those of the mother at birth and disappear from the newborn's circulation by the end of the third month of life. It is important to remember, however, that IgG antibodies offer a fetus little if any protection from herpes acquired when passing through an infected birth canal at the time of delivery.

If a woman contracts a primary or initial genital herpes infection during the first twenty weeks of her pregnancy, she is more apt to experience a spontaneous abortion. TORCH is an acronym for a group of diseases—toxoplasmosis, rubella, cytomegalovirus, and herpes—which are capable of causing similar damage to a fetus when its mother is first infected early in pregnancy. TORCH organisms have been associated with an increased risk of spontaneous abortion, stillbirth, prematurity, and low birth weight, and the newborn may be affected by lethargy, poor feeding, blood coagulation defects, enlargement of the liver and spleen, calcifications of the liver, jaundice, anemia, pneumonia, skin rash, myocarditis (inflammation of the muscle of the heart), cataracts, chorioretinitis (inflammation of the retina and surrounding layer in the eye), and nervous system diseases such as encephalitis, microcephaly (abnormally small head), hydrocephaly (abnormally large head), mental retardation, and calcifications within the skull. But unlike the recommendation for fetuses exposed to rubella, toxoplasmosis, and cytomegalovirus early in pregnancy, most epidemiologists believe that the risk to a fetus exposed to herpes is too low to warrant therapeutic abortion.

What problems may be encountered if a woman has genital herpes during the second half of pregnancy?

If a woman acquires a primary herpes infection after the twentieth week of pregnancy, it has been estimated that she has a 35 percent chance of delivering prematurely and losing her child. Women with chronic recurrent infections are not at this higher risk of giving birth to a premature baby.

Though there are cases in the medical literature of herpesvirus transmission from a mother to her baby via the placenta during the second half of pregnancy, this is extremely rare. Infection of the newborn, in practically all cases, occurs when the infant comes in contact with the virus from the mother's cervix, vagina, or vulva during labor. The amniotic membrane provides the baby with great protection. However, if the membrane ruptures before or during labor, the virus can easily ascend through the cervix and infect the unborn infant within four to six hours.

At least 1,000 babies die each year in the United States as a result of genital herpes transmitted to them at birth by their infected mothers. The risk of a newborn acquiring the virus from an infected mother is about 50 percent. Of those babies who are infected, 60 to 90 percent will either die or develop a severe and permanent disability. HSV-II causes three-fourths of all newborn herpesvirus infections, and HSV-I is responsible for the remaining one-fourth. The severity of infection is equal regardless of which strain the infant contracts. The ability of a doctor to accurately diagnose maternal herpes is complicated by the fact that one-third of infected pregnant women have no externally visible lesions. A common misconception which must be dispelled is that a baby born of a mother having chronic herpes is somehow immune to the infection when the newborn comes in contact with the virus during childbirth. Nothing could be further from the truth! All babies, regardless of whether or not their mothers have primary or recurrent herpes, may become infected and die of herpes if they acquire the disease at this time.

What measures should be taken to protect babies from the damaging effects of herpes?

If a pregnant woman has never been infected with herpes, it is imperative that she avoid unprotected intercourse with a man who has even the slightest evidence of a blister suggestive of herpes. Coitus is probably safe if he wears a condom that completely covers the infectious site. Cold sores in the oral cavity often go unnoticed but, if detected in a man, the couple must avoid cunnilingus. Similarly, a woman with herpes of the mouth may become infected in the genital area after she passes it to the mouth or genitals of her lover. Susceptible pregnant women should avoid close contact with children who may have contracted herpes.

When a woman with visible herpes lesions of the genitals is in labor, the baby can be saved from the dangers of infection if cesarean section is performed. In addition, in the presence of herpes blisters, if the amniotic membrane is ruptured for less than four hours, an immediate cesarean section will usually prevent an ascending infection from passing from the vagina and cervix to the baby. Authorities on this subject doubt that a cesarean section will be preventive if the time from membrane rupture to surgery is greater than six hours. The diagnosis of genital herpes in a patient in labor is probably the only dermatological emergency that I know of. If the blisters are not typical of herpes and the diagnosis is in doubt, an obstetrician should seek immediate consultation from a dermatologist. Obviously, time does not allow for culturing of the virus, though scraping the blisters and looking for multinucleated giant cells and intranuclear inclusions is very helpful. If the diagnosis is still in doubt, cesarean section is preferred to the hazards of vaginal delivery which the infant would be subjected to if herpes is present.

Though at least one-third of women harboring genital herpes at the time of delivery have no symptoms, careful inquiry by a doctor will usually elicit a history of previous genital herpes. Even if the previous infection occurred several years before the present pregnancy, it is vital to remember that the virus may become activated and move down the nerve to the skin at any time. If there is even a remote history of recurrent genital herpes in either sexual partner, or if the man has recurrent oral herpes and has practiced cunnilingus, cultures must be taken from the cervix and vagina each week during the last month prior to the expected date of confinement. If any culture is positive, cesarean section must be performed before or at the onset of labor. Use of a Pap smear instead of the culture is inadequate and will miss at least half of all cases of asymptomatic genital herpes.

Fetal scalp monitors (see chapter 10) should not be used on women who are suspected of having genital herpes until the presence of active herpes infection has been positively ruled out. There are cases in the medical literature of babies contracting neonatal herpes in this manner.

Herpes in the newborn is highly contagious. Infants at even the slightest risk of carrying the infection must be isolated from other babies in the nursery and observed carefully for evidence of infection for two weeks. If the diagnosis of genital herpes is made with certainty in a mother immediately following a vaginal delivery, antiviral ointments should be immediately placed in the baby's eyes in order to prevent a serious infection. These babies should have viral cultures taken from their mouth, eyes, nose, throat, blood, urine, stool, and spinal fluid. As previously mentioned, IgG antibodies against herpes are transferred across the placenta from a mother to her fetus; their presence is no indication of an active infection in the baby. IgM antibodies, on the other hand, are antibodies produced by the fetus which are too large to pass across the placenta. Therefore, if they are found in the baby's umbilical cord blood at birth, they were produced by the infant in response to a specific infection. There are many laboratories which have the capacity to measure elevated IgM antibody levels specific for herpes.

One interesting observation: 10 percent of HSV-I infections occurring in newborns are not associated with a maternal source of contamination. This may mean that some of these infections are transmitted by delivery room and nursery employees.

Cancerous and Precancerous Diseases of the Cervix

Why is cancer of the cervix considered a venereal disease?

The most important single factor in squamous, or epidermoid cancer of the cervix, is intercourse at an early age. During puberty and the teenage years, the young girl's cervix undergoes marked hormonal changes which, for some unknown reason, make its microscopic cells vulnerable to abnormal transformation. The sexual revolution of the 1960s and 1970s has resulted in significantly more women having intercourse at a younger age. As a result, gynecologists have noted an epidemic among young women characterized by abnormal Pap smears and microscopic precancerous changes such as dysplasia and carcinoma in situ. A California study showed that women under twenty-five with carcinoma in situ made up only 30 percent of the total cervical cancer patients in 1951. However, in 1968 these women constituted 93 percent of the total.

How is cervical cancer diagnosed?

The Pap smear, named after its inventor, Dr. George Papanicolaou, and first introduced in the United States in 1943, is a painless, inexpensive screening test used mainly for the detection of cancer of the cervix. To obtain a Pap smear, a cotton applicator or a plastic or wooden spatula is rotated around and against the cervix, and the microscopic cells obtained are transferred to a glass slide, treated with a fixative and sent to a laboratory for examination for abnormal and cancerous cells. The degree of abnormality is then classified on a scale ranging from benign to malignant.

If a Pap smear is abnormal during pregnancy, what is the best method of evaluation and treatment?

Unfortunately, the problem of the abnormal Pap smear during pregnancy is inadequately managed in many areas of the United States. Physicians confronted with this dilemma usually repeat the Pap test with the unrealistic hope that it will revert to normal. Until recently, when the repeat smears remained abnormal, a cone biopsy was performed. This technique involves the removal of a large cone-shaped wedge of tissue from the cervix to determine if microscopic precancerous or cancerous changes were present. Though the cone biopsy technique has a diagnostic accuracy of at least 95 percent, it may cause serious complications for the pregnant woman, including hemorrhage, accidental rupture of the amniotic membranes with subsequent infection and abortion, and incompetent cervix with premature labor. These potential complications, anesthesia risk, and hospital expense can all be avoided by an office examination of the cervix with a low-powered microscope called a colposcope. A doctor skilled at this technique can easily and accurately detect abnormal areas on the cervix and obtain tiny biopsy samples without adversely affecting the outcome of pregnancy. For this reason, it is vital that you insist on colposcopy, rather than cone biopsy, as the initial method of evaluation if your Pap smear is abnormal at any time during pregnancy.

The development of cancer of the cervix evolves slowly over a period of years. Therefore, treatment of precancerous changes, such as dysplasia and carcinoma in situ, can be delayed until several weeks following delivery. Invasive cancer, though extremely rare, is an ominous disease which requires immediate treatment. It is imperative that a doctor determine with certainty that it is not present during pregnancy, since it spreads rapidly and is life-threatening. If invasive cancer is diagnosed during the first six months, it requires immediate treatment with radical hysterectomy or radiation without regard to the fetus. When invasive cancer is found during the third trimester, consideration should be given to the survival of the fetus. Delivery of the baby in the last two months of pregnancy is best accomplished by cesarean section, as soon as it is determined that the infant has a reasonable chance of survival. Radical surgery or radiation for the mother should begin immediately after delivery. Vaginal delivery of a baby through a cervix with invasive cancer will disseminate the disease and hasten the mother's demise.

CMV

What is cytomegalovirus (CMV), and how may it affect the outcome of pregnancy?

Cytomegalovirus, or CMV, is another member of the group of viruses called DNA viruses. Just as herpes has the ability to be transmitted from person to person through sexual and nonsexual contact, so can CMV. The incubation period is one to three months, and most adults who contract CMV are totally unaware that they harbor the infection. When symptoms do occur, they resemble those of infectious mononucleosis and include fatigue and generalized lymph node enlargement. Though few men and women have ever heard of this disease, it is probably the most important infectious cause of birth defects and mental retardation in the United States.

CMV is the most common infection transmitted by blood transfusion. However, that it may also be transmitted sexually is a relatively new finding. Convincing evidence demonstrates that the incidence of this infection increases after puberty as sexual activity increases. In one study the virus was found in the cervix of 29 percent of women attending a venereal disease clinic, compared with 2 percent of women examined in a general gynecology clinic. In addition, CMV has been isolated from the saliva, blood, urine, and semen of sexually active individuals. It is probably more easily transmitted than any other venereal organism, since men and women who harbor it are without symptoms.

It has been estimated that as many as 10 to 15 percent of all women carry CMV in their cervix during pregnancy, and approximately 30,000 newborns each year excrete the virus at birth. Of these, approximately 10 percent have been found with significant evidence of disease. Abnormalities may not be readily apparent at birth in another 2,500 to 8,000 children who will later develop varying degrees of hearing, learning, and neurological disorders. Some researchers believe that CMV may be the leading cause of hearing loss in children in this country.

It is believed that the greatest risk of congenital birth defects caused by CMV occurs among those mothers who are first exposed to the virus just before conception or during the first four months of pregnancy. Congenital defects caused by cytomegalovirus can be varied and devastating, since it is one of the TORCH complex agents (see page 135). Infected newborns are often anemic and have a reduced number of platelets in their blood. Many will have purpura, a hemorrhagic skin rash due to a platelet deficiency. Enlargement of the liver and spleen and pneumonia are also commonly seen. The central nervous system appears to be most vulnerable to attack. Among infants showing symptoms at birth, 50 to 75 percent will be left with permanent and severe neurological disease such as microcephaly, seizures, deafness, blindness, and psychomotor disturbances. There is little doubt that many children are born with an infection that goes entirely unnoticed. These children may, however, constitute a proportion of those individuals who later develop perceptual disorders, learning disabilities, behavior problems, and hearing loss. It can be safely predicted that infected infants who do not show evidence of neurological disease at two years of age are not likely to be significantly affected later in life.

The severity of disease in the newborn infant is dependent upon when in the pregnancy exposure to CMV takes place. Though the greatest damage will occur during first-trimester exposure, the more subtle disabilities are likely to occur when the virus attacks during the second trimester. A fetus is not even safe during the third trimester, since some may experience mild mental retardation, perceptual handicaps, and chronic infections with shedding of the virus. It is of some consolation to know that the damage inflicted by CMV during a mother's primary infection will hardly ever recur and cause damage in subsequent pregnancies, even though she may still have the virus in her body.

An infant may also contract CMV while passing through the infected cervix during labor. Although these babies usually do not develop clinical disease, they may shed the virus for twelve to eighteen months. There are also case reports in which the virus was transmitted to a baby through the breast milk of an infected mother.

How can CMV be prevented and treated?

There is no known medical treatment for cytomegalovirus infections, and since the disease in adults is totally asymptomatic there would be little reason for an otherwise healthy pregnant woman to suspect its existence. Routine culturing of the cervix for cytomegalovirus during the first trimester is not recommended, because the test is performed by very few laboratories. Furthermore, finding CMV does not necessarily help a doctor determine when the first exposure occurred in relation to the date of conception. If the cervical culture is positive for CMV during the first trimester, the only medical treatment that can be offered is a therapeutic abortion, which is most likely to be unnecessary. New blood tests for detecting CMV antibodies are being developed. When available, they should be helpful in identifying actively infected women.

To prevent CMV during pregnancy, one simple but vital precaution that a woman can take is to avoid contact with a new sexual partner when contemplating conception or during the first three months of pregnancy. This would include oral-genital sex, since the virus may be carried in the saliva of infected individuals.

Are there any specific vaccines or medications which can be used against CMV?

Not yet. Prophylactic use of an experimental CMV vaccine made from the weakened virus is now being tried in the United States, Japan, and England.

If a baby is suspected of having cytomegalovirus, how can the diagnosis be made with certainty?

The virus is most likely to be isolated from the baby's urine, though the saliva also contains CMV. Culture samples may take as long as six weeks to show a positive reaction. CMV can also be accurately diagnosed by examination of the urine under an electron microscope. Unfortunately, few laboratories have this expensive instrument or personnel skilled at interpreting the microscopic findings. A more rapid diagnostic method is a blood test which measures the presence of the large IgM (immunoglobin M) antibodies, which are specific against CMV. These antibodies are too large to cross the placenta. Therefore, their presence in the newborn's umbilical cord or bloodstream is significant because they are formed by the baby in response to acute infection.

The most recent advance in the detection of congenital cytomegalovirus has been the use of a quick screening test. For some strange reason, the rheumatoid factor test, available in most hospitals for the detection of rheumatoid arthritis, is also effective in identifying about 40 percent of those infants who are asymptomatic at birth and would otherwise not be detected until much later. One drop of blood from the umbilical cord or heel of the infant is all that is needed to run this simple and inexpensive test. Though a positive test does not necessarily prove that a baby has CMV, it does alert a physician to the possibility so that more definitive studies, such as a urine culture, can be performed.

GB-BHS   **What is GB-BHS, and how is it related to the outcome of pregnancy?**

GB-BHS stands for a bacterium named Group B-beta-hemolytic streptococcus. Though bacteriologists first identified this organism many years ago, it was not until the early 1960s that is was detected in the female urinary and genital tracts. Researchers at that time first reported that GB-BHS could be transmitted through sexual intercourse and was associated with a higher incidence of spontaneous abortion, stillbirth, prematurity, and infection of the newborn. Some bacteriologists believe that GB-BHS is a significant cause of infection and death among newborns. One authority estimates that 12,000 to 15,000 newborns develop streptococcal infections each year, and of these approximately 50 percent die. Though the infection is usually acquired by the baby at the time of labor and delivery, there are several reported cases of the organism's causing infection before the start of labor. This is believed to occur when bacteria enter through the usually protective mucus of the cervix during coitus. Of interest is the finding that the disease more frequently occurs in premature than full-term infants and has a 70 percent likelihood of being fatal in the former group compared to a 33 percent mortality rate among full-term babies.

Delay in diagnosis and treatment is the main reason for the high death rate among newborns infected with GB-BHS. The first sign of infection is usually rapid and labored breathing, which may be mistaken in its similarity to the more common respiratory distress syndrome (see chapter 11). Within hours, this may progress to an overwhelming and irreversible infection. If the bacteria invade the meninges, or covering of the brain and spinal cord, 50 percent of infected babies will be left with permanent neurological damage.

How can GB-BHS of the newborn be prevented?

Some authorities recommend that all pregnant women have cultures taken from the uterus, cervix, and vagina and that antibiotics be prescribed for all culture-positive individuals and their sexual partners. Others have just the opposite view; that cultures are unnecessary and treatment is incapable of completely eradicating the organism from the vagina and cervix. It has recently been demonstrated that a woman's intestinal tract may serve as a reservoir for the organism and the likely source of recurrent vaginal infection. GB-BHS appears to be especially resistant to treatment during pregnancy. It is also interesting to note that the organism, for unknown reasons, disappears from the genital tract without treatment in one-half of all women with positive cultures. Furthermore, though two-thirds of infants born of mothers with positive GB-BHS cultures also have positive cultures, actual infection and illness occurs in less than 1 percent of these newborns. For this reason, many pediatricians prefer to watch culture-positive infants closely and to treat only at the first sign of respiratory difficulty. The policies at most medical centers fall somewhere between these two extremes.

Listeriosis

What is *Listeria monocytogenes,* and how does it affect the outcome of pregnancy?

Listeria monocytogenes is a bacterium which, in the past ten years, has received an increasing amount of attention as a cause of poor pregnancy outcome. The many ways in which this organism may be transmitted are not yet understood; however, there is some evidence to suggest that sexual intercourse is probably one of them.

Recent reports suggest that pregnant women, especially those in the second or third trimesters, have an increased susceptibility to listeriosis. Accurate diagnosis is hindered because there are no specific symptoms which distinguish it from a viral infection or a flu-like illness. Infected women may develop fever, chills, muscle aches, and back pain. Others may experience no symptoms at all.

Maternal listeriosis may severely affect the fetus and newborn infant. There are controversial reports about whether or not listeriosis is responsible for repeated spontaneous abortion. Infected amniotic fluid may lead to premature labor and even fetal death. Some babies, considered healthy at birth, begin to show symptoms of fever, irritability, and poor feeding weeks later. Others may experience immediate and severe respiratory difficulty; hypothermia, or lowered body temperature; enlargement of the liver; circulatory disturbances; and occasionally a rash on the skin or an inflammation of the eyes. In rare cases, the infection may lead to meningitis and death.

How is listeriosis diagnosed and treated?

If doctors do not maintain a high degree of suspicion, the disease is rarely diagnosed. All pregnant women with fever or a flu-like illness and those with a history of repeated unexplained spontaneous abortion should have cultures taken from the vagina, cervix, and blood. *Listeria monocytogenes* grows readily in a culture medium and can be identified within forty-eight hours. Viewing the organism under the microscope, in the absence of cultures, is suggestive but not diagnostic of listeriosis. When the possibility of the disease exists in a newborn, cultures should be taken immediately after the birth from the baby's stomach and pharynx secretions, as well as the blood.

Listeriosis in both the mother and the newborn is easily treated with a variety of antibiotics, including penicillin, ampicillin, kanamycin, and gentamicin. When a baby contracts the infection immediately after birth, it is important to treat with antibiotics for at least three weeks if a recurrence and the late-onset type of infection is to be prevented.

Vaginitis

What causes vaginitis?

Volumes of misinformation have been written about the diagnosis and treatment of vaginitis. As a result, confusion exists as to how a woman contracts different types of vaginitis, what methods should be used to distinguish one type from another, and, most importantly, how each condition should be cured.

Three types of vaginitis may affect the young sexually active woman: trichomoniasis, moniliasis, and nonspecific vaginitis. The organisms are all microscopic. Trichomoniasis is caused by the protozoan *Trichomonas vaginalis,* moniliasis is caused by the yeast-like fungus *Candida albicans,* and nonspecific vaginitis may be caused by one of several bacteria, the most common being an organism named *Hemophilus vaginalis.*

How is trichomoniasis transmitted, and what are its symptoms?

Trichomoniasis, though harmless, is truly a venereal condition, which is transmitted through no other form of lovemaking but intercourse. Also known as "trich," it is by far the most common cause of vaginitis.

The incubation period is usually one to three weeks, and symptoms in a woman consist of a malodorous, bubbly, frothy, white, yellow, or green discharge, usually accompanied by irritation and itching. The vagina and cervix often are red and inflamed.

Though the old claim "I caught it on the toilet seat" does not hold true for most venereally transmitted conditions, it may on rare occasions happen with *Trichomonas vaginalis*. The organism is capable of surviving several hours at room temperature, particularly on moist surfaces, and the vulva and vagina can be contaminated with splashing toilet bowl water, teeming with *Trichomonas vaginalis*, at the time of defecation. The suggestion that women flush a public toilet and wipe the seat carefully before use is an excellent one.

How is the diagnosis of trichomoniasis confirmed, and what is the recommended treatment?

Though the protozoan can be grown in a culture medium, the easiest and quickest method of making the diagnosis is to take a sample of the discharge, add it to a drop of saline, and view it under the microscope. *Trichomonas vaginalis* has a characteristic appearance and can be seen moving in place with the help of its whiplike tail. Women who are embarrassed by the malodorous discharge frequently douche before their gynecological examination. Since douching may temporarily reduce the number of organisms present in the vagina and remove traces of the discharge which is so helpful in making the diagnosis, it is best not to douche for at least three days before the examination.

Metronidazole, more commonly known by its trade name Flagyl, is the only drug that is totally effective against *Trichomonas vaginalis*. All sexual partners must be treated simultaneously to prevent reinfection. Flagyl is not an innocuous drug and should not be casually or routinely prescribed whenever a person becomes reinfected with trichomoniasis. It is capable of decreasing the number of white blood cells which are necessary for fighting infections. Several animal research studies suggest that Flagyl may be carcinogenic, and it should not be taken by those on anticoagulant (blood-thinning) drugs since it can accentuate the effects of these medications and cause bleeding problems. The vast majority of patients tolerate treatment with few if any adverse reactions. If you do not want to take Flagyl, and such reservations are certainly understandable, daily douches with an acidic solution, such as two tablespoons of white vinegar in a quart of warm water, are often helpful in temporarily relieving symptoms, since the protozoan survives best when vaginal secretions are less acidic than normal.

Patients may develop moniliasis (see pages 146–148) following successful treatment of their trichomoniasis. This happens because the normal balance between organisms in the vagina may be disrupted when the "trich" is killed. If the foul-smelling, bubbly discharge of trichomoniasis is replaced by a whitish, sticky, and very itchy discharge which is not malodorous, the diagnosis of moniliasis is a certainty.

What are the effects of trichomoniasis on pregnancy, and how is the condition treated at this time?

Trichomoniasis is usually harmless to both the developing fetus and the newborn as it passes through the vagina during childbirth. Though Flagyl has been taken by hundreds of women during the first three months of pregnancy, without evidence of subsequent fetal abnormalities, it passes from the maternal to the fetal circulation in high concentrations and is approved for use only during the second and third trimesters. However, many obstetricians still refrain from prescribing it at any time during pregnancy, since it is not absolutely essential to a woman's health. If you are treated with Flagyl during the second and third trimester, it is best to use the seven-day regimen rather than the one-day method, since the latter results in higher blood levels reaching the fetal circulation.

Douching is dangerous during pregnancy and should not be used to treat the pregnant woman with trichomoniasis. Creams and vaginal suppositories, such as Vagisec, Sultrin, and AVC, are safe to use but rarely cure the condition or relieve symptoms. Clotrimazole (trade name Gyne-Lotrimin) is a medication that is useful in the treatment of moniliasis during pregnancy (see page 147). Some preliminary studies have suggested that seven days of therapy with clotrimazole cream or vaginal tablets will cure trichomoniasis 50 percent of the time. Until recently, Betadine gel was frequently used to treat vaginitis during pregnancy. However, it has been demonstrated that the iodine in this product rapidly passes through the engorged vaginal wall of the pregnant woman and enters her bloodstream. The high maternal iodine blood levels can then suppress fetal thyroid function and cause iodine-induced goiter and hypothyroidism in the fetus. For this reason, any vaginal disinfectant which contains iodine should not be used to treat vaginitis during pregnancy.

How can a nursing mother treat trichomoniasis?

The nursing woman with trichomoniasis can combine vaginal gels with douching. However, she should avoid Flagyl, since it is secreted in the breast milk in high concentrations, and no one has adequately studied the possible deleterious effects of this medication on the nursing infant. In a 1981 study, nursing women took a single 2-gram dose of Flagyl. Breast milk concentrations of the drug were then measured and found to be highest two to four hours later, followed by a decline over the next twelve to twenty-four hours. The authors of this report concluded that a nursing woman could take Flagyl in a single dose if she temporarily stopped nursing for twelve to twenty-four hours after the drug was taken.

What is moniliasis?

Moniliasis, or "yeast" vaginitis, is an extremely common infection caused by a microscopic fungus named *Candida albicans*. This organism, normally found in the vagina of approximately 30 percent of healthy women, causes symptoms of vaginitis only when it overgrows the other microorrganisms. Monilial vaginitis is characterized by a thick, white, creamy discharge, often resembling dry cottage cheese curd, and intense vulvar itching, swelling, and redness. Intercourse may be painful because of the accompanying vaginal dryness. Unlike trichomoniasis, the discharge of moniliasis is not malodorous.

Are some women more likely to contract moniliasis than others?

Moniliasis may develop whenever the normal microbe population of the vagina is disturbed. This can happen when one takes antibiotics, especially tetracyclines, since, in addition to treating infection, the antibiotics also kill off the usual bacterial inhabitants of the vagina, called Doderlein's bacilli, which maintain the normal pH and prevent a yeast overgrowth. An environment with high concentrations of sugar also favors the growth of *Candida albicans*. For this reason, diabetics are particularly susceptible to recurrent monilial infections, which can be a doctor's first clue that a woman may have diabetes or a prediabetic condition. The hormonal changes of pregnancy are responsible for a significant increase in the incidence of monilial infections. Emotional tension is considered to be a major predisposing factor, and most gynecologists note that this condition is more likely to occur repeatedly among women who live and work under a great deal of stress.

Monilial vaginitis is far more likely to occur when the weather is warm and moist. Women who douche often, take frequent tub baths for prolonged periods of time, wear pantyhose and tight noncotton undergarments, or sit around in wet bathing suits are likely candidates for moniliasis.

Is yeast vaginitis frequently transmitted sexually?

No. An individual susceptibility to the infection is a far more important factor than one's sexual habits, although oral-genital sex may predispose to recurrent monilial infections. Some men will experience redness and penile irritation following coitus with an infected woman.

What are the effects of moniliasis on the fetus and newborn?

Candida albicans in the mother will not affect the developing fetus. However, the baby may contract the infection in its passage through the birth canal during labor. When white patches of the organism are present in the newborn's mouth it is called thrush. The average interval for this to develop following birth is approximately eight days. A dermatitis or inflammation of the skin of the buttocks may also occur. Both conditions are harmless and easily treated. The rare reported cases of severe overwhelming *Candida albicans* infection and pneumonia in newborn infants occurred only in those babies who were already compromised by serious illness or another type of infection.

Is moniliasis common in pregnancy and how is it treated?

Moniliasis is one of the most common problems seen by obstetricians in pregnancy and is certainly the most common type of vaginitis.

The main problem encountered by the woman with genital moniliasis is intense vulvar itching. To relieve this symptom, especially if your pharmacy is closed for the day or you can't immediately reach your doctor, local applications of cool tap water, ice packs, or witch hazel compresses are all helpful. If itching is still not relieved, try a colloid bath: two cups of cornstarch plus one-half cup of baking soda in a tub half filled with warm water. Equally as good is Aveeno colloidal oatmeal added to a half-filled tub of water. This preparation can be purchased without prescription at any pharmacy, and it is an excellent idea to keep it in the house for possible emergencies.

One of the oldest, simplest, and least expensive methods of treating moniliasis is with boric acid capsules and ointment. Capsules containing 600 milligrams of boric acid are placed high in the vagina two times daily for two weeks, and 5 percent boric acid ointment is applied to the irritated areas on the vulva three times daily. In addition to this old but successful method, there is 2 percent micronazole sulfate vaginal cream. The highest cure rates are achieved with this medication. Sold under the trade name Monistat 7, an application of cream or a vaginal suppository is inserted daily for a period of one week. Symptomatic relief is rapid, often occurring within twenty-four to forty-eight hours. Then there is nystatin, an antifungal antibiotic sold as a vaginal tablet under the trade name Mycostatin. Cure rates, though excellent, are not equal to those of Monistat; it is however, considerably less expensive. A tablet is inserted high in the vagina, twice a day, for two weeks. More resistant cases will benefit if treatment is prolonged for a month. Mycostatin ointment and cream are also available for treatment of irritated areas on the outer skin surface of the vulva. If the infection is extensive or if there is reason to believe that the anus and rectum are a source of reinfection, oral Mycostatin tablets in a dose of 500,000 units per tablet should be taken three times daily for one week. Oral Mycostatin will eradicate *Candida albicans* from the mouth and intestinal tract, but, since it is not absorbed into the body, will be of no benefit in treating the vaginal infection. A liquid suspension of Mycostatin, when administered to each side of the newborn's mouth, four times daily, will cure thrush. The great advantage of Monistat and Mycostatin is that both may be used safely during pregnancy and nursing. Another successful agent against *Candida albicans* is clotrimazole. Under the trade name Gyne-Lotrimin, one of these vaginal tablets is inserted daily for seven days. Clotrimazole is also available as a cream which may be applied to the irritated areas of the vulva. While painting of the vulva and vagina with gentian violet preparations is an effective treatment and was quite popular in the past, most doctors now favor the newer medications as less messy to use and not as irritating to the body tissues.

What is nonspecific vaginitis, and how does it affect the outcome of pregnancy?

Nonspecific vaginitis is a sexually transmitted form of vaginitis, not caused by one specific type of bacteria. Anywhere from three to six organisms may be isolated from the vagina, the most common being *Hemophilus vaginalis,* also known as *Corynebacterium vaginale* and *Gardnerella vaginalis.* The most common symptom is vaginal malodor and a yellow-to-gray-green discharge which may be either thick or watery in consistency. Often the discharge is described as having the appearance of a thin paste. Itching or burning of the vagina and pain on urination are reported. The diagnosis is best made by viewing the bacteria under the microscope and taking a culture from a sample of the vaginal discharge.

The most successful treatment is Flagyl, the same medication used to treat trichomoniasis. Less favorable results have been obtained with ampicillin, tetracycline, and cephalosporin antibiotics. To prevent recurrences, all sexual partners must be treated simultaneously. Many doctors have combined oral antibiotics with sulfonamide vaginal creams such as AVC and Sultrin.

Fortunately, nonspecific vaginitis is harmless to both the developing fetus and the baby at the moment of birth. If a woman has this type of vaginitis during her pregnancy, treatment with ampicillin is recommended; use of Flagyl and tetracycline at this time is ill advised.

Genital Warts

What are genital warts, and how are they treated?

Genital warts, also known as *Condyloma acuminata*, are caused by a sexually transmitted virus which is similar to the virus which causes the common skin wart. The average incubation period is about three months, though it may range from six weeks to eight months. In women, the warts most commonly appear over the entire vulva and perineum, where they cause itching but no pain. Less common sites are the cervix and vagina where symptoms may be nonexistent. Some pathologists believe that the condyloma virus may be responsible for abnormal Pap smears and precancerous and cancerous changes of the cervix. The characteristic appearance of genital warts makes diagnosis easy. On rare occasions they may be mistaken for the lesions of secondary syphilis, but this can be simply resolved by a blood test for syphilis or a biopsy of the wart.

The most popular and successful treatment has been to paint the warts with a 25 percent solution of podophyllin in tincture of benzoin or alcohol. If treatment is successful the warts should disappear within two weeks. Quite often retreatment is necessary. Some doctors have reported excellent results with applications of trichloracetic acid and liquid nitrogen. Larger warts can be excised or cut out under local anesthesia, cauterized or burned, treated with cryosurgery or frozen, and most recently burned with a high energy light or laser. For difficult cases, vaccines from the substances of the warts have been used with variable success.

What happens to genital warts during pregnancy, and how are they treated at this time?

Genital warts tend to enlarge dramatically in pregnant women and then regress to their prepregnancy size following delivery. Occasionally, they become so massive that they may actually obstruct the birth canal and interfere with a normal vaginal delivery. No one knows the exact reason for the marked growth of venereal warts during pregnancy, but it has been theorized that the increased vulvar moisture, elevated estrogen levels, and the greater blood supply to the vulva and vagina all contribute to this phenomenon.

The main problem encountered in treating genital warts during pregnancy is that the use of podophyllin is not advisable. There are several reported cases of absorption of the chemical into the bloodstream, harmful both to the mother and fetus. Excision of warts is also difficult because of their large size and the greater risk of hemorrhage during surgery. Most doctors prefer not to treat them during pregnancy or will only excise the smaller warts during the first three months. Others cauterize all warts, regardless of size, at any time. Most warts, regardless of size, do not obstruct the birth canal. If they do, of course, cesarean section is indicated.

Until 1973, it was believed that an infant passing through a birth canal harboring *Condyloma acuminata* was in no danger of contracting the virus. Then, researchers noted a relationship between maternal warts and the development of benign growths, called papillomas, in the larynx or windpipe of some infants born of these women. If a relationship between maternal *Condyloma acuminata* and laryngeal papillomas is established, it is possible that in the future cesarean section for the woman who has genital warts at the time of delivery will be recommended.

Hepatitis

What is hepatitis and how can it be transmitted sexually?

Hepatitis is an inflammation of the liver. Bile pigments which are normally destroyed circulate in the blood, producing jaundice or yellowing of the skin and the whites of the eyes. While hepatitis may result from exposure to chemical or environmental agents, most cases are caused by one of three viruses, appropriately named hepatitis A virus, hepatitus B virus, and non-A and B virus. Hepatitis B is known as serum hepatitis, and for years it was believed to occur only in individuals who received blood transfusions from others with the disease or in drug-addicted persons using contaminated needles. However, as a result of recent studies epidemiologists now believe that hepatitis B is frequently transmitted sexually, while hepatitis A may follow a similar route on rare occasions.

The hepatitis B virus has a very long incubation period (two to six months), and while some individuals with the disease experience few if any symptoms, the majority are quite ill with jaundice, fever, extreme lethargy, loss of appetite, nausea, vomiting, and sometimes generalized body itching and joint pain. The urine is usually dark brown in color and the stools light-colored. About 90 percent of those who contract hepatitis B recover within a few weeks, but in approximately 2 percent the disease is fatal. Estimates vary, but perhaps one out of ten people who acquire hepatitis B remain long-term carriers.

How does hepatitis B affect pregnancy?

When acute hepatitis is contracted by a woman during pregnancy, she is more likely to experience spontaneous abortion, stillbirth, and premature labor. The virus may also pass from mother to fetus across the placenta and cases of neonatal hepatitis have been reported. The placenta may contain extensive yellowish bile pigment throughout its substance.

Women who are asymptomatic carriers of hepatitis B surface antigen usually transmit the antigen and antibodies against the surface antigen to the fetus during pregnancy. The passively acquired antibodies are believed to be of some protection to the infant during the first three months of life. A major concern among epidemiologists is that newborns often acquire the hepatitis B virus from exposure to maternal blood during delivery. This will occur with both vaginal and cesarean section births. A mother may also transmit the disease to her baby through kissing and close contact during the immediate postpartum period. To prevent perinatal hepatitis, a susceptible baby should be treated with hepatitis B immune globulin or hepatitis vaccine immediately after birth.

Whether these mothers should breast-feed is unknown at the present time. However, recent studies suggest that such women may transmit the antigen to their babies in their milk. Most authorities believe that all intimate contact between a susceptible baby and a mother with the hepatitis B antigen in her bloodstream be avoided unless the baby is first given hepatitis B immune globulin or the vaccine.

How can a woman prevent contracting hepatitis B during pregnancy?

Ideally, a woman and her sexual partner should be tested before pregnancy to determine if either carries the hepatitis B surface antigen in the bloodstream. If the man has the antigen but the woman doesn't, she should be immunized with the new and highly successful hepatitis B vaccine. This agent, marketed as Heptavax-B, is composed of highly purified hepatitis B surface antigen from the killed virus. Following two vaccine injections one month apart and a booster six months later, at least 95 percent of all individuals develop antibodies indicative of disease immunity. The woman should also receive the vaccine if she shares a household with a nonsexual contact who is a carrier of the hepatitis B antigen.

The hepatitis B vaccine has not been studied adequately in pregnant or nursing women, though it has been given to a small number of such women without untoward effect to mother or child. If a woman first becomes aware of hepatitis B exposure during pregnancy, the decision on whether or not to receive the vaccine is often a difficult one. Many infectious disease experts believe that the benefits of the vaccine exceed any possible risks since hepatitis may have serious consequences for a woman and her baby. This is especially true for the woman forced to work or live in an area where the chances of contracting hepatitis B appear likely.

An alternative treatment for the susceptible woman exposed to hepatitis B during pregnancy is an intramuscular injection of hepatitis B immune globulin. This antibody substance is derived from the blood of persons who have previously had the disease. It is marketed as H-BIG and Hep-B-Gammagee. Immune globulin prevents the onset of the disease or reduces its severity in over 80 percent of exposed individuals.

Cystitis

What is "honeymoon cystitis," and how is it treated?

"Honeymoon," or postcoital cystitis, is defined as an inflammation of the urinary bladder which occurs approximately thirty-six hours following intercourse. Though not truly a venereal disease, cystitis occurs when bacteria from the urethra, vagina, and external rectal area enter the urethra and are "massaged" into the urinary bladder as a result of penile thrusting and oral and manual stimulation to the vagina and clitoris during lovemaking. Once bacteria enter the urinary bladder, they reproduce rapidly, producing symptoms which include frequency of urination and burning with urination and an urgency to urinate despite the fact that only minimal amounts of urine are passed with each attempt. Hematuria, or the presence of blood in the urine, is commonly observed, and when blood is not present the urine will often have a cloudy appearance. Lower abdominal pain and pain during intercourse are other common symptoms of cystitis.

Cystitis is diagnosed by microscopic examination of the urine and collection of urine for culture which not only identifies the bacterial organism present but tells a doctor which antibiotic is most likely to eradicate the infection.

The most commonly used antibiotic for the treatment of cystitis is a sulfonamide named sulfisoxazole, more commonly known by its trade name Gantrisin. If a woman is sensitive to sulfa, alternative treatment with antibiotics such as ampicillin, tetracycline, and nitrofurantoin may be effectively used. To relieve symptoms immediately, a urinary anesthetic is recommended. It is imperative that repeat urine cultures be taken after the full course of antibiotics is administered.

What is the significance of postcoital cystitis during pregnancy?

Pregnancy alters a woman's immune responses in such a way as to make her more likely to develop a urinary tract infection. The hormonal changes of pregnancy cause the smooth muscles of the urinary bladder and ureter to relax, which is bound to result in a greater frequency of bacterial contamination and infection. Compression of urinary structures, such as the bladder and ureters, by the enlarging uterus also predisposes to poor urine flow and infection.

While postcoital cystitis is diagnosed identically in the pregnant and nonpregnant woman, treatment options are more limited during pregnancy, since some antibiotics and urinary anesthetics are not recommended at this time. Sulfonamides, for example, should not be prescribed during the last four weeks because they can cause jaundice in the newborn.

Many women with a significant number of bacteria in their urine are totally without symptoms of the cystitis. The diagnosis is made only when a routine urinalysis is performed early in pregnancy. This condition, appropriately named asymptomatic bacteriuria occurs in 3 to 7 percent of all pregnant women. If untreated, the bacteria may ascend the ureters and infect the kidneys later in pregnancy or following delivery. It has been estimated that as many as one-third of pregnant women with asymptomatic bacteriuria who are untreated will develop a severe kidney infection, or pyelonephritis, later in pregnancy. Pyelonephritis is characterized by high fever, pain in the side of the back in the area over the kidney, nausea, vomiting, and shaking chills. More importantly, it may precipitate premature labor and lead to silent, progressive kidney damage over a period of several years. For these reasons, asymptomatic bacteriuria should be vigorously treated during pregnancy with the goal of eliminating all bacteria from the urinary tract. If bacteriuria recurs, vigorous antibiotic treatment for several weeks and sometimes throughout the remainder of the pregnancy may be necessary. The urine should be constantly recultured for evidence of bacterial organisms.

Though asymptomatic bacteriuria in the absence of pyelonephritis is considered to be an innocuous condition, there are several carefully controlled studies which conclude that women with this condition may be at greater risk for prematurity and stillbirth. One report showed that 10 percent of patients with untreated or inadequately treated bacteriuria developed toxemia. Among a group of women in which cystitis was treated successfully, the incidence of toxemia was only 4 percent.

If I suspect that I have been exposed to a venereal disease, though I have no symptoms, what should I do?

Venereal diseases may result in serious physical impairment to you and your unborn children if they remain untreated for a long time. Therefore, it is imperative to seek immediate medical attention. Most reasonable physicians will treat you with confidentiality even if you are under eighteen years of age. If you fear that your family doctor will not do this, seek out another physician. Your county medical society can provide you with a list of competent doctors in your area. There are Planned Parenthood Centers in just about every city in the United States where you can be examined for a nominal fee. If you look in the white pages of your telephone directory under your city or county government, there will usually be a listing under the heading of "Health Departments" or "Venereal Disease Clinics."

Finally, there is a toll-free number, called the VD National Hotline. The number is 1-800-227-8922 except for California, where it is 1-800-982-5883. In addition to answering calls about sexually transmitted diseases, reassuring worried callers, and identifying conveniently located sites where diagnostic tests and treatment may be obtained, the trained volunteers of the VD National Hotline are collecting valuable data that document the nature and extent of the venereal disease problem in this country.

6.
Travel

Pregnancy should not stop an otherwise healthy woman from traveling. Unfortunately, many still believe that pregnant women who travel extensively are more prone to premature birth and miscarriage, despite the fact that this has been disproven by as many as five separate studies. Yet, when there are problems with delivery or with the baby, many still attribute this outcome to a particular event such as a long and tedious trip.

Women today are traveling more frequently and going greater distances than ever before, both for business and for pleasure. While it is encouraging to note that so many women are not treating their pregnancies as a pathological condition, the pregnant traveler has unique problems to consider. This chapter addresses these problems and concerns and has some practical and valuable tips for traveling.

Traveling in Automobiles

Can I continue to drive a car or travel in one when pregnant?

Automobile travel, barring accidents, will not harm your pregnancy. In one study of almost 2,000 pregnant drivers, spontaneous abortion and premature labor actually occurred less often than is usually found in the general population.

Though many women find that their coordination and muscular control are decreased during pregnancy, statistics show that the risk of an automobile accident is the same, whether you are pregnant or not. Investigators studying the outcome of hundreds of accidents have concluded that unless there is severe damage to the automobile, the chance of a major life-threatening injury to a pregnant traveler is small. Despite this, the automobile remains the most frequent nonobstetrical cause of maternal death, simply because of the large number of women who drive.

**What are the most common automobile injuries
and how do they affect pregnancy?**

Though the uterus seems extremely vulnerable during pregnancy, the greatest numbers of deaths and disabilities at this time result from blows to the head and injuries to the spleen, liver, kidneys, and intestines. The enlarged uterus actually provides good protection to the organs that lie behind it by absorbing blows to the abdominal wall.

However, when the uterus is damaged, the results may be devastating for both the pregnant woman and her baby. Until the end of the twelfth week, the uterus is well protected by the pubic symphysis bone, and rupture or injury as a result of an automobile accident during this time has never been reported. Beyond the twelfth week, premature separation of the placenta from its uterine attachment, known as abruptio placenta, is the most common injury and the degree of maternal hemorrhage and survival of the infant is determined by how much the placenta becomes detached. Even when less than 25 percent of the placenta is involved, a woman is still at an increased risk of premature labor, and if more than 50 percent of the placenta is separated, the fetus usually dies.

A rupture, or breaking apart, of the muscle of the pregnant uterus is an extremely rare but hazardous situation which may result in death to both a mother and her fetus. Though studies have demonstrated that the uterus may rupture upon impact, with or without a seat belt, it is far more likely to occur when a belt is not worn or is worn improperly.

The most commonly reported fetal injury that is apparent at birth is a skull fracture, often accompanied by a fracture of the mother's pelvic bones. Other common injuries are seen in the collarbone and the bones of the lower leg of the fetus.

Trauma to the uterus at the time of a serious accident may be responsible for a greater number of spontaneous abortions and premature births hours, days, or weeks later. However, the causal relationship between the collision and the unfortunate pregnancy outcome is often difficult to prove.

Should I use a seat belt or shoulder harness in a car?

The lap seat belt reduces the chances of injury to a woman's head and extremities by keeping her from striking the steering wheel and dashboard or being thrown from the vehicle. But a far greater amount of force is directed toward the pregnant uterus when the mother jackknifes over the belt during a sudden stop, so her uterus, fetus, and placenta are more likely to be injured than if she did not wear the belt. However, it is advisable for the pregnant woman to use a lap seat belt since it will keep her from being thrown from the vehicle and protect against the head injuries that are often associated with the highest death rates.

Proper placement of the lap seat belt is of the utmost importance. Too often it is deliberately worn loosely in the mistaken belief that tightening it may harm the uterus or fetus. On the contrary, the belt should be fastened snugly in order to decrease forward motion and injury to the uterus at the moment of impact. Position it at a level as far below the uterine bulge as possible and separate it from the abdominal wall by a small pillow or cushion, which helps distribute the force of the automobile's deceleration. Keep the buckle on the lap belt to one side, rather than centrally located, since this will cause less trauma to the uterus at the moment of impact. Be sure to sit up straight, as slouching can cause the belt to ride up on the abdomen.

The addition of a shoulder harness to the lap belt is now standard equipment in most automobiles. This so-called three-point restraint system should significantly reduce the frequency of maternal and fetal injury by distributing the body force more evenly and by preventing jackknifing of the upper body during a crash. As with seat belts, shoulder restraints should be as tight as possible. Unfortunately, too few women take the time to wear this lifesaving device.

Airplane Travel

How does airplane travel affect the pregnant woman?

Although relatively little is known about the effects of high-altitude jet travel on the pregnant woman and her developing fetus, it would appear that the low levels of noise and vibration found in modern commercial jet aircraft are harmless.

Few people are aware that the humidity in jet aircraft is only about 8 percent, causing passengers to experience a small but significant body water loss. The pregnant woman should compensate by drinking lots of water on long flights and avoid use of diuretics or "water pills," which unfortunately some doctors still prescribe to healthy pregnant women. These medications will only worsen the effects of water loss and cause a greater degree of dehydration.

Edema, or swelling of the ankles, may be accentuated during any trip in which the legs are below the body for prolonged periods of time. You can prevent this by taking frequent walks or elevating your legs on an adjacent seat if one is available. If it is possible to stretch out across two seats, the best position for rest is to lie on your left side. This position takes the weight from the enlarged uterus off the vena cava, the major vein carrying blood to the heart from the pelvis and lower extremities (see chapter 11). Carry a pair of loose-fitting shoes or slippers aboard the plane, since edema of the ankles and feet may be so pronounced at the end of the flight that your original pair of shoes may no longer fit.

Sitting for prolonged periods of time may slow the blood flow in the veins of the legs and pelvis, which in turn may cause clotting or thrombus formation in the veins (phlebs), accompanied by inflammation (itis). Thrombophlebitis involving the superficial or the deep veins of the legs is more common during pregnancy. Superficial thrombophlebitis occurs just beneath the skin in the varicose veins which may develop with childbirth. Few women have serious complications resulting from superficial thrombophlebitis, but thrombophlebitis of the veins deep in the legs and pelvis often presents a real threat to a woman's life. Unfortunately, deep-vein thrombophlebitis may occur without any warning symptoms. When one of these deep clots becomes dislodged from the wall of the vein, it travels through the circulatory system and is called an embolus. If the embolus reaches the lung, it is then called a pulmonary embolus. There, it may block the opening of a large oxygen-carrying blood vessel, causing instant death. Enough said! To prevent this condition, walk about the cabin at least every forty-five minutes for a period of no less then ten minutes.

Most modern passenger-carrying jet aircraft are pressurized to 7,000 feet above sea level. At actual flight levels from 10,000 to 40,000 feet there is a small decrease in the amount of oxygen concentration in the airplane cabin, reducing the amount of oxygen carried from the circulation of a healthy mother to the bloodstream of her baby via the placenta. Most authorities agree that this oxygen reduction is insignificant. On the other hand, travel at altitudes higher than 7,000 feet in nonpressurized aircraft such as private planes, cargo planes, propeller-driven airplanes, and "executive jets" may present a real hazard to the oxygen supply of the developing fetus and are best avoided.

Is it safe for a pregnant woman to be exposed to airport x-ray security machines?

The security machines currently in use at most airports throughout the world emit either low levels of nonionizing radiation or ultrasound waves, rather than the more dangerous ionizing radiation found in x-rays. In the United States, the Energy Research and Development Commission and the Bureau of Radiological Health carefully monitor these systems. Both the hand-held security scanners and the walk-through machines employ nonionizing radiation techniques which, while infinitely safer than ionizing radiation, are not totally innocuous (see chapter 9). It is my belief that a pregnant woman should not have to expose her baby even to this minimal amount of unnecessary radiation. If the security personnel believe that you are carrying a concealed weapon under your maternity dress, you can request a search by a female security guard instead of passing through the security machines.

Are there any additional radiation or environmental hazards which may be encountered inside the aircraft?

Exposure to radiation in an airplane, even at altitudes of 40,000 feet, is very low and should not deter the pregnant traveler from taking as many flights as desired. The National Council of Radiation Protection and Measurements has set the safe limits, exclusive of natural background, such as sun in your backyard, at 170 mrems per year.

Ozone is a colorless gas which is found in greatest concentrations generally between 35,000 and 150,000 feet above sea level and specifically in the northern hemisphere between late February and early May.

In an attempt to decrease fuel costs, many jetliners now fly at higher altitudes where the air is thinner, thereby making it possible to travel more miles per gallon of gas. The average cruising altitude of a plane going from New York to Chicago is 35,000 feet, while the Concorde flies at an altitude of 55,000 feet. Complaints of ozone-related illnesses have been increasing in recent years as fuel supplies have become more expensive.

Symptoms of ozone poisoning include shortness of breath, headache, dizziness, cough, eye irritation, burning of the nose and throat, chest pains, loss of coordination, decreased ability to concentrate, and drowsiness. Though there are no definite studies dealing with the effects of ozone on the developing fetus, the gas does have the capacity to cause abnormal changes in developing cells and produce biochemical alterations in the bloodstream of exposed persons. Some research suggests that flight attendants may have higher rates of miscarriage and give birth to children with greater numbers of birth defects than is found in the general population. Ozone exposure from repeated flights has been proposed as the possible cause. However, such a relationship is still little more than conjecture.

The concentration of ozone in the air which may cause health problems among passengers has not been determined. As of 1981, of all the airlines, only Pan American has taken positive steps to reduce ozone concentrations by installing catalytic converters and charcoal filters in their aircraft. These measures have significantly decreased the number of complaints of ozone intoxication among Pan American passengers.

If a pregnant traveler has a specific disease, how may it be affected by a long-distance flight?

Few patients and physicians are aware of the fact that the dosage of certain medications should be altered on trips in which several time zones are crossed. For example, the insulin needed by a diabetic woman will vary according to the direction in which she is traveling. Eastward travel of five to seven time zones may require a 15 percent decrease, while westward travel often necessitates an increase in dosage. Many other vital drugs, such as cortisone, digitalis, and other medications for heart disease, thyroid medications, anticonvulsives, and medications used for gastrointestinal ulcer therapy, all follow similar principles. It is important for pregnant women who use any of these medications to consult with a knowledgeable physician before departure so that appropriate changes in dosages and scheduling may be planned.

Are there any medical conditions which rule out high-altitude flying for pregnant women?

Pregnant women with a history of heart or lung disease are advised to avoid flights on any aircraft that may attain cruising altitudes between 35,000 and 40,000 feet, heights occasionally reached during long-distance flights. Though the aircraft is pressurized, there will be a slight but significant reduction in the oxygen saturation within the arteries carrying blood from the heart.

When determining oxygen saturation at high altitudes, people often neglect to consider the deleterious effects produced by cigarette smoking. Smoking produces carbon monoxide, which combines with hemoglobin in red blood cells to form a compound called carboxyhemoglobin. Carboxyhemoglobin significantly reduces the amount of hemoglobin in the blood that is available for transporting oxygen. If a pregnant woman smokes, or even sits in the smoking section of a plane, she may have as much as a 5 percent carboxyhemoglobin level in her blood. For a woman with pulmonary or cardiac problems, this decrease in the oxygen available to body tissues may be sufficient to produce such symptoms as shortness of breath and chest pain. Lesser carboxyhemoglobin concentrations resulting from light or moderate smoking at high altitudes may result in impairment of visual acuity and brightness perception, inability to concentrate, faulty manual dexterity and coordination, and the inability to make correct decisions.

Pregnant women often suffer from intestinal gas, which may be intensified by air travel since gases expand when barometric pressure decreases, as it does in modern commercial aircraft. This expansion of gases in the intestinal tract increases discomfort and passage of flatus. To alleviate these problems somewhat, it is best not to eat too quickly or too much before or during a flight, to avoid eating legumes and other gas-forming foods for one to two days before departure, to avoid drinking large quantities of fluid, especially carbonated drinks and beer, and it is best not to chew gum as the plane ascends because when chewing gum you may swallow a great deal of air.

Is it dangerous for some black women to fly during pregnancy?

Some black women may not be able to tolerate high altitudes even in pressurized jets. Ten percent of apparently healthy blacks have a condition called sickle-cell trait. With the exception of a mild anemia, these women are in excellent health, but they may occasionally experience sickling of their blood under conditions causing decreased oxygenation. Microscopic blood clots (thrombi) may form in the arteries supplying blood to various organs, especially the spleen and kidney. When the spleen is involved, the main symptom is severe pain in the left upper quadrant of the abdomen. Hematuria, or blood in the urine, occurs when microscopic thrombi form in the arteries supplying blood to the kidneys. A woman with sickle-cell trait may experience these problems following a flight as short as one hour. Fortunately, symptoms usually subside spontaneously without permanent damage within two to three days.

Since individuals with sickle-cell trait may become quite ill at high altitudes, it is advisable that all blacks be tested for this condition before vacationing at altitudes above 5,000 feet. Even flying in pressurized aircraft at altitudes below 10,000 feet may occasionally precipitate these problems. If susceptible women must fly, it is a good idea for them to breathe supplemental oxygen by mask when altitudes exceed 5,000 feet above sea level.

Sickle-cell anemia, on the other hand, is a very serious disease among a much smaller number of blacks, in whom many of the red blood cells are actually shaped like a sickle. Since pregnancy usually exacerbates this disease travel by those with this sickle-cell anemia is ill advised (see chapter 10).

What specific obstetrical complications make airplane travel hazardous to the fetus?

Though the fetus is much more able to cope with reduced oxygen than the adult, conditions such as chronic hypertension, preeclampsia and toxemia (elevated blood pressure after the twenty-eighth week of pregnancy), diabetes, multiple births, Rh disease, and intrauterine growth retardation, or IUGR (see chapter 10), may significantly reduce the oxygen supply carried across the placenta. With these complications the added insult of even a slight reduction of oxygen caused by high-altitude flying may be all that is needed to permanently damage the developing fetus. Women with a previous history of premature births are also at an increased risk. Though there are no specific rules or guidelines to follow, I personally believe that pregnant women with any of these complications should not fly in pressurized aircraft above 7,000 feet.

How is the traveler affected by jet lag?

Jet lag, or jet-lag fatigue, is a condition caused by rapid air travel through changing time zones. This type of travel has the effect of disrupting our normal twenty-four-hour body cycle, known as the circadian rhythm. At the current speed of air travel, it is not unusual to cross as many as four time zones in as little as four hours. When you land, your body may be four hours off schedule, according to local time. These changes will be more pronounced during transoceanic flights. Research data indicate that this abrupt change of time zones may upset more than a hundred psychological and biological bodily functions. These alterations in circadian rhythm, though short-lived, may be quite serious and include personality changes, lethargy, decreased mental alertness, inability to make rational decisions, defects in memory, diminished physical strength and coordination, digestive disturbances, and changes in body tem-

---

How to Relieve Symptoms of Jet Lag

Although there is no way to completely prevent the disruption of your body rhythms, the following tips prove helpful:

1. A graduated two-week program of conditioning exercises that includes walking up to three miles daily should be instituted.
2. Preset your physiological time schedule and body rhythms before leaving by adopting the time schedule of your new destination. Starting several days before departure, gradually change your eating and drinking schedule. If you're going to be flying west, go to bed an hour later each day and sleep later in the morning. If traveling east, go to bed and arise earlier each day. Also, practice going to sleep in the afternoon.
3. Complete all preparations at least two days before takeoff to allow a period of relaxation. Avoid a bon voyage party, heavy meals, or alcoholic beverages and cigarettes immediately before departure or during the flight.
4. Schedule your flight so that you arrive as close to your regular bedtime as possible. Try to take a nap during the flight.
5. Upon arrival, try to go to bed and sleep through to a reasonable waking hour of the new time zone.
6. Don't schedule important or demanding meetings or lavish entertainment too soon after arrival. Instead, eat a light meal and go to sleep early. Many business failures and errors of judgment have been caused by people suffering from air-travel dysrhythmia. If you have an important meeting at a predetermined time, it is best to arrive at least a day ahead in order to adjust to the new time zone.
7. No drugs have been proved useful in preventing or treating the effects of jet lag, so don't take any. Though some drugs used in psychiatry have shown some promise, the most effective ones, such as lithium, are not safe for use during pregnancy.

perature, pulse rate, respiratory rate, kidney and liver function, and hormonal levels. Scientists refer to these jet-lag changes as "air travel dysrhythmia."

In general, it takes one day of rest to recover following a plane trip in which four to six time zones are crossed, and two days of rest after seven to ten zones are crossed. As crossings approach a complete reversal of the day-night cycle, three days of rest are recommended. However, scientists point out that there is quite an individual variation in sensitivity to time zone changes. Young and physically fit individuals appear to adjust more readily to their new surroundings than do older persons who are not in good physical condition. Pregnant women appear to experience more problems with jet lag than do nonpregnant women.

Travel in a north-south direction does not produce jet lag since no time zones are crossed. Interestingly, it is much easier to adjust to a flight in a westerly direction, in which the traveler lands at an earlier time than the biological clock says it is, than to flights going east.

Sea Voyages

Are there any suggestions that I should follow when traveling by sea?

There is no doubt that the hormonal changes of pregnancy, which increase the likelihood of nausea and vomiting, also bring about a greater susceptibility to motion sickness. Try to plan sea travel for a time of year when storms and rough seas are least likely to occur. A large seaworthy ship with modern stabilizers has less side-to-side roll. Cabin selection is also important; a midship cabin offers the greatest stability and least amount of movement in rough seas, and though many individuals prefer a cabin location high above the main deck, the best cabins for avoiding motion sickness are on the lower middle deck.

Obviously, overindulgence in the lavish meals served aboard cruise ships will contribute to seasickness. Similarly, drinking alcohol even in moderate amounts will add to your discomfort and, more importantly, may be harmful to the developing fetus (see chapter 4).

See also the information on cruise ships on page 161.

Carriers Regulations

What rules govern airline travel by pregnant women?

Airlines are understandably nervous about the possibility of a woman's going into labor in midair, but their rules vary markedly and are always subject to change. When planning a flight, check with the specific airline on which you intend to fly. Most have no restrictions during the first eight months, but a note from your doctor is usually required during the ninth month.

Most airline personnel couldn't tell the difference between a six- and a nine-month pregnancy. In addition, many women appear much larger than their EDC (expected date of confinement) would indicate. It is a good idea to carry a signed letter from your obstetrician when traveling by air during the last four months of pregnancy, giving your EDC, an accurate assessment of your health, and a list of all pertinent medical and obstetrical information.

Do cruise ships have similar restrictions?

Cruise lines also vary in the restrictions they place on pregnant travelers. Most will carry pregnant women up to the seventh month, and then they require a letter releasing them from responsibility in the event of a problem. Check the requirements with the cruise line you plan to use.

Cruise lines usually have elaborate hospital facilities, and all are required to carry a physician abroad. Some even have nurses trained in midwifery and emergency obstetrical care. It is a good idea to investigate these facilities when making your reservations.

What restrictions do bus lines place on the pregnant travelers?

Both Greyhound and Trailways impose no rules or regulations on pregnant women, whether they are traveling short distances or taking cross-country tours. Though there are occasional stories of babies born aboard a bus, remember that drivers have no training in childbirth or first aid, so it is not advisable to plan an extensive tour during the ninth month of pregnancy.

Sunbathing

Does sunbathing intensify "the mask of pregnancy"?

Yes. Exposure to sunlight intensifies chloasma, the name for what is commonly called "the mask of pregnancy." Chloasma is the presence of dark brown pigmented areas on the face. It is often accompanied by a brown coloration of the nipples and the linea nigra, a dark, thin line which runs from the navel to the pubic hairline. These pigmentation changes are caused by the release of large amounts of melanocyte-stimulating hormone (MSH) by the pituitary gland during pregnancy. Though many women with chloasma are often distressed by their appearance, the condition is harmless and improves following childbirth when the output of MSH declines rapidly. The effect of sunlight on chloasma can be reduced to some degree by applying a sun screen to the skin. Once chloasma is well established, the pigmentation can be safely lightened with Eldoquin bleach products. Another product, RV Paque, is recommended for women who have lightened their hyperpigmentation but still need protection from the sun.

Living, Working, or Vacationing at High Altitudes

What effect does high altitude have on pregnancy?

Several studies have demonstrated that the lack of oxygen (hypoxia) at high altitudes is responsible for significantly lower birth weights and other potential pregnancy problems, including a higher death rate among newborns.

People tend to breathe faster, or hyperventilate, at higher altitudes. Hyperventilation causes the body to "blow off" excessive amounts of carbon dioxide. A woman's respiratory rate increases significantly during pregnancy, and the additional demands of higher altitudes tend to exaggerate this phenomenon. Unfortunately, the decrease in a mother's carbon dioxide blood level is passed across the placenta to the baby. There, it produces a metabolic disturbance called metabolic acidosis combined with what is known as a respiratory alkalosis. It is theorized that these metabolic changes may cause the increased mortality they found among infants born 14,000 feet above sea level.

Since mountainous areas in the United States hardly ever approach 14,000 feet, aren't these findings only theoretically significant for most American women?

Doctors at the University of Colorado Medical Center have demonstrated that a baby may be jeopardized at altitudes significantly lower than 14,000 feet. Their findings, published in *Archives of Environmental Health* in 1977, were based on almost 200,000 births which took place in areas of Colorado having three different altitudes above sea level: less than 7,000 feet, 7,000 to 9,000 feet, and greater than 9,000 feet. Infants born at both intermediate and high altitudes were at greater risk of having a lower birth weight and respiratory problems. Both neonatal mortality (death of a live-born infant during the first four weeks of life), and infant mortality (death of a live-born infant during the first year of life) were significantly greater at higher altitudes. Based on these data, it would appear to be best for pregnant women not to live at altitudes of 7,000 feet or more above sea level. Furthermore, I try to discourage pregnant patients from skiing, vacationing, or traveling to these areas. Areas in the national park system with elevations of 7,000 feet or more are given in Table 6–1.

Finding a Doctor Abroad

What should I do if I need medical attention in a foreign city?

One of the greatest fears of all travelers, especially pregnant women is how to seek out a competent physician who speaks one's language. For a one-year personal membership fee of $6 or a family membership of $10 Intermedic, Incorporated (777 Third Avenue, New York, New York 10017), supplies you with an updated, easy-to-carry directory of physicians in more than 200 foreign cities, with special emphasis on those areas most often visited by traveling Americans. Physicians whose names are listed in the directory may be reached day or night. Data on each participating physician, such as medical education, experience, and hospital affiliations, are on file at Intermedic headquarters in New York. In addition, each overseas doctor has certified that he or she speaks English and will respond promptly to calls from Intermedic cardholders. Intermedic physicians have also agreed in writing to a fee ceiling of $25 for an office visit and $40 for a house or hotel call between the hours of 7 A.M. and 7 P.M. The fee ceiling for a house or hotel call between the hours of 7 P.M. and 7 A.M., on weekends, and on local holidays is $50.

The Intermedic directory also includes a two-page Medical Data Form on which you and your doctor can list immunizations, emergency data, allergies or sensitivities, previous illnesses and operations, and other pertinent information. Properly filled out, this form will be of invaluable aid to any doctor treating you overseas.

IAMAT (736 Center Street, Lewiston, New York 14092; telephone 716-754-4883) stands for the International Association for Medical Assistance to Travelers. For a suggested contribution of $5, you will receive a directory listing IAMAT centers in 450 cities and 120 countries throughout the world. These centers furnish the names of English-speaking physicians, a world immunization and malaria risk chart, and a personal clinical record form on which your physician can note any important medical data. All doctors on the IAMAT list have agreed to a fixed fee schedule of $20 for an office visit and $20 for a house or hotel call between 8 A.M. and 8 P.M. From 8 P.M. to 8 A.M. and on weekends and local holidays, the fee increases to $35.

Near Inc. (Oklahoma City, Oklahoma 73127; telephone 405-949-2500) is a relatively new organization. It provides its subscribers with worldwide air-ground ambulance transportation. In addition, if you forward proof of hospitalization coverage to this organization, Near guarantees repayment of hospital charges up to $5,000 anywhere in the world. Near is then reimbursed from your insurance company. The annual fee for this service is $120.

Assist-Card (745 Fifth Avenue, New York, New York 10022) has branches in the United States and fifty-six other countries. This organization provides travelers with legal, medical, and other assistance in emergencies. Medical coverage includes hospital fees up to $3,000 and evacuation by air if necessary.

Another source of help is International SOS Assistance (2 Neshaminy Interplex, Trevose, Pennsylvania 19047). For a fee based on the number of days that you plan to travel, SOS assists in finding a local physician or hospital and provides you with a form that enables you to charge hospital costs to your credit card. If necessary, they also fly you home by chartered aircraft.

Lacking these sources of information, the pregnant traveler with a medical problem can probably receive a competent referral from a local American Express office, U.S. or British consulate, or the nearest medical school or university hospital.

Travelers with medical illnesses such as severe allergies, diabetes, heart disease, epilepsy, and other potentially emergency-producing conditions can register with the Medical Alert Foundation (P.O. Box 1009, Turlock, California, 95380). Members of this worldwide organization receive either a bracelet or necklace bearing a red Medic Alert emblem. This emblem lists the wearer's identification number and gives a brief description of his or her medical problem along with a 24-hour "hot line" number. This service accepts collect calls from physicians or public health officials from all over the world, thereby providing them with the person's full medical history within seconds. The cost of a lifetime membership, including the emblem is only $10. For the financially needy, there is no charge.

How can dental emergencies that arise while traveling be met?

Though many of the organizations mentioned (see pages 162–163) provide a list of dentists throughout the world, you can get temporary relief safely and easily by traveling with a DENT-AIDE Dental Emergency Kit. Developed by a team of practicing dentists, this compact kit comes with an easy-to-follow 56-page instruction

Table 6–1. Areas of National Park System with Elevations of 7,000 Feet or More Above Sea Level

State	Area	Elevation in Feet Above Sea Level
Alaska	Glacier Bay National Monument	0 to 15,300
	Mount McKinley National Park	2,070 to 20,320 (highest road, 3,850)
	Katmain National Monument	0 to 7,585
	Denali National Monument	2,000 to 14,580
	Gates of the Arctic National Monument	0 to 8,800
	Lake Clark National Monument	0 to 10,197
	Wrangell-St. Elias National Monument	0 to 18,000
Arizona	Canyon de Chelly National Monument	5,500 (Visitor Center) to 7,000 (average on So. Rim Drive)
	Chiricahua National Monument	5,160 to 7,300
	Grand Canyon National Park	(Canyon 1,625) South Rim, 7,000; North Rim, 7,970 to 9,165
	Navajo National Monument	7,280
	Saguaro National Monument	2,200 to 8,666
	Sunset Crater National Monument	5,900 to 7,000
California	Death Valley National Monument (also in Nevada)	280 below sea level to 11,049
	Kings Canyon National Park	roads 4,600 to 7,000; back country to 14,000
	Lassen Volcanic National Park	4,822 to 10,457
	Sequoia National Park	1,700 to 14,495
	Yosemite National Park	roads 2,850 to nearly 10,000; back country to 13,000
Colorado	Black Canyon of the Gunnison National Monument	5,500 to 8,500
	Colorado National Monument	4,700 to 7,000
	Curecanti National Recreation Area (also in Montana)	6,500 to 8,800

booklet that is equipped with everything you need for effectively treating dental emergencies such as toothaches, bleeding gums, and lost fillings. It may be purchased by writing to Traveler's Checklist, Sharon, Connecticut 06069.

What medications and first-aid supplies would you recommend for the pregnant traveler?

It is an excellent idea for any traveler to carry a small medical kit for use in an emergency.

If you are taking essential medications such as insulin or cortisone, be sure to have a sufficient supply from your doctor, with full instructions on using the medi-

Table 6–1. Areas of National Park System with Elevations of 7,000 Feet or More Above Sea Level (*continued*)

State	Area	Elevation in Feet Above Sea Level
Colorado cont'd.	Dinosaur National Monument (also in Utah)	5,000 to 9,006
	Florissant Fossil Beds National Monument	8,200 to 9,000
	Great Sand Dunes National Monument	8,200 average elevation of features
	Mesa Verde National Park	8,048 to 9,572
	Rocky Mountain National Park	7,740 to 14,255
	Arapahoe National Wildlife Refuge	7,600 to 12,183
Hawaii	Haleakala National Park	0 to 10,023
Idaho	Craters of the Moon National Monument	4,980 to 7,688
Montana	Glacier National Park	3,190 (Headquarters) to 10,448
New Mexico	Capulin Mountain National Monument	7,280 to 8,182
	El Morro National Monument	7,218 (Visitor Center)
Oregon	Crater Lake National Park	4,824 to 8,926
Texas	Guadalupe Mountains National Park	3,650 to 8,751
Utah	Bryce Canyon National Park	6,620 to 9,091
	Capitol Reef National Park	4,400 to 9,000
	Cedar Breaks National Monument	8,200 to 10,500
	Timpanogos Cave National Monument	5,449 to 8,045
	Zion National Park	4,000 to 8,000
Washington	Mount Rainier National Park	1,342 to 14,410
	North Cascades National Park	2,000 to 9,200
	Lake Chelan National Recreation Area	1,100 to 7,800
	Ross Lake National Recreation Area	400 to 7,400
	Olympic National Park	0 to 7,065
Wyoming	Fossil Butte National Monument	6,669 to 8,084
	Grand Teton National Park	6,330 to 13,770
	Yellowstone National Park (also in Montana and Idaho)	5,314 to 11,358

cation, its proper storage, and how to protect it from damage and deterioration. If you require syringes, be sure to have an adequate number and a letter from your doctor indicating to immigration officials that they are necessary for your medical condition. Women who wear glasses should carry a spare pair or a copy of the prescription, in case glasses are lost or broken. Some areas of travel require special precautions such as insect repellents, special eye ointments, water purification tablets, and electric immersion heaters for boiling water. Prepare for these situations before departure. All items should be packed carefully to avoid breakage. It is best to carry the kit with you rather than subject it to the beating inflicted on most luggage.

For the items I consider most important for the pregnant traveler, see the Pregnant Traveler's Medical Kit in the accompanying box. All recommended medications have been shown to be safe for both mother and fetus.

Pregnant Traveler's Medical Kit

First-aid Kit
Gauze pads, gauze roll, adhesive tape, scissors, tweezers, thermometer, Band-Aids of various sizes, small amount of sterile cotton, antiseptic cream or powder

Medications for Specific Problems
Headache. Acetaminophen (trade names Tylenol or Datril) for mild pain, codeine or acetaminophen with codeine for more severe pain
Constipation. Milk of magnesia
Diarrhea and abdominal cramps. Ginger root capsules for "turista," paregoric for noninfectious diarrhea
Indigestion and hyperacidity. Maalox liquid or tablets
Nausea, vomiting, and motion sickness. Emetrol for mild cases, Dramamine for motion sickness, Phenergan for more severe nausea
Hives, allergic reactions. Benadryl liquid or tablets, epinephrine only if history suggests near-fatal reactions to insect bites
Cough. Robitussin or Phenergan for mild cough, add codeine for more severe cough (Phenergan with codeine or Robitussin A-C)
Sore throat. Chloraseptic or Cēpacol lozenges (antibiotic not recommended unless first evaluated by doctor)
Eye irritation. Visine
Ear inflammation or pain. Auralgan otic solution
Skin irritation. A and D ointment, anesthetic aerosol such as Americaine
Painful or bleeding hemorrhoids. Anusol-HC suppositories
Varicose veins. Jobst elastic stockings (see chapter 3)
Insect bites. Repellent, sleeping net, Calamine lotion for applications to bites
Dermatitis or skin rash from contact with plants such as poison ivy. Ointment or cream containing hydrocortisone applied two to three times daily (concentrations of ½ hydrocortisone or less may be purchased without prescription)
Superficial fungus infections of skin. Lotrimin cream or solution
Sunburn prevention. Suntan lotion with sunscreen protection containing PABA (para-amino-benzoic-acid); SPF (sun protection factor) can range from 15 (for people with very fair skin) to 4 (for dark-skinned individuals)
Cold, nasal congestion. Sudafed tablets or syrup, Afrin nasal spray
Insomnia and nervous tension. Count sheep during the first trimester since all medications are potentially dangerous. After this time, on rare occasions a barbiturate such as Seconal or a minor tranquilizer such as Valium and Librium is probably safe.

Immunizations

Can I be safely vaccinated?

Ideally, if planning to travel to a foreign country, you should receive all required immunizations at least three months before becoming pregnant. Certain vaccines administered after this time may present hazards to the developing fetus.

A vaccine enables an individual to form immunity against an infectious agent without experiencing significant illness. There are three categories of vaccines: toxoids, killed or inactivated bacterial and viral vaccines, and live virus vaccines.

Toxoids are preparations of chemically altered toxins, or poisons, produced by certain bacteria. The combined tetanus and diphtheria vaccine is one example, and there is no evidence to show that the fetus is at risk when this preparation is administered during pregnancy.

Killed vaccines, such as influenza, cholera, plague, and rabies, contain heat or chemically inactivated microorganisms. Though much remains to be learned about the effects of killed vaccines on the fetus, in most cases they are probably harmless. However, a few individuals run a high fever in reaction to killed vaccines which may jeopardize the pregnancy; killed vaccines are best avoided by pregnant women.

Live viruses used for vaccination are either viral strains which are altered in the laboratory or those which are inherently weaker than the virulent wild virus. Live vaccines, such as those for polio, mumps, measles, rubella or German measles, smallpox, and yellow fever, pose the greatest risks to pregnancy because the organisms which they contain may occasionally cross the placenta and infect the fetus. This is especially likely to occur with rubella, measles, and mumps, so these vaccines should never be given during pregnancy or the three months before a contemplated conception. Smallpox, however, is a disease which is known to produce significantly higher mortality rates among pregnant women than among nonpregnant women. Similarly, poliomyelitis has been reported to cause paralysis far more frequently when contracted during pregnancy. Therefore, in these two instances, vaccination would be advisable during pregnancy only if the risk of contracting either of these diseases was strong. Discussing the use of smallpox vaccine during pregnancy has become academic since the disease has been virtually eliminated throughout the world.

Unless the trip is an absolute necessity, a pregnant woman who has not been vaccinated for plague and yellow fever should not go to areas where these diseases are endemic.

Can gamma globulins be safely taken by a pregnant woman to prevent disease and when should they be taken?

Gamma globulins are antibodies which may be detected in a person's bloodstream following exposure to an infectious disease. Though gamma globulin injections are not truly vaccines, they supply antibodies which the person lacks, providing temporary immunity. Unfortunately, they are misused by many physicians for treating colds, allergies, and many other conditions for which they are of no benefit.

There are two types of gamma globulins: standard human immune serum globulin, or HISG, and special human immune serum globulin. Both may be used with complete safety during pregnancy. If an intramuscular injection of HISG is administered to a susceptible woman within forty-eight hours of exposure to measles, it effectively prevents or modifies the disease symptoms. This is particularly important, since measles has been reported to cause spontaneous abortion in up to 50 percent of infected pregnant women and is also associated with an increased rate of congenital malformations and premature labor. While HISG will effectively prevent or modify disease symptoms among women exposed to measles, it is far less likely to be effective in preventing rubella and mumps after exposure and is only recommended following rubella exposure for pregnant women who would not consider therapeutic abortion should they contract the disease.

HISG should also be given to all pregnant women exposed to hepatitis A. Hepatitis A, or infectious hepatitis, is caused by a virus which is similar to hepatitis B (see chapter 4). However, unlike hepatitis B, it is transmitted through contamination of food and water sources, is usually not transmitted sexually, and has a shorter incubation period of two to six weeks. Symptoms include fatigue, weight loss, nausea, headache, joint pains, and fever. Jaundice, or yellowing of the skin and sclera of the eyes, is usually present. Hepatitis A may cause significant maternal illness during pregnancy, and if a woman contracts the disease during the third trimester, she will be more likely to experience premature labor. Hepatitis A may be transmitted to a newborn at delivery if its mother is incubating the virus or is acutely ill with hepatitis at that time. If the disease begins during the first and second trimesters, it will not adversely affect the pregnancy and is not associated with a greater incidence of congenital abnormalities. Pregnant travelers planning to visit areas of the world where hepatitis A is prevalent, such as Africa, Asia, Central America, rural Mexico, the Philippine Islands, the South Pacific Islands, and South America, are advised to receive HISG prior to departure. If you plan an extended stay in one of these areas, the injection should be repeated every three to six months.

The second category of gamma globulins, known as special human immune serum globulins, have a variety of uses. They are given the name "special globulins" because each contains high antibody titres against one specific virus. ZIG, or zoster immune globulin, can prevent or ameliorate chicken pox if given within seventy-two hours of exposure. It is available in limited supplies from the Center for Disease Control, Bureau of Epidemiology, Quarantine Division (Atlanta, Georgia 30333; telephone 404-329-3311) to provide immunity for extremely ill children who would be unable to survive a chicken-pox infection. It is rarely, if ever, given to pregnant women. The one exception would be a woman who has never had chicken pox and is exposed to the disease during the last six weeks of pregnancy. Under such conditions, without ZIG, the virus may cause an overwhelming infection and death of the newborn. Chicken pox contracted during the first trimester increases the likelihood of spontaneous abortion. A distinctive pattern of congenital malformations, including eye defects, skin lesions, and shortening of the limbs, has been reported among infants whose mothers contracted chicken pox during their first and second trimesters.

VIG, vaccinia immune globulin, was formerly administered, along with smallpox vaccination, to individuals likely to be exposed to smallpox. However, this is no longer necessary, since this disease has been virtually eliminated.

RIG and TIG are abbreviations for rabies immune globulin and tetanus immune globulin. Both are effective and safe preparations for use with, but not in place of, tetanus and rabies vaccines.

Information about risks from and need for immunization during pregnancy is summarized in Table 6–2.

Where can I find out about the immunization requirements of a particular country?

Since immunization requirements and the geographic distribution of various diseases is constantly changing, it is vital that travelers—and pregnant women in particular—be provided with the most up-to-date information. In addition to knowing the current immunization requirements of each country you intend to visit, you must not forget those requirements necessary for return to the United States from your travels. This information is available from most state and local health departments, but the Center for Disease Control, Bureau of Epidemiology, Quarantine Division (Atlanta, Georgia 30333, telephone 404-329-3311), is the best national and international resource for information on changing epidemiologic factors and immunization practices. Members of Intermedic (see page 162) can receive current immunization information about any country and a periodic updated list of required vaccinations for various countries throughout the world.

Do you recommend the influenza vaccine for pregnant women?

The influenza vaccine currently in use is a trivalent preparation, comprised of proteins or antigens from three prevalent viruses which have been killed or inactivated. The formulation for each year is determined by which viral strains the experts predict will be most prevalent. (Named each year in a fashion similar to that used for naming famous vintage wines, the components of the 1982–83 influenza vaccine are A/Brazil/78, A/Bangkok/79, and B/Singapore/79.) When the vaccine is correctly matched to the prevalent flu strain, it is about 80 to 90 percent effective in preventing or lessening the severity of the disease.

There is no evidence to suggest that influenza immunization of pregnant women presents any risk to the mother or fetus, and public health officials recommend that doctors use the same criteria for vaccination for both pregnant and nonpregnant individuals.

Studies of previous influenza epidemics of 1918–19 and 1957–58 suggest that pregnant women who contract this illness may have a slightly higher death rate than nonpregnant individuals. An increased risk of congenital malformations and childhood leukemia among children born to women who contracted influenza during pregnancy has been reported but other studies do not support these findings.

If the local risk for influenza appears low, I do not recommend that the vaccine be given during pregnancy. However, if there are many cases in your area, or if you plan to travel to an area which is experiencing an epidemic, if you suffer from heart disease, chronic anemia, diabetes, kidney disease, and pulmonary or lung diseases, such as asthma and chronic bronchitis, you should be immunized.

Specifically, which immunizations are usually required for travel abroad?

The areas most frequented by Americans—Europe, Canada, Mexico, and the Caribbean—do not require vaccinations. However, other foreign countries may require them.

Table 6–2. Immunization During Pregnancy

Immunizing Agent	Risk from Disease to Pregnant Female	Risk from Disease to Fetus or Neonate	Type of Immunizing Agent	Risk from Immunizing Agent to Fetus	Indications for Immunization During Pregnancy	Dose Schedule	Comments
Live Virus Vaccines							
Measles	Significant degree of illness, low death rate; not altered by pregnancy	Significant increase in abortion rate; may cause malformations	Live attenuated virus vaccine	None confirmed	Not recommended (See immune globulins)	Single dose	Vacination of susceptible women should be part of postpartum care
Mumps	Low degree of illness and death rate; not altered by pregnancy	Probable increased rate of abortion in 1st trimester; questionable association of a rare type of heart disease called fibroelastosis in neonates	Live attenuated virus vaccine	None confirmed	Not recommended	Single dose	
Poliomyelitis	No increased incidence in pregnancy, but may be more severe if it does occur	Fetal damage caused by a lack of oxygen; 50% death rate in newborns with this disease.	Live, attenuated virus (OPV) and inactivated virus (IPV) vaccine*	None confirmed	Not routinely recommended for adults in U.S., except persons at increased risk of exposure	*Primary:* 3 doses of IPV at 4–8 week intervals and a 4th dose 6–12 months after the 3rd dose; 2 doses of OPV with a 6–8 week interval and a 3rd dose at least 6 weeks later, customarily 8–12 months later. *Booster:* Every 5 years until 18 years of age for IPV	Vaccine indicated for susceptible pregnant women traveling in endemic areas or in other high-risk situations

Disease	Effect of pregnancy on disease	Effect on fetus	Type of vaccine	Effect of vaccine on fetus	Indicated during pregnancy	Dose schedule	Comments
Rubella	Low degree of illness and death rate; not altered by pregnancy	High rate of abortion and congenital rubella syndrome	Live attenuated virus vaccine	None confirmed	Not recommended	Single dose	Teratogenicity of vaccine is theoretical, not confirmed to date; vaccination of susceptible women should be part of postpartum care
Yellow Fever	Significant degree of illness and death rate; not altered by pregnancy	Unknown	Live attenuated virus vaccine	Unknown	Not recommended except if exposure unavoidable	Single dose	Postponement of travel preferable to vaccination, if possible

Inactivated Virus Vaccines

Disease	Effect of pregnancy on disease	Effect on fetus	Type of vaccine	Effect of vaccine on fetus	Indicated during pregnancy	Dose schedule	Comments
Influenza	Possible increase in degree of illness and death rate during epidemic of new antigenic strain	Possible increased abortion rate; no malformations confirmed	Inactivated type A and type B virus vaccines	None confirmed	Usually recommended only for patients with serious underlying diseases; public health authorities to be consulted for current recommendation	Consult with public health authorities since recommendations change each year	Criteria for vaccination of pregnant women same as for all adults
Rabies	Near 100% fatality; not altered by pregnancy	Determined by maternal disease	Killed virus vaccine	Unknown	Indications for prophylaxis not altered by pregnancy; each case considered individually	Public health authorities to be consulted for indications and dosage	

NOTE: *Inactivated polio vaccine (IPV) recommended for unimmunized adults at increased risk

Table 6–2. Immunization During Pregnancy *(continued)*

Immunizing Agent	Risk from Disease to Pregnant Female	Risk from Disease to Fetus or Neonate	Type of Immunizing Agent	Risk from Immunizing Agent to Fetus	Indications for Immunization During Pregnancy	Dose Schedule	Comments
Inactivated Bacterial Vaccines							
Cholera	Significant degree of illness and death rate; more severe during 3rd trimester	Increased risk of fetal death during 3rd trimester maternal illness	Killed bacterial vaccine	Unknown	Only to meet international travel requirements	2 injections, 4–8 weeks apart	Vaccine of low efficacy
Meningococcus	No increased risk during pregnancy; no increase in severity of disease	Unknown	Killed bacterial vaccine	No data available on use during pregnancy	Indications not altered by pregnancy; vaccination recommended only in unusual outbreak situations	Public health authorities to be consulted	
Plague	Significant degree of illness and death rate; not altered by pregnancy	Determined by maternal disease	Killed bacterial vaccine	None reported	Very selective vaccination of exposed persons	Public health authorities to be consulted for indications and dosage	
Pneumococcus	No increased risk during pregnancy; no increase in severity of disease	Unknown	Polyvalent polysaccharide vaccine	No data available on use during pregnancy	Indications not altered by pregnancy; vaccine used only for high-risk individuals	In adults 1 dose only	
Typhoid	Significant degree of illness and death rate; not altered by pregnancy	Unknown	Killed bacterial vaccine	None confirmed	Not recommended routinely except for close, continued exposure or travel to endemic areas	*Primary:* 2 injections, 4 weeks apart; *Booster:* single dose	

Toxoids

Agent	Risk from disease to pregnant woman	Risk from disease to fetus or neonate	Type of immunizing agent	Risk from immunizing agent to fetus	Indications for immunization during pregnancy	Dose schedule	Comments
Tetanus-Diphtheria	Severe degree of illness, tetanus mortality 60%, diphtheria mortality 10%; unaltered by pregnancy	Neonatal tetanus mortality 60%	Combined tetanus-diphtheria toxoids preferred: adult tetanus-diphtheria formulation	None confirmed	Lack of primary series, or no booster within past 10 years	*Primary:* 2 doses at 1- to 2-month interval with a 3rd dose 6–12 months after the second; *Booster:* single dose every 10 years, after completion of the primary series	Updating of immune status should be part of antepartum care

Immune Globulins: Hyperimmune

Agent	Risk from disease to pregnant woman	Risk from disease to fetus or neonate	Type of immunizing agent	Risk from immunizing agent to fetus	Indications for immunization during pregnancy	Dose schedule	Comments
Hepatitis B	Possible increased severity during 3rd trimester	Possible increase in abortion rate and prematurity. Neonatal hepatitis can occur if mother is a chronic carrier or is acutely infected	Hepatitis B immune globulin (HBIG)	None reported	Postexposure prophylaxis	.06ml/kg immediately and 1 month later of HBIG	Infants to HBsAg-positive mothers should receive 0.5 ml of HBIG as soon after birth as possible and the same dose repeated 3 and 6 months later
Rabies	Near 100% fatality; not altered by pregnancy	Determined by maternal disease	Rabies immune globulin (RIG)	None reported	Postexposure prophylaxis	20 IU/kg in one dose of RIG	Used in conjunction with rabies killed virus vaccine
Tetanus	Severe degree of illness; mortality 60%	Neonatal tetanus mortality 60%	Tetanus immune globulin (TIG)	None reported	Postexposure prophylaxis	250 units in one dose of TIG	Used in conjunction with tetanus toxoid

Table 6–2. Immunization During Pregnancy   (continued)

Immunizing Agent	Risk from Disease to Pregnant Female	Risk from Disease to Fetus or Neonate	Type of Immunizing Agent	Risk from Immunizing Agent to Fetus	Indications for Immunization During Pregnancy	Dose Schedule	Comments
Varicella	Possible increase in severe varicella pneumonia	Can cause congenital varicella with increased mortality in neonatal period; very rarely causes congenital defects	Varicella-zoster immune globulin (VZIG)	None reported	Not routinely indicated in healthy pregnant women exposed to varicella	1 vial/kg in one dose of VZIG, up to 5 vials	Only indicated for newborns of mothers who developed varicella within 4 days prior to delivery or 2 days following delivery. Approximately 90–95% of adults are immune to varicella
Immune Globulins: Pooled							
Hepatitis A	Possible increased severity during 3rd trimester	Probable increase in abortion rate and prematurity. Possible transmission to neonate at delivery if mother is incubating the virus or is acutely ill at that time	Pooled immune globulin (IG)	None reported	Postexposure prophylaxis	.02ml/kg in one dose of IG	IG should be given as soon as possible and within 2 weeks of exposure. Infants born to mothers who are incubating the virus or are acutely ill at delivery should receive one dose of 0.5 ml as soon as possible after birth
Measles	Significant morbidity, low mortality; not altered by pregnancy	Significant increase in abortion rate; may cause malformations	Pooled immune globulin (IG)	None reported	Postexposure prophylaxis	.25 ml/kg in one dose of IG, up to 15 ml	Unclear if it prevents abortion. Must be given within 6 days of exposure

Of all currently available immunizations, only cholera, yellow fever, and small-pox vaccines are required by the local health departments of various countries in order to prevent the introduction and spread of these potentially epidemic diseases. Although other vaccines are recommended for the personal protection and well-being of the traveler, they are not required. Interestingly, for fear of discouraging tourism, many tropical countries where yellow fever is present do not require vaccinations as a condition for entry, but you may be stopped when you leave such a country and try to enter another which is free of yellow fever. When planning such an itinerary, read "Vaccination Certificate Requirements for International Travel," published by the World Health Organization.

If an arriving traveler does not meet the immunization requirements of a country, they may, under World Health Organization authority, be subject to quarantine and even vaccination. Yellow fever vaccination is not recommended during pregnancy and smallpox vaccination has its potential hazards (see page 168), and while some countries may not enforce these regulations if risks are minimal, other nations regularly and periodically enforce them. Fortunately, you can avert these problems because most countries accept a written statement from a personal physician confirming that you are pregnant and that the vaccine in question should not be given. This letter must be dated, signed, and written on stationery bearing the physician's letterhead. Although this usually allows you to avoid vaccination, it may not be enough to prevent your isolation or quarantine at the time of an epidemic.

Any immunization against smallpox, cholera, and yellow fever you have received before pregnancy should be recorded on an International Certificate of Vaccination form by your doctor, and validated by a city, county, or state health department. Without properly validated certificates, you may encounter serious difficulties and delays later in your travels. Vaccination certificates for cholera are valid for a period of six months before revaccination is necessary. Smallpox immunization lasts three years; yellow fever is valid for a period of ten years.

Do today's travelers risk contracting malaria and how does malaria affect pregnancy?

In recent years, there has been a staggering increase in the worldwide incidence of malaria. It is hard to convince people that malaria occurs not only in exotic far-off lands but may be found in such places commonly visited by tourists as the Dominican Republic, Mexico, Central America, and South America.

The disease is transmitted by the bite of the female Anopheles mosquito that is infected with the Plasmodium protozoan, the causative microbe. The incubation period, defined as the time from the mosquito bite to the appearance of symptoms of chills and fever, varies from eight to twenty-eight days.

The symptoms recur every few days over a period of four to six weeks. After this time, the organisms reside in the liver and cause unpredictable periodic relapses, anemia, and enlargement of the liver and spleen. The deadly strain of the disease, *Plasmodium falciparum*, may attack blood vessels in the brain and other internal organs. Symptoms may include severe headache, coma, convulsions, profuse vomiting and diarrhea, and circulatory failure.

Epidemiologists have noted that the acute attack of malaria is likely to be more severe for the pregnant woman. In addition, the stress of pregnancy and labor is more likely to activate a quiet or latent case of malaria. There are several reports in the medical literature in which a fatal collapse occurred immediately following delivery. The fetus may also be jeopardized by the extremely high maternal fevers during the first trimester. During the second and third trimester, malaria causes placental swelling, hemorrhage, and edema which is responsible for a significantly greater incidence of prematurity, stillbirths, and newborn deaths. In rare cases, the organism may migrate to the fetus. Symptoms of congenital malaria appear in the newborn two to three days after birth and include fever, vomiting, convulsions, jaundice, and enlargement of the liver and spleen. Death may occur from respiratory failure. Congenital malaria is most likely to take place during a mother's first attack of the disease and not when it is in its chronic form.

The diagnosis of malaria in the newborn, as well as in the adult, requires finding Plasmodium organisms within the red blood cells when viewed under the microscope.

How can malaria be prevented and treated?

Since there is no vaccine against malaria, the only sure preventive is to avoid travel to areas where the disease is prevalent. There are a host of antimalarial drugs that are recommended for travelers to such areas. These drugs suppress the multiplication of Plasmodium in a person's red cells but do not prevent entry of the organism into the body. With continued use of these medications, the organism is eventually eliminated from the body and symptoms of malaria are prevented. Unfortunately, most antimalarial preparations are not recommended during pregnancy because they may be responsible for causing birth defects. The one exception is chloroquine, which has been proven safe in pregnancy. If you must travel to an area of the world where the malaria risk is significant, chloroquine should be taken at weekly intervals, starting one week before arriving and continuing for at least four weeks after departure, in order to completely eliminate the organism from the bloodstream. This course of suppressant therapy is also essential for a short visit of only a few hours in an airport or harbor in a malarious region. This is especially true if the visit is likely to occur between sunset and dawn, when the mosquito is most apt to bite. Side effects of chloroquine include nausea, diarrhea, headache, and blurring of vision. Chloroquine is deposited in high concentrations in the liver and white blood cells and should be used with caution in persons having liver disease and blood disorders.

Motion Sickness

Are antimotion sickness medications safely taken during pregnancy?

While I share the concern of pregnant women that medication be taken only when absolutely necessary, it is also true that the persistent vomiting associated with mo-

The International Association for Medical Assistance to Travelers provides its members with detailed charts listing the sanitary conditions of the water, milk, and food in all areas of the world.

How can travelers' diarrhea be treated?

Doxycycline hyclate (trade name Vibramycin) is an antibiotic which has gained popularity as a preventive for travelers' diarrhea. Since it is a type of tetracycline, it should not be taken during pregnancy (see chapter 7). Other antibiotics such as ampicillin have also been recommended for this purpose. Most infectious disease experts, however, discourage use of antibiotics in this fashion since they may actually increase a person's susceptibility to more serious intestinal ailments, such as salmonella and shigella, by killing off protective bacteria in the intestine. Furthermore, by upsetting the normal bacterial flora of the intestine, antibiotic therapy may actually cause diarrhea. Considering that travelers' diarrhea is a self-limited condition which is usually not serious, it is probably best not to take antibiotics as a preventive.

Iodochlorhydroxyquin (trade names Diodoquin and Enterovioform) is a drug which was widely used in the past to prevent and treat travelers' diarrhea. This is an extremely dangerous medication which is no longer available in the United States. However, you may be sold it over the counter in many other countries, such as Mexico. In a recent visit to Mexico City, I was shocked to find that chloramphenicol, a potentially lethal drug (see chapter 7), was also sold without prescription as a preventive against traveler's diarrhea.

When turista strikes, the natural tendency is to prescribe medications which will control the symptoms. Until recently, standard treatment consisted of nonspecific antidiarrheal agents such as Lomotil (diphenoxylate hydrochloride and atropine sulfate), Kaopectate (kaolin and pectin), Imodium (loperamide), and paregoric. Though these medications have the capacity to decrease cramps and diarrhea, many doctors now believe that they actually produce more harm than good, since diarrhea is the body's way of ridding the intestine of harmful bacteria and toxins. Antidiarrheal agents, by slowing the movement of the intestine, actually prolong the time that these poisons remain in the body.

The most promising and least toxic method of preventing and treating traveler's diarrhea is with bismuth subsalicylate, better known by its familiar trade name Pepto-Bismol. In a 1980 study published in the *Journal of the American Medical Association*, researchers at the University of Texas confirmed their earlier observations that Pepto-Bismol in doses of 2 ounces taken every six hours will prevent traveler's diarrhea at least 75 percent of the time. For the person suffering with traveler's diarrhea, a dose of 1 to 2 ounces every thirty minutes for eight doses will significantly reduce the episodes of diarrhea and bring subjective relief from abdominal cramps within twenty-four hours. One drawback of the Pepto-Bismol treatment plan is that a traveler will consume an 8-ounce bottle each day. A couple traveling to Mexico for a three-week visit would have to pack forty-two 8-ounce bottles of Pepto-Bismol. That would hardly leave room for a bathing suit.

Another more serious concern about the use of Pepto-Bismol is that it contains a form of salicylate, the same compound found in aspirin. The recommended daily dosage of Pepto-Bismol for the treatment of traveler's diarrhea is equivalent to about eight aspirin tablets. Aspirin ingestion in pregnancy, especially during the last month, may be associated with fetal complications (see chapter 7). Though it has been theorized that prolonged ingestion of the bismuth in Pepto-Bismol may cause neurological toxicity, to date there are no known reports of such an occurrence.

Regardless of the cause of the diarrhea, the most important rule of therapy is to replace the water, sodium chloride, potassium, and bicarbonate that is lost in the stool. In mild and moderately severe cases, rehydration with broths, carbonated drinks, or preparations such as Gatorade usually suffice. A solution, sold in many countries under the brand names ORS or Oralyte, is also recommended. For more severe diarrhea, fluids should contain sugar, which helps in the absorption of sodium and chloride from the intestine into the bloodstream.

Both the Center for Disease Control and the World Health Organization have established formulas for fluid replacement in the treatment of moderately severe diarrhea. These solutions can be made up readily with materials found in even the most remote markets or stores. If either of these treatment schedules is followed,

Formulas for Treatment of Diarrheal Disease

Very mild
Any convenient source of drinkable water, Gatorade if available.

Moderate

World Health Organization regimen:
   Sodium chloride (table salt), 3.5g (4 tsp.)
   Sodium bicarbonate (baking soda), 2.5g (3 tsp.)
   Potassium chloride, 1.5g
   Glucose, 20g, or sucrose, 40g
   Instructions: Dissolve in 1 liter drinkable water. Drink 2 to 5 liters per day

Center for Disease Control regimen:
   Prepare one glass each of the following:

Glass No. 1
8 oz. apple, orange, or pineapple juice
½ tsp. honey or corn syrup
1 pinch table salt

Glass No. 2
8 oz. boiled or carbonated water
½ tsp. baking soda

Instructions: Drink alternately from each glass and supplement with carbonated beverages or water and tea made with boiled or carbonated water as desired. Avoid solid foods and milk until recovery occurs.

Severe
Hospitalization and intravenous fluids recommended.

intraveneous fluid replacement is rarely required. These formulas are given in the accompanying box.

The pregnant woman must be especially careful in taking antibiotics for acute traveler's diarrhea. *Escherichia coli*, the most common cause of traveler's diarrhea, rarely requires antibiotic therapy. However, for those severe cases in which the organism invades the intestinal wall, ampicillin has been found to be safe during pregnancy provided there is no history of penicillin allergy. Ampicillin is also valuable in the treatment of shigella and salmonella. Tetracyclines and a combination of trimethoprim and sulfamethoxazole (trade names Bactrim and Septra) are excellent medications for treating shigella but should never be taken during pregnancy (see chapter 7). Similarly, chloramphenicol is effective against salmonella but should not be prescribed during pregnancy. Metronidazole (trade name Flagyl) or quinicrine (trade name Atabrine) are equally effective in the treatment of giardia. Of the two quinicrine is preferred for use during pregnancy. Furozolidone, another effective medication against giardia, is not recommended during pregnancy. Paromomycin is the name of a new antibiotic which recently has been used to safely and effectively treat giardiasis during pregnancy. If these preliminary reports can be confirmed, it will become the drug of choice for this condition. Quite often, giardia causes minimal if any symptoms, and treatment can usually be delayed until after delivery. Since there is no reasonably acceptable alternative in the treatment of a potentially dangerous amebiasis infection during pregnancy, Flagyl must be given together with diiodohydroxyquin (trade name Iodoquinol).

7.
Medications

Until the early 1960s, doctors and their patients were not as aware as they should have been that medications given to a mother might adversely affect her baby. A tranquilizer named thalidomide changed all that. This drug, first used in Germany, was responsible for the birth worldwide of 5,000 to 10,000 children with limb deformities.

Another drug, diethylstilbestrol, or DES, used since the 1940s to prevent miscarriage, has recently been associated with characteristic abnormalities of the genital tract of both female and male offspring born of these pregnancies. In addition to a greater likelihood of pregnancy complications, DES daughters must live with the fear of contracting an unusual and potentially lethal form of vaginal and cervical cancer (see questions on the "morning-after" pill, page 15).

Although these events have made us aware of the effect medicine has on the mother and the fetus, an estimated 90 percent of all pregnant women take at least one medication during the course of their pregnancies. Furthermore, it is estimated that 75 percent take drugs that are not prescribed and that the average pregnant woman uses approximately four different medications throughout her pregnancy. The most commonly prescribed drugs are analgesics for pain relief and antiemetics for relief of morning sickness.

Almost all chemical substances can cross the placenta and become concentrated in the fetus. Whether or not a drug causes harm depends on many factors, including the genetic makeup of mother and fetus, the specific chemical structure of the drug, the month of pregnancy in which the drug is used, and the total dose. There are a host of medications that damage the fetus only during early pregnancy, when organ and limb formation take place. Others cause harm only during the last three months, while a third group appears to be most dangerous when administered immediately before delivery.

During the past few years, both drug manufacturers and the FDA have been criticized for rushing products on the market before their safety has been determined with certainty. Unfortunately, it is impossible to be absolutely sure that any drug is safe before it is marketed. Even after extensive clinical testing, relatively little is known about the prenatal effects of most drugs, because some fetal defects are so rare that they only surface after thousands of pregnant women have been treated. We are faced with a dilemma: on the one hand it is ethically wrong to perform extensive clinical trials of a new drug on pregnant women, but it is just as irresponsible to allow a relatively untested drug on the market. Laboratory studies on pregnant animals, even when they are extensive, are still poor predictors of what will happen when a pregnant woman is given the same drug.

Effects of medications on the baby do not end at childbirth since many harmful substances can be rapidly transmitted from mother to nursing infant via the breast milk. Concentrations in the milk vary, again depending on the drug's chemical structure. While some medications appear only in trace amounts, others are highly concentrated and potentially harmful to the infant, particularly during the baby's first month, when certain enzyme systems which normally metabolize and detoxify drugs are not fully developed.

The list of potentially harmful drugs is expanding daily, and though a cause-and-effect relationship has not been clearly defined in all instances, the prudent woman should avoid all medication during pregnancy and nursing unless absolutely necessary. On the other hand, many medications have been proven to be safe for use during pregnancy and the postpartum period. To refuse treatment even when it is medically indicated and necessary is as dangerous as to use drugs indiscriminately. This very important chapter evaluates the various categories of drugs which may be prescribed for the pregnant woman, providing an up-to-date reference for the concerned woman who wants to be sure that any medication she takes is safe for her and her baby.

Antibiotics

How safe are antibiotics for pregnant and nursing women?

Too often, antibiotics are prescribed for inappropriate reasons, such as colds and viral sore throats. When the diagnosis is in doubt, your doctor should obtain a culture for bacterial growth before beginning treatment.

Of all antibiotics prescribed, **penicillin** is one of the safest for use during pregnancy. In addition, there are the **synthetic penicillins**—ampicillin, amoxicillin, mezlocillin, piperacillin and bacampicillin—which are sold under a variety of trade names. These drugs, unlike penicillin, are effective against a broad spectrum of bacteria, such as those commonly associated with urinary and respiratory tract infections. Patients who are allergic to penicillin are likely to experience a similar reaction to these medications, however, so individuals with this type of allergy should not take them.

It has been reported that ampicillin and amoxicillin, when administered during the third trimester, may lower the concentration of estriol in the plasma and urine by 30 to 50 percent. Estriol measurement is used as a method of determining fetal well-being during the last two months of pregnancy. Though ampicillin and amoxicillin do not harm the fetus, they may lower the urinary estriol concentration to the point where the test may be invalid. An obstetrician who is unaware of the relationship between ampicillin use and low estriols may intervene unnecessarily in a healthy pregnancy.

Penicillin, ampicillin, and amoxicillin are rapidly transferred to the breast milk.

Babies born with a genetic susceptibility to develop a serious penicillin allergy at a later time may become initially sensitized to these medications while nursing. There are reports in the medical literature of babies who have developed skin rashes, itching, and diarrhea problems following breast-feeding when their mothers have been taking these drugs. For this reason, it is imperative that nursing infants whose mothers are being treated with these antibiotics be carefully and continuously observed for early signs of a drug reaction.

Other newer penicillin derivatives such as oxacillin, methicillin, carbenicillin, piperacillin, and hetacillin are usually reserved for serious infections that threaten the life and health of the pregnant woman. The safety of these preparations for use during pregnancy has not been documented, but they do appear to be safe for the developing fetus and nursing infant.

Cephalosporins are a group of antibiotics which have been used extensively by practicing physicians in recent years. Studies show that in the usual therapeutic doses they cross the placenta and produce significant blood levels in the fetus. To date, however, no toxic effects have been reported, so cephalosporins are considered acceptable for use by pregnant women.

There are many antibiotics in the cephalosporin group, with newer, more effective, and safer drugs being introduced each year. Examples of cephalosporins are cefazolin (trade names Ancef and Kefzol), cephradine (trade names Anspor and Velosef), cephalexin (trade name Keflex), cephalothin (trade name Keflin), cefoxitin (trade name Mefoxin), cefadroxil (trade name Ultracef, Duracef), cefaclor (trade name Ceclor), and cephapirin (trade name Cefadyl). Cefamandole nafate (trade name Mandol), cefoperazone (trade name Cefobid), moxalactam (trade name Moxam), and cefotaxime (trade name Claforan), are relatively new and popular drugs which are similar to the cephalosporins in chemical structure and antibacterial activity, so they are included here.

All the cephalosporins are excreted in the breast milk during lactation. To date, laboratory animal studies and human experience have not demonstrated adverse effects on the nursing infant.

Erythromycin is a popular antibiotic which is often prescribed for individuals who are allergic to penicillin. It crosses the placenta in far lower concentrations than does penicillin, and to date there have been no reports of fetal abnormalities or illness resulting from its use during pregnancy. The fact that so little of this antibiotic reaches the fetus is both an advantage and a source of concern to doctors who use this drug in the treatment of syphilis during pregnancy (see chapter 5).

Though erythromycin is generally a very safe antibiotic, it may cause impaired though reversible liver dysfunction and a condition called cholestatic hepatitis. Of the erythromycin compounds, erythromycin estolate (trade name Ilosone) is most often associated with this complication. The symptoms, jaundice, severe generalized itching of the skin, weakness, nausea, vomiting, abdominal cramps, and fever subside when the antibiotic is stopped.

The hormonal changes of pregnancy can cause changes in the liver similar to those produced with Ilosone and some susceptible women suffer with what is termed recurrent cholestasis during each pregnancy, with symptoms ranging from mild discomfort to severe itching and marked jaundice. Erythromycins in general, and Ilosone in particular, are best avoided by these women and by any women with a history of liver disease. For the pregnant women who does not have a history of liver disease, erythromycin preparations other than Ilosone should be used.

Sulfonamides such as sulfisoxazole, more commonly known by its trade name Gantrisin, are very effective in treating urinary tract infections during pregnancy. If taken in the last month, however, sulfonamides can cause jaundice in the newborn infant. Since a woman's expected date of confinement may be inaccurate, and since premature labor is always a possibility, sulfonamides should not be used during the last eight weeks of pregnancy, nor should they be prescribed for women who intend to nurse their babies, because sulfonamides rapidly cross the placental barrier and are excreted in the breast milk.

Some of the newer sulfonamide preparations are combined in a single tablet with another drug named trimethoprim. The trade names of this combination are Septra and Bactrim. Convincing reproductive studies in rats and rabbits have demonstrated a significant increase in the incidence of cleft palate and fetal death among fetuses exposed to trimethoprim. Septra and Bactrim should not be given during pregnancy. Trimpex, and Proloprim, which contain only trimethoprim, were introduced recently as urinary antibacterial agents. Naturally, they too should be avoided during pregnancy and nursing.

Novobiocin, a seldom-used antibiotic, produces jaundice in a fashion identical to that of the sulfonamides and may also cause an abnormally low platelet count (thrombocytopenia) in infants whose mothers are given this antibiotic before delivery.

Pyridium and Urised are the trade names of two urinary anesthetics which are used to relieve symptoms of painful urinary tract infections. Pyridium, or phenazopyridine hydrochloride, turns the urine into a beautiful reddish-orange color. It is available combined with sulfonamides in a single tablet, such as Azo Gantanol and Azo Gantrisin. Urised is composed of six different compounds. It changes the appearance of the urine to a characteristic striking blue color. Either drug can safely be taken during pregnancy or breast feeding.

Though **tetracyclines** are popularly used to treat infections in nonpregnant individuals, they are among the most dangerous drugs when prescribed during pregnancy. Deaths from liver failure have been reported for pregnant women given large doses of intravenous tetracyclines as treatment of severe kidney infections.

Tetracyclines rapidly cross the placenta and, when prescribed during the last half of pregnancy, may cause a yellow-green discoloration of the baby teeth, underdevelopment of tooth enamel, and a decrease in the growth of the long bones of the fetus. After years of exposure to light, the yellow-green tooth color becomes gray to brown. Experimental studies on laboratory animals given tetracycline early in pregnancy have suggested that it is also toxic at this time.

Tetracyclines are excreted in breast milk and may hinder tooth development and normal tooth coloration in the nursing infant. Women who intend to breast-feed their babies must not take tetracyclines. Since tooth development may be adversely affected until the eighth year of life, it is also best to avoid this drug when treating childhood infections.

There are several types of tetracyclines, including Achromycin, Aureomycin, Declomycin, Minocin, Sumycin, Terramycin, Tetrex, Vibramycin, and Vectrin. All are equally dangerous.

Chloramphenicol (trade name Chloromycetin) is a potent broad-spectrum antibiotic which is metabolized well by the mother but poorly handled by the infant. A high concentration of this drug in a newborn, especially a premature infant, may result in the "gray baby syndrome," also known as the "gray syndrome." Manifestations of this disorder include abdominal distention, labored respirations, circulatory collapse, and death of 40 percent of affected infants within a few hours after the onset of symptoms. When the fetus is in utero, the maternal liver enzyme system is able to metabolize the drug, and "gray baby syndrome" usually does not occur. Despite this, there are far safer alternative medications for use during pregnancy, and chloramphenicol is best avoided. Since chloramphenicol also appears in the breast milk, it should not be given to a nursing woman.

Nitrofurantoin (trade names Macrodantin and Furadantin) is a drug commonly used for treating urinary tract infections. Though the safety of nitrofurantoin during pregnancy and nursing has not been established, there have been only a few case reports of hemolytic anemia in newborns following maternal use of the drug immediately before delivery. As a result, it is not recommended during the last weeks of pregnancy. A hemolytic anemia is one in which the red blood cells are destroyed too rapidly. This results in an accumulation of blood pigments in the skin which cause jaundice. Fortunately, the hemolytic anemia subsides once exposure to the drug is eliminated following delivery.

Nalidixic acid is another popular urinary antibiotic which is more commonly known by its trade name NegGram. Though the drug has not been studied extensively during the first trimester, reports of its use during the second and third trimesters have all been favorable.

On rare occasions, infants treated with this drug in high doses have experienced neurological disturbances such as headaches, agitation, and even convulsions. These symptoms subsided as soon as the drug was discontinued. It is highly unlikely that the reduced concentrations of nalidixic acid in breast milk can cause similar problems for the nursing infant. However, if a safe alternative urinary antibiotic is available, I would advise that it be substituted.

Clindamycin hydrochloride (trade name Cleocin HCl) is a new antibiotic which is unique in its ability to destroy a variety of anaerobic bacteria, which live and reproduce within necrotic tissue and abscesses containing no oxygen. The most infamous anaerobic bacterium, named *Bacteroides fragilis,* is the culprit in many life-threatening infections. A small percentage of patients using this drug will develop a severe form of colitis which may even prove fatal.

Experience with clindamycin among pregnant women is quite limited, and as a result its safety during pregnancy is not known. It has been detected in significant concentrations in breast milk, however so the prudent suggestion would be to discourage breast-feeding among mothers who require this antibiotic.

Lincomycin is a drug similar in structure to clindamyin but lacking both its potency and its toxic effects. Two studies involving 600 patients indicated no detectable increase in fetal or perinatal complications when Lincomycin was used. Lincomycin appears in the breast milk but is believed to be harmless to the infant.

The **aminoglycosides** are a group of potent antibiotics which are frequently used to treat serious bacterial infections. They are administered intramuscularly and intravenously and are therefore practically always limited to use within the hospital. Streptomycin is the oldest of the group; while still used in the treatment of tuberculosis, it has been replaced in most other instances of infection by newer aminoglycosides such as amikacin sulfate (trade name Amikin), gentamicin sulfate (trade name Garamycin), kanamycin sulfate (trade name Kantrex), and tobramycin sulfate (trade name Nebcin).

All aminoglycosides readily cross the placenta and have the capacity to damage the infant's eighth cranial nerve in the brain. This nerve, named the auditory nerve, is responsible for hearing and balance. To date, there have been more than thirty cases of hearing deficit and auditory nerve damage in infants exposed to streptomycin in utero. Streptomycin has also been implicated in causing spinal cord and bone abnormalities in experimental animals and human beings. The other aminoglycosides have not been similarly indicted.

As expected, the longer that the fetus is exposed to aminoglycosides, the more likely is the risk of auditory nerve damage. If these antibiotics must be used—and often there is no adequate substitute—they should be administered at the lowest possible effective dose for as short a time as possible. Since aminoglycosides can be transferred to an infant in the breast milk, I would advise against nursing if these drugs must be used.

Are there any other commonly prescribed antiinfective agents which may adversely affect either pregnancy or nursing?

Metronidazole (trade name Flagyl) has been mentioned as a valuable drug in the treatment of trichomoniasis (see chapter 5) and a variety of parasitic diseases. Though it is also effective in the management of certain bacterial infections, its potential for producing abnormalities makes its use inadvisable, especially during the first trimester. When administered to nursing women, Flagyl is secreted in the breast milk. The subsequent effects on the infant are unknown but some researchers theorize that it could cause loss of appetite, vomiting, and a lowering of the white blood cell count. As previously mentioned (see chapter 6), when a single oral dose of Flagyl is taken by a nursing woman it reaches maximum concentrations in her breast milk two to four hours later. Recent studies suggest that Flagyl can probably be taken if nursing is delayed for twelve to twenty-four hours, when the levels in the milk are minimal.

Antituberculosis drugs may also pose problems. Isoniazid (trade name INH), although the most popular, should be prescribed during pregnancy only when absolutely necessary, since it has been associated with a higher spontaneous abortion rate in laboratory animals. Though the use of INH is not restricted if a woman is breastfeeding, the manufacturer cautions that babies be carefully observed for adverse effects which include vomiting, hepatitis, and neurological abnormalities. My own

Table 7–1. Safety of Antibiotics During Pregnancy and Nursing

Drug Class	Generic and Trade Names of Drugs*	Suggestions for Pregnancy	Suggestions for Nursing
Aminoglycosides	amikacin (Amikin), gentamycin (Garamycin), kanamycin (Kantrex), streptomycin (Streptomycin) tobramycin (Nebcin)	All aminoglycosides readily cross the placenta and may cause damage to the auditory nerve of the fetus: streptomycin may be responsible for a higher rate of spinal cord and bone abnormalities; use only if absolutely necessary	Aminoglycosides found in breast milk; best not to nurse if they are used
Cephalosporins	cefaclor (Ceclor), cefamandole nafate (Mandol), cefazolin (Ancef, Kefzol), cephalexin (Keflex), cephalothin (Keflin), cephapirin (Cafadyl), cephradine (Anspor, Velosef)	Safe for use	Safe for use
Chloramphenicol	chloramphenicol (Chloromycetin)	"Gray baby syndrome" may occur in newborns; should not be taken in pregnancy	Found in significant concentrations in breast milk: not to be taken if nursing
Clindamycin	clindamycin (Cleocin HC1)	No known harmful effects	Discourage breast feeding, though no known harmful effects
Erythromycins	erythromycin (Ilotycin, Pediamycin, Pediazole, Robimycin, E-Mycin), erythromycin estolate (Ilosone), erythromycin ethylsuccinate (E.E.S., E-MycinE, WyamycinE), erythromycin stearate (Erythrocin, Bristamycin, Ethril, SK-Erythromycin, Pfizer-E Film Coated Tablets)	Erythromycins, especially erythromycin estolate, may cause liver disorders and cholestatic hepatitis; may lower estriol levels	Avoid if woman has history of liver disease
Lincomycin	lincomycin (Lincocin)	Extensive use in pregnancy has demonstrated no adverse fetal effects; safe for use	Appears in breast milk without ill effect to the nursing infant
Nalidixic acid	nalidixic acid (NegGram)	No harmful effects reported during pregnancy; considered safe	1 reported case of hemolytic anemia in nursing infant with G6PD deficiency; some infants tolerate drug poorly; best avoided
Nitrofurantoins	nitrofurantoin (Furadantin, Macrodantin, Nitrex)	Safe for use	Safe for use though rare cases of hemolytic anemia in babies with G6PD deficiency

Table 7–1. Safety of Antibiotics During Pregnancy and Nursing *(continued)*

Drug Class	Generic and Trade Names of Drugs*	Suggestions for Pregnancy	Suggestions for Nursing
Penicillins	penicillin G (Bicillin, Pentids, Pfizerpen, SK-Penicillin G, Crysticillin, Duracillin, Wycillin) penicillin V (Betapen, Ledercillin, Pen. VeeK, Robicillin, Veetids, V-Cillin K, Uticillin, SK-Penicillin VK)	Safe for use	Safe for use
Sulfonamides	sulfacytine (Renoquid), sulfadiazine (Suladyne), sulfamethizole (Microsul, Thiosulfil), sulfamethoxazole (Azo Gantanol, Gantanol), sulfasalazine (Azulfidine), sulfisoxazole (Gantrisin, Azo Gantrisin, SK-Soxazole)	Should not be taken during last 4 weeks of pregnancy; may cause jaundice in newborn	Should not be taken while nursing; may cause jaundice in baby
Sulfonamide combinations	sulfamethizole and tetracycline (Azotrex, Urobiotic)	See information on tetracyclines	See information on tetracyclines
	sulfamethoxazole and trimethoprim (Septra, Bactrim)	Laboratory animals exposed to trimethoprim demonstrate high incidence of cleft palate and fetal death. Sulfonamides in last 4 weeks may cause jaundice in newborn	Should not be taken when nursing
Synthetic penicillins	amoxicillin (Amoxil, Larotid, Polymox, Robamox, Trimox, Wymox), ampicillin (Amcill, Omnipen, Pen A Capsules, Penbritin, Pensyn, Polycillin, SK-Ampicillin, Totacillin, Principen), oxacillin (Bactocill, Prostaphlin), methicillin (Celbinin, Staphcillin), carbenicillin (Geocillin, Pyopen)	No harmful effects during pregnancy but may lower estriol levels: safe for use	Safe, but nursing infant may develop skin rash, itching, and diarrhea on rare occasions
Tetracyclines	tetracycline (Achromycin, Aureomycin, Declomycin, Minocin, Sumycin, Terramycin, Tetrex, Vectrin)	If taken during the last half of pregnancy, will cause discoloration of baby teeth, underdevelopment of tooth enamel, and decrease in growth of long bones	Normal tooth development and color hindered in nursing infant; should never be taken when nursing
Trimethoprim	trimethoprim (Trimpex)	As above	As above

NOTE: *All prescription drugs.

feeling is that these potential problems are too serious to justify breast-feeding by women taking INH.

Rifampin (trade names Rifadin, Rifamate, and Rimactane) is one of the newest drugs used in the treatment of tuberculosis. Experimental studies have shown anomalies of the spine and cleft palate in rats and mice exposed to rifampin in utero. Human experience is limited but encouraging—in one report of 313 tubercular women treated with rifampin during pregnancy, there was no evidence of congenital anomalies—but too little is known about rifampin to recommend its use during pregnancy. Since only a very small percentage of rifampin given to a woman enters the breast milk, it is probably safe for nursing mothers.

Ethionamide (trade name Trecator-SC) is used in the treatment of active tuberculosis when the usual medications fail to adequately eradicate the disease. If at all possible, it should be avoided during pregnancy. In one human study, seven of twenty-three infants born of mothers treated with ethionamide had anomalies, most commonly of the brain and spinal cord.

Ethambutol (trade name Myambutol) is a drug which has gained popularity in the treatment of tuberculosis. Ethambutol's ability to cause abnormalities in experimental animals, including cleft palate as well as heart, vertebral column, and central nervous system abnormalities, is well established. Exposure to this drug in human pregnancy has not been associated with fetal abnormalities or evidence of growth retardation. Ethambutol is excreted in the breast milk, but its effects on a nursing infant are unknown at the present time.

Paraaminosalicylic acid is no longer as frequently used to treat tuberculosis, but most experts agree that it is not harmful to the pregnant woman or her fetus.

Analgesics

Analgesics, medications used to relieve pain, are undoubtedly the most commonly prescribed class of drugs during pregnancy, labor and delivery, and the postpartum period.

How safe is aspirin during pregnancy?

Until recently aspirin and aspirin-containing products were consumed by approximately 80 percent of all pregnant women. This is no longer true, and I now caution my pregnant patients to strictly avoid aspirin and products which contain aspirin. Unfortunately, too many women refuse to heed this advice.

Laboratory studies on rats and mice given extremely high doses of aspirin early in pregnancy have demonstrated a greater incidence of malformations, although evidence of human malformations is still considered circumstantial. There are other controversial reports about the effects of aspirin during pregnancy. In one study, doctors determined that the weights of infants whose mothers took aspirin throughout pregnancy were significantly lower than for those whose mothers took no drugs at all, and the incidence of stillbirths and neonatal deaths was significantly higher in the aspirin-treated group. Another report, however, found no relationship between prenatal aspirin use and these complications.

When a woman takes excessive amounts of aspirin during the last two weeks of pregnancy, a newborn may experience salicylate or aspirin intoxication. When the concentration of aspirin in the blood declines, withdrawal symptoms will usually be noted in the baby within forty-eight hours. These include a generalized increase in muscle tone, irritability, agitation, and a shrill cry.

Prostaglandins are chemical substances produced by the body which have the capacity to stimulate strong uterine contractions. Aspirin is one of several drugs which are classified as prostaglandin inhibitors (see chapter 10). When aspirin is taken late in pregnancy, it may actually delay both the onset and completion of labor by preventing prostaglandin release. Prostaglandin inhibitors, including aspirin, have also been implicated in causing the premature closure or narrowing of a fetal blood vessel near the heart named the ductus arteriosis. This vessel usually remains open until immediately after birth. If it closes when the infant is still in utero, it may lead to a serious heart and lung disease in the newborn named pulmonary hypertension.

In addition to aspirin, other prostaglandin inhibitors commonly used for pain relief must also be avoided during pregnancy. This would include ibuprofen (trade name Motrin), mefenamic acid (trade name Ponstel), naproxen (Anaprox and Naprosyn), indomethacin (Indocin), diflunisal (Dolobid), zomepirac (Zomax), sulindac (Clinoril), tolmetin (Tolectin), and meclofenamate (Meclomen).

A potentially more serious complication of aspirin use late in pregnancy is alterations in blood platelet adhesiveness, resulting in a higher incidence of maternal bleeding both before and after delivery, as well as a greater risk of intracranial hemorrhage and death in the newborn infant. Though this is especially likely to occur when aspirin is used chronically in significant amounts of more than ten tablets per day, research has shown that maternal ingestion of as little as one aspirin may cause abnormal platelet changes which could last for four to seven days. Premature infants are especially susceptible to intracranial hemorrhage if their mothers took aspirin.

Although aspirin is excreted in breast milk, in normal therapeutic doses the effects on a nursing infant would appear to be minimal. However, high maternal doses of more than fifteen aspirins per day may cause a baby to develop a generalized body rash and respiratory distress. If a nursing mother uses aspirin, the risk to her infant will be minimized if she takes it just after nursing, since most of the drug will be metabolized by the next feeding several hours later.

Unfortunately, too few patients and doctors realize that aspirin is an ingredient in a great number of analgesics, including A.P.C., Anacin, Ascriptin, Empirin, Arthritis Strength and regular Bufferin, Arthritis Pain Formula, Darvon Compound, Darvon Compound-65, Equagesic, Fiorinal, and Percodan. Excedrin, a very popular over-the-counter preparation, contains salicylamide, which is closely related to the salicylic acid found in aspirin and should not be taken during pregnancy either.

What safe alternatives are there to aspirin for pain relief during pregnancy?

Acetaminophen (trade names Tylenol, Datril, and Phenaphen) does not produce the adverse reactions associated with aspirin use. It is a safe nonprescription analgesic for use during all trimesters of pregnancy and while nursing.

Propoxyphene is the scientific name for one of the most commonly used and abused analgesics prescribed in the United States. Medications which contain propoxyphene include all compounds containing the name Darvon and Darvocet. Wygesic, another frequently used pain medication, contains propoxyphene and acetaminophen. The safety of propoxyphene during the first two trimesters of pregnancy has not been established. However, there are case reports in the medical literature in which chronic use by pregnant women has resulted in withdrawal symptoms in their newborns: tremors, high-pitched cry, irritability, hyperactivity, sweating, diarrhea, weight loss in the presence of a ravenous appetite, and seizures. Most researchers conclude that this will not occur if the drug is taken in normal therapeutic doses.

Pentazocine (trade name Talwin) is a nonnarcotic analgesic which relieves moderate to severe pain. Although pentazocine is often used as a substitute for patients who are addicted, sensitive, or allergic to narcotics, drug dependence may develop following prolonged use. The safety of pentazocine during pregnancy has not been established. However, animals studied have not produced offspring with deformities. Chronic maternal use during pregnancy has resulted in the birth of addicted newborns. Withdrawal symptoms in these babies include tremors, inability to feed, and hyperactivity. Women given this drug only during labor have experienced no adverse effects. Similarly, their newborns have fared well. Despite this, the manufacturer of pentazocine suggests that the drug be used with caution in women delivering premature infants who are less able to metabolize and inactivate this drug.

Interestingly, pentazocine is not excreted in the breast milk, so it is an ideal analgesic for the nursing woman who is experiencing moderate to severe pain.

Zomepirac sodium (trade name Zomax) is a nonaddicting analgesic recently introduced for the treatment of mild to moderately severe pain. Too little is known about this drug to recommend its use during pregnancy or nursing.

Phenacetin is an analgesic which may cause a condition named methemoglobinemia in certain sensitive newborns. With other safer medications available, phenacetin is certainly not the analgesic of choice for pregnant women. Medications which contain phenacetin include A.P.C., Fiorinal, Percodan, Percodan-Demi, and Synalgos-DC.

What are ergot alkaloids, and how can they affect the outcome of pregnancy and lactation?

Ergot alkaloids are a group of drugs commonly used for the relief of vascular and migraine headaches. Popular trade names are Cafergot (ergotamine tartrate and caffeine) and Sansert (methysergide maleate). They should not be taken during pregnancy because they can cause severe uterine contractions, lack of fetal oxygen, and miscarriage.

Ergot preparations have been reported to enter the breast milk in high concentrations and produce ergotism, or ergot poisoning, in nursing infants. Symptoms of ergotism include weakness, vomiting, diarrhea, weak pulse, and an unstable blood pressure. These drugs also significantly decrease the amount of breast milk.

Ergonovine maleate (trade name Ergotrate Maleate) and methylergonovine maleate (trade name Methergine) are ergot preparations which, by contracting the muscles of the uterus, help to decrease the amount of blood loss following abortion and childbirth. Their use following childbirth, however, should be restricted to women who do not intend to nurse.

How safe are the narcotic analgesics during pregnancy and labor?

Though the hazards of narcotic abuse on the outcome of pregnancy have been discussed in chapter 4, several of these drugs have been used with great success in the treatment of moderate to severe pain during pregnancy, labor, and the postpartum period. When taken in the correct therapeutic doses during the first two trimesters of pregnancy, no increased incidence of fetal loss, chromosomal damage, or physical abnormalities has been noted.

Codeine is probably the most commonly prescribed narcotic during the first eight months of pregnancy. An even greater degree of pain relief may be safely obtained during pregnancy when codeine is combined with acetaminophen in a single pill. Empracet with Codeine, Phenaphen with Codeine, and Tylenol with Codeine are examples of this safe and effective analgesic combination.

There is no known relationship between codeine use during the first two trimesters and fetal deaths or abnormalities. Though codeine is transmitted through the breast milk, when it is taken in normal therapeutic doses it will not depress the reflexes or respirations of the nursing infant.

Oxycodone hydrochloride is described in the pharmaceutical literature as a semisynthetic narcotic. It is the main ingredient of a pill named Percodan, one of the most abused drugs in the United States. There are no studies which demonstrate either the safety or potential harm of oxycodone on the developing fetus or nursing infant. However, the other ingredients of Percodan, aspirin, phenacetin, and caffeine, should discourage a nursing woman from using this medication. The same may be said for Percodan-Demi, even though the dose of oxycodone is one-half that found in Percodan. Percocet-5 is probably a safer alternative during pregnancy, since it contains only oxycodone and acetaminophen rather than aspirin, phenacetin, and caffeine. To thoroughly confuse the consumer, Endo Laboratories manufactures a nonprescription tablet named Percogesic for the relief of mild to moderate pain. It contains acetaminophen and phenyltoloxamine citrate, but not oxycodone as one would expect, so it is safe for use during pregnancy and the postpartum period.

All narcotics pass rapidly from the maternal to the fetal circulation and brain tissues via the placenta. Unfortunately, the fetus metabolizes these drugs and transfers them back to the maternal circulation at a far slower rate than they are received. Narcotics used inappropriately during labor have caused respiratory depression, poor muscle tone, slowing of the heartbeat (bradycardia), and lowered body temperature (hypothermia) in the newborn infant.

When sedatives and tranquilizers are used in combination with narcotics (to enhance the narcotic's action) the depressive effects on the baby may be greater.

Nor is there much evidence to support the value of this practice. On the contrary, research suggests that barbiturates may actually reduce the analgesic effects of narcotics.

The use of narcotics during labor should be restricted in women with specific pregnancy problems such as prematurity and fetal growth retardation since their infants are known to be more sensitive to these drugs. The reason for this is that the placenta of a fetus in difficulty is unable to transfer the metabolized narcotic back to the maternal circulation as rapidly as that of a healthy fetus.

Do not pressure your obstetrician into using more medication during labor than is safe. All analgesic preparations have the capacity to cross the placenta and cause respiratory depression. Since this is most likely to occur if an infant is delivered at the moment the drug is at peak concentrations, your doctor will try to coordinate the narcotic dose with your anticipated time of delivery. Unfortunately, predicting the time of birth is often difficult if not impossible, and occasionally a baby may be born with more than the desired amount of medication in its bloodstream. This situation may be remedied by injecting a so-called narcotic antagonist named naloxone hydrochloride (trade name Narcan) intramuscularly or directly into the blood vessels of the umbilical cord.

The analgesic selected for use during labor is often based on your doctor's personal experience with a particular agent. Meperidine (trade name Demerol) is by far the most popular, though some doctors prefer the shorter duration of action of alphaprodine hydrochloride (trade name Nisentyl). Most obstetricians have abandoned the use of morphine during labor because it is more likely than other narcotics to produce maternal nausea and infant respiratory depression. Hydromorphone hydrochloride (trade name Dilaudid) was once popular, but recent pharmacological studies suggest that significant levels of this drug may be found in the body for at least fourteen hours after it is given. This would obviously be extremely dangerous for a newborn infant whose mother received the drug during labor.

Butorphanol tartrate (trade name Stadol) is a new and potent analgesic which is stronger than meperidine and has the advantage of being nonaddicting. It is also far less likely than other analgesics to cause respiratory depression in the newborn. Since butorphanol is such a new drug, its safety for use in pregnancy and labor has not been established. The manufacturer cautions that at the present time butorphanol is not recommended for nursing women because it is not known if the drug is excreted in the breast milk. Despite these warnings, the reports available to date on its safety are very encouraging.

Nalbuphine hydrochloride (trade name Nubain) is another new analgesic which, unlike butorphanol, is addicting. Since nalbuphine is a new product, its safety for use during early pregnancy has not been confirmed. However, animal reproductive studies have not uncovered any harmful fetal effects. Though this drug has been used with success in the relief of pain during labor, it does cross the placenta and may be responsible for causing respiratory depression in the newborn. The safety of nalbuphine for the nursing infant remains unknown at the present time.

Can narcotic analgesics affect the length of labor and the tests that monitor fetal well-being during labor?

The latent or early phase of labor is characterized by the presence of uterine contractions without accompanying dilatation of the cervix. It is generally believed that narcotic analgesics administered at this time diminish the strength and frequency of uterine contractions and unnecessarily prolong the latent phase.

The active phase of labor is characterized by contractions which produce rapid cervical dilatation. Some investigators believe that once this phase is reached, medications exert little effect on slowing uterine activity and may sometimes enhance it. However, a 1976 study of labor patients given either morphine, meperidine, or alphaprodine, concluded that all these agents were more likely to reduce uterine activity than to increase it.

Use of narcotic analgesics during labor may alter the fetal heart rate pattern as it is observed on the electronic fetal monitor. Variability of the fetal heart rate is an encouraging sign that a baby is healthy. However, in a 1978 study of pregnant women receiving either intravenous meperidine, alphaprodine, or morphine during labor, doctors found a disturbing and significant decrease in fetal heart rate variability. Another ominous heart rate abnormality noted on a fetal monitor is the sinusoidal pattern (see chapter 10). In one study of forty women receiving alphaprodine for relief of labor pain, this pattern appeared in seventeen women and lasted an average of sixty minutes. However, these changes were not associated with obvious depression of the baby at birth.

Antinauseants and Antiemetics

What can I do about morning sickness?

Nausea and vomiting in early pregnancy is an extremely common occurrence which, until 1980, was most frequently treated with a medication named Bendectin. It has been estimated that 3 million women worldwide have taken Bendectin since its introduction in 1956, and that 20 percent of pregnant women in the United States have used it to combat morning sickness.

Originally, Bendectin contained three ingredients: dicyclomine to prevent stomach spasm, an antihistamine named doxylamine succinate, and pyridoxine, or vitamin B6, which has antinauseant properties. In 1976, dicyclomine was eliminated from Bendectin because it was found not to add to the drug's effectiveness.

Although many studies of women and laboratory research performed on rats and rabbits have produced no evidence to suggest that use of this drug by pregnant women is associated with an increased risk of birth defects, the FDA has in its files over 100 reports by physicians in which a woman who took Bendectin gave birth to a child with deformities. However, upon evaluating these cases in detail, no direct association could be established, since many of these women had other complicating medical conditions or used other drugs throughout their pregnancies. Claims have been made that this medication is responsible for defects of the heart and limbs, though the manufacturer vehemently denies the allegations and many impartial

Table 7–2. Safety of Antinauseants and Antiemetics During Pregnancy and Nursing

Generic and Trade Names of Drugs	Route of Administration	Suggestions for Pregnancy	Suggestions for Nursing
chlorpromazine (Thorazine)	capsules, tablets, liquid, intramuscular and intravenous injection; prescription required	Reported instances of jaundice, retinal damage, and delay in the onset of crying and breathing in newborn infants whose mothers had received chlorpromazine; studies on rodents show increased rate of fetal and newborn deaths; use in pregnancy only when absolutely necessary	Excreted in breast milk though no harmful effects reported; drug may actually increase amount of breast milk
cyclizine lactate (Marezine)	tablets and intramuscular injection; no prescription needed for tablets	Associated with fetal anomalies when given to pregnant rats, mice, and rabbits; best avoided	Effects on nursing infant unknown
dimenhydrinate (Dramamine)	tablets, liquid, suppositories, intramuscular and intravenous injection; no prescription needed for tablets and liquid	Safe for use in pregnancy	Effects on nursing infant unknown; probably safe
diphenhydramine (Benadryl)	capsules, liquid, intramuscular and intravenous injection; prescription required	No reports of harmful effects to fetus: considered safe; when used with narcotic medications during labor, may enhance narcotic effect and depress the newborn	Best avoided when nursing; may cause adverse reaction in the baby
doxylamine and pyridoxine	tablets; prescription required	Questionable association with birth defects; avoid use until more is known	Drug not indicated for use other than during pregnancy
hydroxyzine hydrochloride (Vistaril, Atarax)	capsules, liquid, intramuscular and intravenous injection; prescription required	Drug not to be used during pregnancy because of association with fetal abnormalities when given early in pregnancy to rats, mice, and rabbits; when used with narcotics in labor, may enhance narcotic effect and depress the newborn	Not recommended for nursing women
levulose, dextrose, and orthophosphoric acid (Emetrol)	liquid; no prescription needed	Safe for use in pregnancy	Unlikely to enter breast milk; safe for use
meclizine hydrochloride (Bonine, Antivert)	chewable tablets; no prescription needed	Contradictory reports; associated with birth defects in some studies; best avoided	Effects on nursing infant unknown

Table 7–2. Safety of Antinauseants and Antiemetics During Pregnancy and Nursing (*continued*)

Generic and Trade Names of Drugs	Route of Administration	Suggestions for Pregnancy	Suggestions for Nursing
perphenazine (Trilafon)	tablets, intramuscular and intravenous injection; prescription needed	Safe use of this drug and others in the phenothiazine group not established: contradictory results; some studies show increase in incidence of birth defects when used in first trimester; if given intravenously, may lower blood pressure, prolong labor and cause postpartum hemorrhage; best avoided	Phenothiazines excreted in breast milk, though no harmful effects reported; may actually increase amount of breast milk
prochlorperazine (Compazine)	tablets, capsules, suppositories, intramuscular and intravenous injection; prescription needed	This drug a phenothiazine; see above	Phenothiazines excreted in breast milk, though no harmful effects reported; may actually increase amount of breast milk
prochlorperazine and isopropamide iodide (Combid)	capsules; prescription needed	Suggestions as above for phenothiazines plus iodide could cross the placenta and alter fetal thyroid function; best avoided	Should not be taken by nursing women; isopropamide may inhibit lactation and iodide may depress fetal thyroid gland function
promethazine (Phenergan)	tablets, liquid, suppositories, intramuscular and intravenous injection; prescription needed	Probably safe; however, in 1 study possible association between its use and congenital hip dislocation reported; in another small study of women given this drug in labor, ¾ delivered infants with temporary blood platelet dysfunction: when used with narcotics in labor, may enhance the narcotic effect and depress the newborn; a phenothiazine (see suggestions above)	Effects on nursing infant unknown
thiethylperazine (Torecan)	tablets, suppositories, intramuscular injection; prescription needed	Should not be taken during pregnancy	Should not be taken when nursing; if must be prescribed, nursing should be stopped
trimethobenzamide hydrochloride (Tigan)	capsules, suppositories, intramuscular injection; prescription needed	Experimental studies on rats and rabbits show no birth defects, but higher stillborn rates; no adequate human pregnancy studies; best avoided	Effects on nursing infant are unknown; best avoided

studies, including an extensive 1979 survey conducted by the Center for Disease Control, do not support these claims.

It is not now possible to state positively that Bendectin is free of risk to the fetus. Until more conclusive findings are available, I have advised my patients not to use Bendectin during the first trimester of pregnancy. Safer alternatives such as eating dry crackers, chewing ice chips, and drinking only liquids which are very hot or very cold greatly alleviates symptoms and reduces the need for medication.

Antacids and Antispasmodics

Should I use antacids during pregnancy?

Well-known antacids such as Maalox, Amphojel, Mylanta, Mylicon, milk of magnesia, Gelusil, Titralac, and Camalox may all be safely used during pregnancy for the relief of heartburn and hyperacidity. Many of these compounds contain, or are combined with, antiflatulents for the relief of excessive gas.

Alka-Seltzer is not recommended during pregnancy since each tablet contains 276 milligrams of sodium, or salt.

Tagamet is the trade name for cimetidine, the newest and most popular drug used for treating conditions which are characterized by hyperacidity. Unlike other drugs, cimetidine acts by blocking the effects of histamine, the body chemical responsible for the release of acid from the stomach lining. Since the drug is so new, there has been little experience to date with the use of cimetidine by pregnant women. Though animal studies have demonstrated that it rapidly crosses the placenta to reach the fetus, there is no evidence that it causes developmental abnormalities. It is not known if cimetidine is excreted in human milk. Until more is learned about this excellent medication, it is best to avoid using it during pregnancy or while breast-feeding.

What other medications are there for the relief of gastrointestinal distress during pregnancy?

Some very popular medications which are prescribed for intestinal disorders are best avoided during pregnancy. One such example is Donnatal, a drug which contains a mixture of ingredients designed to decrease intestinal secretions, spasm, and motility. Unfortunately, each Donnatal capsule, tablet, and liquid teaspoonful contains 16 milligrams of phenobarbital, a barbiturate which may be associated with an increase in fetal abnormalities when taken during the first trimester of pregnancy. When taken late in pregnancy, phenobarbital may be responsible for drowsiness, respiratory depression, and withdrawal reactions in the newborn. Since this drug may pass into the breast milk, it is possible that a nursing infant may be adversely affected. Atropine sulfate, another ingredient of Donnatal, is a valuable agent in decreasing excessive intestinal and bronchial secretions. Though atropine is harmless to the developing fetus, when given to a nursing woman it can inhibit lactation.

Other nonrecommended products which contain phenobarbital and atropine are Donnazyme Tablets, Donnatal Extentabs, and Donnatal #2 Tablets. Bellergal, Bellergal-S, and Bentyl with Phenobarbital contain phenobarbital without atropine and should also be avoided. Donnagel, which has atropine but not phenobarbital, is probably safe for use during pregnancy.

Bentyl is the trade name for an antispasmodic named dicyclomine hydrochloride. It is available with and without phenobarbital; obviously, the latter is preferred during pregnancy. However, women who intend to nurse should be aware that dicyclomine hydrochloride may inhibit lactation.

Isopropamide iodide is an antispasmodic which is combined with the antinauseant prochlorperazine (trade name Compazine) in a capsule named Combid. I do not recommend this drug during pregnancy, since the iodide it contains may cross the placenta and, theoretically, could inhibit fetal thyroid function after the twelfth week of pregnancy. Isopropamide also has the capacity to diminish lactation in nursing women.

Pro-Banthine is the trade name for a popular drug named propantheline bromide. It has the dual capability of slowing excessive gastrointestinal motility and spasm while reducing stomach acid secretions. Experience among pregnant women treated with propantheline bromide over many years has not revealed evidence of fetal toxicity or abnormalities. Limited studies on nursing women suggest that there is no significant excretion of the drug in the breast milk. As with other antispasmodics, however, propantheline bromide may inhibit lactation.

Since many gastrointestinal disorders such as spastic colon, colitis, and peptic ulcer are often associated with significant degrees of anxiety and tension, manufacturers have combined the antispasmodic medications with the so-called minor tranquilizers in a single pill. Examples include Librax (chlordiazepoxide, trade name Librium, and clidinium bromide), Milpath (meprobamate, trade names Miltown, Equinal, and tridihexethyl chloride), and Pathibamate, which has the identical ingredients of Milpath. These preparations are mentioned only to be condemned. They should never be taken during pregnancy, especially during the first trimester. I also urge nursing women to avoid using minor tranquilizers or medications which contain minor tranquilizers.

How should I treat constipation during my pregnancy?

For most women, constipation is an annoying problem throughout pregnancy. It occurs because there is a relaxation of the smooth muscles of the intestinal tract at this time, thereby interfering with the forward wavelike movement, called peristalsis. Vitamin preparations which contain iron only serve to worsen this problem. Fortunately, none of the commonly used laxatives and stool softeners have ever been reported to cause harm to the developing fetus.

The woman who is breast-feeding, however, should select a laxative with care since some may cause increased bowel activity and diarrhea in the nursing infant. Preparations which contain cascara, such as Peri-Colace and Kondremul with Cascara, are best avoided. Similarly, laxatives with danthron, such as Doxidan, Modane, Laxatyl, Dorbantyl, Dorbane, and Doctate-P, should not be used. Stool softeners, saline catheretics, bulk-forming laxatives, mineral oil, and milk of magnesia are all harmless. Laxatives which contain senna, such as Senokot, Glysennid, and X-Prep

Liquid, will cause no problems for the nursing infant when administered in therapeutic doses. However, diarrhea has been reported in infants of mothers who have taken greater than normal amounts of senna. Phenolphthalein is the chemical found in many nonprescription laxative products such as Ex-lax, Argoral, Trilax, and Sarolax. While reports concerning the effects of these products on the nursing infant's bowel habits are contradictory, the general conclusion is that they are safe to use if taken in normal therapeutic doses.

Nasal Decongestants and Allergy and Asthma Drugs

What precautions should be taken in treating nasal congestion and allergic symptoms during pregnancy?

Considering the frequency with which obstetricians are asked to treat nasal congestion, allergic reactions, and bronchial asthma during pregnancy, there is an appalling lack of adequate research on the safety to medications used to relieve these conditions. Antihistamines and decongestants are prescribed with far greater frequency during pregnancy, since many women with no previous allergic history will suffer from a condition called "vasomotor rhinitis and sinusitis." This harmless though annoying problem is characterized by nasal stuffiness, mucous congestion, and postnasal secretions. Symptoms may appear at any time during pregnancy, only to mysteriously disappear within one or two days following delivery. Though the cause of vasomotor rhinitis and sinusitis during pregnancy is unknown, doctors believe that it is related to the many hormonal changes which affect women at this time.

Antihistamines are useful in the treatment of hives, adverse reactions to medications, sinusitis, and allergic rhinitis or inflammation of the membranes of the nose due to hay fever and specific agents such as dust or molds. In a 1977 epidemiologic study of thousands of women treated with antihistamines during the first five months of pregnancy, researchers concluded that brompheniramine, the chemical found in Dimetane, was statistically more likely than other agents to be associated with abnormalities in the newborn. Antihistamines containing diphenhydramine (trade name Benadryl), tripelennamine (Pyrobenzamine and PBZ), pheniramine (trade name Triaminic) and chlorpheniramine (trade name Chlor-Trimeton) were found to be safe when used judiciously during pregnancy, although the authors were quick to point out the many variables and tenuous conclusions of their studies.

Bronchial dilators are a group of medications which dilate or open, the respiratory passages. They are often used effectively in the treatment of bronchial asthma and may be combined with other medications in pills, liquids, and nasal sprays.

Theophylline (trade names Slo-Phyllin, Elixophyllin) is probably the most popular bronchial dilator. However, doctors have noted recently that there may be some problems associated with its use during pregnancy. A 1979 report found that asthmatic women receiving theophylline therapy had a longer average duration of labor than did untreated women. This is undoubtedly due to the muscle-relaxing action of this drug. In another article published in 1979, doctors found that two newborns and their mothers had comparable theophylline blood levels at the time of birth. While neither infant had any serious symptoms, it does demonstrate a baby's inability to metabolize and excrete this drug. Transient mild jitteriness and a rapid heart rate have been observed among some newborns whose mothers were found to have high levels of theophylline in their blood.

Cromolyn (trade name Intal) is a medication which, when used regularly, prevents flare-ups of severe bronchial asthma. It is especially beneficial for individuals in whom the frequency and intensity of asthmatic attacks are totally unpredictable. It is not a bronchial dilator or antihistamine and is of no benefit in treating an acute attack of asthma. It is used by being inhaled into the nasal passages with a special inhalator. Animal studies have demonstrated no adverse fetal affects of cromolyn at normal therapeutic levels. Though experience with the use of cromolyn in human pregnancy is limited, observations to date have shown no damaging effects on the fetus. Most experts consider cromolyn to be a safe drug for use during pregnancy.

Whereas many medications are dangerous to the fetus when administered during the first trimester, those which contain iodides pose their greatest risk when taken after the twelfth week of pregnancy. The reason for this is that the fetal thyroid gland begins to function and take up iodides after the twelfth week. As a result, iodides given to a mother may cross the placenta and induce congenital goiter formation and hypothyroidism in her newborn. In some instances, the enlarged goiter can actually block the infant's airway and cause respiratory distress. In addition to avoiding the usual saturated solution of potassium iodide, more commonly known as SSKI, pregnant women are advised not to use Elixophyllin-KI Elixir, Isuprel Compound Elixir, Mudrane GG Elixir and Tablets, Mudrane Tablets, or Quadrinal Tablets and Suspension. Iodides are excreted into breast milk in small quantities. Even though a nursing infant would receive a small dose, it might be enough to inhibit thyroid function and produce hypothyroidism and goiter.

How safe is cortisone in the treatment of asthma during pregnancy and nursing?

Cortisone is just one of several structurally related chemicals called corticosteroids. In pill and injectable form they are invaluable in the treatment of severe attacks of bronchial asthma which are resistant to other forms of therapy. In addition, they have been used successfully in treating allergic conditions and such serious diseases as adrenal gland insufficiency; the so-called collagen diseases, rheumatoid arthritis and lupus erythematosis; certain kidney diseases; chronic ulcerative colitis; dermatological and eye disorders; shock; and specific types of leukemia and cancer.

There is no doubt that corticosteroids should be administered at any stage of pregnancy if it is determined that they are needed to successfully treat a serious disorder. However, these agents can create some undesirable side effects: fluid and chemical inbalance, abnormal glucose tolerance and diabetes, susceptibility to infections, peptic ulcers which may bleed or perforate, osteoporosis or loss of the minerals of the bones, elevation of the blood pressure, generalized muscle weakness, and psychiatric disturbances. High doses of corticosteroids used for long periods of time are responsible for a person's developing a characteristic "moon face," obesity of the body but not of the arms and legs, the so-called "buffalo hump" protrusion over the

Table 7–3. Safety of Some Commonly Used Bronchial Dilators During Pregnancy and Nursing

Generic and Trade Names of Drugs	Route of Administration	Suggestions for Pregnancy	Suggestions for Nursing
aminophylline (Somophyllin)	liquid, capsules, suppositories, intravenous	Considered safe; many asthmatics treated without adverse fetal effects	Effects on nursing infant are unknown
diphylline (Neothylline)	tablets, liquid, intramuscular injection	Safety for use during pregnancy not established	Effects on nursing infant are unknown
ephedrine hydrochloride, theophylline, and phenobarbital (Tedral)	tablets, liquid	Best avoided; phenobarbital use during first trimester may be associated with higher rate of fetal anomalies; use before labor may cause respiratory depression: theophyllin may prolong length of labor	Effects on nursing are unknown. One case in the medical literature of sleepiness in a nursing infant following maternal barbiturate use
ephedrine sulfate, guaifenesin, theophylline, and phenobarbital (Bronkolixir, Bronkotabs)	the first available as liquid, the second as tablets	Same warning as above	Same warning as above
ephedrine sulfate, theophylline, ethyl alcohol, hydroxyzine hydrochloride (Marax)	tablets, liquid	Should not be used during pregnancy; hydroxyzine hydrochloride may be associated with fetal anomalies when taken early in pregnancy; when used in labor with narcotics, may depress newborn; alcohol not advised during pregnancy; theophylline may prolong length of labor	Not recommended
epinephrine (Medihaler-EPI)	aerosol spray	Should not be used during the first 4 months; may be associated with higher incidence of malformed infants	Effects on nursing infant are unknown
isoproterenol hydrochloride, ephedrine sulfate, theophylline, potassium iodide, alcohol, phenobarbital (Isuprel Compound Elixir)	liquid	Should not be taken during pregnancy because of 3 potentially dangerous ingredients: phenobarbital, potassium iodide, and alcohol	Not recommended

Table 7–3. Safety of Some Commonly Used Bronchial Dilators During Pregnancy and Nursing (*continued*)

Generic and Trade Names of Drugs	Route of Administration	Suggestions for Pregnancy	Suggestions for Nursing
isoproterenol sulfate (Medihaler-ISO)	aerosol spray	No known harmful effects on fetus; if taken late in pregnancy or during labor, may stop contractions (see chapter 10)	Effects on nursing infant unknown
metaproterenol sulfate (Alupent, Metaprel)	aerosol spray, tablets, liquid	Studies on mice, rats, and rabbits show no fetal anomalies at doses 310 times daily aerosol dose and 31 times daily human oral dose; in rabbits, fetal loss and congenital defects observed at higher doses	Effects on nursing infant unknown
oxymetazoline hydrochloride (Afrin)	nasal spray, nose drops	Probably safe during pregnancy	Effects on nursing infant unknown
pseudoephedrine sulfate (Afrinol)	tablets	Probably safe during pregnancy	Effects on nursing infant unknown
terbutaline sulfate (Brethine)	tablets, injection under the skin	No adverse effects on fetal development noted in animal studies; if taken in the last trimester, may stop uterine contractions (see chapter 10)	Effects on nursing infant unknown
theophylline (Slo-Phyllin, Elixophyllin)	capsules, liquid, Slo-Phyllin also in tablets	Considered safe; many asthmatics successfully treated without adverse fetal effects; recent reports suggest may prolong length of labor by inhibiting uterine contractions	Drug known to accumulate in the body of a nursing infant whose mother is taking therapeutic doses though no infant side effects have been reported
theophylline and potassium iodide (Elixophyllin-KI)	liquid	Same precautions as above for theophylline; potassium iodide should not be taken after week 12; may reduce fetal thyroid function	Should be avoided because of the small risk of potassium iodide altering fetal thyroid function

Table 7–4. Safety of Commonly Used Antihistamines During Pregnancy and Nursing

Generic and Trade Names of Drugs	Route of Administration	Suggestions for Pregnancy	Suggestions for Nursing
brompheniramine (Dimetane, Dimetapp)	tablets, liquid	Associated with possible increase in birth defects if taken during first 5 months	Should not be taken while nursing because newborns, and premature infants in particular, very sensitive to this drug
chlorpheniramine maleate (Chlor-Trimeton, Histaspan, Teldrin)	Chlor-Trimeton available as tablets, liquid, and intravenous, intramuscular, and injection under the skin; Teldrin and Histaspan available as time-release capsule	Probably safe during pregnancy	Should not be taken while nursing
dimenhydrinate (see table 7–2) (Dramamine)	tablets, liquid, suppositories, intramuscular and intravenous injection	Safe during pregnancy	Probably safe
diphenhydramine (see table 7–2) (Benadryl)	capsules, liquid, intramuscular and intravenous injection	Safe for use throughout pregnancy: when used with narcotics during labor, may enhance effect of narcotic and depress newborn	Small amounts excreted in breast milk but no adverse effects reported
phenylpro-panolamine hydrochloride, pheniramine maleate, pyrilamine maleate (Triaminic)	tablets, syrup	Should not be used during pregnancy because phenylpropanolamine associated with higher incidence of birth defects if taken during the first 5 months	Should not be taken while nursing
promethazine (Phenergan)	See table 7–2	See table 7–2	Probably safe
pseudoephedrine hydrochloride (Sudafed)	tablets, capsules, and liquid	Safe for use throughout pregnancy	Best avoided since newborns may be sensitive to this drug
pyrrobutamine and cyclopentamine (Co-Pyronil)	pulvules, liquid	Inadequate information available to endorse its use	Avoid if nursing
tripelennamine (PBZ)	tablets and liquid	Probably safe	Safety for the nursing infant has not been established
triprolidine hydrochloride and pseudoephedrine hydrochloride (Actifed)	tablets, liquid	Experience with this drug too limited to endorse its use during the first 5 months; probably safe during last 4 months	Nursing women should not use this drug because newborns, and premature infants in particular, very sensitive to it

top of the back, striae or purple stretch marks of the skin, acne, and an overabundance of facial and body hair. These serious and distressing side effects are more apt to occur when corticosteroids are administered orally, intramuscularly, or intravenously for prolonged periods of time. Though there is no clinical information on the safety of corticosteroid nasal sprays and inhalators, such as dexamethasone and beclomethasone, most experts believe that they are less likely to cause these unpleasant complications. Therefore, it is best to first try corticosteroid sprays and aerosols for nasal congestion and asthma before resorting to more potent treatments. Corticosteroid creams and gels will rarely be responsible for any of these serious side effects, since only a small fraction of the total amount is absorbed from the skin into the bloodstream.

Once corticosteroids are taken for more than two or three days, use should taper off gradually to avoid a withdrawal reaction caused by acute adrenal gland insufficiency. Early symptoms of this potentially dangerous condition are fever, muscle weakness, and joint pain. Furthermore, the ability of the adrenal gland to respond normally to stressful situations such as labor and surgery, may be inhibited for several months after corticosteroids are discontinued. For this reason, doctors often administer a booster injection of corticosteroids to individuals who have been given these drugs within six months prior to stressful events such as labor or surgery.

Most reports in the medical literature attest to the safety of even high doses of corticosteroids during pregnancy. However, there are some notable exceptions. These medications may pose definite risks to both a mother and her fetus and should be prescribed only when absolutely necessary. In addition to a corticosteroid user's diminished capacity to respond to the stress of labor, anesthesia, or surgery, she may encounter other problems related to the altered blood sugar, sodium retention, and elevated blood pressure.

Laboratory studies on rabbits suggest that the use of corticosteroids may be associated with a higher incidence of cleft palate and cleft lip, but this has not been substantiated in humans. However, a disturbing article from England in 1968 reported that of thirty-four pregnant women who took the steroid prednisolone, eight had stillbirths and another nine showed evidence of fetal distress prior to delivery. And in a 1978 study, researchers found that prenatal exposure to prednisone resulted in a significant number of full-term newborns weighing less than 5½ pounds.

In recent years, costicosteroids have been given with far greater frequency to mothers who are likely to deliver premature infants. These drugs are thought to be capable of stimulating the production of a substance in the baby's lung named surfactant which prevents respiratory distress in these small babies (see chapter 10). When used in this manner for short periods of time, corticosteroids are unlikely to cause adverse maternal or fetal complications. Follow-up studies of seven-year-old children, given corticosteroids to mature their lungs in utero, show that their physical development, reading skills, motor coordination, intelligence, and psychological maturity were all normal when compared to a group of children who received no medication.

Corticosteroids given in very high doses to a pregnant woman may cause an abnormal lowering of the levels of estriol hormone which are used for measuring the well-being of the fetus. Though a baby may be in excellent condition, the test may falsely suggest fetal distress.

Studies have demonstrated that corticosteroids are transmitted in breast milk, but no side effects have been reported in infants whose mothers used these drugs.

How safe is allergy immunotherapy during pregnancy?

Immunotherapy is the process by which a doctor periodically administers small skin injections of allergens, substances to which a person is allergic to slowly build immunity or resistance to the offending agent. If a pregnant woman needs, or is already receiving, allergy immunotherapy, it should be administered cautiously to avoid severe reactions. This is especially true during the first trimester, when the smallest amount of allergen should be given. Children born of allergic mothers are 50 percent more likely than other children to develop allergies. For this reason, some doctors are of the opinion that if a mother continues taking allergy shots during pregnancy, her baby may be less sensitive to allergies later in life.

Allergy skin testing is the initial step taken by an allergist to determine the allergens to which a person is most susceptible. As with immunotherapy, caution should be exercised during allergy skin testing. Ideally, allergy and asthma management should begin well in advance of a contemplated pregnancy so that the disorder can be controlled with a minimal amount of medication or immunotherapy.

Sleeping Pills

Are there any sleeping pills which may safely be taken during pregnancy?

Medications which we commonly refer to as sleeping pills are actually a class of drugs called sedative-hypnotics. There are several categories, and I advise my patients to avoid them all during pregnancy.

Barbiturates are easily the most commonly prescribed sedative-hypnotics. They are available under a variety of trade names such as Tuinal (secobarbital and amobarbital), Seconal (secobarbital), Nembutal (pentobarbital), Butisol Sodium (sodium butabarbital), Phenobarbital (phenobarbital), and Amytal (amobarbital). In both animal experiments and studies of pregnant women, there is evidence to suggest that barbiturate use during the first three months of pregnancy may be associated with a significant increase in the incidence of fetal abnormalities. All barbiturates rapidly cross the placenta and are stored in the fetal liver and brain. A fetus may encounter difficulty because its kidneys are unable to eliminate barbiturates rapidly. As a result, the concentration of these drugs is often higher than it is in the mother.

If barbiturates are taken within eight hours of delivery, they can pass across the placenta and cause sleepiness and respiratory depression in the newborn. This type of medical problem is one of the most difficult for doctors to treat because, unlike narcotics, there are no effective antidotes to newborn barbiturate depression other than artificial respiration. Barbiturate withdrawal symptoms have also been observed in babies born of mothers who have taken large doses of these drugs throughout pregnancy or in the last trimester.

Though barbiturates are known to pass into the breast milk, there is only one report in the medical literature of questionable drowsiness of a nursing infant. Despite this, manufacturers of barbiturates suggest that women stop nursing if these drugs are prescribed.

Glutethimide (trade name Doriden) has not been studied adequately to recommend its use during pregnancy or nursing. However, withdrawal symptoms have been exhibited by infants born to mothers dependent on this drug, and reports suggest that it may have prolonged adverse neonatal effects.

Chloral hydrate (trade name Noctec) is an effective sedative which was popularly used as a rectal suppository in years past to allay apprehension during the early stages of labor. It is no longer recommended for this purpose. There is no known association between its use and fetal anomalies, and for this reason it would be preferred over the barbiturates if sedation was necessary during pregnancy. Though chloral hydrate is excreted in breast milk, the amount is not significant to depress an infant if used in the normal recommended doses.

Ethchlorvynol (trade name Placidyl) is an excellent drug for the treatment of insomnia. However, pregnant rats given ethchlorvynol have shown a higher percentage of stillbirths and a lower survival rate of infants beyond the neonatal period. For this reason, heed the manufacturer's suggestion that this drug not be used during the first and second trimesters. During the third trimester, ethchlorvynol has been associated with central nervous system depression and withdrawal symptoms in the newborn. There are not enough data available to endorse its use by a nursing mother.

Dalmane is the trade name for flurazepam hydrochloride, a relatively new drug which is replacing barbiturates as the most popular "sleeping pill." Although flurazepam has not been studied adequately to determine whether it may be associated with fetal abnormalities, its structure is derived from the minor tranquilizers, so it should always be avoided during pregnancy.

Though the scientific name of methaqualone and its trade name Mequin may sound unfamiliar to most readers, the more common trade name of Quaalude has gained nationwide notoriety as an overly prescribed and abused sedative-hypnotic. Methaqualone is absolutely not recommended for women who are pregnant or planning to become pregnant. It has been associated with developmental bone abnormalities in offspring of laboratory animals given high doses of this drug. Though there is no information about its effects on a nursing infant, its extreme potency would preclude its use.

Methyprylon (trade name Noludar) is a sedative-hypnotic about which too little is known to recommend its use during pregnancy or while breast-feeding.

Tranquilizers and Drugs Used in Psychiatry

What are minor tranquilizers?

The minor tranquilizers are a group of drugs that are used medically for the relief of acute anxiety and nervous tension. Unfortunately, they are indiscriminately abused by too many people who are either unaware or unconcerned that these medications may be habit-forming and a cause of emotional and physical dependence. It has become commonplace in our society to take a tranquilizer as a cure for each minor stress of everyday life, as proven by the fact that diazepam, better known by its

Table 7–5. Safety of Commonly Used Psychiatric Drugs During Pregnancy and Nursing

Generic and Trade Names of Drugs	Classification	Indications for Use	Suggestions for Pregnancy	Suggestions for Nursing
amitriptyline hydrochloride (Elavil, Amitril)	tricyclic	Relief of depression	Animal studies inconclusive and human experience inadequate to recommend its use; best avoided if possible	Probably safe; in one recent study, none detected in the bloodstream of a nursing infant whose mother took this drug
amitriptyline hydrohloride and chlordiazepoxide (Limbitrol)	combination of Elavil and Librium	Treatment of depression and anxiety	Suggestions as for Elavil; Librium should not be taken during first trimester because of higher incidence of birth defects; it can depress newborn if taken during labor	Best avoided if nursing
amitriptyline hydrochloride and perphenazine (Triavil)	combination of Elavil and Trilafon	Relief of anxiety and depression associated with psychiatric disorders	Suggestions as for Elavil; safety of Trilafon not established; chemically similar drugs have been associated with birth defects	Excreted in breast milk though no harmful effects reported; drug may actually increase amount of breast milk
chlorpromazine (Thorazine)	phenothiazine	To control excessive anxiety and agitation and in the treatment of manic-depression and other psychotic disorders	Reported instances of jaundice, retinal damage, and delay in the onset of crying and breathing in newborn infants whose mothers had received chlorpromazine; studies on rodents show increased rate of fetal and newborn deaths; use in pregnancy only when absolutely necessary	As above
desipramine hydrochloride (Norpramin, Pertofrane)	tricyclic	Relief of depression	Research on mice, rats, and rabbits has revealed no fetal anomalies, but no information available about effects on human pregnancy; use only if absolutely necessary	No information available about its concentration in breast milk or its effects on the nursing infant; therefore, best not to nurse if drug must be taken
doxepin hydrochloride (Sinequan, Adapin)	tricyclic	Psychotic and neurotic disorders characterized by depression and anxiety, manic-depressive disorders	Reproductive studies on rabbits, monkeys, and dogs show no fetal damage; no studies on pregnant women using this drug; therefore, avoid if possible	Laboratory studies of drug concentrations in breast milk vary from practically none to levels about equal to those in mother's plasma; nursing should probably be avoided

Generic and Trade Names of Drugs	Classification	Indications for Use	Suggestions for Pregnancy	Suggestions for Nursing
fluphenazine (Prolixin)	phenothiazine	Schizophrenia	Results contradictory; some studies show an increase in the incidence of congenital anomalies, especially heart defects, when phenothiazines are used in the first trimester; other studies show no harmful effects; if given intravenously, may cause a marked lowering of the blood pressure, prolonged labor, and postpartum hemorrhage; use in pregnancy only when absolutely necessary	Phenothiazines excreted in breast milk, though no harmful effects reported; drug may actually increase amount of breast milk
haloperidol (Haldol)	butyrophenone	Psychotic disorders	Rodents given high doses show increase in pregnancy loss and cleft palate; in humans, 2 cases of limb malformations in offspring of mothers who took this drug between day 25 and 37 of pregnancy; avoid if possible, especially in first trimester	Manufacturer suggests women not nurse when taking this drug
imipramine hydrochloride (Tofranil, Presamine, Antipres, SK-Pramine, Imavate, Janimine)	tricyclic	Relief of depression	Effects on the fetus inconclusive; isolated reports of skull, facial, nervous system, and limb deformities among infants exposed to drug in utero; however, several large studies refute these findings; use only if absolutely necessary	1 recent study showed very high levels in breast milk; avoid if nursing
lithium carbonate (Eskolith, Lithane, Lithobid, Lithonate, Lithotabs)	alkali-metals	Manic-depression	Best avoided throughout pregnancy, especially in the first trimester since severe abnormalities of the heart, nervous system, and ears have been reported in exposed infants; may be toxic to pregnant women if salt is restricted	Drug excreted in breast milk in high concentrations; best avoided since it may cause goiter and chemical imbalance in a nursing infant

Table 7–5. Safety of Commonly Used Psychiatric Drugs During Pregnancy and Nursing *(continued)*

Generic and Trade Names of Drugs	Classification	Indications for Use	Suggestions for Pregnancy	Suggestions for Nursing
nortriptyline hydrochloride (Aventyl, Pamelor)	tricyclic	Relief of depression	Animal reproduction studies have yielded inconclusive results; use only if absolutely necessary	No information available about its concentration in breast milk or effect on nursing infant; avoid if possible
perphenazine (Trilafon)	phenothiazine	Psychotic disorders and relief of nausea and vomiting	See information for other phenothiazines	See information for other phenothiazines
phenelzine (Nardil)	MAO inhibitor	Treatment of severe depression	In experimental studies, pregnant mice given this drug had a significant decrease of viable offspring; no reports of its safety in human pregnancy, but avoid if possible	Drug excreted in breast milk but no information about its safety; best not to nurse if taking this drug
protriptyline hydrochloride (Vivactil)	dibenzocycloheptene derivative	Treatment of depression	In 1 study of mice, rats, and rabbits given high doses, no apparent ill effects; experience with human pregnancy insufficient to endorse its use	No information available about concentration in breast milk or effect on the nursing infant; best not to nurse if drug must be taken
thioridazine hydrochloride (Mellaril)	phenothiazine	Psychotic disorders, agitation, depression, tension	See information for other phenothiazines	See information for other phenothiazines
tranylcypromine sulfate (Parnate)	MAO inhibitor	Treatment of severe depression	Drug known to cross placenta and enter fetal circulation; data insufficient, but no known anomalies reported in humans or experimental animals; use only for severe depression which does not respond to less potent drugs	Drug found in breast milk but no information about its safety; best not to nurse if taking this drug
trifluoperazine hydrochloride (Stelazine)	phenothiazine	To control excessive anxiety and agitation and treat psychotic disorders	See information for other phenothiazines	See information for other phenothiazines

trade name Valium, is the most frequently prescribed medication in the United States. Other popular minor tranquilizers are meprobamate (trade names Equanil and Miltown), chlordiazepoxide hydrochloride (trade names Librium and Libritabs), clorazepate dipotassium (trade name Tranxene), oxazepam (trade name Serax), prazepam (trade names Verstran and Centrax), and lorazepam (trade name Ativan). Though all these drugs are classified as minor tranquilizers, they have the capacity to cause major problems during pregnancy.

What is thalidomide and how did it affect the outcome of pregnancy?

One of the great tragedies of obstetrical history occurred with the minor tranquilizer named thalidomide. This drug, first used in Germany, attained popularity in 1960s. Unfortunately, 5,000 to 10,000 infants were born with serious malformations when their mothers were given thalidomide between the twentieth and fortieth day following conception. The most frightening observation of the thalidomide story is that the drug passed considerable animal testing on mice, rabbits, and rats before it was released. However, these animals were somehow insensitive to its malforming effects. After the tragedy was discovered, laboratory studies were performed on primates, such as baboons and marmosets, and the human abnormalities were easily reproduced. This has led researchers to conclude that tests on primates have far greater validity in evaluating drugs for abnormalities than do those on rats, mice, and rabbits. Unfortunately, none of the minor tranquilizers available today have undergone this type of rigid laboratory scrutiny, and therefore they are best avoided during pregnancy.

How can the currently used minor tranquilizers alter the outcome of pregnancy, and what effect can they have on a nursing infant?

In a report published in 1974, doctors studied the incidence of severe birth defects in children whose mothers had received either meprobamate or chlordiazepoxide during the first six weeks of pregnancy. The rate of abnormalities per 100 live births was 12.1 and 11.4 in the meprobamate and chlordiazepoxide groups respectively, compared to only 2.6 per 100 among women who used no medications. The most frequently found abnormalities involved the heart, though joint and skull defects were also reported. Other studies have linked first trimester meprobamate and diazepam use with a significant rise in the incidence of cleft lip and cleft palate. Clorazepate dipotassium (trade name Tranxene) is a new and very popular minor tranquilizer. In a 1980 report, a woman who had taken a large dose of Tranxene during the first trimester gave birth to an infant with limb deformities similar to those induced with thalidomide.

If a woman uses relatively high doses of Valium over a prolonged period of time during the third trimester, her newborn infant may experience agitation and other withdrawal symptoms when the drug is no longer in the bloodstream following birth.

The use of intravenous and intramuscular diazepam as a tranquilizer for women in labor is ill advised since the drug readily crosses the placenta and may depress the baby. Effects on the newborn may last for as long as eight to ten days following delivery and are more likely to occur among premature infants.

Especially hazardous is the use of narcotics combined with tranquilizers, since the depressant effects of both drugs may be exaggerated. If this combination is used, the usual narcotic dose should be reduced by at least one-third. Whereas the depression caused by narcotics may be reversed with a narcotic antagonist such as Narcan, there is no specific antidote for reversing the harmful effects caused by tranquilizers.

One sign of fetal well-being during labor is a continual variability or changing of its heart rate. This so-called "beat-to-beat variability" may be lost when tranquilizers are given to a mother during labor. Researchers theorized that this occurs because these drugs depress the nerves which control fetal heart function.

Conduction anesthetics such as epidural, spinal, and saddle block may occasionally cause abnormal lowering of the blood pressure (hypotension). This in turn may increase the risk of fetal distress, since less oxygen will pass from mother to child across the placenta. Tranquilizers administered during labor may potentiate this harmful hypotensive reaction.

It is very important that a breast-feeding woman be aware of the fact that the concentration of meprobamate is two to four times greater in her breast milk than in her bloodstream. Chlordiazepoxide and diazepam, on the other hand, are transmitted to breast milk in lower concentrations, and it is unlikely that a nursing infant will be adversely affected if its mother ingests these preparations in therapeutic doses. Nevertheless, the manufacturer of diazepam recommends that women should stop nursing if the drug is prescribed.

Which drugs are used to treat the more severe emotional disorders, and how can they affect the outcome of pregnancy?

Unfortunately half the medications used to treat severe emotional disorders and various forms of psychotic and deranged behavior are prescribed by nonpsychiatrists who often fail to recognize their potentially harmful effects on the pregnant woman.

Manic-depressive psychosis is a fairly common and very serious psychiatric disorder characterized by unpredictable and dangerous mood swings. It is treated with lithium carbonate. Lithium, however, causes severe abnormalities and its use should be avoided by pregnant women and women likely to conceive. Studies of infants exposed to lithium carbonate during the first trimester of pregnancy have revealed a 9 percent incidence of severe anomalies of the heart and its great vessels and defects of the central nervous system and the external ears have been noted. The most vulnerable period for the fetus is between the eleventh and ninetieth day following conception. As a result of the severity of these abnormalities, a registry of lithium-exposed babies has been established in order to determine more precisely the types of anomalies that may be associated with the use of this drug.

Women receiving lithium therapy during the last two trimesters of pregnancy should not restrict their sodium or salt intake and should not take diuretics. When sodium intake is restricted, lithium excretion is reduced and lithium intoxication may result. If at all possible, avoid the drug in the last month of pregnancy, since it may cause infant toxicity—poor muscle tone and thyroid dysfunction—at birth. Lithium is excreted in breast milk at a quarter to half the concentrations of maternal serum levels. Therefore, it is advisable to discourage breast-feeding by mothers receiving lithium therapy.

Many antipsychotic agents are derived from a basic chemical class called phenothiazines. Examples of popular phenothiazines are chlorpromazine (trade name Thorazine), promazine (trade name Sparine), trifluoperazine (trade name Stelazine), thioridazine (trade name Mellaril), and fluphenazine (trade name Prolixin). Studies have not clearly demonstrated whether these drugs cause malformations. There have been a few reports, however, of abnormal neuromuscular reactions in newborns following use of phenothiazines late in pregnancy. Women taking phenothiazines can probably safely nurse their babies since, even in high doses, only very small amounts enter the breast milk.

Haloperidol (trade name Haldol) is a drug which is frequently used to treat psychotic disorders. There have been occasional cases of severe limb malformations following maternal use of haloperidol early in the first trimester. Haloperidol is secreted in breast milk in slightly higher concentrations than the phenothiazines.

The newest class of drugs, called tricyclic antidepressants, have not been subjected to adequate clinical investigation. Though reproduction studies in rats have shown no fetal abnormalities, these medications are still not recommended for use during pregnancy. Withdrawal symptoms in newborns have been reported in a few instances during the first thirty days of life when their mothers were taking tricyclic antidepressants late in pregnancy. These babies experienced shortness of breath, poor color, rapid heart rate, irritability, profuse sweating, and urinary retention. Most studies have found little or no excretion of tricyclics in breast milk, and suggest that nursing need not be discontinued by women taking these drugs. A minority of reports, however, have noted tricyclic levels in a woman's breast milk to equal those in her bloodstream. Amitriptyline (trade name Elavil), desipramine (trade name Norpramin), doxepin (trade name Sinequan), nortriptyline (trade name Aventyl, Pamelor), imipramine (trade name Tofranil, Imavate), and protriptyline (trade name Vivactil, Triptil) are all examples of tricyclic antidepressants.

Very little is known about the fetal effects of another group of antidepressants known as monoamine oxidase (MAO) inhibitors. Unlike the tricyclics, which increase the supply of breast milk, these drugs will suppress lactation and should not be used by a woman who is attempting to nurse her baby. Isocarpoxazid (trade name Marplan), phenelzine (trade name Nardil), and tranylcypromine (trade name Parnate) and popular MAO inhibitors.

Anticonvulsants

What problems may be encountered during pregnancy by a woman who is treated for seizure disorders?

Obstetricians and neurologists caring for the pregnant epileptic often face difficult decisions. Anticonvulsant medications, while invaluable in the control of seizures, may involve a greater risk of fetal damage, while discontinuing the medication may precipitate seizures which could cause even greater harm to the pregnant woman and her fetus. Studies suggest that seizure frequency is increased in 45 percent, unaltered in 50 percent, and decreased in only 5 percent of pregnant women.

Dilantin is the trade name of the most commonly prescribed anticonvulsant. It is generically named phenytoin and belongs to a class of drugs called hydantoins. Mephenytoin (trade name Mesantoin) is another popular hydantoin. Amazingly, it was not until 1970 that a relationship between hydantoin use and congenital malformations was first reported, despite the fact that this drug had been used extensively for many years. Cleft palate, cleft lip, and congenital heart disease have now been documented in both animal and human reproductive reports. The incidence of congenital heart disease in the general population is approximately 5 per 1,000 births, and that of cleft palate and cleft lip is 2 per 1,000 births. In the children of women with epilepsy who use anticonvulsants, the incidence of both conditions increases to 10 per 1,000 births.

In addition to these problems, some authors have described a group of abnormalities termed "the fetal hydantoin syndrome." This occurs in 11 percent of infants exposed to hydantoins in utero and consists of prenatal and postpartum growth deficiency, an abnormally small head (microcephaly), and mental retardation.

Fatal hemorrhage in newborns has been reported following maternal anticonvulsant therapy with hydantoins. Studies show that newborns suffering from this form of hemorrhage lack vitamin K which is associated with clotting of blood. Bleeding usually occurs within twenty-four hours of birth and may involve the brain, lungs, and abdominal organs of the infants.

Hydantoins, when used in normal therapeutic amounts, are transmitted to the breast milk in one-fourth the concentration found in the mother's bloodstream. This amount is probably too low to adversely affect the infant, and most authorities believe that a woman may continue to nurse while using these medications.

Phenobarbital, a barbiturate, is often prescribed in the treatment of epilepsy. As previously mentioned, use of phenobarbital is associated with an increased rate of birth defects. However, the incidence of major malformations, such as cleft palate, cleft lip, and congenital heart disease, is believed to be significantly lower than it is with hydantoin. Phenobarbital use during the last trimester and the postpartum period presents other problems (see question on sleeping pills, page 206).

Trimethadione (trade name Tridione) is used to control mild seizures called petit mal. The relationship between fetal exposure and malformations is more firmly established with this drug than for any other anticonvulsant and it should never be used during pregnancy. Equally as dangerous is paramethadione (trade name Paradione), which is also used in the treatment of petit mal; in one study, doctors reported thirteen prenatal deaths among fifty-three women using trimethadione or paramethadione during pregnancy. As with hydantoins, maternal use of trimethadione has been associated with severe infant bleeding during the first twenty-four hours of life. This occurs because the drug causes a defect in vitamin K-dependent clotting factors. The safety of trimethadione for use during lactation is unknown at the present time.

Carbamazepine (trade name Tegretol) is a new, popular, and potent drug which has been used successfully in the treatment of epilepsy. Information about the effects of Tegretol on pregnancy outcome is quite limited, but in one report of only three human pregnancies, doctors noted carbamazepine use was associated with abnormalities in two of the offspring. Until further information is available, I would avoid use of this drug during pregnancy and breast-feeding.

Depakene is a trade name for valproic acid, an anticonvulsant used to treat brief and usually mild seizures. The effects of valproic acid on human pregnancy are unknown, but animal studies on rats and rabbits have proven that the drug is easily transferred across the placenta to the fetus. Animals exposed to valproic acid in utero have demonstrated higher rates of rib and vertebral abnormalities, fetal death, and delay of the onset of labor, and when valproic acid was administered during the nursing period, postpartum growth and survival was adversely affected.

What advice do you have for the pregnant woman with a convulsive disorder?

Ideally, you should have a full evaluation by a neurologist before you try to conceive. It is sometimes discovered that a particular medication you are taking is unnecessary, especially if you have been free of seizures for many years. Sometimes, the medication you are taking can be changed to another that is less likely to cause fetal abnormalities. If you are taking trimethadione or paramethadione it should be discontinued before a contemplated pregnancy and replaced with a safer alternative. You should be aware of the fact that even if you take no medications and experience no seizures during pregnancy, your chances of giving birth to an infant with anomalies may still be slightly greater than average. Modern methods of detecting fetal abnormalities are of very limited help in this particular situation.

If you require hydantoins, be assured that you have a 90 percent chance of giving birth to a normal child. If you are taking phenobarbital, your risk of giving birth to a deformed infant is probably significantly less than the 10 percent figure quoted for hydantoins. If you doctor decides that these medications must be taken during pregnancy, you should heed this advice since the risk of maternal and fetal damage may be greater if severe and uncontrolled convulsions occur. On occasion, the dose of anticonvulsant needed to control seizures may actually increase as pregnancy progresses.

Be sure that your baby receives an intramuscular injection of vitamin K (trade name AquaMEPHYTON, generic name phytonadione) in the delivery room if you have been treated with hydantoins or barbiturates before delivery. This will prevent a bleeding disorder caused by a depletion of coagulation factors by the anticonvulsant. Some doctors administer vitamin K during labor and in the last months of pregnancy to prevent this complication, though the benefits of this treatment method have not been proven. One distinct drawback of administering vitamin K injections prior to delivery is that it may cause jaundice in the baby shortly after birth.

After delivery, your baby should be carefully examined for congenital malformations and the nursery alerted to perform clotting factor and platelet counts every two to four hours during the first twenty-four hours of life. Infants exposed to phenobarbital should be observed for drowsiness and barbiturate withdrawal symptoms.

Anticoagulants

What are anticoagulants, and how may they cause problems during pregnancy?

Anticoagulants are lifesaving medications which prevent the clotting of blood. A thrombus is defined as a clot attached to the wall of an artery or vein. When in a vein (phleb), it is often accompanied by inflammation (itis). Thrombophlebitis is most common in the veins of the legs and pelvis and may be either superficial or deep. The superficial variety is located just beneath the surface of the skin in the varicose veins which may develop with childbirth. Few women have serious complications from superficial thrombophlebitis, but thrombophlebitis of the veins deep in the legs and pelvis often presents a real threat to a woman's life. Unfortunately, deep thrombophlebitis may occur without any warning symptoms at all. When one of these deep clots becomes dislodged from the wall of the vein, it travels through the circulation and is called an embolus (plural, emboli). If this embolus reaches the lung, it is then called a pulmonary embolus. There, it may block the opening of a large oxygen-carrying blood vessel, causing instant death. Anticoagulants are invaluable in preventing the formation and spread of thrombophlebitis and pulmonary emboli. They are also essential in the prevention and treatment of certain types of stroke and heart disease.

Anticoagulants are either oral or injectable. Examples of oral preparations are warfarin (trade name Coumadin, Panwarfin) and bishydroxycoumarin (trade name Dicumarol). The injectable anticoagulant is heparin sodium. Heparin may be administered intravenously or subcutaneously. It should not be given intramuscularly because it may produce a blood clot (hematoma) at the injection site. During the first trimester, oral anticoagulants may cause the "fetal warfarin embryopathy syndrome." This occurs in 15 to 25 percent of exposed infants and is characterized by underdevelopment of the cartilage of the nose, stippled cartilage on x-ray examination of the vertebral column and long bones, small fingers and hands, atrophy of the nerves of the eye, cataracts leading to blindness, retarded physical and mental development, and an abnormally small head (microcephaly). If oral anticoagulants are taken by a mother in the second trimester, fetal hemorrhage may occur along with developmental defects, such as microcephaly, blindness, and mental retardation. Fetal and placental hemorrhage have been reported following maternal use of oral anticoagulants during the last trimester.

If anticoagulant therapy is necessary during pregnancy, heparin is preferred, but it may not be totally innocuous. Despite the fact that heparin does not cross the placenta to damage the fetus, in one study, maternal use of this drug was associated with a 12 percent incidence of stillbirths and a 30 percent rate of prematurity. However, this poor pregnancy outcome might not have resulted from the use of heparin but from the underlying disease conditions which demanded its use. Osteoporosis is an abnormal loss of minerals from the bones, which may be aggravated with prolonged use of heparin. When osteoporosis is severe it can cause fractures of the bones of the vertebral column. Recent studies from England suggest that pregnant women may be more prone to this complication than nonpregnant women. In the days immediately following delivery, heparin use may be associated with a 50 percent risk of postpartum hemorrhage.

Most medical textbooks advise against the use of oral anticoagulants while breast-feeding for fear that they will anticoagulate the baby. However, recent studies have clearly demonstrated that warfarin does not enter the breast milk and cannot possibly cause harm to the nursing infant. Heparin is known to be safe because its large molecule does not readily pass from a woman's bloodstream into her breast milk.

Antihyper-
tensives

Which medications should be avoided and which may be safely used in the treatment of hypertension during pregnancy?

Hypertension is an abnormal elevation of the blood pressure which occurs in approximately 5 to 10 percent of the adult population. The cause of the high blood pressure is unknown 90 percent of the time. There is a form of hypertension which occurs specifically after the twentieth week of pregnancy, known as preeclampsia, eclampsia, and toxemia. Pregnancy-induced hypertension completely subsides following childbirth.

A wide variety of antihypertensive agents have been advocated for use during pregnancy. Of these, some are less than ideal and others are unquestionably a poor choice.

Reserpine is the perfect example of a popular antihypertensive medication that should not be used during pregnancy. In addition to causing too sudden a drop in the blood pressure during exercise or change in position, it may also be responsible for an increase in stomach acid secretion, peptic ulcer, and frequent bowel movements. One unusual maternal complication resulting from reserpine use is nasal stuffiness due to dilatation of small arteries in the nose. Interestingly, reserpine also crosses the placenta to cause the same nasal changes in the fetus. The difference, however, is that the newborn will demonstrate severe nasal congestion associated with excessive mucus production and respiratory distress. Other unpleasant fetal effects are lethargy, poor appetite, and bradycardia, or an abnormally slow pulse. These effects may be lessened if the drug is not taken within one day of delivery—a bit of information that is of little practical use, since it is usually difficult if not impossible to predict the onset of labor. Reserpine is excreted in significant quantities in breast milk and has been reported to cause lethargy, diarrhea, and nasal stuffiness in nursing infants.

Popular antihypertensive brands that contain reserpine are Regroton, Diupres, Diutensen-R, Exna-R, Hydra-Es, Hydromox R, Hydropres, Hydroserp, Hydrotensin, Hyser Plus Tablets, Metatensin, Naquival, Rau-Sed, Renese-R, Reserpine Tablets, Ropres, Ruhexatal with Reserpine, Salutensin, Sandril, Ser-Ap-Es, Serpasil, Unipres, Harmonyl, Raudixin, and Rauzide.

Inderal is the trade name for propanolol, a drug used in the treatment of hypertension. Propanolol and other drugs of similar chemical structure are classified as beta-blockers. They have been used successfully in Europe to treat hypertension during pregnancy. However, American physicians have been reluctant to prescribe beta-blockers during pregnancy because of isolated case reports of fetal growth retardation, a higher stillbirth rate, prolonged labor, and, following delivery, respiratory distress, abnormally low blood sugar (hypoglycemia), and an abnormally slow heart rate (bradycardia) for as long as three days. Unfortunately, there are no large controlled studies that have tested the safety of beta-blockers during pregnancy.

The breast milk concentration of propranolol is believed to be less than 40 percent of its concentration in the maternal bloodstream. In 1979, researchers calculated that a nursing infant would absorb only 1/100 of a normal pediatric dose, and that this amount was safe. However, the authors did advise close observation of nursing infants for signs of respiratory depression, hypoglycemia, and bradycardia.

Clonidine (trade name Catapres) is an antihypertensive agent that must undergo considerably more study before it can be recommended for use during pregnancy. Reproduction studies on animals have not shown this drug to produce malformation, but they did show a higher incidence of early fetal loss. Maternal problems encountered with Clonidine—such as sodium and fluid retention, bowel disturbances, drowsiness, and abnormal lowering of the blood pressure—may discourage pregnant women from using this drug. The safety of Clonidine for the nursing infant has yet to be established.

Diazoxide (trade name Hyperstat) is a potent antihypertensive agent which is given intravenously in combating severe hypertensive emergencies. The unpleasant maternal side effects such as severe hypotension, salt and water retention, and elevation of the blood sugar limits its usefulness. Studies in pregnant monkeys and sheep demonstrate that diazoxide readily crosses the placenta, with fetal concentrations of the drug equaling maternal levels one to two hours after injection. Prolonged hyperglycemia, or abnormal elevations in the blood sugar, have been noted, believed to be caused by the drug's capacity to destroy the insulin-producing cells in the fetal pancreas. In a report of a neonatal death published in the *Journal of the American Medical Association* in 1980, a hypertensive woman treated with diazoxide immediately prior to delivery gave birth to an infant with severe and prolonged hyperglycemia. At the present time, the effects of diazoxide on the nursing infant are unknown.

The two safest and most effective antihypertensive agents for use during pregnancy are hydralazine (trade names Apresoline and Dralzine) and methyldopa (trade name Aldomet).

Though some of the reported side effects of hydralazine in adults have included sodium and water retention, weight gain, flushing, nasal congestion, headaches, dizziness, and palpitations, most patients tolerate the drug extremely well. There are conflicting reports in the medical literature on the effects of hydralazine on the blood flow to the uterus and placenta. This is an important determination because the amount of oxygen received by the fetus is directly related to the amount of blood reaching the uterus and placenta. The majority of research conducted on pregnant sheep seems to indicate that hydralazine increases the uterine blood flow. Animal studies on mice and rabbits indicate that hydralazine may produce cleft palate and malformations of the facial and skull bones. Extensive clinical experience in human pregnancy, however, has not revealed any such abnormalities. There is no information available to document either the safety or hazards of hydralazine use by breast-feeding women.

Methyldopa has been endorsed by most medical authorities as an ideal antihypertensive agent for long-term use during pregnancy because it does not impair the flow of blood and oxygen to the uterus. Methyldopa's safety to the fetus has been documented in several clinical trials involving hundreds of pregnancies. Compared to hypertensive patients who are untreated, those receiving methyldopa have lower abortion rates, increased birth weights of their babies, fewer premature deliveries, and decreased neonatal mortality. However, in a 1981 study from England, doctors found that infants born to mothers treated with methyldopa during pregnancy had a significantly reduced blood pressure during the first two days of life. There was no evidence that the infants were compromised by this temporary condition. The drug is not without maternal side effects such as drowsiness, depression, salt retention, and constipation.

In addition to its high concentration in breast milk, methyldopa has been found to stimulate the secretion of prolactin hormone from the pituitary gland. This may have the positive effect of increasing the quantity of breast milk. The safety of methyldopa in lactating women, however, has not been documented in any large clinical studies.

Diuretics

How safe are diuretics—"water pills"—during pregnancy?

Diuretics are agents which increase the amount of urine excreted. Better known as water pills, diuretics are medically valuable in the treatment of hypertension, heart failure, and a variety of disorders which are characterized by edema, the swelling of tissues with fluid. Premenstrual edema is often successfully relieved with diuretics.

In the past, diuretics were frequently used to relieve the normal physiological edema which accompanies pregnancy. Some doctors even proposed that they be used prophylactically to prevent the development of toxemia. However, convincing research has demonstrated that the routine use of diuretics during normal pregnancy exposes a mother and her fetus to unnecessary hazards while in fact doing nothing to prevent toxemia. Unfortunately, diuretics are still extensively prescribed for pregnant women in this country.

Edema during pregnancy is rarely a cause for concern. The so-called dependent edema of pregnancy is characterized by swelling of the ankles and results from restriction of blood flow through the veins of the legs and pelvis by the enlarged uterus. The vena cava is a huge vein which carries blood to the heart from the lower part of the body. It runs behind and to the right of the enlarged pregnant uterus. Often, the only treatment necessary to relieve edema during pregnancy is to lie on your left side in bed for several hours at a time. This will prevent the floppy uterus from falling against the vena cava, thereby increasing the amount of blood that is carried from the lower extremities. Other helpful measures in reducing edema are elevating the legs and wearing support stockings. When these simple measures fail, and edema is severe enough to cause great discomfort in the legs or numbness and pain in the hands, a short course of diuretic therapy is occasionally appropriate.

Of all diuretics, the thiazide group of drugs is the most commonly prescribed during pregnancy. Popular thiazides are chlorothiazide sodium (trade name Diuril), hydrochlorothiazide (trade names HydroDIURIL and Esidrix), trichlormethiazide (trade names Naqua, Metahydrin, and Metatensin), bendroflumethiazide (trade name Naturetin), Methyclothiazide (trade name Enduron), Benzthiazide (trade names Exna and Aquatag), Cyclothiazide (trade name Anhydron), Methyclothiazide (trade name Aquatensen), and Polythiazide (trade name Renese). Aldactazide, Diutensen, and Enduronyl are trade names of compounds which contain thiazides in combination with other drugs.

Though often casually prescribed, thiazide diuretics may occasionally create serious problems for the pregnant women who use them. One of these is a chemical imbalance caused by excessive loss of potassium and sodium. These chemical changes may be transmitted to the fetal circulation, where they may cause heart rate irregularities. Maternal pancreatitis (inflammation of the pancreas), hyperglycemia (abnormal elevation of the blood sugar), and hyperuricemia (abnormal elevation of the blood uric acid level) have all been reported following use of thiazides during pregnancy.

Though thiazides have not been associated with congenital abnormalities, fetal complications have included low birth weight, salt and water depletion, abnormally low blood sugars, and depression of blood cell formation in the bone marrow. Thrombocytopenia is a decrease in the number of platelets which are vital to the normal blood-clotting mechanism. A small percentage of newborns will experience this life-threatening complication following use of thiazides by their mothers. Thiazides are best avoided during lactation, since they are found in significant concentrations in the breast milk and may also decrease the quantity of the breast milk.

Furosemide (trade name Lasix) is a very potent diuretic. In human experience to date, no abnormalities have been reported among infants whose mothers were given furosemide. However, animal reproductive studies have shown that the drug may cause fetal abnormalities, and it is also known to decrease uterine blood flow. Probably the only two valid reasons for using this potent diuretic during pregnancy are severe congestive heart failure and kidney disease requiring immediate and massive excretion of urine. Furosemide, like other diuretics, will decrease the quantity of breast milk. Its concentration in breast milk and its effects on the nursing infant have not been adequately studied.

Ethacrynic acid (trade name Edecrin) is a potent diuretic which has quickly achieved wide acceptance because of the rapid and massive urine flow it produces. However, little is known about its safety during pregnancy, and the manufacturer states that it is not recommended for nursing mothers. There is some evidence that Edecrin may cause uterine contractions.

Spironolactone (trade name Aldactone) is not as potent a diuretic as ethacrynic acid. It has been found to cross the placenta, but its effects, if any, on the fetus have not been determined. A metabolite of spironolactone, named canrenone, appears in the breast milk. Though its effects on the nursing infant are unknown, the manufacturer recommends that women stop nursing if they require treatment with spironolactone.

Cardiac Drugs

How can drugs which are used to treat abnormal heart rhythms alter the outcome of pregnancy?

Digitalis and its derivatives are frequently prescribed in the treatment of heart failure and other cardiac conditions characterized by an abnormal heart rate and rhythm. Some of the more popular drugs in this group are digoxin (trade name Lanoxin), lanatoside (trade name Cedilanid), digitoxin (trade name Cystodigin), and gitalin (trade name Gitaligin). Since digitalis preparations are so essential to the health of the person being treated, it is a relief to know that they have been given to a large number of pregnant women for varying periods of time without any reports of fetal ill effects or anomalies. All digitalis preparations readily pass from the maternal to the fetal circulation and, theoretically, they could cause abnormal slowing of the fetal heart rate. However, with the exception of one fetal death in the medical literature resulting from a maternal digitoxin overdose, this does not appear to be a problem. In the unlikely event that digitalis intoxication of the fetus is to occur, it is most likely to happen during the eighth month of pregnancy.

Quinidine is another commonly prescribed drug used in the treatment of abnormalities of the cardiac rate and rhythm. Some popular trade names of quinidine preparations are Duraquin, Quinaglute, Cardioquin, Quinidex, and Quinora. It is not known if the use of quinidine can adversely affect the outcome of pregnancy. Approximately 40 percent of the drug found in a mother will diffuse across the placenta to her uterus. Most doctors conclude that if a woman requires the drug she can be reasonably certain that it will not adversely alter the outcome of pregnancy. Quinidine has been shown to freely pass into the breast milk in a concentration similar to that found in the mother's bloodstream. Since this drug may accumulate in the immature liver of a newborn, most doctors believe that continued exposure to quinidine via breast-feeding should be avoided.

Antidiabetic Medications

How safe are the medications used for treating diabetes during pregnancy?

Since the pregnant diabetic is at significantly greater risk of delivering a baby with congenital anomalies or a stillbirth, the detrimental effects produced by medications may be difficult to distinguish from those caused by the diabetic condition. As is the case with anticoagulants, there are two classes of medications used to control diabetes: oral hypoglycemics and injections of insulin.

Tolbutamide (trade name Orinase), the most popular oral hypoglycemic, acts by stimulating the synthesis and release of insulin from the pancreas. It should not be used during pregnancy, since animal studies have demonstrated a high incidence of fetal death and congenital anomalies. Given to a mother at the end of pregnancy, tolbutamide passes into the fetal circulation and stimulates the fetal pancreas to secrete excessive amounts of insulin, which may cause a dangerous lowering of the newborn's blood sugar.

Chlorpropamide (trade name Diabinese) is an oral hypoglycemic which, in addition to the problems caused by tolbutamide, may produce respiratory distress and a lowering of the blood platelet count in newborn infants. Two other hypoglycemics, acetohexamide (trade name Dymelor) and tolazamide (trade name Tolinase), are also not to be used during pregnancy.

There is no evidence to show that insulin produces abnormalities in humans, and it is unquestionably the drug of choice for treating diabetes during pregnancy. Insulin taken by a diabetic mother will not enter her breast milk and therefore will pose no hazards for the nursing infant.

Thyroid Medications

What problems may be encountered when using medications to treat thyroid disease during pregnancy and nursing?

Since uncontrolled thyroid gland disease will worsen a woman's chances for a successful pregnancy outcome, it is imperative that the diagnosis be made and treatment begun as early as possible, ideally before pregnancy. Normal pregnancy induces a number of changes in thyroid function studies, some of which may confuse the unenlightened physician interpreting these laboratory tests. As a result, medications are too often prescribed when they are not really needed.

The chances of a pregnancy in a woman with an underactive thyroid gland (hypothyroidism) ending in spontaneous abortion are greatly increased. The obvious treatment for a poorly functioning thyroid gland is thyroid hormone replacement therapy. Thyroid extracts containing the two natural hormones of the thyroid gland, thyroxine and triiodothyronine, are the most popular. Thyroid hormones appear to cross the placenta very poorly if at all, and as a result one is never sure if the fetus is receiving adequate amounts of this medication during pregnancy. In spite of widespread use of thyroid hormone, there have been only a few isolated case reports of children born with congenital malformations following maternal use of these preparations, and most authorities consider thyroxine and triiodothyronine to be extremely safe.

Examples of some natural and synthetic thyroid medications are levothyroxine sodium (trade names Synthroid and Levothyroid), thyroid tablets derived from natural extracts of animal thyroid glands, liothronine sodium (trade name Cytomel), liothyronine sodium and levothyroxine sodium (trade name Thyrolar), and thyroglobulin (trade name Proloid). Periodic thyroid function tests throughout pregnancy are invaluable in determining if the dose of thyroid hormone has to be adjusted.

Both thyroxine and triiodothyronine are not excreted in breast milk in significant amounts, and a woman using these medications can safely nurse her infant. If a hypothyroid newborn is not promptly treated with adequate amounts of thyroid hormone, permanent mental retardation and cretinism may develop. Thyroxine and triiodothyronine, when ingested by nursing women, have actually helped prevent permanent damage to infants born with severe hypothyroidism. In one study, twelve of fifteen nursing infants born with hypothyroidism had average intelligence compared to only twelve of thirty-two formula-fed infants.

The treatment of maternal hyperthyroidism, or excessive thyroid activity, is far more complex and unpredictable than that of hypothyroidism. Though the details of the various treatment regimens endorsed by different specialists is beyond the scope of this discussion, the most popular method involves suppression of excessive maternal thyroid function with either Propylthiouracil or methimazole (trade name Tapazole). Unfortunately, both drugs readily cross the placenta and have the capacity to induce severe hypothyroidism and even cretinism in the developing fetus. Therefore, these drugs should be used at the lowest dose capable of maintaining thyroid function at its upper limits of normal. Under ideal conditions, the drug can be stopped completely two to three weeks prior to delivery in order to minimize the risks to the fetus.

Use of Propylthiouracil during pregnancy has not been associated with fetal anomalies, but methimazole has been linked to a specific ulcerlike scalp defect among exposed infants. For this reason, Propylthiouracil is preferred for suppression of thyroid gland hyperactivity during pregnancy. Many older medical textbooks state that women who take Propylthiouracil should not nurse their infants. However, a 1980 report from Denmark clearly demonstrated that it is not concentrated in breast milk to any significant degree and women taking this drug can safely breast-feed their babies.

Propranolol (trade name Inderal) is an antihypertensive medication which is gaining popularity in the treatment of hyperthyroidism. However, the safety of its use during pregnancy has been questioned (see page 217).

Iodides have also been used to suppress thyroid activity. Ingestion of iodides after the twelfth week of pregnancy is not recommended since they may cause hyperthyroidism and goiter in the fetus. Needless to say, use of radioactive iodine as a diagnostic test of thyroid function or in the treatment of thyroid disease is absolutely not recommended during pregnancy.

Tapazole is excreted into the breast milk in concentrations which are three to twelve times higher than those found in the maternal bloodstream. Mothers who require Tapazole should not nurse because the drug will inhibit the infant's thyroid function. Iodides are also excreted in breast milk but in much lower concentrations. However, since milk ingestion by the baby could theoretically depress the functioning of its thyroid gland, women who use iodides should not nurse.

Sex Hormones   **What are the dangers of fetal exposure to sex hormones in pregnancy?**

Fetal exposure to natural and synthetic estrogens and progestogens early in pregnancy is associated with a significantly greater risk of fetal anomalies. These preparations must never be used as a means of bringing on a late period unless a negative pregnancy test is first obtained. The administration of hormones as a means of preventing spontaneous abortion is mentioned only to be deplored. Estrogens in birth control pills will diminish the quantity of breast milk, while progestins will adversely affect its quality.

For a full discussion of the adverse effects of female sex hormone use in pregnancy, including that of DES, see chapter 1. The effects of hormones on the nursing woman and her baby are discussed in chapter 11.

Danazol (trade name Danocrine) is a relatively new synthetic hormonal preparation, similar in structure to the male hormone testosterone, which has been used effectively in the treatment of endometriosis. This benign condition occurs when fragments of endometrium from the lining of the uterine cavity are found in other locations such as the ovary or pelvis. Endometriosis is associated with infertility and danazol is often effective in improving a woman's chances of conception. If a pregnancy does occur while a woman is taking danazol, the drug may masculinize the genitals of her female fetus.

Vitamins

How does use of vitamins affect pregnancy?

Too many or too few vitamins may significantly change the outcome of pregnancy. The vitamins most often associated with a poor pregnancy outcome, when used in doses above those which are recommended, are vitamin A and vitamin D. Two cases of urinary tract malformations have been reported in infants exposed to excessive amounts of vitamin A during the first trimester. In a 1972 study, researchers noted a higher maternal vitamin A level in mothers of infants with central nervous system malformations when compared to a control group. Similarly, excessive maternal intake of vitamin D has been linked to infantile hypercalcemia, or pathologically high levels of calcium in the bloodstream. In addition, stenosis or narrowing of the aorta, the largest artery in the body, has been associated with excessive maternal intake of vitamin D during pregnancy.

A full discussion of vitamin use and nutritional requirements during pregnancy is presented in chapter 8.

8.
Nutrition

During the past ten years there has been a great interest in the subject of nutrition during pregnancy. It's hard to believe that only a short time ago obstetricians pontificated about the importance of strict weight control and salt restriction in preventing toxemia. Patients dutifully followed this erroneous advice, often to the detriment of their pregnancies. Most pregnant women today are better informed and more inquisitive than their predecessors, and many are shocked to discover that they know more about nutrition than their obstetricians. This is not surprising, since most medical schools and residency training programs devote little, if any, time to this vital subject.

Weight

How much weight should I gain during pregnancy?

Animal experimentation and studies of human gestation clearly demonstrate that the weight of a baby at birth is directly related to two independent factors: the mother's weight before pregnancy and her weight gain during pregnancy. The growth of the fetus requires energy, and this can only come about through adequate intake of calories by its mother.

Most nutritionists concur that the optimum weight gain during pregnancy is probably between twenty-four and twenty-eight pounds, two to four pounds during the first trimester and twelve pounds during each of the last two trimesters. This translates to a weekly weight gain of almost a pound during the last six months of pregnancy. Most of the weight gain for the baby takes place over the last three months, while that for the mother is more evenly distributed throughout pregnancy. Of the total weight gain during normal pregnancy, slightly less than half is gained in the fetal compartment, consisting of the fetus, placenta, and amniotic fluid.

It is unrealistic for you to expect that your weight increase will follow the ideal textbook pattern. More often than not, the number of pounds gained varies significantly from one prenatal visit to the next, and weight gains as high as thirty-five pounds are not necessarily harmful and may even be beneficial for some underweight women. However, total disregard for sensible eating habits and the abandoning of all dietary restraints should not be encouraged; maternal overeating may have an adverse effect on the fetus, and it can make labor and delivery more difficult.

It is unwise for your doctor to strictly preset the maximum amount of weight that you may gain during pregnancy since you may reach your limit well before your expected date of confinement (EDC). Under such conditions, intentional weight control may be harmful to the fetus. It has been estimated that a baby gains one ounce a day and its brain develops most rapidly during the last eight weeks of pregnancy. During this time, more calories and nutrients are required than at any other time, and restricting the mother's caloric intake may compromise fetal growth and brain cell development.

Of great concern is the woman who gains little weight or loses weight the third trimester despite an adequate caloric intake. This may signify a poorly functioning placenta and a distressed infant. Equally as disconcerting is the woman who has a sudden and marked weight gain over a short period of time during the last trimester. This may be an early indication of impending preeclampsia. For this reason, weigh yourself at weekly intervals and report significant deviations from your normal pattern of weight gain to your doctor.

Assuming that the ideal prepregnancy caloric intake is about 2,000 calories per day for most adult women and 2,300 calories per day for growing teenagers, the recommended intake necessary to achieve an adequate weight gain should be increased by at least 300 calories per day to 2,300 and 2,600 calories respectively. This adds up to a caloric cost of pregnancy equal to approximately 84,000 calories (300 × 280 days). Many authorities believe that the minimum daily caloric intake for all women during the last trimester should be at least 2,600 calories. It is important to remember that the extra calories you consume count toward the extra nutrients you need. Therefore, avoid so-called empty calories such as potato chips and soft drinks since they contain virtually no nutritional value and will only diminish your appetite for more substantial foods. During the postpartum period, women who nurse their babies will need an extra 750 calories a day above the usual 2,000 calories needed by women who bottle-feed their infants.

Often a woman's greatest concern about gaining weight during pregnancy is that she will be unable to shed her excess pounds following delivery. In actuality, however, the weight is quickly lost. Approximately twelve to fourteen pounds disappear immediately at the moment of delivery if one adds the average weight of the baby, placenta, and amniotic fluid. Over the next six weeks, reduction in the size of the uterus (involution) is accompanied by the loss of excessive body fluid and body fat. It has been found that breast-feeding women tend to lose their pregnancy body fat at a faster rate than women who do not nurse their babies. The most pleasant surprise for many women at their six-week postpartum visit is that they have no more than five or ten pounds to lose in order to achieve their normal prepregnancy weight.

Should these same recommendations be made for underweight and malnourished women?

When a woman's prepregnancy weight is 5 percent or more below the ideal weight for her given height, she will be at a significantly greater risk of giving birth to an infant of low birth weight, one weighing less than 5½ pounds. Researchers demonstrated that a prepregnancy weight of 120 pounds or less combined with a total gestational weight gain of under 11 pounds resulted in the birth of even greater numbers of low birth weight infants, and they recommend that underweight women try to reach their ideal weight before becoming pregnant.

Sadly, the consequences of being born to a mother who is underweight may never be reversed. Most authorities believe that women under 120 pounds should be encouraged to eat according to appetite and that weight gain should be at least 1 pound per week for the first three months of pregnancy. If, by the twentieth week of pregnancy, a gain of at least 10 pounds has not occurred, a woman must be strongly urged to eat more.

Should an obese woman go on a reducing diet when she becomes pregnant?

No. The overweight woman has a greater likelihood of diabetes and hypertension, as well as an increased risk of difficult labor and the birth of an infant weighing more than nine pounds, but though the natural tendency for doctors is to insist that these individuals diet during pregnancy, the correct advice is to prevent them from losing weight. The babies of overweight mothers who gained little during pregnancy were found to be twice as likely to die shortly before or after birth than the babies of heavy women who gained more than twenty pounds during the course of their pregnancies. Dieting during pregnancy can deprive the baby of an adequate supply of protein and other essential nutrients which could impair development of its brain and body. Furthermore, the breakdown of fat, which occurs when a person loses weight, releases toxic ketone bodies which can harm the fetus. In a 1982 report, doctors at Northwestern University Medical School in Chicago observed that even minor dietary deprivation, such as one missed meal, during the third trimester could cause ketone bodies to form in the bloodstream. This occurred in both lean and obese women and pointed out the necessity for all pregnant women to eat at least three meals a day.

Though it would seem logical that an obese woman would naturally gain more weight during her pregnancy than a woman of normal weight, a 1980 study showed that the opposite is true. Most nutritionists agree that the overweight woman should not lose weight during pregnancy, but few have suggested an ideal amount of weight that these individuals should gain. Based on the statistics of more than 13,000 pregnancies, doctors from the University of Pittsburgh concluded that obese women follow the same recommended weight gain of twenty-four to twenty-eight pounds made for women of normal weight.

Protein Intake   ### How much protein is necessary during pregnancy, and which foods are protein-rich?

Protein forms the basic structure of every cell in the body and is vital to the normal development of fetus and placenta. An increase in the intake of protein is required during pregnancy to provide for fetal needs and to allow for the necessary maternal bodily changes such as an expansion of the blood volume, growth of the breasts, and enlargement of the uterus. While the recommended daily protein intake for a non-pregnant woman is 45 grams, the minimum daily amount needed during pregnancy is 75 grams. Some women, especially those in their teens, will fare better with 100 grams of protein daily. If a woman elects to breast-feed, she will usually require 20 grams of protein above her prepregnancy total of 45 grams.

Few people are aware of the amount of protein in various foods. Potatoes, for example, are usually considered to be high in carbohydrates and poor in protein content. In fact, a potato is only slightly higher in calories than an apple, but each potato contains three grams of protein. Similarly, it's difficult for some people to appreciate that protein-rich foods, such as beef, may contain a significant number of calories. In general, carbohydrates and proteins provide 4 calories per gram of weight compared to 9 calories per gram of weight for fats.

Proteins are made up of smaller elements called essential amino acids. During pregnancy there appears to be an active transfer of amino acids across the placenta to accommodate fetal protein synthesis. Amino acids are found in greatest abundance in animal proteins such as meat, fish, milk, cheese, and eggs. Animal proteins also supply iron, phosphorus, zinc, iodine, vitamin E, and B vitamins, such as riboflavin, niacin, vitamin B6, and vitamin B12. About two-thirds of the protein consumed during pregnancy should be of this high biologic quality. Vegetables contain significantly less protein than meat, but they are valuable because they supply the pregnant woman with iron, thiamin, folic acid, vitamin B6, vitamin E, phosphorus, magnesium, and zinc. Vegetables with the most abundant source of protein are lima beans, kidney beans, lentils, tofu or soy bean curd, soybeans and other dried beans, peas, nuts, and sunflower seeds. Vegetable protein is enhanced in nutritional value when it is served at the same meal as animal protein. Fruits usually have insignificant amounts of protein.

What are the effects of maternal protein deprivation on the fetus?

It is often difficult to distinguish between the harm caused by a deficiency in total nutritional content and that which results strictly from protein deprivation. However, it has been demonstrated that a reduced protein intake during pregnancy decreases the availability of amino acids for the fetus, which, in turn, may affect its mental and motor development. Unlike the situation which occurs with other nutrients, when a pregnant woman experiences protein malnutrition, her protein stores will not be entirely sacrificed for the sake of her baby. Instead, her body retains some protein for herself at the expense of the fetus.

Animal experimentation and human experience has shown that protein restriction adversely affects fetal and placental size. Litter sizes among protein-starved animals are often significantly reduced, while implantation of the fertilized egg into the uterine cavity may also be impaired. Protein-deficient women are more likely to give birth to shorter babies with reduced birth weights.

Doctors are usually able to clinically recognize several distinct types of growth-retarded babies. When the cause of the problem is a poorly functioning placenta, the babies will characteristically have a reduction in size of all their organs except the brain, which will maintain a normal number of cells. If, however, the cause of fetal growth retardation is protein malnutrition, the number of brain cells will be diminished by at least 15 percent.

Following childbirth, protein deprivation in the newborn will lead to a 20 percent reduction in the number of brain cells. When a combined prenatal and postpartum protein restriction occurs, the reduction in the number of brain cells will be approximately 60 percent, rather than the expected total of 35 percent. The reason for this exaggerated reaction is unknown. However, it is an especially tragic type of mental disability since it is totally preventable.

Preeclampsia is a condition characterized by an elevation of blood pressure during the last three months of pregnancy. Other features include the presence of protein in the urine as well as marked swelling of the face and hands. When preeclampsia becomes more severe it may be associated with convulsions or coma. If this occurs, it is called eclampsia or toxemia. Preeclampsia remains an enigma despite the fact that many doctors have devoted their lives' work to determining its cause. One popular theory is that a dietary deficiency of protein is responsible, because it has been known for many years that the incidence of this disease is far greater among indigent women and those who eat practically no protein during pregnancy.

Salt

Should I limit my salt intake?

I always seem to encounter a look of skepticism whenever I tell my prenatal patients that they need not restrict their dietary salt intake. Until very recently, obstetricians preached that sodium was the cause of toxemia, but this theory has been totally discredited and it is now known that sodium is essential for the normal expansion of the pregnant woman's tissues and blood volume. If anything, restriction of dietary salt may actually hasten the onset of toxemia by decreasing the volume of fluid in the circulatory system (hypovolemia), thereby causing a greater concentration of blood cells in relation to plasma (hemoconcentration). While we often use the words "salt" and "sodium" interchangeably, the salt we add to our food contains 40 percent sodium and a variety of other chemicals. It is important that you use only iodized or sea salt, since this will prevent goiter or abnormal enlargement of thyroid gland caused by a lack of iodine.

A regimen of restricting sodium and taking diuretics, or water pills, serves only to compound the circulatory problems that could lead to toxemia. It is generally agreed that diuretic therapy in pregnancy is of no benefit but carries multiple risks. If you are receiving prenatal care from a doctor who believes in the implementation of a low salt diet and the use of diuretics, please find another obstetrician. If you experience swelling of the hands and legs, bedrest on your left side for twenty-four hours at a time will prove remarkably effective in alleviating the problem. There is some controversy as to whether salt should be restricted once a woman has developed preeclampsia. Most authorities now believe that salt restriction is of little if any benefit in the treatment of this disease and that use of salt will not precipitate a toxemic crisis.

A common treatment for nonpregnant women with chronic hypertension is sodium restriction and long-term diuretic therapy. Whether these women should continue this treatment during pregnancy is controversial, but there is some evidence that kidney and uterine blood flow may be affected if this treatment is continued. Instead, a more logical approach would be to discontinue the diuretic and use specific antihypertensive drugs (see chapter 7) only if they are absolutely necessary. While it may not be essential to totally eliminate salt from the diet of a chronic hypertensive during pregnancy, foods which contain a high salt content should be used sparingly. These foods are listed below.

Foods Containing Large Quantities of Salt

Asparagus (canned)	Milk (more than 2 glasses a day)
Bacon	Milk chocolate
Beets (canned)	Mustard
Bouillon	Olives (green and ripe)
Broth	Oysters (frozen)
Butter (salted)	Peanuts (salted)
Calves' liver	Peas (canned)
Carrots (canned)	Pickles
Catsup	Pizza
Cheese (including cottage)	Popcorn, salted
Chili sauce	Potato chips
Corned beef (canned)	Pretzels
Corn (canned)	Relish
Corn chips	Salmon (canned pink)
Frankfurters	Sardines (canned in oil)
Green beans (canned)	Sauerkraut
Ham (especially cured)	Sausage
Lima beans (canned and frozen)	Soy sauce
Lobster	Tomatoes (canned)
Luncheon meats	Tuna (canned in oil)
Margarine (salted)	Waffles (enriched)
	Worcestershire sauce

Caffeine

How dangerous is caffeine consumption for the pregnant woman and her fetus?

Research linking high doses of caffeine with limb reduction abnormalities, delayed bone growth, cleft palate, and other birth defects in rats, mice, and rabbits has received much publicity. Based on these studies, the FDA issued a warning to pregnant women to moderate or stop their consumption of coffee and other caffeine-containing beverages and foods, but the FDA also stated that the evidence linking caffeine to birth defects in humans is inconclusive and that rat experiments do not necessarily apply to human pregnancies.

Although it is difficult, if not impossible, to apply laboratory results in rodents to human experience, it is known that caffeine does cross the human placental barrier and is distributed to all fetal tissues. The fetus's ability to clear or remove caffeine from its bloodstream is far less efficient than that of its mother. Studies from France have clearly demonstrated that the caffeine levels in the umbilical cord blood of the baby at birth are almost twice as high as those detected in the mother's bloodstream. Furthermore, caffeine stays in the bloodstream of the fetus and newborn almost fifteen times longer than it does in the adult. These differences are especially pronounced among premature infants. In a 1978 study from the University of Washington, researchers tested hundreds of newborns for behavioral and physical condition on the first day of life. They found that heavy maternal caffeine use during the first five months of pregnancy was responsible for the birth of babies who had poorer than average muscle tone and who were less active at birth. Mothers who reported the highest caffeine use were more likely to give birth to babies with the lowest scores. A recent study of 190 mothers of malformed children in Belgium found that nearly 25 percent drank eight or more cups of coffee a day compared with only 13 percent of mothers with normal babies. In contrast, doctors at the Boston Hospital for Women recently studied the medical records of 12,000 births and found no relationship between heavy coffee consumption during pregnancy and major birth defects. In another important epidemiological study, conducted in 1982, researchers compared coffee consumption in mothers of 2,742 infants with a variety of birth defects. They found no relationship between the amount of coffee consumed and the presence of anomalies. Limb reduction defects, which were associated with heavy coffee consumption in animal studies, were not linked with coffee consumption in this study.

Based on available information, most authorities would conclude that ingestion of one cup of coffee or a caffeine-containing drink per day should cause no harm to the developing fetus. However, I do not feel confident in recommending amounts greater than this, and I am disturbed by the knowledge that 60 percent of the United States adult population drinks an average of two cups of coffee and that 13 percent of pregnant women, or 4,000,000 women each year, drink five or more cups of coffee per day.

Often, recommendations on caffeine use are made without a true understanding of how much caffeine is present in various products. These approximate amounts are listed in table 8–1.

Cola syrup, often taken to relieve morning sickness, contains caffeine. "Pepper" drinks and many noncola soft drinks, some of which contain citrus flavors, may also have significant amounts of caffeine. Sprite, 7-Up, RC-100, and Cragmont Cola are popular sodas which contain no caffeine. Ginger ales, club sodas, tonic waters, root beers and most fruit-flavored drinks contain no natural or added caffeine. If caffeine is added, it must be listed on the label. Carefully read the labels of all beverages which you purchase during pregnancy.

Decaffeinated coffee is a logical and safe alternative coffee substitute, since each cup is estimated to contain only 1 to 6 milligrams of caffeine.

How much caffeine is secreted in breast milk?

Doctors at the Washington University School of Medicine have shown that caffeine rapidly enters the breast milk and achieves peak levels sixty minutes later. They

Table 8–1. Approximate Caffeine Content of Commonly Used Products

Cola	15 to 30 milligrams per 8-ounce can (FDA estimate is 30 to 65 milligrams per 12-ounce can)
Cocoa or hot chocolate	Up to 50 milligrams per 5-ounce cup (FDA estimate is 2 to 40 milligrams per 5-ounce cup)
Chocolate bar	25 milligrams (6 milligrams per ounce) of solid milk chocolate
One cup of brewed coffee	80 to 120 milligrams (FDA estimate is 75 to 155 milligrams)
One cup of instant coffee	66 to 100 milligrams
One cup of leaf tea	30 to 75 milligrams
One cup of bagged tea	42 to 100 milligrams (FDA estimate is 9 to 50 milligrams)
One cup of instant tea	30 to 60 milligrams
One cup of freeze dried coffee	66 milligrams

calculated that a liter of breast milk, collected during the first hour after a woman ingests one cup of coffee, would contain only about 1.5 milligrams of caffeine, an amount that is safe for the nursing infant. They do point out that with repeated maternal caffeine ingestion the risk of caffeine accumulation in the infant would depend upon a variety of factors, such as the volume of breast milk ingested, the infant's clearance rate for caffeine, and the average concentration of the drug in a woman's serum and breast milk. There have been reports of restless, wakeful babies after the ingestion of large amounts of caffeine by breast-feeding mothers.

Are there any caffeine-containing medications which the pregnant and nursing woman should avoid?

Yes. Caffeine is present in a variety of over-the-counter analgesics (Midol, Anacin, Excedrin, Stanback, Vanquish), diet pills (Bio Slim T, Dexadiet II, and Dexatrim), decongestants, (Coryban-D), cold preparations (Dristan), and medications used as stimulants for maintaining mental alertness (No Doz). For a more complete list, see table 8–2. As stated in chapter 7, it is best to avoid these and all other medications during pregnancy and nursing unless absolutely necessary.

Can a nursing mother drink herbal teas or cocoa?

Herbal teas need to be used judiciously by nursing mothers. Many herbal teas contain active ingredients that a woman may secrete in her milk in sufficient amounts to affect her infant. Cathartics, such as buckthorn bark and senna, when present in herbal teas, may cause cramps and watery diarrhea. Camomile tea can cause an allergic reaction in someone who is sensitive to ragweed pollen. Herbal tea manufacturers are not required to list the ingredients of their products on labels, so nursing mothers must be cautious about the possible side effects of the use of these teas.

Recent studies show that a chemical found in cocoa passes freely into human milk, and this may cause a number of adverse reactions such as diarrhea, constipation, eczema, irritability, and sleeplessness.

Besides its caffeine content, are there other problems associated with drinking tea?

Drinking tea with meals may contribute to iron-deficiency anemia during pregnancy. The tannins in tea inhibit the absorption of iron from the intestinal tract, and this is especially likely to occur if the diet is rich in vegetables. However, iron absorption is not affected when meat is regularly eaten.

Vitamins

Why is folic acid necessary during pregnancy, and what is its recommended daily allowance?

Folic acid, also referred to as folate and folacin, is a B vitamin which is essential in the synthesis of a vital cellular protein named deoxyribonucleic acid, or DNA. DNA is found in the nucleus of all cells of the body, especially those undergoing rapid division. For this reason, the fetus, placenta, and maternal bone marrow would all be primarily affected by a folic acid deficiency. Folic acid also enables red blood cells to carry oxygen to cells of the body which require it.

The daily folate requirement for adults ranges between 200 and 400 micrograms, and most authorities believe that this amount should be doubled during pregnancy. While one would assume that a well-nourished woman will easily meet these requirements in her daily diet, there is some evidence to show that the amount of folate supplied by normal diets may vary significantly from one meal to the next, and subtle deficiencies may exist. For this reason, most obstetricians in the United States routinely prescribe prenatal vitamins containing between 300 and 1,000 micrograms of folic acid. There are no known harmful consequences resulting from an excess of folic acid during pregnancy.

Folic acid is abundant in many foods, especially liver, kidney, green leafy vegetables, broccoli, asparagus, peanuts, mung bean sprouts, cow peas, wheat germ, wheat bran, kidney beans, peas, lima beans, soybeans, and garbanzo beans. Surprisingly, chocolate is a fairly good source of folic acid; whole milk, rice, corn, cereals, and processed foods are notably poor.

Aside from individuals with dietary inadequacies, which women should be most carefully observed for folate deficiencies during pregnancy?

Among healthy individuals, folic acid is readily and efficiently absorbed from the small intestine. For most women, this mechanism is not altered significantly during pregnancy. Excessive vomiting during pregnancy, also known as hyperemesis gravidarum, is probably the most common reason for poor folate absorption. A small number of otherwise healthy women are incapable of absorbing folic acid during pregnancy and require intramuscular supplements in order to maintain their normal blood levels of this vitamin. Several rare intestinal diseases, known as malabsorption

Table 8–2. Caffeine-Containing Drugs

Nonprescription Brand	Use	Milligrams of Caffeine per Tablet	Comments
Anacin Analgesic Tablets, Anacin-3, Anacin Maximum Strength	Pain relief	32.0	Avoid if possible, since Anacin contains aspirin
Aqua-Ban	Diuretic (medication to relieve fluid retention)	100.0	Do not use during pregnancy
Bio Slim T	Aid in weight reduction	140.0	Dieting not recommended during pregnancy and nursing
Cope	Pain relief	32.0	Avoid if possible, since it contains aspirin
Coryban-D	Relief of nasal congestion and runny nose	30.0	Contains phenylpropanolamine, which may cause birth defects (see chapter 7)
Dexadiet II and Dexatrim and Dietac	Aid in weight reduction	200.0	Contains phenylpropanolamine, which may cause birth defects, and dieting is not recommended during pregnancy
Dristan Decongestant, Dristan A-F Decongestant Tablets	Relief of cold symptoms, sneezing, nasal congestion, aches, minor pains	16.2	Avoid if possible, since it contains aspirin
Excedrin	Relief of pain of headache, sinusitis, muscular aches, minor pain	64.8	Contains aspirin-like medication, which is best avoided
Goody's Headache Powders	Relief of pain and headache	32.5 (per dose)	Avoid if possible, since it contains aspirin
Midol	Pain relief	32.4	Avoid if possible, since it contains aspirin
No Doz	Stimulant to maintain alertness and prevent sleep	100.0	Avoid if possible

Table 8–2. Caffeine-Containing Drugs   (*continued*)

Nonprescription Brand	Use	Milligrams of Caffeine per Tablet	Comments
Prolamine	Weight control	140.0	Contains phenylpropanolamine, which may cause birth defects, and dieting is not recommended during pregnancy
Sinapils	Cold and allergy symptoms	32.4	Contains phenylpropanolamine
Stanback Analgesic Powders	Relief of headache, muscular aches, other pain, control of fever	15.0 (per dose)	Avoid if possible, since it contains aspirin
Triaminicin	Relief of cold and allergy symptoms	30.0	Avoid because it contains aspirin and phenylpropanolamine
Vanquish	Relief of headache, muscular aches, other pain, control of fever	33.0	Avoid if possible, since it contains aspirin
Vivarin Tablets	Stimulant to maintain alertness and prevent sleep	200.0	Avoid if possible
Prescription Drugs			
Apectol	Sedative and pain reliever	40.0	Should not be taken because it contains aspirin, barbiturate, and phenacetin (see chapter 7)
Cafergot	Relief of migraine headache	100.0	Contains ergotamine tartrate, which may cause dangerous uterine contractions and constriction of blood vessels
Darvon Compound	Relief of mild to moderate pain	32.4	Contains propoxyphene hydrochloride, which has not been proved safe in pregnancy, and withdrawal symptoms in newborns have been reported
Esgic Tablets and Capsules	Sedative and pain reliever	40.0	Avoid because it contains a barbiturate

continued

Table 8–2. Caffeine-Containing Drugs   (*continued*)

Nonprescription Brand	Use	Milligrams of Caffeine per Tablet	Comments
Fiorinal	Pain relief, especially for tension headache	40.0	Avoid because it contains aspirin, barbiturate, and phenacetin
Migral	Vascular headaches, especially migraine	50.0	Avoid because it contains ergotamine tartrate and cyclizine, which may cause fetal anomalies (see table 7–2)
Migralam	Migraine headache	100.0	Contains isometheptene mucate, which may cause dangerous uterine contractions and constrict blood vessels
Soma Compound	Pain reliever and muscle relaxant	32.0	Contains carisoprodol, a muscle relaxant—effect on fetus unknown—and contains phenacetin, which should be avoided

syndromes, also cause a decrease in folate absorption; celiac disease is an example. Phenytoin (trade name Dilantin), a drug which is commonly prescribed in the treatment of epilepsy, also interferes with folate absorption into the body from the intestinal tract. Alcoholic women, too, are more likely to experience a folic acid deficiency, as a result of their inadequate food consumption.

Various blood disorders characterized by premature destruction, or hemolysis, of red blood cells create a greater demand for folic acid; examples are chronic hemolytic anemias, sickle-cell disease, G6PD deficiency, and thalassemia, the last most common among individuals of Mediterranean origin. All these disorders require a supplement of at least one milligram of folic acid daily during pregnancy.

The increased maternal blood volume combined with the growing fetus and placenta are all responsible for creating a greater need for folic acid during pregnancy. Maternal bodily stores are the source of much of this folic acid, and women with two or more pregnancies in rapid succession have less time to replenish their folate stores. Similarly, women experiencing a multiple birth deplete more of their folic acid in meeting the greater fetal and placental demands.

What are the symptoms of a folic acid deficiency and how is it diagnosed?

Though folic acid deficiency during pregnancy is quite common, it develops slowly and most women with this condition are without symptoms. Overt disease, characterized by severe anemia and bone marrow abnormalities, is usually apparent if the deficiency has been long neglected.

When a person with a previously adequate diet is suddenly deprived of folic acid, it takes approximately three weeks for the serum folate levels to reflect this decline. While the serum folate test is the earliest method of detecting a folic acid deficiency, it is never routinely performed during pregnancy.

At seven weeks following folate deprivation, a type of circulating white blood cell, called a neutrophil, will demonstrate a greater number of segments in the lobes of its nucleus. These characteristic changes can easily be viewed under the microscope and represent a simple and highly specific test for diagnosing a folic acid deficiency. A good laboratory technician should be able to make the diagnosis while performing the routine prenatal blood count. However, if the diagnosis is missed at this point, it will take fourteen weeks of folate deprivation for a urine test to detect the disease. This test measures the concentration of a chemical substance named formiminoglutamic acid, also known by the acronym FIGLU. Under normal conditions, FIGLU is converted to a chemical named glutamic acid by folic acid. However, with a folate deficiency, this reaction cannot take place, and FIGLU accumulates in the urine.

Two weeks after a positive FIGLU test laboratory studies will show a decrease in folic acid levels within red blood cells.

The severe and symptomatic stages of folic acid deficiency will occur approximately eighteen to twenty weeks following its removal from the diet. These include bone marrow abnormalities, severe anemia characterized by abnormally large and bizarre red blood cells, and a pronounced platelet deficiency (thrombocytopenia).

How will a folic acid deficiency affect pregnancy?

In the rare event that a folic acid deficiency is neglected to the point of anemia and thrombocytopenia, the pregnancy will be adversely affected. Severe anemia is associated with a higher incidence of fetal loss, premature birth, and perinatal complications, while a low platelet count may cause life-threatening maternal hemorrhage during pregnancy, labor, and the postpartum period. Both situations can be treated and prevented by adequate supplements of folic acid.

Studies which have attempted to correlate folic acid deficiency with recurrent spontaneous abortion and congenital abnormalities have come to conflicting conclusions. Congenital abnormalities are known to be higher among women treated for cancer during the first trimester of pregnancy with medications known as folic acid antagonists. Similarly, women with epilepsy who are treated with Phenytoin are more likely to give birth to abnormal infants. It has been theorized that both drugs produce their ill effects by diminishing folic acid levels in the fetus.

It was first theorized in 1966 that a relationship existed between folate deficiency and the presence of severe fetal neural tube defects such as anencephaly and hydrocephaly (see chapter 10). Though the chances of giving birth to a baby with a neural tube defect are quite small, once this misfortune occurs a woman will be at a 2 to 5 percent risk of its happening again. For unknown reasons, women in the United

Kingdom and Ireland are more likely to give birth to infants with these abnormalities than women living in the United States. In a 1980 study from England, doctors gave multivitamins to 178 nonpregnant women who had previously given birth to infants with neural tube defects and wished to become pregnant again. The vitamins were begun at least twenty-eight days before conception and continued through the critical first eight weeks of pregnancy when neural tube formation occurs. Of this group, 137 women conceived and only one gave birth to an infant with a neural tube defect. This recurrence rate of only 0.6 percent was far below the expected incidence of 2 to 5 percent. Among a control group of 187 women with identical pregnancy histories, 13, or the expected 5 percent, gave birth to infants with neural tube defects. The only difference was that this group did not receive vitamin supplements either before or during pregnancy. As a result of these studies, a number of other investigative teams throughout the world will be conducting their own tests to confirm the validity of these potentially significant findings. Reports from Great Britain have claimed that a woman with a folate deficiency will incur a fivefold greater risk of hemorrhage due to premature separation of the placenta from the uterine wall. A relationship between folate deficiency and other causes of pregnancy bleeding as well as toxemia has also been proposed. At the present time, however, most authorities doubt that an asymptomatic folic acid deficiency can be implicated as a major cause for a poor pregnancy outcome.

Finally, as previously mentioned in chapter 5, a folic acid deficiency may be associated with a falsely abnormal Pap smear suggestive of cervical cancer. By providing folic acid supplements, rather than surgery, the astute obstetrician can cure this condition without unnecessary surgical intervention.

Aside from folic acid, how essential are other B vitamin supplements during pregnancy?

While the requirements for folic acid are doubled during pregnancy, the need for all other vitamins increases only slightly. Contrary to what the pharmaceutical companies may tell you, these requirements are easily met through the normal diet. Despite this knowledge, it is customary in the United States for doctors to prescribe prenatal vitamins to practically all pregnant women. Though these vitamin supplements do not cause harm when taken in the normal dosage, the fact is that they are most often unnecessary. Furthermore, too many women mistakenly rely on vitamins as a quick and easy substitute for good nutrition and proper dietary habits.

The B vitamins are numbered 1 through 12. In general, the requirements for all B vitamins may be met with adequate servings of milk, meat, poultry, eggs, fish, whole grain bread and cereal, wheat germ, and brewer's yeast.

Thiamine, or vitamin B1, is essential for a healthy appetite, normal digestion, and good muscular tone of the gastrointestinal tract. Though it is needed for bodily growth and lactation, a maternal deficiency will not necessarily be harmful to the fetus. In one report, a thiamine deficiency was noted in 30 percent of pregnant women studied, but selective transport of this vitamin across the placenta was proven by the fact that all the newborn infants had normal thiamine levels. Especially good sources of thiamine are pork and pork products, liver, heart, kidney, peas, beans, and wheat germ. Since this vitamin is not stored in the body, it is important that pregnant women maintain an adequate diet each day in order to prevent its depletion.

Riboflavin, or vitamin B2, is necessary for the normal growth and development of the fetus. A deficiency of this vitamin may be manifested by skin dryness, cracking of the lips and corners of the mouth, inflammation of the tongue, and eye problems such as burning, itching, poor vision, and light sensitivity. A good source of riboflavin is milk, and four cups of milk or milk products a day will meet all of the pregnant woman's requirements. Beef and calf liver also contain large amounts of riboflavin. Several studies have shown that women who use birth control pills are more likely to be deficient in riboflavin. This deficiency is greatest among those on the Pill for the longest periods of time. For this reason, a woman who conceives shortly after stopping the Pill should be made aware of the importance of adequate riboflavin intake.

The United States RDA for riboflavin is 1.5 milligrams. It has been suggested that an additional 0.3 milligram be added during pregnancy and 0.5 milligram for nursing.

A recent study from Cornell University found that people who engage in regular, vigorous physical exercise may need more riboflavin than the current recommended RDA. For the woman who remains active during pregnancy, this would indicate a greater need than that currently advised.

Niacin is an important B vitamin which is found in abundance in peanuts and brewer's yeast and also in canned tuna, beef, and pork. It is vital in the building of brain cells and also prevents infection and bleeding of the gums. Early signs of a niacin deficiency are loss of appetite, nausea, vomiting, abdominal pain, headache, dizziness, and burning, numbness, and weakness of the hands and feet. As with riboflavin, women who use birth control pills prior to conception will be more likely to be deficient in niacin.

The RDA for niacin is approximately 15 milligrams for women fifteen to eighteen years of age and 13 milligrams among those in the eighteen-to-thirty-five-year age group. Suggested increases for pregnant and nursing women are 2 and 7 milligrams respectively.

Pyridoxine, or vitamin B6, is essential for the metabolism of fat and fatty acids and for the production of antibodies. Labels on food packages and supplements may list B6 as pyridoxine, pyridoxal, or pyridoxamine. For practical purposes, all these names may be thought of as being identical. Symptoms of a vitamin B6 deficiency are mental depression, lethargy, fatigue, impaired glucose and insulin metabolism, numbness and tingling of the arms and legs, loss of balance, and anemia. A pyridoxine deficiency during pregnancy has been implicated as the cause of depression which some women experience at this time. Milk, cereals, yeast, liver, and wheat germ contain abundant amounts of pyridoxine. Other sources are grains, beans, nuts, and dried fruits. If a woman restricts her intake of high carbohydrate foods, she may not take in enough of vitamin B6 in her diet.

A number of investigators have reported a vitamin B6 deficiency among women using birth control pills, In one study, doctors were able to demonstrate abnormal pyridoxine metabolism in 80 percent of those who stayed on the Pill for six months or longer. For this reason, some physicians have recommended a daily 25-milligram supplementation of vitamin B6 for all women using birth control pills. This dose is ten times the usual RDA for pyridoxine.

Researchers from Purdue University have recently expressed concern that some pregnant women may need significantly more vitamin B6 than the daily 25 milligrams which is currently recommended. They concluded that vitamin B6 levels be checked at the fifth month of pregnancy and that additional supplements be given if necessary.

Though a 0.5 milligram increase in the RDA for pyridoxine is currently recommended during lactation as well as pregnancy, there has been great controversy in the past two years as to the wisdom of this policy. A minority of researchers have claimed that pyridoxine will reduce the quantity of a woman's breast milk. However, from the available reports, I would surmise that pyridoxine, in the currently recommended amount of 2.5 milligrams daily, would be an unlikely cause of inhibited or faulty lactation.

Vitamin B12, also known as cobalamin and cyanocobalamin, is essential for the normal development of red blood cells. A severe deficiency of this vitamin causes pernicious anemia, a very rare condition, occurring in only 1 out of every 10,000 women of reproductive age. Since a woman with pernicious anemia will also have diminished fertility, it is unlikely you will have this problem.

As previously stated, most nutritionists endorse the use of folic acid supplements during pregnancy. In addition to preventing and treating anemia caused by a lack of folic acid, these supplements will also correct the red blood cell abnormalities associated with pernicious anemia caused by a vitamin B12 deficiency. However, folic acid will not correct the progressively worsening neurological defects associated with pernicious anemia and may even delay the accurate diagnosis of this condition. As with some of the other B vitamins, the levels of vitamin B12 may be significantly reduced among users of oral contraceptives. This should be emphasized to all women who conceive following prolonged use of the Pill.

The RDA for vitamin B12 has been set at 5 milligrams, with increased increments of 3 milligrams and 1 milligram recommended for pregnancy and lactation respectively.

Biotin is a B vitamin which is found in an infinite number of foods. While milk, egg yolk, meats, cereals, legumes, and nuts are especially rich in this vitamin, it is also produced in the human intestine by microorganisms. A naturally occurring isolated biotin deficiency has never been reported. The RDA for biotin is set at 0.3 milligram, though this is probably twice the amount actually needed. Pregnancy and lactation do not alter the body's biotin needs.

Pantothenic acid is a B vitamin found in just about all foods. Especially good sources of pantothenic acid are liver, kidney, eggs, peanuts, and wheat bran, though even poor diets usually contain adequate amounts of this vitamin. As with biotin, a pure pantothenic acid deficiency has only been created under experimental conditions. The RDA for pantothenic acid is 15 milligrams. Since the bodily requirements for this vitamin are unchanged during pregnancy and lactation, it would be difficult to justify the use of pantothenic supplements during these times.

What are the recommended daily allowances for vitamin A during pregnancy?

Retinol, or **vitamin A**, builds resistance to infection, is necessary for maintaining visual acuity, strengthens mucous membranes, plays a role in the formation of tooth enamel, hair, and fingernails, and is also responsible for proper functioning of the thyroid gland. Vitamin A greatly contributes to the development of fetal eyes, skin, and glands. Claims have been made that Vitamin A will relieve skin diseases, warts, sinusitis, ulcers, and stretch marks. There is no scientific justification for these supposed benefits.

The usual RDA for nonpregnant women is 5,000 International Units (IU) of vitamin A. This is increased in pregnancy to 6,000 IU, while 8,000 IU are recommended during lactation. A woman's serum levels of vitamin A will usually decline in early pregnancy and then begin to rise between the thirteenth and sixteenth weeks. At thirty-six weeks, vitamin A levels reach an average of one and a half times normal.

Several experimental animal studies and one report of a human pregnancy have confirmed that very large overdoses of vitamin A, in the range of five to ten times the RDA, may be associated with greater risks of kidney abnormalities in the fetus. The potential for birth defects with amounts considerably less than this is probably nil. Animal studies have shown that both a deficiency of vitamin A, as well as an excess, may be associated with fetal abnormalities. It is believed that several factors, one of which is a deficiency of vitamin A, may be linked in some way to the development of cancers of the colon, stomach, esophagus, breast, liver, and uterus.

Fortified whole milk, cream, ice cream, fortified margarine, butter, egg yolks, fish, liver oils, liver, kidney, green leafy and yellow vegetables, such as green or red peppers, kale, pumpkins, spinach, sweet potatoes, and carrots and cantaloupe are all excellent sources of vitamin A. Good sources include apricots, broccoli, tomatoes, watermelons, and winter squash.

What are the vitamin C requirements during pregnancy and lactation?

Vitamin C, or ascorbic acid, has very important functions. In addition to helping in the formation of body connective tissues and hemoglobin, it also plays a role in the metabolism of folic acid, the strengthening of capillary and cell walls, improving resistance to infection, the removal of body toxins or poisons, the absorption of iron from the intestine, the acidification of the urine, wound healing, and the repair of fractures.

A person's vitamin C levels will often depend on several factors. Bodily stress, infection, and fever will deplete stores of vitamin C. Alcohol, smoking, aspirin, and birth control pills will all interfere with vitamin C absorption from the intestinal tract. Excessive cooking of vegetables in too much water will cause a significant loss of dietary vitamin C.

Though a severe vitamin C deficiency will result in a rare and serious disease called scurvy, a lesser deficiency of this vitamin may manifest itself as swollen, reddened gums which readily bleed, bruise easily, and have a greater susceptibility to infection.

Ever since chemist Linus Pauling began to extol the benefits of vitamin C, researchers have been trying to determine whether large amounts of this vitamin can prevent colds or lessen their severity. The few preliminary studies in support of Pauling's hypothesis have been notably lacking in proper research design and technique. Unfortunately, the public has been too ready to accept as fact the supposed benefits of vitamin C megadoses. Of the many who have taken up the fad of using vitamin C in this manner, few are aware of its potential dangers. It is known, for example, that large doses of vitamin C can cause diarrhea, excessively acid urine, kidney stones, interference with the germ-fighting ability of the body's white blood cells, high blood cholesterol levels in rats and some humans and the blockage of the activity of certain drugs.

Doses of vitamin C in excess of 1 gram (1,000 milligrams) daily may also be harmful to the fetus. Vitamin C readily crosses the placenta from the maternal circulation. When a woman ingests excessive vitamin C during pregnancy, it stimulates the enzyme system of the fetus to metabolize this increased amount. Following birth, normal amounts of vitamin C may be insufficient to satisfy the overly stimulated enzyme system of the newborn. As a result, these babies may experience a severe vitamin C deficiency and even scurvy.

The United States RDA for vitamin C is approximately 55 to 60 milligrams for the nonpregnant woman, though many knowledgeable nutritionists are convinced that one-half to two-thirds of this amount is more than adequate. It has been suggested that an additional 5 to 20 milligrams should be added for pregnancy, and 5 to 40 milligrams during lactation. These modest increases can be readily provided in the diet, and the traditional practice of incorporating supplements of approximately 90 milligrams of vitamin C in most prenatal vitamins would appear to be both excessive and unnecessary. The best natural source of vitamin C is citrus fruits, though spinach, cantaloupes, strawberries, broccoli, green and red peppers, kale, tomatoes, white and sweet potatoes, cauliflower, parsley, watermelon, brussels sprouts, cabbage, turnips, asparagus, okra, green beans, and lima beans are all sources of this vitamin.

What specific obstetrical benefits have been attributed to vitamin C?

As a result of several nonscientific anecdotal claims made by vitamin C enthusiasts, there is a widely held belief that megadoses of this vitamin can improve many aspects of pregnancy and childbirth. Supposed benefits of using 10,000 or more milligrams of vitamin C daily include a lower rate of miscarriage and bleeding, shorter and less painful labor, a marked reduction in the incidence of lacerations and tearing during delivery, fewer stretch marks (striae), a lower number of complications such as postpartum hemorrhage and retention of placental tissue, and a quicker maternal recovery following delivery. Vitamin C enthusiasts have also claimed that babies born of megadose-treated women have higher Apgar scores (see chapter 11), are healthier during the first few weeks of life, and are less likely to experience sudden death in childhood.

Though all these superlatives attributed to vitamin C use might sound impressive, they are not supported by substantial scientific data.

How much vitamin D is required in pregnancy?

Vitamin D is essential in the metabolism and deposition of calcium and phosphorus in teeth and bones. This vitamin crosses the placenta freely, and its concentrations in the fetus are directly dependent on maternal levels. A vitamin D deficiency in late pregnancy may be associated with low calcium levels (hypocalcemia) in the newborn's circulation. More severe maternal deprivation can cause enamel defects of the teeth and irreversible deformities of the fetal skeleton. Premature infants born of mothers with little or no prenatal care are far more likely to have a vitamin D deficiency and hypocalcemia.

At the opposite extreme, too much vitamin D may also be harmful. Of all vitamins, D is probably the easiest to take inadvertently in toxic excess. Studies suggest a possible association between excess maternal vitamin D and severe infantile hypercalcemia, skull and facial abnormalities, and stenosis or narrowing of the aorta and pulmonary artery of the newborn. For this reason, I discourage all women from indiscriminately taking vitamin D supplements during pregnancy.

There are two sources of vitamin D: ingested food and sunlight. Most nutritionists concur that the RDA for vitamin D during pregnancy and lactation should remain unchanged from the 400 International Units (IU) per day suggested for non-pregnant women. This is the amount contained in one quart of vitamin D-fortified milk. All doctors do not share this view, however, and some research conducted at the University of Edinburgh in 1980 suggests that pregnancy supplements of vitamin D should be as high as 500 to 700 IU daily. Further research is required before these recommendations can be endorsed.

In addition to vitamin D-fortified milk, other good sources are fish, liver oils, mackerel, salmon, tuna, sardines, and herring. Curiously, this vitamin is very scarce in most other foods.

When the ultraviolet light of the sun comes in contact with the skin's surface, a chemical reaction takes place and vitamin D is formed. A woman can receive her entire daily allowance of vitamin D in this fashion, depending obviously, on the amount of skin surface exposed to the sun. Therefore, women who are pregnant during the summer months and those living in warm climates are more apt to have adequate vitamin D derived from sunlight. A dark-complexioned woman needs more sun exposure than a fair-skinned person, because the melanin pigment of her skin offers better protection against the sun's rays.

Several studies, including one conducted in 1980, clearly demonstrate that breast-fed infants have lower vitamin D concentrations than bottle-fed babies. As a result, many nutritionists now recommend that breast-fed newborns be given a supplement of vitamin D.

What is the function of vitamin E?

It has been stated sarcastically that the E in **vitamin E** stands for "excess" because at one time or another it has been acclaimed as a cure or preventive for just about every disease and ailment. Contrary to the claims, vitamin E supplementation of the ordinary diet will not cure ignorance, impotence, frigidity, sterility, heart disease, skin disorders, wrinkles, or ulcers. It will not prevent spontaneous abortion, alleviate burns or minimize their scars, increase resistance to infection, delay the aging process, or prevent crib death in infants. The known and accepted functions of vitamin E, or alpha tocopherol, are its ability to aid in the metabolism of vitamin A, promote healing, and develop healthy red blood cells. Vitamin E is also a potent antioxident. This means that it helps govern the amount of oxygen the body uses and prevents oxygen from combining with, and prematurely breaking down, important substances in the body cells. The life of these cells may be shortened in a person whose diet is deficient in vitamin E.

Though vitamin E is thought of as a very exotic and rare vitamin, in actual fact it is found in essentially every food. Its wide distribution in vegetable oils, cereal grains, corn, peanuts, eggs, and animal fats makes a deficiency of vitamin E in humans extremely unlikely. Therefore, the use of vitamin E supplements should be restricted to very unusual situations such as premature infants with low vitamin E stores and women with cystic fibrosis and other intestinal fat-absorption diseases. Vitamin E is a fat-soluble vitamin along with vitamins A, D, and K. All may be deficient in the presence of one of these rare diseases.

The United States RDA for vitamin E has been set at 30 IU, although one-half of this amount easily satisfies a person's nutritional requirements. Although vitamin E enthusiasts have endorsed amounts as high as 800 to 1,000 IU daily, there is absolutely no evidence that these high doses are of any benefit. While it is commonly stated that there are no known harmful consequences of vitamin E megadoses, some animal studies do not support this claim. Some physicians have claimed that hypervitaminosis E in humans may be associated with dangerous coagulation disorders, thrombophlebitis (clots and inflammation in the veins), hypertension, fatigue, headache, dizziness, nausea, diarrhea, intestinal cramps, muscle weakness, and a variety of other problems. The long-term effects of vitamin E supplementation have never been adequately tested, and until more is known, its use should be discouraged.

What are the vitamin K requirements of pregnancy?

Vitamin K is vital for normal coagulation of the blood. It is synthesized in the intestinal tract by bacteria and does not come from a specific food source.

A baby born with a deficiency of vitamin K–dependent clotting factors is at a great risk of serious and even fatal hemorrhage. This complication is far more common than is currently realized and is especially likely to occur when convulsions such as those of epilepsy are treated with Phenytoin. Neonatal hemorrhage in susceptible newborns can be prevented by treating them with an intramuscular injection of vitamin K. However, the administration of vitamin K injections to a pregnant woman may lead to jaundice in her newborn and is usually not recommended. Oral anticoagulants, such as warfarin (Coumadin) and bishydroxycoumarin (Dicumarol) are known to cross the placenta and inhibit vitamin K and clotting factors dependent on vitamin K. As a result, fetal and neonatal hemorrhage may occur. For this reason, oral anticoagulants are not recommended for use during pregnancy. The continued use of antibiotics may kill intestinal bacteria which are responsible for vitamin K production and in this manner may create a deficiency. Increased serum levels of vitamin K–dependent clotting factors have been found among women using oral contraceptives. It has been suggested that this is the reason for the higher incidence of abnormal blood clotting among these women.

Minerals

How essential are iron supplements during pregnancy?

The body's requirements for **iron** increase tremendously during pregnancy, and there is no doubt that supplemental iron is essential. Without iron, a woman is unable to make red blood cells which are so vital to the transfer of oxygen to both maternal and fetal body cells. Unfortunately, the nonpregnant American woman stores an average of only 300 milligrams of iron in her bone marrow. This amount is totally inadequate in meeting the great demands imposed by pregnancy. In addition, previous pregnancies and menstrual blood loss only tend to further reduce iron stores and intensify this problem.

As the pregnant woman's plasma volume increases, her erythrocyte, or red blood cell count, will also expand but at a much slower pace. It has been calculated that a total of 500 milligrams of iron is needed during pregnancy to satisfy the expanded maternal blood volume. The development of the fetus and placenta requires an additional 300 milligrams of iron. This, combined with the previously mentioned 500 milligrams, will give a total iron requirement for pregnancy of about 800 milligrams. If the iron obtained is all at the expense of the pregnant woman's limited reserves, she may easily become anemic. It has been estimated that as many as one-half of all pregnant women who do not receive supplemental iron will be anemic at the time of delivery.

To meet the 800-milligram iron requirement for pregnancy, a woman must take daily supplements in quantities that will result in her absorbing 4 to 5 milligrams of iron per day throughout the latter half of pregnancy. Despite exaggerated claims and often misleading advertising, the most commonly prescribed and least expensive supplemental iron preparation remains ferrous sulfate. Since only 10 to 20 percent of dietary iron is absorbed from the intestine, and since ferrous sulfate contains about 20 percent elemental iron, tablets in a dose of 150 milligrams to 300 milligrams (30 to 60 milligrams of elemental iron) per day would allow absorption of the needed quantity of supplemental iron. It is interesting to note that the elevated iron content of several commonly used preparations varies significantly. For example, products containing ferrous gluconate will have only 11 percent elemental iron, while preparations with ferrous fumarate will contain a high of 30 percent elemental iron. Therefore, though ferrous fumarate preparations may be more expensive than generic ferrous sulfate, you do get more elemental iron for your money with this product. There is some evidence to show that iron absorption is enhanced when it is given with vitamin C, in doses of 100 to 200 milligrams daily.

Taking iron may cause nausea, diarrhea, or constipation. Bowel movements also become black in color. Iron therapy is not necessary during the first trimester, when intolerance to this medication is most likely. In fact, iron supplementation in the first eight weeks has been implicated as a possible cause of malformations in the fetus though this has not been substantiated in any large studies. If a woman is unable to tolerate iron preparations throughout her pregnancy, periodic intramuscular iron injections can be administered. Most authorities recommend that iron supplements be maintained for two to three months postpartum in order to replenish iron stores which may have been diminished during pregnancy.

Good sources of dietary iron include dried fruits, liver, kidney, prune juice, dried beans, lima beans, dark molasses, fish, egg yolk, raisins, varieties of bread and cereal fortified with iron, and vegetables, such as spinach, broccoli, kale, and greens. Certain substances such as carbonates, phosphates, oxalates, fiber-rich foods, and tannates in tea may all be responsible for inhibiting iron absorption from the intestine.

How much calcium do I require?

Calcium is a necessary mineral for proper fetal bone and tooth development. The calcium content of the newborn's skeleton is approximately 30 grams, with most of the accumulation occurring during the last trimester. Even if a woman has an inadequate calcium intake, her fetus is still able to obtain sufficient amounts by extracting it from her bony skeleton. The parasitizing of a mother's bony skeleton by her fetus sounds worse than it really is, since only about 2.5 percent of her total body content of calcium is sacrificed for the sake of the fetus. This small amount will rarely if ever create a negative calcium balance in a well-nourished woman. Though most women's serum calcium levels will be lower during pregnancy, it does not necessarily mean a calcium deficiency. Instead, it merely shows that the calcium is distributed more thinly through greater blood volume which occurs during pregnancy. Research actually shows that calcium absorption and storage are enhanced during pregnancy.

The United States RDA for calcium is 1,200 milligrams for nonpregnant women fifteen to eighteen years of age and 800 milligrams for those nineteen years of age and older. An additional 400 milligrams is recommended during pregnancy and lactation. Milk is unquestionably the best source of calcium, and four glasses daily will satisfy the entire pregnancy RDA. Skim milk has just as much calcium as whole milk and low-fat milk. If you don't enjoy drinking milk, add it in liquid or powdered form to puddings, soups, baked goods, hot cereal, casseroles, and other prepared foods. If you are unable to drink large quantities of milk, it's helpful to know that other dairy products, such as 1 cup of yogurt, 1½ ounces of hard unprocessed cheese, such as cheddar and Swiss, 1¾ cups of ice cream, or 2 cups of cottage cheese all supply an amount of calcium equal to that found in 1 glass of milk. Though there are other natural foods which contain calcium, it is virtually impossible to meet the 1,200-milligram daily allowance without the use of dairy products. Fairly good non-dairy sources of calcium include oysters, salmon, sardines, dark green and leafy vegetables, such as broccoli, kale, and mustard greens, and dried figs, dates, and apricots. The active and useful form of calcium is the free or unbound variety.

There are a significant number of women who can't tolerate regular milk because they are unable to digest lactose, the milk sugar. Symptoms of this condition, named lactose intolerance, are abdominal pain, bloating, and diarrhea following milk ingestion. For unknown reasons, it is more common among blacks, Asians,

Mediterraneans, Jews, central Europeans, and American Indians. The problem of lactose intolerance may be remedied by drinking acidophilus milk, in which the lactose is predigested by bacteria. Another option is to treat regular milk with enzymes that break down lactose. One product which does this is Lact-Aid, available through your pharmacist or the Sugarlo Company (P. O. Box 111, 600 Fire Road, Pleasantville, New Jersey, 08232). Cultured dairy products such as yogurt, buttermilk, sour cream, and hard cheese contain very little lactose. Soy milk, rather than cow's milk, is also recommended for the pregnant woman who is unable to tolerate lactose.

If these suggestions fail, calcium supplements in the form of calcium gluconate or calcium lactate pills should be taken. To assure maximum absorption from the intestine, these supplements should be eaten on an empty stomach, preferably with either a dairy product or a citrus fruit or juice. The former contains high amounts of vitamin D, while the latter is rich in vitamin C. Both aid in calcium absorption from the intestinal tract.

Early symptoms of a calcium deficiency include sleeplessness, irritability, muscle cramps in the legs, and exaggerated pain over the ligaments supporting the uterus.

What can a woman do to relieve leg cramps caused by lower calcium levels?

The characteristic sudden cramps in the back of the calf which some women experience in the last half of pregnancy are believed to be caused by declining serum levels of free calcium obtained with a rise in serum phosphorus. A natural response is to drink more milk. Actually, milk intake should be reduced, because milk contains large amounts of phosphorus as well as calcium. Calcium tablets should be taken, but any product containing calcium phosphate should be avoided because it will lower free calcium levels and increase phosphorus concentrations. It is for this reason that many pharmaceutical companies have changed their calcium supplements from calcium phosphate preparations to those which contain calcium lactate and calcium carbonate. Another valuable suggestion in relieving leg cramps caused by low calcium levels is to ingest aluminum hydroxide on a daily basis. Trade names of products which contain aluminum hydroxide include Aludrox, Gaviscon, Mylanta, Camalox, Gelusil, Maalox, and Amphojel. Aluminum hydroxide has the effect of lowering phosphate levels by forming inactive aluminum phosphates which are not absorbed into the body from the intestine.

What other minerals are important?

Phosphorus metabolism is intimately related to that of calcium, and a proper balance between these two minerals is necessary for normal bone and tooth development. Phosphorus is also important in energy production and the use of proteins. While both phosphorus and calcium are found in great amounts in milk, there are many foods which lack calcium but supply lots of phosphorus. The RDA for phosphorus is approximately 800 milligrams for the nonpregnant woman, with 1,200 milligrams recommended during pregnancy and lactation. Some representative food servings and their phosphorus contents are: a serving of liver—300 milligrams; a hamburger—165 milligrams; a serving of fish—200 milligrams; and a shredded wheat biscuit—100 milligrams. With these high amounts in many foods, a phosphorus deficiency is never really a nutritional concern for the pregnant woman.

Zinc is an important constituent of enzymes which are vital to the body's metabolism. It aids in protein digestion and in the synthesis of insulin, and plays a role in increasing the blood volume to the brain and other organs of the body. Zinc also speeds the healing of wounds and helps white blood cells fight infection. An adult's RDA for zinc is 15 milligrams, with an additional 5 and 10 milligrams added for pregnancy and lactation, respectively. Most diets which contain adequate amounts of animal protein will easily meet these requirements. Fish, oysters, meat, eggs, and milk are the best sources of zinc. Occasional zinc deficiencies have been noted among vegetarians and others who consume large amounts of unprocessed grains, bran, beans, and whole wheat products, since the large amount of phytic acid in these products binds zinc and prevents the body from using it.

The potential dangers of a zinc deficiency have not been fully elucidated. When a zinc deficiency is artifically induced in experimental pregnant animals, offspring are at greater risk of prematurity, stillbirth, and major fetal malformations. There is also evidence to suggest that a zinc deficiency may be a contributing factor in emotional disorders of children.

Magnesium is an essential nutrient, an important constituent of bone and tissues, and an activator of various enzyme systems in the body. Articles in popular magazines to the contrary, a magnesium deficiency only occurs under unusual circumstances such as prolonged starvation, chronic malnutrition, alcoholism, diseases causing poor intestinal absorption, and severe kidney disease. Magnesium is found in just about all foods, though fresh fruits and vegetables supply the greatest amounts. The United States RDA for magnesium during pregnancy is 450 milligrams, or 150 milligrams above that recommended for nonpregnant adults.

Iodine is found throughout the body but is concentrated in the thyroid gland. In the past, iodine deficiencies and subsequent goiter formation were noted in a number of states in which inhabitants ingested diets deficient in this mineral. Today, with the use of iodized salt, this is no longer a problem. The United States RDA for nonpregnant women is about 125 to 150 micrograms, with an additional 25 micrograms recommended during pregnancy. The nursing woman is advised to ingest 175 to 200 micrograms per day of iodine. However, it is important to remember that too much iodine can suppress thyroid function. For this reason, the recommended daily requirement during pregnancy should not exceed 225 micrograms. Iodine-rich supplements, such as kelp, can bring the pregnant woman dangerously close to this limit.

Copper, along with zinc, plays an important role in the body's metabolism. The United States RDA for copper is 2 milligrams. Cereal grain, organ meat, cocoa, peas, beans, shellfish, and nuts are all excellent sources of copper. Surprisingly, women who use birth control pills have increased serum levels of copper, leading some nutritionists to suggest that they may have a decreased dietary need for copper. It is not known if pregnant women require greater or lesser amounts of copper than nonpregnant women. Cow's milk and mother's milk have notoriously low amounts of copper, and it is for this reason that copper deficiencies have been detected in infants but not in adults.

Symptoms of a copper deficiency include anemia, scurvy-like bone changes, and a smaller number of the blood's white blood cells. Some animal research suggests that when the amount of copper in the body is reduced in relationship to the concentration of zinc, potential harmful body changes may occur. In a 1977 report, doctors at Los Angeles County Harbor General Hospital compared serum copper levels in fourteen patients with premature rupture of the amniotic membranes prior to the onset of labor to twelve women in a control group. The first group had significantly lower serum copper levels, leading the doctors to speculate that a maternal copper deficiency could in some way weaken the amniotic membranes.

Manganese is a mineral which abounds in many foods. In experimental pregnant animals, a deficiency will cause irreversible neurological defects in the newborn. A manganese deficiency may also be a possible cause of impaired bone and cartilage growth as well as diabetes. However, further research is necessary to confirm this association.

Fluoride

What are the advantages and risks of using fluoride supplements during pregnancy?

It is believed that fluoridation of public water supplies is a safe, effective, and practical way of preventing dental caries and reducing the cost of dental care among children and nonpregnant adults. At the present time, less than one-half of our population, or 105 million Americans, are supplied with fluoridated water. If you want to find out whether or not your water is fluoridated, simply call your city or state department of health.

While most authorities endorse the use of fluoride supplements during childhood, there is some controversy as to the advantages and safety of these preparations when they are given prenatally. In a 1971 study, researchers documented increased fluoride concentrations in the primary teeth of infants whose mothers received a fluoride supplement during pregnancy. One recently published study, conducted by Dr. Frances Glenn, a pediatric dentist, compared the teeth of children born of three different groups of mothers who were started on fluoride in their third month of pregnancy. The women and their children were followed for the remarkably long period of fifteen years. The first group drank normally fluoridated water, and on long-term follow-up 23 percent of their children had teeth which were free of caries. In a second group, called the "vitamin-fluoride group," mothers took a tablet containing 1 milligram of fluoride each day; 69 percent of their children had caries-free teeth. The third group of women took a 2.2 milligram fluoride tablet from the third to the ninth month and also continued to give their children fluoride tablets from birth to their teen years. An impressive 97 percent of these children were free of caries. In addition, their primary and permanent teeth were pearly white in color, were without structural defects, and were less likely to develop plaque. Children in this group also had fewer potentially pathological bacteria surrounding their teeth. As a result of her studies, Dr. Glenn has enthusiastically referred to prenatal fluoride as "the prenatal tooth vaccine that we have been searching for." Unexpected obstetrical findings of her report were that prenatal fluoride supplementation was associated with a heavier birth weight and longer birth length, slightly fewer birth defects, and a significantly lower prematurity rate.

A number of prominent obstetricians have viewed Dr. Glenn's report cautiously because at the present time too little is known about the possible abnormality-producing effects of fluoride on the unborn infant. It is known, for example, that fluoride rapidly passes from the maternal to the fetal circulation and achieves equal concentrations in both bloodstreams. The safe limits of maternal fluoride use remain unknown at the present time. However, the FDA, the AMA, and the American Dental Association have already taken a position supporting the safety of fluoride supplementation during pregnancy. While enthusiasts claim that fluoride prevents tooth decay in the fetus by being incorporated into a calcium-containing complex in dental enamel, other dentists believe that preeruptive tooth buds of the fetus have amounts of calcium which are too insignificant to be affected by maternal fluoride use. These dentists also claim that further studies will refute Dr. Glenn's conclusions. Until more research is available, I would assume that most obstetricians will not prescribe fluoride supplements for women who have adequate concentrations of fluoride, or approximately 0.7 parts per million, in their drinking water. However, in the absence of adequate fluoride in the drinking water, a daily supplement of 1 to 2.2 milligrams is harmless and is probably beneficial.

What is the relationship between the use of anesthesia and fluoride supplementation?

Few doctors and dentists are aware of the very important relationship between the use of two general anesthesics, methoxyflurane (Penthrane) and enflurane, and fluoride poisoning. Several studies in the medical literature have documented that blood fluoride levels increase in the fetal and maternal circulation as a result of the chemical breakdown of these agents during anesthesia. In a 1980 review dealing with this subject, doctors at the University of Tennessee noted that very high levels of fluoride caused by prolonged methoxyflurane anesthesia had the capacity to produce a severe form of kidney failure. More alarming is the fact that this same type of problem has been noted when these anesthesics are administered for relatively short periods of time, as with a delivery. Obviously, the potential for kidney failure affecting a woman or her baby will be greatest if prenatal fluoride supplementation is combined with the use of one of these two anesthesic agents.

Planning Meals

What does an ample basic food plan for a pregnant woman contain?

Though many complex nutritional formulas and charts have been devised, a simple and basic approach is to plan meals according to the four major food groups:

Group 1: Protein
Two or more servings are recommended daily during the first half of pregnancy, and three or more servings are recommended in the last half of pregnancy and dur-

ing lactation. This group can include lean meats, chicken, fish, dried beans, and nuts. Cheaper grades of meat are just as nutritious as the more expensive ones. A serving is defined as 2 to 3 ounces of lean cooked meat, fish, or poultry without bones. The following servings of foods will contain equivalent amounts of protein:

¼ pound cooked hamburger
1 medium fish or meat patty
2 frankfurters
2 slices of liver
2 slices of meat loaf
2 medium chicken drumsticks
1 chicken leg, including thigh
1 medium fish steak
1 slice roast meat or poultry 2¼ inches x ¼ inch

Substitutes for the above are:

½ cup cottage cheese
3 ounces cheddar, Monterey jack, swiss, munster, brick, or longhorn cheese
1 cup cooked dried beans, peas, or lentils
½ cup shelled peanuts
4 tablespoons peanut butter
3 eggs

Group 2: Milk and Milk Products

Four or more cups of milk are recommended each day. Whole milk, skim milk, buttermilk, reconstituted dried milk, yogurt, and custard are of equal value. The following amounts of cheese equal 1 cup milk:

1-inch cube cheese
1⅓ cups cottage cheese
1½ slices (equals 1½ ounces) cheese

Group 3: Fruits and Vegetables

Four or more daily servings are recommended, and one serving is equal to any of the following:

½ to ¾ cup of apple, orange, potato, grapefruit, or cantaloupe
1 apple, 1 orange, 1 potato, ½ grapefruit, or ½ cantaloupe

Group 4: Bread and Cereal

At least two to three daily servings during the first half of pregnancy and four to five servings during the second half are recommended. A serving of whole-grain and enriched bread consists of one of the following:

1 slice enriched or whole grain bread
½ to ¾ cup cooked whole-grain cereal, such as cracked wheat, oatmeal, brown rice, or rolled wheat

½ to ¾ cup cooked enriched cereal, such as grits or cornmeal
½ to ¾ cup enriched noodles, macaroni, or spaghetti
¾ cup enriched ready-to-eat cereal
½ to ¾ cup rice, enriched or converted
1 large enriched flour tortilla
2 small corn tortillas

To ensure an adequate daily food intake, plan to eat one serving of each of the four groups at breakfast, lunch, and dinner. This allows you an additional serving as a snack each day from Groups 2, 3, and 4 throughout pregnancy, and an additional serving from Group 1 during the last five months. Though eating three small meals and three snacks daily may seem excessive, food is more easily digested when served in this manner. It is not healthy for you or your baby to go without food for eight or more hours. In addition to these recommendations, it is important that you not restrict salt intake and that you use only iodized salt.

You do not have to follow this meal outline fanatically. Some women will need additional calories from extra servings or from fat such as butter, margarine, mayonnaise, or salad oil. Discuss your food intake and weight gain with your obstetrician during your prenatal visits.

Liquids are also important, and the drinking of four to six cups of water, broth, tea (1 cup maximum daily), or coffee (1 cup maximum daily) each day should be encouraged. When shopping for snacks, buy nutritious foods, such as raisins, raw vegetables, nuts, and fruits, and avoid high-calorie, low nutrition foods, such as candy, cookies, pies, and soft drinks. Processed and refined carbohydrates, such as foods with large amounts of table sugar, provide more "empty calories" than natural carbohydrates. Try not to cook all fruits and vegetables because it will only reduce their vitamin C content.

Can a vegetarian receive adequate nutrition during pregnancy?

Since there is a growing popularity of vegetarian diets, it is imperative that obstetricians learn to work with, assist, and encourage the vegetarian rather than criticize her. Many uninformed individuals are quick to ridicule the vegetarian, but there is evidence which suggests these diets may prove critical in the prevention of diseases, such as heart disease, cancer, obesity, and osteoporosis, or loss of bone density. In my private obstetrical practice, I have been impressed by the excellent health, knowledge of nutrition, and pregnancy outcome of the vegetarians under my care.

A total vegetarian is defined as one whose diet is based solely on plant food sources, while a lactovegetarian will eat dairy products in addition to plant foods. Lacto-ovovegetarians are individuals who will use both eggs and dairy products in addition to plant foods. While a successful pregnancy outcome can easily be achieved by all three groups, it is obvious that the total vegetarian will be least likely to meet all the nutritional requirements of pregnancy.

The main concern is that the vegetarian receive adequate amounts of good-quality protein. The quality of a protein is determined by the amount that is available to the body for use and the number of eight smaller units, called amino acids, which it contains. Protein foods of animal origin are called high-quality proteins because they contain these eight amino acids in optimum amounts which are easily available to the body. Cereal grain proteins favored by vegetarians are considered to be "low-quality" because they lack one of the eight important amino acids, lysine. Fortunately, legumes such as dried beans and peas contain large amounts of lysine, but they are also low-quality proteins because they are deficient in an amino acid named methionine. If cereal and legume proteins are eaten together, the vegetarian will be ingesting a protein of better quality than if either product is eaten alone. If this mixing of proteins is carried out throughout pregnancy, the nutritional value obtained will approach that of the high-quality animal protein eaten by the nonvegetarian. The more liberal vegetarian diets can provide adequate protein with two daily servings of eggs and dairy products. Two daily servings of high-protein nuts and peanut butter are recommended for the stricter vegetarian.

In addition to eating vegetables and grains, the total vegetarian can obtain more daily protein by eating one of the following:

1 cup soybeans plus 12 ounces soymilk or soy yogurt
½ pound tofu and 1 pint soymilk or soy yogurt
1 quart soymilk or soy yogurt and ½ cup soybeans
1 cup hydrated TVP (texturized vegetable protein) and 1 cup soymilk or soy yogurt

Additional protein for the lactovegetarian is more easily obtained by daily amounts of the following:

2 cups cottage cheese
1 quart skim milk, low-fat yogurt, or buttermilk

The diet of a total vegetarian may be deficient in calcium, iron, riboflavin, vitamin B12, vitamin D, and zinc. While it is important to try to meet the pregnancy demands for these vitamins and elements with substitute foods, the amounts obtained from available food sources are often inadequate. For this reason, it is important that all vegetarians, and total vegetarians in particular, take supplements containing the important vitamins and minerals.

The greatest risk to a vegetarian comes from dependence on the limited nutritional benefits of a single food source. Macrobiotic enthusiasts, whose diets consist mainly of grain and vegetables, are at great risk of protein, iron, and calcium deficiencies. It is especially important that such individuals take vitamin and mineral supplements throughout pregnancy. As with all foods eaten during pregnancy, vegetarian diets should not contain excessive amounts of "empty calories" as are found with refined fats and oils, starchy foods, refined sugars, and alcohol.

Where can I get good nutritional advice if I suspect that I know more about nutrition than my doctor?

Many obstetricians' nurses or receptionists know more about nutrition then they do, and some hurried doctors do not take the time to adequately advise about diet. If

Table 8–3. Nutritional Value of Some Fast Foods

	Wt (g)	Energy (kcal)	PRO (g)	CHO (g)	Fat (g)	Vitamins A (IU)	B_1 (mg)	B_2 (mg)	Nia. (mg)	B_6 (mg)	B_{12} (µg)	C (mg)	D (IU)	Minerals Ca (mg)	Fe (mg)	K (mg)	P (mg)	Na (mg)
Arby's®																		
Roast Beef	140	350	22	32	15	X	0.30	0.34	5	—	—	X	—	80	3.6	—	—	880
Beef and Cheese	168	450	27	36	22	X	0.38	0.43	6	—	—	X	—	200	4.5	—	—	1220
Super Roast Beef	263	620	30	61	28	X	0.53	0.43	7	—	—	X	—	100	5.4	—	—	1420
Burger Chef®																		
Hamburger	91	244	11	29	9	114	0.17	0.16	2.7	0.16	0.26	1.2	—	45	2.0	208	106	—
Cheeseburger	104	290	14	29	13	267	0.18	0.21	2.8	0.17	0.36	1.2	—	132	2.2	218	202	—
Double Cheeseburger	145	420	24	30	22	431	0.20	0.32	4.4	0.31	0.73	1.2	—	223	3.2	360	355	—
Fish Filet	179	547	21	46	31	400	0.23	0.22	2.7	0.04	0.10	1.0	—	145	2.2	271	302	—
French Fries, small	68	250	2	20	19	0	0.07	0.04	1.7	—	0	11.5	—	9	0.7	473	62	—
French Fries, large	85	351	3	28	26	0	0.10	0.06	2.4	—	0	16.2	—	13	0.9	661	86	—
Vanilla Shake (12 oz)	336	380	13	60	10	387	0.10	0.66	0.5	0.1	1.77	0	—	497	0.3	622	392	—
Chocolate Shake (12 oz)	336	403	10	72	9	292	0.16	0.76	0.4	0.1	1.07	0	—	449	1.1	762	429	—
Dairy Queen®																		
Frozen Dessert	113	180	5	27	6	100	0.09	0.17	X	—	0.6	X	—	150	X	—	100	—
DQ Cone, regular	142	230	6	35	7	300	0.09	0.26	X	—	0.6	X	X	200	X	—	150	—
DQ Cone, large	213	340	10	52	10	400	0.15	0.43	X	—	1.2	X	8	300	X	—	200	—
DQ Malt, regular	418	600	15	89	20	750	0.12	0.60	0.8	—	1.8	3.6	100	500	3.6	—	400	—
DQ Malt, large	588	840	22	125	28	750	0.15	0.85	1.2	—	2.4	6	140	600	5.4	—	600	—
DQ Float	397	330	6	59	8	100	0.12	0.17	X	—	0.6	X	X	200	X	—	200	—
Brazier® Chili Dog	128	330	13	25	20	—	0.15	0.23	3.9	0.17	1.29	11.0	20	86	2.0	—	139	939
Brazier® Dog	99	273	11	23	15	—	0.12	0.15	2.6	0.08	1.05	11.0	23	75	1.5	—	104	868
Jack in the Box®																		
Hamburger	97	263	13	29	11	49	0.27	0.18	5.6	0.11	0.73	1.1	20	82	2.3	165	115	566
Cheeseburger	109	310	16	28	15	338	0.27	0.21	5.4	0.12	0.87	<1.1	20	172	2.6	177	194	877
Regular Taco	83	189	8	15	11	356	0.07	0.08	1.8	0.14	0.5	<0.9	6	116	1.2	264	150	460
French Fries	80	270	3	31	15	—	0.12	0.02	1.9	0.22	0.17	3.7	<1	19	0.7	423	88	128
Vanilla Shake	314	342	10	54	9	440	0.16	0.47	0.5	0.18	1.1	3.5	44	349	0.4	536	318	263
Chocolate Shake	317	365	11	59	10	380	0.16	0.60	0.6	0.18	0.98	<3.2	38	350	1.2	633	332	294
Kentucky Fried Chicken®																		
Original Recipe® Dinner*																		
Wing & Rib	322	603	30	48	32	25.5	0.22	0.19	10.0	—	—	36.6	—	—	—	—	—	—
Wing & Thigh	341	661	33	48	38	25.5	0.24	0.27	8.4	—	—	36.6	—	—	—	—	—	—
Drum & Thigh	346	643	35	46	35	25.5	0.25	0.32	8.5	—	—	36.6	—	—	—	—	—	—

Extra Crispy Dinner*

Wing & Rib	349	755	33	60	43	25.5	0.31	0.29	10.4	—	—	36.6	—	—	—	—	—	—
Wing & Thigh	371	812	36	58	48	25.5	0.31	0.35	10.3	—	—	36.6	—	—	—	—	—	—
Drum & Thigh	376	765	38	55	44	25.5	0.32	0.38	10.4	—	—	36.6	—	—	—	—	—	—
McDonald's®																		
Big Mac®	204	563	26	41	33	530	0.39	0.37	6.5	0.27	1.8	2.2	33	157	4.0	237	314	1010
Cheeseburger	115	307	15	30	14	345	0.25	0.23	3.8	0.12	0.91	1.6	13	132	2.4	156	205	767
Hamburger	102	255	12	30	10	82	0.25	0.18	4.0	0.12	0.81	1.7	12	51	2.3	142	126	520
Quarter Pounder®	166	424	24	33	22	133	0.32	0.28	6.5	0.27	1.88	<1.7	23	63	4.1	322	249	735
Quarter Pounder® w/Ch	194	524	30	32	31	660	0.31	0.37	7.4	0.23	2.15	2.7	25	219	4.3	341	382	1236
Filet-O-Fish®	139	432	14	37	25	42	0.26	0.20	2.6	0.10	0.82	<1.4	25	93	1.7	150	229	781
Regular Fries	68	220	3	26	12	<17	0.12	0.02	2.3	0.22	<0.03	12.5	<1	9	0.6	564	101	109
Chocolate Shake	291	383	10	66	9	349	0.12	0.44	0.5	0.13	1.16	<2.9	44	320	0.8	580	335	300
Vanilla Shake	291	352	9	60	8	349	0.12	0.70	0.3	0.12	1.19	3.2	26	329	0.2	422	314	201
Taco Bell®																		
Bean Burrito	166	343	11	48	12	1657	0.37	0.22	2.2	—	—	15.2	—	98	2.8	235	173	272
Beef Burrito	184	466	30	37	21	1675	0.30	0.39	7.0	—	—	15.2	—	83	4.6	320	288	327
Taco	83	186	15	14	8	120	0.09	0.16	2.9	—	—	0.2	—	120	2.5	143	175	79
Wendy's®																		
Single Hamburger	200	470	26	34	26	94	0.24	0.36	5.8	—	—	0.6	—	84	5.3	—	239	774
Double Hamburger	285	670	44	34	40	128	0.43	0.54	10.6	—	—	1.5	—	138	8.2	—	364	980
Single w/Cheese	240	580	33	34	34	221	0.38	0.43	6.3	—	—	0.7	—	228	5.4	—	315	1085
Double w/Cheese	325	800	50	41	48	439	0.49	0.75	11.4	—	—	2.3	—	177	10.2	—	489	1414
Chili	250	230	19	21	8	1188	0.22	0.25	3.4	—	X	2.9	—	83	4.4	—	168	1065
French Fries	120	330	5	41	16	40	0.14	0.07	3.0	—	—	6.4	—	16	1.2	—	196	112
Frosty	250	390	9	54	16	355	0.20	0.60	X	0	—	0.7	—	270	0.9	—	278	247
Pizza Hut® *serving size: 2 slices of medium (13″) pizza/4 servings per pizza																		
THIN 'N CRISPY®																		
Standard Cheese	—	340	19	42	11	600	0.45	0.51	4	—	—	X	—	500	3.6	190	—	900
Standard Pepperoni	—	370	19	42	15	700	0.45	0.43	4	—	—	X	—	400	3.2	225	—	1000
THICK 'N CHEWY®																		
Standard Cheese	—	390	24	53	10	800	0.75	1.19	8	—	—	X	—	600	4.5	290	—	800
Superstyle Cheese	—	450	31	54	14	1000	0.83	0.68	8	—	—	1.2	—	950	4.5	295	—	1000

* Includes two pieces of chicken, mashed potato and gravy, cole slaw, and roll.
Dashes indicate no data available. X = less than 2% US RDA; tr = trace.

your doctor does not provide you with up-to-date information about nutrition and pregnancy, you can obtain three excellent pamphlets on the subject: "Assessment of Maternal Nutrition," "Food, Pregnancy and Family Health," both published by the American College of Obstetricians and Gynecologists (1 East Wacker Drive, Chicago, Illinois 60601); and "Partners in Growth During Pregnancy," published by National Dairy Council (Rosenat, Illinois 60018).

How nutritious are the meals purchased at fast-food restaurants?

Fast-food restaurants line the approaches to just about every city and town in the United States. Though the words "junk food" are often used to describe the products sold in these establishments, I am certain that a good percentage of pregnant women eat one of these convenient and inexpensive meals at least once during their pregnancy.

Though I do not endorse the frequenting of fast-food restaurants, I do believe that if you carefully select your meals, some nutritional benefits are possible. Pizza, for example, is a well-balanced food that derives 50 percent of its calories from protein, 27 percent from fat, and the rest from carbohydrates. It is also rich in calcium and several D vitamins. When a Burger King's Whopper or a McDonald's Big Mac is eaten with french fries and a vanilla shake, a woman's protein, calcium, vitamin A, iron, and vitamin C intake will be significantly greater than it would be following the typical meal of a hamburger, french fries, and a cola drink. A soft drink contributes no nutrients to the diet, but a "shake" will increase the calcium and phosphorus value of the meal. The "shakes" sold at these establishments are not called milk shakes because they do not contain milk. However, they do contain calcium phosphorus and protein, along with the gums used for thickening. Cheeseburgers are better than hamburgers because of the calcium, phosphorus, and protein contained in the cheese. Table 8-3 lists the relative nutritional content of some popular "fast-food" meals.

The two notable drawbacks of fast-food meals are their low fiber and high salt content. Though fiber is believed by some doctors to play an important role in prevention of colon and rectal cancer, on a more practical level it is also an effective preventive and treatment for constipation. This common problem of pregnancy can only be made worse by frequent fast-food meals. These foods have a very high sodium or salt content, and though salt need not be restricted during pregnancy, the amounts are still excessive, particularly for the woman with hypertension or heart disease. The average meal provided by fast-food establishments will usually contain between 2,000 and 4,000 milligrams of sodium. When ordering french fries, ask that no salt be added. Sauces and pickles put on sandwiches also have large amounts of salt and are best avoided. Though shakes are more nutritious than soft drinks, they do contain twice the amount of sodium found in milk (see table 8-3).

9.
Environmental and Occupational Hazards of Pregnancy

Over the past twenty years, the pregnant woman has become painfully aware of many contaminants in the environment which threaten her health and the health of her unborn baby. We seem constantly to be besieged by shocking news bulletins reporting the release of a toxic chemical, herbicide, pesticide, or radioactive substance, and we have come to realize that just about all these contaminants can cross the placental barrier.

While the overwhelming majority of pregnant women are fortunate to have less dramatic concerns than the Love Canal and Three Mile Island inhabitants, many still encounter serious problems related to a wide variety of toxins in their home and work environments. Insulating a house or painting and preparing a room for a baby brings with it questions about the effects of these chemicals on the developing fetus. Misconceptions about the dangers of radiation released by microwave ovens and television sets often add to the pregnant woman's anxiety, as do fears that she must put a beloved pet cat, bird, or turtle to sleep to be sure that the potentially serious diseases which are carried by these animals will not harm the fetus.

Based on known fertility rates, over one million pregnancies can be expected among working women every year. Exposure to cigarette fumes, noxious chemicals, noise pollution, and radiation post definite hazards to a pregnant woman. Knowledge of these hazards and the methods for preventing or at least minimizing their effects is invaluable to the outcome of a successful pregnancy.

Practical medical and financial concerns, such as limiting activity at work and when to begin and terminate maternity leave must also be addressed.

Your medical history is not complete unless your obstetrician asks where you and your partner presently work and where you have worked during the past five years. Hobbies and outside activities must also be investigated to find out if you are exposed to possible pollutants. This chapter deals with the many questions and concerns about the home and occupational environment of the pregnant woman.

Cigarette Smoke

How does smoking affect pregnancy?

Despite the overwhelming evidence linking cigarette smoking to harmful maternal and fetal complications, as many as one-fourth of American women continue this self-destructive habit throughout pregnancy, usually fully aware that their physical dependence on tobacco is unwholesome. Such women often experience feelings of guilt throughout pregnancy and the years following childbirth because they know that they have not given their babies the best possible start in life.

The well-documented detrimental effects of smoking which are shared equally by men and women include an increased risk of such diseases as chronic bronchitis, emphysema, and lung cancer. While lung cancer was formerly far more common among men, female lung cancer death rates have increased dramatically in the past thirty years as the number of women smokers has approached that of male smokers. (According to the U.S. Public Health Service, in the past decade the number of adult male smokers declined by 14 percent, while only 2.6 percent of women smokers gave up their habit.) Cardiovascular diseases—such as arteriosclerosis, myocardial infarction (heart attack), and impaired circulation in the extremities—are all problems more readily experienced by chronic smokers. Although heart attacks are still relatively uncommon among women, 75 percent of heart attacks occurring in women under forty-five have been attributed to smoking. There is also evidence suggesting that peptic ulcer and cancer of the urinary bladder are more common among smokers. As expected, the incidence of all these diseases is directly related to the length of time that one smokes and the number of cigarettes smoked each day. Smoking may also affect a woman's ovarian function. There are a number of studies which clearly demonstrate that the onset of menopause occurs significantly earlier in women who smoke a pack of cigarettes a day or more over several years.

Of the more than 4,800 separate chemicals that have been identified in cigarette smoke, the most harmful are nicotine, carbon monoxide, hydrogen cyanide, tars, resins, and several carcinogens—cancer-causing agents such as diazobenzopyrene. While all chemicals in tobacco smoke are potentially harmful, nicotine and carbon monoxide are the two which are most detrimental to the outcome of pregnancy. In both animal experimentation and human experience, nicotine has been noted to stimulate the release of body substances known as catecholamines. These in turn cause a narrowing of the blood vessels to the uterus. As a result, there is a decrease in the amount of blood flowing to the uterus and a reduction in the concentration of oxygen in the fetal circulation. Researchers now believe that this constriction of blood vessels in the uterus may permanently damage them and affect the outcome of future pregnancies (see page 263) and is the most likely reason why smokers give birth to smaller babies. Nicotine can cause a frightening temporary decrease, and even stopping, of fetal movement, along with alterations in the breathing rate, immediately after a woman smokes as little as one cigarette. The higher number of stillbirths and neonatal deaths among infants born of smoking mothers may be attributed, in part, to this phenomenon.

Carbon monoxide is a poison which is found in significant concentrations in tobacco smoke. It readily crosses the placenta and has been found in the umbilical cord of infants born of smoking mothers. The danger of carbon monoxide is that it combines with hemoglobin in both the maternal and fetal bloodstreams to form a compound called carboxyhemoglobin. Carboxyhemoglobin reduces the blood's oxygen-carrying capacity. One pack of cigarettes smoked per day will raise the maternal blood carboxyhemoglobin level by 4 or 5 percent. Fetal carboxyhemoglobin concentrations are directly related to those of the mother, and under conditions of continuous smoking they may be 10 to 15 percent higher than maternal levels. Scientists fear that the carbon monoxide in cigarette smoke is a more significant cause of permanent and disabling fetal growth retardation than is nicotine or any of the other pollutants.

Regardless of which particular chemical in cigarette smoke is most responsible for a poor fetal outcome, the overwhelming evidence supports the view that smokers are subjecting their unborn infants to cruel and unusual punishment. For example, smokers give birth to babies whose weights are on the average 10 to 15 percent below optimal weight, with smaller head circumferences and body lengths. This difference in weight becomes even greater as the number of cigarettes smoked increases. The smaller size of these tobacco-exposed infants is in part due to the fact that they are born prematurely, but more significant than this is their retarded growth in utero. Such infants are referred to as "small-for-dates." Women who smoke more than one pack of cigarettes a day are almost twice as likely to give birth to a baby weighing less than 5½ pounds than women who smoke less than one pack a day, and nonsmokers are much less likely to experience this complication.

The risk of a child's contracting pneumonia and bronchitis during the first year of life is higher if its mother smoked during pregnancy. The reasons for this remain unknown, though Dr. Richard L. Naeye, director of the 1979 U.S. Collaborative Perinatal Project, theorizes that a greater frequency of bacterial infections in the amniotic fluid of smokers permits the unborn infant to draw infected fluid into its lungs, thereby causing pneumonia. Dr. Naeye also believes that infection of the amniotic fluid contributes small-for-dates babies.

The U.S. Collaborative Perinatal Project found that smoking increases the frequency and severity of Rh disease. An Rh-negative woman, one who is lacking the Rh factor, may form antibodies which destroy the red blood cells of her Rh-positive fetus. The destroyed red blood cells are unable to carry adequate amounts of oxygen to the fetal tissues, and carbon monoxide from inhaled cigarette smoke is believed to further impair this oxygen transport system.

Several studies have concluded that smoking mothers are also more likely than nonsmokers to experience spontaneous abortions and to give birth to infants with lower IQ scores, congenital malformations, hyperactivity, and reading and learning disorders, although whether some of these intellectual and physical inadequacies are permanent has not been established. The follow-up assessment of the Collaborative Perinatal Research Project demonstrated no differences at age eight in IQ or motor development between offspring of smokers and those of nonsmokers. However, equally impressive studies conclude that the children of smoking mothers do *not* catch up with the offspring of nonsmokers. In one report, the incidence of children with hyperactive-impulsive behavior at the age of seven was twice as great if their mothers smoked during pregnancy. The hyperactivity rates were also higher in families where the mother smoked two or more packs of cigarettes per day than in those in which one pack of cigarettes was smoked daily. Most recently, it has been found that the likelihood of crib deaths, also known as sudden infant death syndrome, or

SIDS, is increased by 52 percent among infants born of mothers who smoke.

It is of interest to note that infants of smokers experience an accelerated growth rate during the first six months of life when compared to infants of nonsmoking mothers. This probably occurs because they are removed from their toxic, growth-inhibiting in utero environment.

The harmful effects of smoking affect all babies, regardless of their mothers' otherwise normal or above-normal nutrition and weight: a smoker, regardless of her weight, will give birth to smaller infants than a nonsmoker of equal weight. This relationship applies even when the food intake and the pregnancy weight gain is identical between the smoker and the nonsmoker.

In addition to these risks to the fetus, smoking may increase the incidence of serious complications for the mothers. In one study, it was found that premature separation of the placenta from the uterine wall (abruptio placenta) occurred with significantly greater frequency in smokers than in nonsmokers. Among moderate smokers, the risk increased by 24 percent, while in heavy smokers it climbed to 68 percent. Placental infarcts are areas of unoxygenated dead tissue in the placenta which are caused by an inadequate supply of oxygen-bearing blood. Researchers have found that placental infarcts occur more frequently among heavy smokers.

During the last trimester of pregnancy, the placenta is usually attached to the upper part of the uterine cavity. However, on rare occasions it may attach in an abnormally low position and partially or completely cover the cervix. This condition is called placenta previa, and it may be responsible for profuse bleeding during the third trimester. The incidence of placenta previa has been reported to increase by 25 percent in moderate smokers and by 92 percent among heavy smokers.

How have the effects of cigarette smoking on the fetus been studied?

One of the most alarming aspects of cigarette smoking is the temporary aberrations of fetal movements, breathing patterns, and fetal heart rates which are noted immediately after a woman smokes. With the help of continuous ultrasound monitoring, doctors at Oxford University in England recorded the fetal breathing patterns of ten pregnant volunteers after they smoked two cigarettes within a period of fifteen minutes. Within five minutes from the start of smoking, a significant increase in the rate of fetal breathing was noted. This persisted for sixty minutes. The women recorded the number of fetal movements they felt before and after they smoked; the number decreased markedly in the hour after the two cigarettes were smoked. Since fetal activity has become an important method of detecting fetal well-being, this diminution of movement is somewhat disconcerting.

The nonstress test, or fetal-acceleration determination (FAD), has been demonstrated to be an important method for assessing fetal status in high-risk pregnancies. In this test, an amplifier is placed on the mother's abdomen and the fetal heart rate is recorded on a strip of monitoring paper. A woman is instructed to immediately push a button, which she holds in her hand, whenever she detects a fetal movement. This is recorded on the monitor along with the fetal heart rate. Under normal conditions, most women will experience four or more fetal movements within a twenty-minute period with the heartbeat of the baby accelerating by at least fifteen beats per minute in the fifteen seconds immediately after the fetal movement is detected. When the fetus responds in this fashion, it is termed a reactive nonstress test, indicating that it is in no distress. However, a nonreactive nonstress test, in which the heart rate does not accelerate adequately, may indicate a compromised infant.

In a report published in the *American Journal of Obstetrics and Gynecology* in 1980, a comparison of the nonstress tests of 128 smoking and 350 nonsmoking pregnant women with high-risk pregnancies showed, significantly, that 20.8 percent of smokers had nonreactive nonstress tests while only 13.2 percent nonsmokers experienced this reaction.

Ultrasonic visualization of the fetal skull throughout pregnancy enables doctors to determine if growth is being retarded. The distance between the two large parietal bones of the skull, called the biparietal diameter, is the most commonly employed measurement. In one recent study, doctors found that the biparietal growth rate of fetuses of smokers was consistently slower than those of nonsmokers, starting with the twenty-first week of pregnancy.

Are any congenital malformations associated with cigarette smoking during pregnancy?

Despite innumerable studies, it cannot be stated with certainty that a relationship exists between maternal cigarette smoking and congenital malformations. In the largest study to analyze the relationship between maternal smoking and congenital anomalies, published in the *British Medical Journal* in 1979, doctors studied the outcome of 67,609 pregnancies among mothers who were divided into three categories: nonsmokers, light smokers (one to nine cigarettes per day), and heavy smokers (more than twenty cigarettes per day). They found that the overall incidence of congenital malformations was about 2.8 percent in both smokers and nonsmokers, and no correlation was found between smoking habits and malformations of the cardiovascular, gastrointestinal, genitourinary, or skeletal system. A slightly higher incidence of cleft palate, cleft lip, or both was noted in infants of moderate to heavy smokers, though this was not considered to be statistically significant. Only neural tube defects, such as anencephaly and spina bifida, were found to relate significantly to smoking; heavy smokers were the most likely to give birth to infants with these defects.

In an attempt to correlate neural tube defects and smoking with a woman's social class, the doctors found the fewest neural tube defects in children born to professional and managerial nonsmokers and the most in those whose mothers were semiskilled and unskilled, regardless of smoking habits. This led the investigators to speculate that social class may be more important than smoking in accounting for congenital malformations.

In a 1979 report from Sweden, the smoking habits of the mothers of sixty-six infants with cleft palate and cleft lip and another sixty-six infants with neural tube defects were studied. While women who gave birth to infants with cleft palate and cleft lip were heavy smokers, no such relationship was noted for neural tube defects.

Are smoking complications of pregnancy less likely with reduced-tar-and-nicotine cigarettes?

It has been demonstrated that the risk of lung cancer may be significantly reduced among women who smoke low-tar-and-nicotine cigarettes. However, there is no evidence that these cigarettes can reduce the complications caused by smoking during pregnancy or that they lower the risk of cardiovascular diseases, emphysema, and bronchitis. To replace the flavor lost by cutting tar and nicotine levels, cigarette manufacturers have added such substances as shellac, caramel, eugenal, some of which produce carcinogens when burned. Some epidemiologists fear that these new additives may eventually prove to be more dangerous than the chemicals they replaced.

While the reduced concentrations of nicotine found in the newer brands of cigarettes should diminish fetal toxicity to a degree, the concentrations of carbon monoxide, the most harmful constituent of cigarette smoke, has remained virtually unchanged. As a result, the amount of carboxyhemoglobin formed in the fetal bloodstream from the low-tar-and-nicotine cigarettes should be equal to that produced by most of the other brands.

If a woman is a nonsmoker, can her health suffer as a result of breathing the cigarette smoke produced by others?

Yes. So-called passive smokers who inhale this "sidestream" or "secondhand" smoke have received great attention recently. In a 1981 study reported in the *British Medical Journal,* doctors found that women who did not smoke but were exposed to their husbands' cigarette smoke developed lung cancer at a much higher rate than nonsmoking wives of nonsmoking husbands. Women whose husbands smoked more than a pack a day were found to have a risk of lung cancer two times higher than women whose husbands did not smoke. If the husband smoked one to nineteen cigarettes a day, the risk was 1.6 times higher than for the wives of nonsmokers. One frightening statistic is that nonsmoking wives of men who smoke die on the average four years sooner than they would if their husbands did not smoke.

Pregnant women who work are often exposed to the noxious chemicals produced by cigarette smoke, especially during the winter months when windows and doors of office buildings are made as airtight as possible in order to conserve energy. This lack of adequate ventilation may prolong the time that pollutants, such as nicotine and carbon monoxide, remain in the air. Women who work where smoking is not restricted are most likely to suffer the effects of passive smoking. There is some evidence to suggest that these individuals may be at greater risk of experiencing a stillbirth or perinatal death. Thiocyanate is a metabolic byproduct of tobacco smoke. In a 1982 study, reported in the *American Journal of Obstetrics and Gynecology,* doctors found elevated levels of thiocyanate in the umbilical cord blood vessels of newborns whose nonsmoking mothers were exposed to cigarette smoke throughout pregnancy.

If you are a pregnant nonsmoker who is suffering because of the smoking habit of your husband or another household member, stand up for your rights and the rights of your unborn baby and prohibit smoking in your home. If this can't be achieved, ask that all smoking be done as far away from you as possible, near an open window and in an area of the house that is well-ventilated. If you work next to someone who smokes, demand that your employer prohibit smoking on the job or, at the least, isolate smokers from other employees.

Aside from cigarette smoke, how can the pregnant woman inhale noxious carbon monoxide fumes?

Carbon monoxide concentrations are heaviest in the air around big cities. In one recent survey, it was found that in the South Pole the carbon monoxide concentration was 0.02 parts per million, compared to 13 parts per million in midtown Manhattan. On occasion, levels in high traffic areas in New York City have been reported to be as high as 40 parts per million. In some sections of Los Angeles, carbon monoxide levels have reached an amazingly high 100 parts per million.

Even low levels of carbon monoxide, absorbed repeatedly, could deprive the fetus of some of the oxygen needed to develop normally. For this reason, pregnant women should not work around cars and trucks, near furnaces, or in any confined space where there is heavy smoke or fumes. A job as a toll booth attendant would appear to be extremely hazardous during pregnancy.

The rising costs of home heating fuel have resulted in the widespread use of energy-efficient kerosene heaters. However, a report published in the October 1982 issue of *Consumer Reports* has concluded that these devices are responsible for the release of dangerous amounts of toxic chemicals such as carbon monoxide, carbon dioxide, nitrogen dioxide, and sulfur dioxide. Of the eighteen kerosene models studied, investigators found that all exceeded the Environmental Protection Agency's air standards for air pollution by significant amounts. With respect to the carbon monoxide levels, the *Consumer Report*'s medical consultants determined that several hours' exposure to a kerosene heater was especially hazardous to people with heart disease, pregnant women and their fetuses, newborns, and those with respiratory disease. Though the kerosene heater companies have disputed these findings, several have taken steps to market heaters that can force their emissions outdoors through a vent. Unfortunately, these vented heaters are significantly more expensive than the portable models.

Do ex-smokers have any greater pregnancy risks than women who never smoked?

Based on the 1979 Collaborative Perinatal Project of over 50,000 pregnancies at twelve United States medical centers, it is now believed that even if a woman gives up smoking before becoming pregnant, her previous habit will increase the risk of certain pregnancy complications. Researchers theorized that smoking before pregnancy may permanently damage the small arteries of the uterus of some women. This in turn can result in a higher incidence of spontaneous abortion, placental infarcts (areas of dead and nonfunctioning tissue caused by an inadequate blood supply of oxygen), placenta previa (low implantation of the placenta), and infant death. These complications are more apt to occur among women who were heavy smokers over a prolonged period of several years.

The conclusions of this study should in no way promote a fatalistic attitude on the part of a woman who finds that she is pregnant and still has not given up the habit. It is never too late to quit! Many benefits are realized the moment after the last cigarette is smoked. For example, if you finally stop smoking as late as the early stages of labor, you will still be less likely to transfer measurable amounts of toxic chemicals, such as carbon monoxide and nicotine, to the bloodstream of your baby than if you smoke during this time. In the event of a complicated pregnancy, in which the fetus shows evidence of distress, the cessation of smoking during the last few days may spell the difference between a successful or tragic pregnancy outcome.

If you can break your habit before the fourth month, you will have the added advantage of giving birth to a baby whose weight is equal to that of a nonsmoker, since the maximum amount of growth retardation associated with maternal smoking takes place during the last six months of pregnancy. Therefore, while it is best that you never start smoking, you will realize positive benefits whenever you break this unwholesome habit.

Isn't there evidence which proves that it is the personality and behavior of the person who smokes, rather than the smoking itself, which is responsible for the low birth weight of infants?

While at least fifty different studies have noted a cause-and-effect relationship between cigarette smoking during pregnancy and impaired fetal growth and development, a few investigators, most notably Dr. J. Yerushalmy, claim that it is the personality, behavior, socioeconomic status, and physical makeup of the person who smokes, rather than the smoking itself, which is responsible for the low birth weight of their infants.

Dr. Yerushalmy found that the incidence of low-birth weight infants in the pregnancies of women who were nonsmokers during pregnancy but who later became smokers was similar to that of women who smoked in every pregnancy. When compared to mothers who smoked during all their pregnancies, ex-smokers had significantly fewer babies of low birth weight.

Some of the investigative techniques used by Dr. Yerushalmy and others supporting this theory have been criticized, and it is important to emphasize that the majority of researchers do not support these views. The present consensus is that maternal smoking before pregnancy and during the first trimester will not influence a baby's birth weight, provided the habit is stopped before the fourth month.

What are the effects of smoking on breast-feeding?

Reports attempting to determine the relationship between cigarette smoking and the quantity and quality of breast milk have been both inconclusive and contradictory.

The two largest studies suggested that smokers may have a less adequate milk supply than nonsmokers, but both reports have many scientific deficiencies. One investigator observed a shorter average nursing period for smokers than for nonsmokers among women who nursed for at least two months. Of special note was the fact that mothers who stopped smoking during the last three months of pregnancy nursed as long as nonsmokers. In one experiment, mothers who smoked seven cigarettes in two hours noted a marked reduction in milk quantity.

Experiments show that most of the chemicals in tobacco smoke are transmitted to the breast milk. When sensitive chemical assays are employed, nicotine can be detected in the milk of all women who smoke. However, deleterious fetal effects are rarely seen. In one case report, an infant whose mother smoked twenty cigarettes per day was noted to have symptoms of a nicotine overdose, characterized by restlessness, vomiting, diarrhea, and a rapid heartbeat. These symptoms subsided spontaneously when the mother stopped smoking.

Though the reasons remain unknown, infants who are nursing from mothers who smoke appear to be at increased risk of gastrointestinal disturbances.

Too little attention has been given to the unfortunate baby who lives in an environment in which adults are smoking. Such an infant unwittingly becomes a passive smoker by inhaling tobacco fumes in its environment. As a result, these infants are at greater risk of contracting bronchitis and pneumonia during the first year of life. This is especially true if both parents are heavy smokers.

Stress

Do stress and anxiety affect pregnancy?

Though there is little scientific data available on this subject, several clinical investigations have concluded that anxiety-prone women are more likely to experience spontaneous abortion and stillbirth and to produce babies of diminished birth weight. This information is especially relevant today because greater numbers of women are experiencing job-related anxieties.

Based on animal research, scientists have theorized that the anxious pregnant woman releases an abundance of epinephrine and norepinephrine. These body chemicals, classified as catecholamines, enter the circulation of susceptible women and narrow the uterine arteries which carry oxygen to the fetus. They also increase the uterine muscle tone, and this further reduces the amount of oxygen transmitted to the fetus.

Several reports of human pregnancy tend to support some of the observations and conclusions reached in laboratory experiments. In one study, published in 1970, doctors evaluated the "anxiety-proneness" of 150 women tested on the Taylor Manifest Anxiety Scale; the more anxiety-prone women gave birth to smaller babies. There are also isolated and less scientific reports in which extreme maternal anxiety resulted in habitual abortion and fetal death. Doctors have reported successful pregnancies among habitual aborters after they were treated with psychotherapy. This suggests that the alleviation of stress in anxiety-prone individuals will improve their fetuses' prognosis for survival.

While childbirth education classes, the support of family and friends, an understanding doctor and hospital nursing staff, and a homelike environment in the labor room all help to allay fears of pregnancy, there still remains a small group of women who are simply unable to rid themselves of these fears, and the fear of labor in particular. For such women, the stress of labor will trigger excessive catecholamine release and jeopardize fetal well-being. Anesthesia techniques, such as epidural and caudal, eliminate perception of pain during labor and delivery and provide a more favorable environment for the infants of anxiety-prone individuals. One very important study from Yale University compared the relationship between a woman's psychological characteristics, as tested during the last trimester of her first pregnancy, and the amount of pain medication and sedation which she received during labor. Among the sixty-four women studied, it was found that the amount of medication which was administered by an obstetrician during labor was based more on the woman's psychological state during pregnancy than her actual requirements during labor, those demonstrating high anxiety during pregnancy tended to receive the largest amounts of analgesics and sedatives during labor even though they did not necessarily require medication. If, as we believe, an anxiety-ridden woman is more apt to give birth to a compromised infant, the added insult of unneeded medication can only worsen the chances of survival.

Since maternal anxiety levels appear to be a determinant of pregnancy outcome, one would anticipate that a woman who lives in complete tranquility will be more likely to have a successful pregnancy. A 1974 report from the World Health organization appears to bear this out. Natives of the South Pacific islands of Fiji and Western Samoa were found to have an incredibly low number of pregnancy complications. Their 5.4 percent of premature births was found to be lower than any other of the twenty-three populations reporting to the World Health Organization and appeared to be related to their physical and emotional relaxation combined with their generous food intake during pregnancy.

Noise Pollution

Can excessive environmental noise adversely effect the outcome of pregnancy?

There is increasing scientific evidence that exposure to noise, especially unexpected and uncontrollable noise, is associated with hearing loss, high blood pressure, heart disease, insomnia, and nervous disorders. As with other forms of stress, "noise pollution" may also increase maternal catecholamine release and decrease fetal oxygenization. This has special significance for pregnant women living in populated cities or other areas where extensive highway, factory, or construction noise is present. Studies conducted as early as 1941 noted that maternal emotional agitation induced by harsh sound profoundly decreased the fetal heart rate. Though fetuses have never been interviewed, it is known that they hear some of the sounds to which their mothers are exposed. However, the protective uterine and amniotic fluid environment screens out most of the noise.

In studies on the effects of noise on the outcome of pregnancy conducted on pregnant women living near busy airports, it was found that babies born of women living in close proximity to Los Angeles International Airport had a higher incidence of birth defects such as anencephaly, spina bifida, abdominal hernia, cleft lip, and cleft palate; the stillbirth rate was higher among women living closest to Heathrow Airport; and expectant mothers living near Osaka International Airport had lower levels of human placental lactogen (see chapter 10) and gave birth to babies with lower birth weights than pregnant women living in quieter areas of Japan.

Recently, doctors have used sound stimulation as a test of fetal well-being. When a speaker is placed on the maternal abdomen and a measured amount of pure sound is applied for ten seconds, a healthy fetus responds with an acceleration of its heart rate by fifteen beats per minute for at least two minutes. An impaired infant shows no such response. Studies from England and Brazil suggest that a responsive sound test is a good predictor of fetal well-being, and that a nonresponsive sound test accurately reflects fetal compromise (see chapter 10).

Hair Dyes

What are the dangers involved if a woman uses hair dyes during pregnancy?

Studies suggest that hair dyes may be associated with an increased incidence of cancer and birth defects. Many of the hair dye ingredients are classified as aromatic amines and diamines, chemicals which are closely related to known carcinogens, such as benzidine and beta-naphthylamine. Chemists have concluded that at least eighteen different chemicals found in hair dyes may be carcinogenic, and a good half of these may also be responsible for birth defects in the offspring of mothers who use them.

In 1975, Dr. Bruce N. Ames of the University of California studied the effects of 169 commercial hair dyes including those with and without peroxide, on the genetic characteristics of a bacterium named *Salmonella typhimurium*. He found that 150 of the dyes changed the genetic characteristics of the bacterial organism. Though it might seem that tests on bacteria have little application to humans, this test is regarded as a sensitive initial method of screening chemical and consumer products for possible toxic effects. In support of Dr. Ames's research, at least two other laboratory studies have demonstrated that cultured cells from mammals undergo chromosomal damage when exposed to constituents of hair dyes.

Human experience with hair dyes, though incomplete, is somewhat disconcerting. For example, when a woman dyes her hair, the chemicals in the dye are absorbed through her skin, enter her bloodstream, and then are excreted in her urine. Hair dyes may also be absorbed through the skin of the hands. In a 1978 published report from England, doctors tried to determine if chromosomal damage was more likely to occur among sixty male and female professional hair colorists than in a group of individuals involved in other occupations. Despite the fact that occupational exposure was substantial, and ranged over a period of one to fifteen years, no significant differences in chromosomal damage was found between the two groups. However, when the women of the study were regrouped according to whether or not their own hair was dyed, there was a statistically significant excess of chromosomal damage and breaks among those who dyed their hair. One explanation for this difference is that most hair colorers and tinters wear gloves when applying hair dyes to the scalps of others. This prevents absorption of the dyes through the skin of the hands. The authors of this report claim that, even without gloves, absorption through the skin of the hands is probably less than that through the skin of the scalp because of the smaller surface area, the thicker skin layer of the hands, and the lack of sebaceous or oily glands in the palm. The scalp contains numerous sebaceous glands which aid in the absorption of hair dye chemicals. If it is substantiated that chromosomal damage is more likely among men and women with dyed hair, it is disturbing to know that the potential exists for transmitting these abnormalities to the fetus.

It should come as no surprise that studies sponsored by the hair color industry have failed to note an association between hair dye use and cancer or complications of pregnancy. Based on these conflicting reports it is difficult, if not impossible, for a woman to decide whether or not to use hair dyes during pregnancy or before a planned pregnancy. Considering that 33 million Americans regularly use hair dyes, it is vital that an honest and accurate conclusion about their potential hazards be reached. Many potential harmful carcinogens and mutation-inducing agents remain in all hair dye formulas. The public should not feel secure until the laws are changed so that the chemicals in cosmetics and hair dyes undergo the same premarket testing and FDA approval policies as those in foods and drugs.

What hair dyes can a pregnant woman use?

Those who use hair dyes usually know little about the contents of the hair dyes which they use. Thanks to research by *Consumer Reports,* many of these questions can now be answered.

Coal-tar chemicals are found in permanent, semipermanent, and temporary hair dyes. While none are safe, permanent dyes have the greatest potential for harm. These products are usually advertised as "shampoo-in" dyes and are sold in two-part kits which contain coal-tar chemicals in one bottle and hydrogen peroxide "developer" in the other. The two liquids are mixed together just before use and shampooed into the hair shaft. The color lasts until the hair grows out in about four to six weeks.

Semipermanent hair dyes do not contain peroxide but have chemicals that penetrate the hair shaft. The color generally lasts for three to four weeks. Though these products are probably safer than the permanent hair dyes, their coal-tars still penetrate the skin and may be absorbed into the bloodstream.

Temporary hair dyes, also known as rinses, contain coal-tar dyes that coat rather than penetrate the hair shafts. As a result, there is less of a likelihood for absorption of the dyes into the scalp. These products are usually removed with the next shampooing. This should not lull the consumer into a sense of security, since *Consumer Reports* investigators encountered a great deal of secrecy surrounding the exact ingredients of these products. Chemicals in temporary hair dyes, bearing names such as Direct Brown 1:2, Direct Blue 6, and Acid Black 107, when traced to their laboratory origins, were found to contain several coal-tar derivatives that have long been suspected of causing cancer and chromosomal damage.

Henna is a dye which has the advantage of being a plant substance rather than a coal-tar chemical. It is generally applied as a "pack" in which the ground leaves and stems are made into a paste with hot water and left on the hair for various lengths of time. Henna products are carefully regulated by the FDA. These products are perfectly safe, but the only color produced is an orange-red. If any henna-containing products boast that they can produce colors other than orange-red, check the label to be sure that coal tars have not been added to it.

Metallic dyes, known as "progressive dyes," are applied daily and cause a gradual darkening of the hair. These products contain a metallic salt, such as lead acetate, which reacts with sulfur to produce a pigment that colors the hair.

In evaluating the safety of lead acetate, the Food and Drug Administration has concluded that the amount which penetrates the skin and is absorbed into the body is far too little to produce toxic effects. However, it is important that these products not be used if there is a cut or abrasion of the scalp because too much of the chemical may then be absorbed into the body. The effects of lead on the outcome of pregnancy can be quite significant.

Since the safety of all hair dyes has been questioned, the best advice is to avoid these products if you are pregnant or are of childbearing age. This is especially true for products which contain coal-tar chemicals, since there is no doubt that they have the potential to damage chromosomes and cause cell changes or mutations. Theoretically, changes produced in a woman's immature unfertilized ovarian follicles could be transmitted to her offspring at a later date.

If you insist on using hair dyes, products containing henna would appear to be the safest. Unfortunately, not everyone wants to have orange-red hair. Metallic dyes are probably safer to use during pregnancy. Of the products which contain coal-tars, I would surmise that the permanent hair dyes are the most dangerous, followed closely by the semipermanent dyes. Temporary dyes are theoretically less likely to be absorbed from the scalp because they coat rather than penetrate the hair shafts. If you want to use a hair dye, use a technique that involves minimal contact between the dye and your scalp. Frosting, tipping, streaking, and painting involve less scalp contact than permanent dyes applied in the form of shampoos.

Anesthetic Gases	**Is it true that pregnancy complications are more common among operating room nurses and other hospital employees who are exposed to anesthetic gases?**

Since 1967, reports form Russia, Denmark, Great Britain, and the United States have concluded that women who are continually exposed to trace amounts of anesthetic gases when working in operating rooms are at greater risk of aborting or giving birth to babies with congenital abnormalities. In two of these reports, it was noted that there was a higher incidence of infertility among women anesthesiologists when compared to a control group of women physicians. In the largest study, published in 1974 by a committee of the American Society of Anesthesiologists, 50,000 operating room professionals were surveyed. When compared to a control group who were not exposed to anesthetic gases, it was found that 30 percent of pregnancies among operating room nurses ended in spontaneous abortion as compared with 9 percent in the control group. Women anesthesiologists had a 28 percent spontaneous abortion rate compared to 10 percent in a control group to which they were compared. While wives of male anesthesiologists showed no greater incidence of spontaneous abortion, they did have a 25 percent increased risk of giving birth to an abnormal child. This suggests that trace amounts of anesthetics in the operating room may damage sperm cells, as well as developing and fertilized eggs. In addition, female anesthesiologists and anesthetists and operating room nurses are considerably more likely than unexposed women to give birth to babies with congenital anomalies.

Research at New York University College of Dentistry suggests that dentists, wives of dentists, and dental technicians may also be threatened by the effects of anesthetic gases. Many dentists use nitrous oxide, or "laughing gas," as an office anesthetic. In this study, it was found that the incidence of liver disease was 70 percent higher among dentists who used nitrous oxide than among those who did not. Furthermore, the rate of spontaneous abortion was 11 per 100 among wives of dentists who used this gas and only 6.7 per 100 for wives of dentists not using it. Heavily exposed dental technicians gave birth to more babies with birth defects and had a spontaneous abortion rate of 17.5 per 100, compared to 7.6 per 100 for technicians who were not exposed.

Other investigators have reached different conclusions. In a 1979 report from Sweden, when 494 women who worked in operating rooms for varying periods of time during their pregnancies were compared with a control group, the women exposed to anesthetic gases did not show any differences in their risks of threatened abortion, reduced birth weights, perinatal deaths, or congenital abnormalities.

At the present time, no one can say with certainty if continued employment in an area in which general anesthesia is used is detrimental to the outcome of pregnancy. However, since doubt exists, it would be wise for the pregnant operating room nurse or aide to transfer to a different area of the hospital, especially during the first trimester. Women employed as dentists and dental technicians are best advised to stay out out of rooms in which nitrous oxide anesthesia is being used. Similarly, if you need extensive and prolonged dental work during pregnancy, you should select a local anesthetic, such as Novocain (procaine) or Xylocaine (lidocaine), rather than nitrous oxide.

The concentration of anesthetic gases in a dental office or an operating room can be easily measured and can be reduced to concentrations of less than 1 percent by use of modern scavenging systems which remove the gas through the ventilation system. If you are a pregnant operating-room employee, it is not unreasonable to insist on knowing the concentration of anesthetic gases in your working area. If the levels are above 1 percent, you should demand that corrective measures be taken to improve the situation.

Can dental personnel experience pregnancy-related problems other than those caused by anesthetic gases?

Aside from exposure to x-rays, which are totally preventable (see pages 277–84), few people are aware of the fact that exposure to mercury vapors is an occupational hazard for dentists and dental assistants. These vapors are produced in the preparation of mercury amalgams used for filling cavities. Analysis of the air in a dental office will confirm their presence or absence. Theoretically, chronic inhalation of mercury can cause mercury poisoning, which is characterized by permanent nervous system and kidney damage. In actual practice, there are less than a handful of documented cases of mercury poisoning among dentists and their technicians, but it is well documented that mercury easily passes through the placenta to the fetus, and that the fetus is far more sensitive to its toxic effects than is its mother. Though this problem is extremely rare, it you work in a dental office you can ask to have the air analyzed for mercury vapors.

Phenolic Germicides

What is hexachlorophene and how can it cause pregnancy complications among medical and dental personnel?

Hexachlorophene, better known by the popular trade name of pHisoHex, is a potent antibacterial disinfectant which was first introduced in the United States in 1941. It rapidly gained popularity throughout the world and was soon added to soaps, face lotions, hair tonics, acne medications, antiperspirants, and toothpaste. A University of Washington study which found that brain damage occurred more frequently among newborn infants who were routinely washed with hexachlorophene solutions led the FDA to restrict the marketing of hexachlorophene to physician and hospital use. Several studies have confirmed hexachlorophene's unusual ability to rapidly penetrate the unbroken skin, enter the bloodstream, and migrate quickly into the cells of the brain, liver, and other organs. In a report from France, infants accidentally exposed to high concentrations of hexachlorophene in talcum powder suffered severe brain damage. Interestingly, one 1972 report suggested that women may absorb hexachlorophene into their bloodstreams at a more rapid rate than men.

During pregnancy, hexachlorophene easily passes from mother to fetus via the placenta. In 1978, Swedish doctors reported that severe congenital malformations occurred fifty times more frequently in newborn infants born of hospital workers who washed their hands with a 1 to 3 percent of hexachlorophene soap from ten to seventy times daily during the first three months of pregnancy. Subsequent research on laboratory animals in the United States has confirmed the relationship between hexachlorophene use and birth defects.

Based on these data, it would seem prudent for medical, nursing, and dental personnel to avoid use of pHisoHex soap during pregnancy. This should present no problems, since there are many other excellent disinfectants that can be substituted. Burdeo is the trade name of a lotion which also contains hexachlorophene and must not be used by the pregnant woman. Newborns should be washed with germicides other than pHisoHex, unless there is a contagious bacteral infection in the nursery which is resistant to all other disinfectants.

Unlike many pesticides and toxic chemicals which remain in the body for prolonged periods of time, hexachlorophene is believed to pass out of the body within seventy-two hours. Therefore, birth defects will result only if exposure occurs during pregnancy, and especially in the first three months. A woman who last washes with pHisoHex five days before conception is at no greater risk of harming her fetus than someone who has never used this product.

Parasites from Pets

Does a cat present risks to the pregnant woman?

Yes. Of all diseases caused by household pets, none has aroused more attention and concern among pregnant women than toxoplasmosis. This disease, caused by a microscopic protozoan named *Toxoplasma gondii,* is commonly transmitted by contact with infected cat feces or by the handling or eating of infected raw meat. Adults who contract the disease usually have no symptoms and never know they have acquired it. When symptoms are present, they consist of a mild illness characterized by a low-grade fever, cough, headache, lethargy, and lymph node enlargement. Unfortunately, during pregnancy the organism crosses the placenta in 45 percent of all cases and severely damages or kills the fetus. Though many people consider toxoplasmosis to be a rare disease, the alarming truth is that it is the most common worldwide human parasitic infection, and one-third of all pregnant women will have antibodies in their blood suggestive of previous exposure to *Toxoplasma gondii.* Epidemiologists have determined that a woman's chances of contracting toxoplasmosis for the first time during pregnancy are approximately 1 in 1,000. In addition, over 3,000 infants are born with toxoplasmosis each year.

Toxoplasmosis is one of a group of diseases which cause similar defects in the developing fetus. They have been given the acronym TORCH complex, with the TO standing for toxoplasmosis. The other members of the infamous group are rubella (R), cytomegalovirus (C), and herpesvirus (H) (see chapter 5). If a woman contracts toxoplasmosis during the first trimester of pregnancy, it is estimated that her fetus will have a 17 percent risk of becoming infected. Of this 17 percent, 80 percent will be stillborn or show severe manifestations of the disease such as microcephaly (abnormally small head), hydrocephaly (abnormally large head), cerebral calcifications, blindness due to destruction of the retina, and convulsions. Blood platelet deficiencies and abnormal enlargement of the liver and spleen are also frequently seen. For women infected during the second trimester, 25 percent of their infants will be infected and 30 percent of this group will have severe defects. Among women infected during the third trimester, 65 percent of the fetuses will become infected but few will show obvious problems at birth although problems may develop later.

Toxoplasma gondii undergoes a complex life cycle. The adult form of the organism invades body cells, multiplies and then forms cysts within body tissues. If these cysts rupture, protozoa are released and the life cycle is repeated. Scientists have discovered that the cat intestine is unique among all animal species because it is here that little sacs, called oocysts, are formed. These oocysts are filled with *Toxoplasma gondii* organisms, and once formed they are passed daily in a cat's feces. This potential for disease dissemination may persist throughout the lifetime of the cat. If its feces are disturbed, the oocysts may become airborne and inhaled into the mouth or nose of a susceptible person. A household cat left to roam outdoors in the company of other cats will easily contract the disease and introduce it in the home.

Cockroaches and flies are also capable of transmitting oocysts from cat feces to exposed foods.

A woman who has been previously exposed to toxoplasmosis before pregnancy, or from a previous pregnancy, will develop antibodies and immunity against reinfection and will rarely, if ever, transmit the disease to the fetus of her present pregnancy. The diagnosis of previous exposure to toxoplasmosis can be ascertained by an antibody blood test. However, the results and interpretation of these tests are occasionally confusing and misleading. If doubt exists, other more sophisticated blood tests are available in a very few specialized laboratories in the United States.

What steps should I take to avoid contracting toxoplasmosis?

There is no need to throw out the family cat as soon as the diagnosis of pregnancy is confirmed. However, extreme caution should be taken to avoid infection. While it is best that other family members empty the litter box, you can do this provided that it is done at least once each day. The reason for this is that the oocysts in the cat feces are not infectious for the first twenty-four hours. Oocysts have the capacity to survive in soil and water for as long as eighteen months and, if the litter box is not completely and carefully emptied, infection after the first twenty-four hours is possible. Periodically disinfect metallic litter boxes for five minutes with nearly boiling water to help to kill oocysts, but assign this job to another family member. Wear gloves when handling litter boxes or other materials that may be contaminated with cat feces. This is especially important when gardening in an area where cat feces may have been deposited. Whenever you touch your cat, wash your hands thoroughly. Handwashing should also be thorough before each meal, since oocysts can be transmitted from the hands to the mouth. Keep house cats indoors, away from possible sources of infection such as infected mice and other animals. In addition, do not feed cats raw meat. Since outdoor cats have a higher risk of acquiring toxoplasmosis, it is best that they be kept outdoors and away from the immediate environment of the pregnant woman. Pregnancy is not the time to introduce a stray cat into the household.

Most cases of toxoplasmosis are acquired by eating raw or poorly cooked meat. Smoking or curing meats in brine are effective against *Toxoplasma gondii* oocysts. It is a good idea to wear gloves when handling raw meat, but if you don't, be sure to avoid touching the mucous membranes of your mouth and eyes at these times. Always wash your hands and all kitchen surfaces after they come in contact with raw meat.

A woman with a high toxoplasmosis antibody titre prior to pregnancy need not take these precautions, because her fetus will not be in jeopardy.

What steps can doctors take to diagnose and treat toxoplasmosis during pregnancy?

Since the disease in adults is usually without symptoms, its prenatal detection is extremely difficult. Certain high-risk women, such as cat owners, meat handlers, and individuals working in veterinary hospitals, should be tested as early in pregnancy as possible. Ideally, testing of all women just prior to pregnancy could identify those without antibodies who are at risk. If a woman does not have antibodies on this initial test but continues to be exposed to possible sources of infection, the test should be repeated at the twentieth week of pregnancy. A high antibody titre at this stage indicates an acquired acute infection, and the decision must then be made to either treat the infection or terminate the pregnancy with a therapeutic abortion.

Most authorities have not endorsed routine toxoplasmosis antibody screening of all pregnant women because of the small yield of active cases and the unavailability of laboratories to test the specimens. It has also been argued that routine testing will only add to the escalating costs of prenatal care. However, some doctors believe that mass screening for toxoplasmosis during pregnancy is useful and feasible.

Though information is limited, it is now believed that if a woman is treated early, it will reduce the incidence of congenital disease and the spread of infection to her fetus. Unfortunately, one never knows until after the baby is born if treatment was initiated early enough. For this reason, most women opt for therapeutic abortion when the disease is diagnosed with certainty during the first twenty-four weeks of pregnancy. If a woman elects to be treated, she must understand that pyrimethamine, one of the drugs used to treat toxoplasmosis, has been associated with congenital birth defects when administered during the first trimester. Spiramycin, a less toxic agent, is available in other countries but has not been approved for use in the United States.

What is tularemia and how can it affect the outcome of pregnancy?

Tularemia is an infectious disease of wild animals which domestic pets may contract during forays outdoors if they kill or feed on infected animals. Humans may contract the disease if scratched or bitten by an infected domestic cat or dog. Symptoms of tularemia include fever, ulcerative lesions of the skin, lymph node enlargement, and an enlarged spleen.

Little is known of the effect of tularemia on a woman and her fetus, though most women who have had the disease during pregnancy have delivered normal infants. However, there is a report in the medical literature of a woman who contracted tularemia in the eighth month and delivered an infected infant that subsequently died. There is also a recent report of a woman who received tularemia immunization with the live vaccine before realizing she was pregnant. Though her infant suffered no ill effects, vaccination during pregnancy is not recommended. Tularemia may be safely treated with antibiotics during pregnancy, though keeping your pet under close supervision is probably the best preventive.

What problems may be encountered by the pregnant dog owner?

Assuming that your dog is not rabid (see rabies in chapter 6, table 6–2) and you are not one of the 1.5 million humans bitten each year in this country, you should be able to safely enjoy the company of your canine friend during pregnancy. It should be noted, however, that an increasing number of recent medical reports have dealt with the growing problem of parasitic diseases that may be passed to humans from woman's best friend.

One such disease, named toxocariasis, is caused by the roundworm *Toxocara canis*. (In the cat, this organism is equally as infectious and is named *Toxocara cati*.) Though this disease is relatively unknown, public health officials estimate that it may be one of the more common parasitic infections in the United States. *Toxocara canis* eggs contain infective-stage larvae which are passed with the dog's feces and may be found in streets, soil, sandboxes, lawns, and gardens. As the number of unwanted and poorly supervised pets has increased, the droppings of infected animals in public locations has created a serious form of environmental pollution and a great health hazard. Though all age groups are at risk, the disease is most prevalent among children one to fourteen years of age. Although previously considered a mild disease, there is growing concern that severe damage to the eyes, brain, lungs, liver, and other organs may occur. Nothing is known about its effect on the outcome of pregnancy. However, one must assume that a mother's debilitation resulting from this disease can only mean trouble for her baby.

Heartworm, another dog infection, can also be transmitted to humans. This disease, named dirofilariasis, is caused by a parasite named *Dirofilaria immitis*. Transmission to humans takes place when one of several types of mosquitoes, infected with the microscopic larvae while feeding on the blood of infected dogs, bites the human skin surface. Pregnant women are advised to have their pet dogs examined for parasites at regular intervals by a veterinarian. Dogs that run loose are more likely to contract a parasitic disease, and therefore more careful supervision is necessary during pregnancy. Pregnancy is not the time to adopt a stray.

What are the health hazards associated with owning other pets?

Pet turtles are known to be a frequent source of salmonella bacterial infections in humans. Salmonella is the same organism which causes food poisoning. It has been estimated that almost 15 percent of the nearly 300,000 cases of salmonella-associated infections reported in the United States each year result from contact with contaminated turtles or the water in which they live. Most cases occur in children who handle the turtles and then touch their hands to their mouths. However, salmonellosis in adults may also be contracted in this manner. If you own a pet turtle or plan to buy one, make sure to do it through a reputable dealer who is willing to certify that the animal is free of salmonella. If you have young children, discourage them from touching the turtles or the water in which they swim. When you are pregnant, it is probably best to wear gloves when cleaning the tank, changing the water, or handling the turtles.

Psittacosis, or ornithosis, commonly known as parrot fever, is an infectious disease of birds caused by a microscopic parasite named *Chlamydia psittaci*. Transmission of the infection to humans often occurs following contact with infected pets, such as parrots and parakeets, though all birds, including pigeons, ducks, turkeys, and chickens, may also infect humans. Psittacosis is almost always transmitted to humans by inhalation of the organism into the respiratory tract. On rare occasions it may be acquired from the bite of a pet bird, though there are no cases of infection acquired through eating poultry products. In the lungs, *Chlamydia psittaci* causes inflammation or pneumonitis, fever, and a generalized weakness. From this site it may spread to the liver and spleen and also enter the bloodstream.

Psittacosis is considered to be an occupational disease of individuals employed in pet shops, poultry breeders and processors, taxidermists, and zoo attendants, but you can contract the disease by spending only a few minutes in an environment previously occupied by an infected bird. As with other infectious diseases of this type, the best advice is to avoid contact with infectious birds. If you contract psittacosis, the odds are that your doctor will not make the diagnosis unless he or she has a high index of suspicion. The treatment of choice for this disease is tetracycline antibiotics. However, their use is not recommended during pregnancy, and less predictable antibiotic alternatives must be employed.

Nonionizing Radiation

How dangerous is the radiation emitted by household appliances such as microwave ovens, radios, and television sets?

Radio waves and microwaves are forms of invisible penetrating waves of energy known as nonionizing radiation. Both are used extensively for communication, in industry, for medical purposes, and in the home. In addition to the microwave oven, other sources of nonionizing radiation include word processors, CRT terminals, radios, televisions, long-distance telephone and telegraph transmissions, citizens band (CB) radios, radar, taxi dispatch lines, high-voltage power lines, certain burglar alarms, "electronic" garage door openers, and electric toys. It has been estimated that microwave and radiowave use has increased by approximately 15 percent each year over the past few years, and at the present time there are more than 10 million microwave ovens and 40 million CB radios in use in the United States.

Unlike the ionizing radiation produced by x-ray machines, nuclear weapons, and nuclear power plants, nonionizing radiation does not generally have enough energy to cause serious mutations or genetic damage. This is not to imply, however, that scientists are unconcerned about the safety of this increasingly popular form of energy. Research conducted to date has been inconclusive and controversial. It has been suggested, but not proven, that high levels of nonionizing radiation in humans may be associated with a greater incidence of cancer, nervous disorders, cataracts, sterility, genetic damage, heart disease, and even death.

The FDA has the authority to regulate the levels of nonionizing radiation emitted from consumer products. Microwave ovens manufactured after 1976 have had to meet rigid requirements, so that all of these release amounts of radiation well within the limits of safety. If you were to use your microwave oven ten times daily, standing at a distance of two inches from the door, you would still not reach the total daily limit for nonionizing radiation. However, you can remove all risks of microwave exposure during pregnancy by standing away from the oven when it is in use. Microwave ovens manufactured before 1976 will sometimes develop gaps between the door and the frame which will allow higher emissions of radiation. If doorframes are not kept clean during use, radiation can leak out. Unfortunately, these leaks can only be detected with sophisticated laboratory equipment which is not available in homes.

Color television sets emit more nonionizing radiation than black and white sets. The original models released far greater amounts than those manufactured during the past five years. If a pregnant woman avoids other unnecessary radiation hazards, it is highly unlikely that her color TV could emit enough radiation to cause problems during pregnancy.

Is there a limit recommended for exposure to nonionizing radiation?

Yes. The United States Occupational Safety and Health Administration has recommended that exposure to nonionizing radiation for workers be limited to 10 milliwatts per square centimeter, or 10 mW/cm². Sadly, this standard is not mandated by law, and many workers are exposed to amounts significantly higher. In one study, levels as high as 21mW/cm² were found in the upper floors of office buildings located close to radio and TV transmitters. In another report, it was found that 90 percent of radio-frequency equipment operators and nearby workers were exposed to levels equal to or higher than 10mW/cm². The highest exposure level found was 1,000mW/cm². Amounts of nonionizing radiation in this range would, in the opinion of most scientists, pose significant hazards to maternal and fetal health. If you are pregnant and work with radio-frequency equipment, it is not unreasonable to ask your employer or union representative to verify that the suggested standard of 10mW/cm² is being met. The same advice applies to women working in the upper floors of office buildings which are in close proximity to radio and TV transmitters.

How much radiation is released at the new indoor suntanning centers?

Indoor suntanning centers have gained great popularity in this country over the past few years. Under names such as Plan-A-Tan, Tantrific Sun, and Sum Tan, these establishments give customers courses of treatment with ultraviolet light cabinets that surround the user with high-intensity sunlamps. Although ultraviolet radiation may burn a pregnant woman's skin and may be associated with precancerous and cancerous diseases of the skin, premature wrinkling, skin plaques, skin atrophy, and pigment abnormalities, it will not cause the chromosomal damage or congenital defects associated with ionizing radiation. Those who are taking medications such as sulfonamides, diuretics, chlorpromazine, or tetracyclines and women with light-sensitivity diseases such as porphyria cutanea tarda and lupus, may also suffer adverse effects from this type of light exposure.

Ionizing Radiation

How can ionizing radiation in the form of diagnostic x-rays affect the developing fetus?

Unless it is absolutely essential all diagnostic x-rays should be avoided during pregnancy especially during the first trimester, when the rapidly dividing and differentiating fetal tissues are most susceptible to radiation damage. Despite innumerable warnings and prominently placed signs in radiology offices and hospital x-ray departments, too many fetuses continue to be inadvertently radiated before the diagnosis of pregnancy is confirmed. Excessive amounts of radiation administered between the third and twelfth week of pregnancy may be associated with abnormalities of the central nervous system, microcephaly (abnormally small head), and mental retardation of the fetus. Similar doses given during the first two weeks of pregnancy are unlikely to cause fetal anomalies but may be more apt to result in a spontaneous abortion. Exposure to high doses of diagnostic radiation during the last two trimesters, though less likely to cause malformations, are certainly not innocuous. The central nervous system, gonadal system, and teeth continue to grow and develop until the moment of birth, and too many x-rays may lead to a significant degree of permanent growth retardation. Fortunately, the risk of producing fetal abnormalities is slight when diagnostic x-ray procedures are used judiciously and conservatively during pregnancy.

A rad is defined as a measurement of radiant energy absorbed in body tissues, while a rem actually measures the amount of tissue damage produced by one rad of x-rays. These differences are of no relevance to your understanding of this discussion, and for our purposes the rad and rem may be considered identical. Radiologists have calculated that the hypothetical risk of a fetal malformation from diagnostic radiation is approximately 1 to 5 per 1,000 births for each rad of radiation exposure. While it is theoretically possible for any dose of radiation to cause anomalies if administered at a critical time during the first trimester, a high incidence of malformations is only likely when doses greater than 20 rads are absorbed by the fetus. To receive this dangerous amount, a woman would have to undergo several diagnostic x-ray procedures directed at her lower abdomen (see table 9–1).

Unfortunately the damage caused by radiation cannot always be measured by the presence of an obvious fetal abnormality. Even if a baby appears perfectly normal at birth, radiation can cause mutations or changes in the structure of the genes and chromosomes within its body cells. No statistics are available which accurately show the probability of inducing a mutation in humans at specific radiation doses, and chromosome and gene changes have been found in human embryos after only minimal radiation exposure. Therefore, it is best to assume that there is probably no safe dose with respect to mutation induction, and even the lowest levels of radiation have the potential to cause fetal genetic change. This is especially relevant because mutations induced in the immature germ cells of a fetal ovary and testes may be passed to succeeding generations where they may appear as obvious defects and abnormalities.

It has been estimated that significant exposures of 5 to 10 rads increases an adult's risk of cancer by less than 1 percent. Cancers most commonly associated with ionizing radiation are leukemia, thyroid, breast, and lung cancer, though cancer of the stomach, esophagus, urinary bladder, and lymph nodes also occur. The fetus may be more sensitive to radiation-induced cancer than the adult. Several epidemiological studies of large numbers of pregnancies suggest that radiation exposure in utero significantly increases the risk of childhood malignancy. While all types of cancers have been reported, leukemia is by far the most common, and even fetal

Table 9–1. Estimated Radiation Doses to the Fetus from Commonly Used X-ray Procedures

Examination	Reported Range (in millirads)
A. Low-dose group	
1. Dental	.03 to 0.1
2. Upper spine	8 to 55
3. Chest	0.2 to 43
B. Moderate-dose group	
1. Upper G.I. series	5 to 1230
2. Gallbladder study	14 to 1600
3. Lower thigh	1 to 50
C. High-dose group	
1. Lumbar spine (mid back)	20 to 2900
2. Lumbosacral (lower back)	73 to 1780
3. Pelvis	40 to 1600
4. Hip and upper thigh	50 to 1000
5. Intravenous pyelogram (IVP)	50 to 4000
6. Lower G.I. series	20 to 9200
7. Abdomen	18 to 1400
8. Pelvimetry	160 to 4000

doses as low as 0.2 to 0.5 rads have been implicated. In one report of almost 20,000 pregnant women, it was noted that the death rate from leukemia in white offspring of mothers exposed to x-rays was three times higher than in white children born of mothers who were not exposed. The children of irradiated black women showed no increased leukemia risk. It should be noted that some studies, including one of almost 40,000 pregnant women, have shown no association between diagnostic radiation during pregnancy and later childhood cancer.

Because of the unpredictability of radiation effects on the fetus, some authorities have suggested that a woman be offered a therapeutic abortion if more than 1 rad is received by her fetus in early pregnancy. Others maintain that as many as 5 rads may be considered safe. Following a fetal exposure of 5 to 10 rads, therapeutic abortion should be strongly encouraged. This level is harder to reach than is commonly realized. For example, if you were to receive dental x-rays, a chest x-ray, and an upper gastrointestinal series, the total dose to your fetus would still be less than 2 rads.

In table 9–1 I have listed the amount of radiation in millirads (1/1,000 rad) which is absorbed by the fetus during various x-ray procedures. There is a wide range of radiation doses for each procedure. Rather than refuse all x-rays during pregnancy, be sure that the radiologist uses the most modern equipment and the most meticulous technique, in which the fewest number of x-rays are taken. The use of high-speed films helps to cut exposure time in half. X-ray machines found in the offices of most general physicians do not meet the high standards of those used by radiologists.

Can x-rays taken before pregnancy affect subsequent births?

A 1980 study from the University of Hawaii, as well as earlier studies, show that x-ray exposure before conception more than doubled the chances that subsequent offspring would develop cancer. Though less extensively studied, it has been noted that benign tumors of childhood, such as polyps, papillomas, lipomas or fatty tumors, fibromas, adenomas of the kidney, hemangiomas, neurofibromas, and dermoid cysts of the ovary, occur more often among children born of women who had been irradiated before pregnancy. There is some evidence to suggest that preconceptual radiation of a man also increases the risk of benign and malignant tumors in his offspring.

The researchers from the University of Hawaii theorize that diagnostic x-rays induce damage and changes in the immature sperm and egg cells prior to fertilization. These defects are then passed on to the susceptible fetus at the time of fertilization.

**What is x-ray pelvimetry, and why is there
so much controversy surrounding its use?**

Simply stated, pelvimetry is a measurement of the maternal pelvis. While a doctor may obtain a general idea of the size of a woman's pelvis by careful physical examination and palpation of the pelvic bones, the use of an anteroposterior (front to back) and lateral (side) x-ray is by far the most accurate method of achieving this. Ultrasonic techniques have replaced x-ray procedures for the diagnosis of a wide variety of pregnancy complications, but it is of no value in accurately assessing the diameters of the maternal birth canal.

X-ray pelvimetry is often used by obstetricians before and during labor to determine the relative size and shape of a woman's pelvis in relation to the size of the baby. For some doctors, these measurements are crucial in determining whether or not a cesarean section is necessary. Pelvimetry is also helpful in deciding if a baby in a breech position (buttocks or feet first) should be delivered vaginally or by cesarean section. Other abnormal positions of the baby, as well as congenital abnormalities, may be detected through the use of this technique. It has been estimated that approximately 7 percent of women in labor will undergo pelvimetry, though its use will vary from a low of 1.8 percent in some hospitals to a high of 16 percent in others.

While some obstetricians have endorsed pelvimetry use, others have completely abandoned it despite its advantages because of the amount of radiation to which the fetus is subjected. Even with the best technique and the finest equipment, the fetus will still receive a minimum of 160 millirads from the two x-rays which are taken. The amount of ionizing radiation received by the fetus is far greater with the anteroposterior x-ray film than it is with the lateral film. Occasionally, the x-rays have to be repeated because of the difficulties encountered in properly positioning a woman on the x-ray table during active labor. If repeated x-rays are required, it may subject the fetus to as many as 4,000 millirads. Significantly lower doses of radiation have been associated with childhood cancer among exposed infants.

In addition to concerns about the radiation risks of pelvimetry, some doctors have questioned the clinical value of the information acquired. In an excellent 1979 review of this subject, Drs. John J. Barton and John A. Garbaciak of Illinois Masonic Medical Center in Chicago concluded that pelvimetry was of little prognostic value in determining which women would require cesarean section. Almost half of the women who underwent cesarean section because of poor progress in labor were noted to have adequate pelvic measurements on x-ray.

While most obstetricians would not agree that we should totally abandon x-ray pelvimetry, there is no doubt that its use should be limited to a very small percentage of women. When x-rays are absolutely necessary, one lateral film of the pelvis will usually provide enough information at a fraction of the dose of the anteroposterior view.

In my own practice, I have probably ordered three x-ray pelvimetry examinations in the last five years. If a woman's contractions are of adequate quality and frequency but her labor is not progressing, a cesarean section is indicated even if the x-ray tells me that the dimensions of her pelvis are adequate for a vaginal delivery. And if a 9-pound baby is in a breech position during a woman's first labor, there is no need to routinely order pelvimetry because a cesarean section is a certainty.

If your doctor determines that you need x-ray pelvimetry, it is not unreasonable to discuss your concerns and to voice your objections. Remember, the overwhelming majority of these examinations will not influence the outcome of your labor, but will create a slight though significant cancer risk to your baby.

What other sources of ionizing radiation may the pregnant woman be exposed to?

Low levels of background radiation and fallout account for an average of approximately 125 millirads per year of radiation exposure for every United States resident. However, many people are exposed to levels far greater than this amount.

The damage to humans caused by environmental accidents such as the Three Mile Island nuclear power plant leak in 1979 is difficult to assess. While initial evaluation of women who were pregnant and living within a ten-mile radius of the accident has detected no increase in infant mortality rates, long-term studies of up to twenty-five years are needed before definite conclusions can be reached. Workers at nuclear reactor sites are exposed to significantly higher levels of radioactivity than the general public. Pregnant women and others in the reproductive age group should not seek employment in or around a nuclear power plant. Young men must also be wary of this type of work because the testes are especially vulnerable to ionizing radiation, and sperm damage may occur at exposure levels which often exist in nuclear power plants. A man working in these facilities should be advised to avoid procreation for at least six months after he leaves the job in order to rid his body of damaged and abnormal sperm. Lead-lined jock straps should be mandatory for all male nuclear power plant workers.

Many women are exposed to ionizing radiation through jobs, such as medical and dental x-ray technicians and nurses. Those employed in industries that manufacture radioisotopes for medicine, science, and industry are also vulnerable. Laboratory technicians working with electron microscopes receive low levels of ionizing radiation, as do thousands of female physicists and research technicians who work with high voltage x-ray machines on a daily basis. Though hospital rules governing the use of radioactive materials are quite specific and restrictive, occasionally a female employee may unknowingly receive radiation when, for example, she holds a baby that is being x-rayed or comes in close proximity to a patient receiving radium or radioactive material in the treatment of cancer.

In contrast to rigid hospital regulations, the monitoring of dentists, dental technicians, dental hygienists, and radiologists and x-ray technicians in private offices is almost nonexistent.

Radiation is greatest at higher altitudes, and women who work as flight attendants throughout pregnancy receive greater exposure than women working on the ground or those taking infrequent flights. It has been estimated that cosmic radiation at 30,000 feet is about seven times that at sea level. This translates to an extra 160 millirems (1 rem = 1,000 millirems) per year for the average flight attendant. According to the National Council on Radiation Protection and Measurements, this amount should be harmless for the developing fetus. The council has recommended that nonoccupationally exposed individuals receive no more than 170 millirems per year, exclusive of natural background and deliberate medical x-rays. However, most knowledgeable radiologists would concur that there is no level of radiation that is completely safe. Some scientists believe that as little as 20 millirems may increase the risk of genetic damage. While the internationally established upper limit of safe radiation exposure has been set at 5 rems to the whole body per year per individual radiation worker, such doses would in my opinion be catastrophic for the pregnant woman and her fetus.

Ozone is found in high concentrations in the upper atmosphere as a result of the interaction of solar radiation with oxygen. Industry and the automobile also contaminate the environment with ozone. It has been estimated that flight personnel may be exposed to three to five times higher levels of ozone than the National Institute of Occupational Safety and Health permits. There are unconfirmed reports of higher spontaneous abortion rates and birth defects among flight attendants resulting from chronic exposure to high altitude ozone. Further studies are required before this relationship can be confirmed (see chapter 6).

Aside from employment, some pregnant women may be exposed to significant amounts of radiation in their immediate environment. For example, some of the drinking water in states, such as Utah, Colorado, and New Mexico, contains radioactive elements leached by rainfall running from uranium mines. Utah residents have had the additional misfortune of higher infant death rates among children exposed in utero to radiation fallout following supposedly safe nuclear tests in the 1950s and 1960s. In parts of Colorado, uranium slag has been used for building roads and house foundations. For the past twenty-five years, the Tennessee Valley Authority has been selling radioactive slag to companies for fabricating cinder blocks used to construct homes and schools throughout the South, East, and Midwest. As recently as April 1981, New York residents were shocked by the announcement that radioactive water leaked from a shut-down nuclear power plant and

Table 9–2. Number of Workers in Various Occupations Exposed to Radiation and Estimated Annual Dose Rate

Source	Number of Workers Exposed	Percent Women	Average Dose Rate (mrems/year)
Medical x-rays	195,000	80	300–350
Dental x-rays	171,000	85	50–125
Radiopharmaceuticals	100,000	20	260–350
Commercial nuclear power plants	67,000	5	400
Fuel processing and fabrication	11,250	10	160
Particle accelerators	10,000	—	Unknown
X-ray diffraction units	10,000–20,000	—	Unknown
Electron microscopes	4,400	60	50–200
Airline crew and flight attendants	40,000	90	160

drained into the nearby Hudson River. Despite assurances by Consolidated Edison Company that the spill of this water into the river presented no danger to health, the perpetuation of these accidents afford us reasons to be skeptical.

What can I do to prevent unnecessary exposure to ionizing radiation?

Diagnostic medical and dental x-rays are easily the greatest source of ionizing radiation to which the pregnant woman is subjected. More than 240 million x-ray examinations are performed in the United States each year. Government radiation experts estimate that 30 percent of these x-rays are unnecessary, and many that are performed during pregnancy could be omitted or postponed without adversely altering the outcome of treatment.

Often x-rays are taken when a woman is unaware that she is pregnant. Tell your doctor if you are in the second half of your menstrual cycle and there is a chance that you may be pregnant. It is always safest to have all elective x-ray examinations performed before ovulation, or during the first ten days of the menstrual cycle (day number 1 is the first day of your menstrual flow).

There is nothing wrong with asking your doctor or dentist to explain why an x-ray is necessary before submitting to it. And, of course, inform your doctor that you are pregnant, when you are. If necessary request the opinion of another doctor or dentist. In the case of x-ray pelvimetry, you're in a difficult bargaining position during labor, and it is much easier to resolve this question during your initial prenatal visits.

If you agree with your doctor that an x-ray procedure is clearly necessary, insist on consulting with a radiologist before taking the films. Techniques can be modified so that the maximum amount of information may be achieved with the lowest number of exposures. Films exposed between rapid rare-earth screens yield the lowest amounts of ionizing radiation. To protect your fetus and your ovaries from scattering of rays, be sure to request a lead shield or apron over your abdomen when your x-ray examination involves parts of the body other than the lower abdomen and pelvis.

While it is often more convenient to be x-rayed with the archaic equipment used by most family physicians, the machines found in modern radiology offices and teaching hospitals can give more accurate information with considerably less exposure to ionizing radiation. In 1979, the FDA published the results of a forty-five state survey in which the safety of x-ray units was determined. Of over 35,000 dental x-ray machines studied, 36 percent had exposures which were excessively high. Of the 3,000 breast x-ray units checked, 46 percent were similarly inaccurate.

Women exposed to ionizing radiation in medical and industrial settings should wear film badges for monitoring. These badges, read at three-month intervals, determine the amount of radiation accumulated during the preceding three months. A woman working in such a setting and planning a pregnancy should request a monthly badge reading to ensure that her dose has remained within safe limits. The most commonly quoted safe limit for industrial radiation exposure during pregnancy is 1.5 rems. This is roughly equivalent to a dose of 0.5 rem (500 millirems), since the maternal abdominal wall absorbs much of the radiation before it reaches the fetus. However, as previously stated, any dose of ionizing radiation is too much for the fetus and efforts should be directed toward lowering these levels to zero. Pregnant personnel should be constantly alert to potential dangers of ionizing radiation in their environment.

Heavy Metals

How can exposure to heavy metals affect the pregnant woman?

In discussing exposure to heavy metals, we are mainly concerned with lead, mercury, and cadmium. Nickel and selenium have not yet been proved to be harmful to the human fetus.

It is commonly believed that **lead** poisoning is limited to babies and young children who eat particles of lead paint peeling from the walls in old buildings. However, the problem greatly affects adults who are employed in industries which use lead. Though inhalation is the most important route of lead intake, exposed workers may also accidentally ingest significant amounts from contaminated dust on fingers, lips, and cigarettes, through water and in contaminated foods. The industries presenting the greatest risks of lead poisoning are lead smelting, storage battery manufacturing, ship breaking, paint manufacturing, printing, ceramics, ammunition, glass manufacturing, and pottery glazing. If you or your husband are employed in these industries, you should ask your employer for proof that concentrations of lead in the air have met federal safety standards. If not, use of a respirator is required until the standards are met. Other safety precautions include the wearing of protective clothing, changing clothes and washing hands before eating, and never eating in the work area. Washing thoroughly and changing clothes before leaving work would prevent the introduction of lead dust particles into the home. It is probably much easier for the pregnant woman to ask her employer for a temporary transfer to a safer work area.

Women who live near heavily traveled roads, drive or bicycle a great deal in heavy traffic, or work as tollbooth attendants may have elevated blood lead levels. Water may be a source of lead contamination where it is acidic or where old lead pipes are still in use. In addition, it has become fashionable to buy and renovate old homes. Many of these homes have lead-base paints. Removing and handling these paints can increase the pregnant woman's lead exposure. It has been scientifically demonstrated that lead easily crosses the placenta and enters the fetal bloodstream, brain and liver. Pregnant women exposed to high levels of lead are at risk of a spontaneous abortion or stillbirth. Surviving infants are more likely to suffer from birth defects, chromosomal anomalies, prematurity, mental retardation, and convulsions. The effects may be more subtle and take the form of permanent learning disabilities. Lead is also secreted in breast milk and has been shown to result in paralysis and other neurological impairments in exposed laboratory animals who nurse.

Fortunately, there is a simple blood test, called the erythrocyte protoporphyrin, or EP test, which detects early signs of lead poisoning. Women who fear they may have been exposed to excessively high levels of lead can have this test performed. If it is positive, more specific studies for blood lead levels may then be carried out.

Mercury has been responsible for several tragedies in the past, when pregnant women ate food contaminated with mercury from polluted waters or pesticides sprayed on farm produce. Mercury vapors may be inhaled in the work environment of dentists, dental hygienists, dental technicians, laboratory technicians, and laboratory workers. In a 1979 study reported in the *Archieves of Environmental Health*, scientists studied the chromosomes of workers in a chemical plant who were exposed to mercury vapors. Although these individuals appeared to be in good health, they were found to have a relatively high incidence of chromosomal breaks and gaps. Some of these abnormalities persisted long after the high concentrations of mercury in their bloodstream returned to normal.

High levels of mercury may on rare occasions cause severe neurologic and kidney disease in an adult, but most individuals do not experience symptoms. The fetus, however, is extremely sensitive, and mercury readily passes into its bloodstream and brain to cause damage. Some reports show that the average mercury level in the baby's umbilical cord blood is 20 to 30 percent greater than the corresponding mercury concentration in maternal blood. Cerebral palsy, severe mental retardation, tremors, seizures, and kidney and liver disease have been noted among many infants whose mothers showed no symptoms of illness. In some instances, infantile poisoning worsened following the taking of mercury-contaminated breast milk. The diagnosis of elevated mercury levels can be determined by a blood or urine test, and concentrations of mercury dust and vapors in the working environment can also be measured with special instruments.

In the mid-1970s there was a great deal of publicity and concern about dangerously high levels of mercury in swordfish and canned tuna. Even today, women continue to ask if these popular foods are safe for consumption during pregnancy. Research has proven that the mercury levels in these two saltwater fish are no different than they were before the use of mercury in industry many years ago. These levels are minute when compared to concentrations needed to cause maternal or fetal problems. The FDA has set 0.5 part per million as the maximum tolerable level of mercury in canned tuna and swordfish.

Cadmium is another heavy metal which may affect the fetus. It is often discharged into sewage systems by the electroplating industry and into the air by deterioration of rubber tires, and is a constituent of tobacco smoke. Cadmium may cause severe toxicity in the form of liver, kidney, heart, and lung disease. Abnormalities in the body's blood cells are also frequently observed. Chronic cadmium exposure may increase a woman's risk of cancer, reduce fertility, and lead to anomalies in her offspring. All this is easily avoided if air standards for cadmium levels in fumes and dust are met. If you work in a factory where cadmium is used, you can have the concentrations of the metal in your urine checked to be sure that your working environment is safe.

Halogenated Hydrocarbons

What are halogenated hydrocarbons and how can they affect the outcome of pregnancy?

Halogenated hydrocarbons are a group of agricultural and industrial chemicals which are known to be toxic to the liver and kidneys. Members of this group include the infamous polychlorinated and polybrominated biphenyls (PCBs and PBBs), vinyl chloride, trichloroethylene, perchlorethylene, vinylidine chloride, oxychlordane, heptachlor epoxide, and many other compounds of similar chemical structure. Geneticists are concerned because the percentage of children born with congenital defects has doubled in the past twenty-five years, and they believe this is from the PCBs and the more than 2,000 other mutation-causing agents currently in our environment. As a result of a woman's increased metabolic rate during pregnancy, it is believed that she may be more susceptible to absorption of these agents at this time. Halogenated hydrocarbons readily enter the breast milk and may increase the nursing infant's risk of chemical toxicity and cancer.

PCBs are used as plasticizers, heat-exchange fluids, and insulation material in transformers and other electrical devices such as capacitors. Other common products which utilize these compounds include lubricants, pesticides, cutting oils, adhesives, wax extenders, inks, sealants, caulking compounds, and paper coating. Although the production of PCBs was officially terminated by the Environmental Protection Agency in 1979, federal regulations do not prohibit the use of existing supplies. As a result, there are still thousands of transformers and capacitors in use that contain PCBs. Since the useful life of this equipment is ten to twenty years, surveillance for PCB contamination and appropriate environmental disposal of these chemicals must continue for many more years. In anticipation of the ban on PCBs, many manufacturers stockpiled them, so that even though their manufacture is discontinued, products containing PCBs will continue to be marketed.

Industrial and electrical plants have discharged their PCBs into nearby sewers and streams, thus contaminating them. The chemical leaks into underground water supplies from junkyards and dumps and is released from supposedly safe sewage treatment plants.

PCBs may enter the body by ingestion or inhalation or through the pores of the skin. Excessive amounts of PCBs in the body cause a characteristic "cola-colored" complexion. One study of ten affected newborns found that their mothers had used a specific brand of cooking oil during pregnancy, and the source of contamination was in the manufacture of the cooking oil, from the erosion of pipes containing PCBs used for heat transfer. Although the "cola-colored" complexion faded these children were smaller in size and shown more likely to have eye defects and other abnormalities when compared to children who were not exposed to PCBs. Some affected infants later displayed premature tooth eruption and overgrowth of their gums. In addition to these problems, PCBs have been suspected of causing liver cancer, reproductive failure, allergic skin diseases and acne-like eruptions, nausea, dizziness, eye and nasal irritation, and asthmatic bronchitis. The transfer of PCBs via breast milk is quite significant, and nursing infants may appear lethargic and lacking in muscle tone. In a study conducted by the Environmental Protection Agency, it was found that 31 percent of 1,038 samples of breast milk contained measurable amounts of PCBs. Interestingly, the milk of women from Kansas, Michigan, New York, Texas, and Wisconsin had the highest levels of PCBs.

The FDA has set the maximum level of PCBs in fish shipped in interstate commerce at 5 parts per 1 million. Not all states have adopted this standard for the sale of fish within state borders. The great variety of patterns of migration and of life for different fish makes the determination of PCB levels impossible in the absence of a chemical test on every fish purchased. In addition, some species of fish absorb higher amounts of PCBs than others. Eels, for example, have been found with PCB levels as high as 700 parts per million because, as bottom-feeders, they ingest the silt where PCBs are in greatest concentrations. Freshwater fish, such as bass, carp, whitefish, trout, pike, and catfish, and some saltwater fish, such as flounder and sole, are most frequently contaminated. Ocean fish such as cod, red snapper, halibut, and haddock are usually free of PCBs. A diet that limits potentially contaminated varieties of fish can prevent accumulation of PCBs during pregnancy.

PBBs, or polybrominated biphenyls, are similar in chemical structure to PCBs. They were manufactured as a fire-retardant by the Michigan Chemical Corporation and sold under the name of "firemaster" PB-6. This product is no longer being produced. While some researchers have theorized that persons who ingested PBBs in breast milk as infants may be more susceptible to cancer as adults, there are no data at the present time to support this supposition.

Vinyl chloride is probably one of the most widely used chemicals in the United States. This halogenated hydrocarbon has its greatest use in the manufacture of plastic plumbing pipes and conduits. It is also used for wire cables in electrical systems but may be found in such diverse products as flooring, garden hoses, and clothing. Significantly, almost 5 million workers are exposed to vinyl chloride gas in factories throughout the United States. Until it was recently banned, vinyl chloride monomer, or VCM, was used as a propellant for hundreds of household and cosmetic products. Users of these products, mostly women, may have been exposed to this agent in closed rooms such as bathrooms and laundry rooms even if they were well ventilated. Susceptible women included beauticians and cosmetologists who used hair sprays extensively and household workers who used cleaning and furniture polishing products. Trace amounts of VCM have also been detected in cigarette smoke.

Vinyl chloride can induce brain, liver, lung, and lymph node cancers among workers exposed to its vapors. Exposure during pregnancy to vinyl chloride and chloroprene, a chemically similar compound used in the synthetic rubber industry, may be associated with higher rates of birth defects. In some studies, chromosomal aberrations have been found, and increased fetal mortality was noted among wives of vinyl chloride workers.

Trichlorethylene and vinylidine chloride are two halogenated hydrocarbons which are suspected of being cancer-inducing agents. The former is occasionally used in inhalers for the relief of pain during labor. It also serves as a degreasing agent for metals and as an extractant in foodstuffs. Vinylidine chloride is widely employed in the manufacture of plastics.

What advice would you give to the nursing woman who is concerned about contamination of her breast milk with PCBs?

While animal studies and human experience have demonstrated that high doses of PCBs in a woman's body are hazardous to her nursing infant, there is no proof that trace amounts of these chemicals are detrimental. PCBs are everywhere in our environment. Of the 1,038 samples of breast milk studied by the Environmental Protection Agency, only 9 were totally free of PCBs.

I would concur with the La Leche League's recommendation that nursing mothers avoid exposure to PCBs if at all possible. General precautions suggested for nursing mothers are that they avoid eating freshwater fish, or at least limiting such meals to one per week, and that they not work at jobs involving possible exposure to PCBs. Nursing women are also advised not to lose great amounts of weight over a short period of time. The reason for this is that PCBs are stored in a person's body fat, and rapid weight loss through crash diets might release greater amounts from the body fat to the breast milk.

Some scientists have recommended that all women planning to nurse their infants first have the PCB levels measured in their milk. Women whose milk contains more than 1 part per million are advised not to nurse. Unfortunately, such analyses are not widely available at this time and are often too expensive to order routinely. Analysis of breast milk samples for PCBs and a wide variety of insecticides is performed by Hazelton-Raltech Inc. (3301 Kinsman Boulevard, Madison, Wisconsin 53703, telephone 608-241-4471). The fee for this service is now $69.

Pesticides, Insecticides, and Herbicides

How can exposure to pesticides and insecticides alter the outcome of pregnancy and nursing?

Of the hundreds of pesticides and insecticides currently registered in this country, at least one-fourth are suspected of causing toxicity, sterility, and chromosomal changes among individuals who are exposed to relatively high concentrations. Infants exposed in utero to these toxins will suffer from a higher incidence of birth defects. The effects of exposure to low concentrations of pesticides and insecticides are unknown at the present time. Many of these chemicals, especially the chlorinated hydrocarbons, such as benzene hexachloride, are readily transmitted to a nursing infant in the breast milk.

Of all the chemical agents that have ever been marketed, only heptachlor, chlordane, DDT, mirex, and DBCP have been restricted. Since the use of DDT was banned, there has been a steady decline in its concentration in both breast and cow's milk. Most babies are exposed to DDT and other pesticides before birth via placental transfer. At birth, a newborn already has more insecticide stored in its body than it is likely to acquire from breast-feeding.

A commonly used pesticide in the textile, adhesive, and automobile industries is 2,4,5-TCP. It has been investigated by the Environmental Protection Agency because of its possible toxic effects. This compound contains a chemical contaminant named dioxin, which is suspected of causing birth defects and cancer in humans. There is concern that workers in the industries that use 2,4,5-TCP might be exposed to unsafe amounts through skin contact or by breathing its vapors. The chemical is manufactured by Dow Chemical Company under the trade name Dowicide 2 and is similar in structure to the infamous herbicide named 2,4,5-T (see page 290).

In a 1979 report, the General Accounting Office of the U.S. Government found that 14 percent of the dressed meat and poultry sold in supermarkets contained illegal residues of chemicals and pesticides. Of the 143 drugs, pesticides, and insecticides studied by the GAO, 20 were suspected of causing birth defects and 6 of causing chromosomal changes. It takes from six to twenty-five days to complete the chemical analyses of meat samples taken at a slaughterhouse, but the animal is divided into wholesale cuts and shipped out twenty-four hours after slaughter. Until technology is sufficiently advanced to permit instant analysis of chemical residues in meat at the slaughterhouse, pregnant women will continue to be exposed to insecticide and pesticide residues in the meat and poultry they eat.

To protect yourself and your babies from the effects of pesticides on foods, avoid use or exposure to pesticides in a home garden, lawn, or greenhouse. If you must use one of these agents, scientists recommend that you wear gloves and a disposable face mask. A pregnant or nursing woman should consciously try to avoid foods that are suspected of containing pesticide residues. Fruits and vegetables should be peeled or thoroughly washed. Some scientists have suggested that women have their milk tested for pesticide and insecticide content. However, recent studies suggest that there is often a dramatic variance between specimens collected on two different days. With such variations, single tests would be inconclusive, and in most cases the repeated testing and careful analyses required to give meaningful results would be extremely expensive and time consuming.

How should household pesticides be used during pregnancy?

There are no known studies linking normal use of household pesticides with an increased incidence of birth defects. However, to be on the safe side, it is best to wait until after the first trimester to spray pests such as roaches, fleas, spiders, flies, and ants within your home. In addition to delegating the job of spraying to someone else, be sure to completely cover all food and do not allow spraying of your clothing. You should stay out of your house for at least twenty-four hours in order to allow the pesticide to settle. Ideally, someone other than yourself should come in and scrub down all the eating surfaces in your home and air out the house before you go back in.

What harmful effects may be associated with herbicide exposure?

Herbicides are chemicals which destroy vegetation. They often contain a poisonous substance named dioxin, a chemical classified by the Environmental Protection Agency as one of the most toxic known. Dioxin is actually a manufacturing impurity that contaminates many industrial products including wood preservatives and sealants. TCDD is a potent dioxin derivative. In laboratory studies, pregnant rhesus monkeys exposed to this agent showed a marked increase in the rate of spontaneous abortion, massive hemorrhage, and birth defects such as cleft palate and kidney abnormalities. In 1971, an industrial explosion in Italy dispersed TCDD over a wide area and exposed thousands of people to this chemical. Some research suggested that this accident resulted in higher rates of spontaneous abortion and fetal malformations.

Agent Orange is the most notorious product ever to be manufactured. It consists of the dioxin-laden herbicides 2,4-D and 2,4,5-T. Following Agent Orange's widespread use in defoliating jungles in Vietnam, women inhabitants exposed to this chemical experienced significant increases in spontaneous abortions, stillbirths, and malformed infants. Vietnam veterans who worked with Agent Orange have suffered from higher cancer rates, and their children have been found to be more susceptible to birth defects. During the 1970s, large quantities of 2,4,5-T were sprayed in parts of Oregon to increase the productivity in commercial forests by killing off vegetation competing for light with trees that were planted. An Environmental Protection Agency study which was completed in 1979 demonstrated spontaneous abortions occurring at three times the normal rate throughout the area that was sprayed. Dioxin levels in breast milk were also significantly elevated among nursing women living in the sprayed areas. As a result of these studies, the Environmental Protection Agency has placed a ban on 2,4,5-T and Silvex, a related chemical used by homeowners as a weed killer for lawns and gardens. As of March 1, 1979, the use of these agents has been prohibited on forest lands, pasturelands, and utility and railroad rights-of-way in the United States. Continued use, however, is permitted on rangelands and rice fields. I do not understand why 2,4,5-T is not banned on rangelands where cattle graze, since some studies have found dioxin in the flesh of beef cattle in the Middle West. Also curious is the Environmental Protection Agency's decision not to ban 2,4-D since it is so chemically similar to 2,4,5-T. This should be a source of concern to all citizens, since over 1,500 products with 2,4-D are used in this country to kill undesirable plants in lawns, forests, rangeland, pastures, and aquatic areas.

In the interest of fair reporting, it should be mentioned that not all studies have found an association between dioxin exposure and adverse fetal effects. It will be several more years before researchers will be able to offer the public additional meaningful information.

Urea Formaldehyde Foam Insulation

What problems may be encountered if I want to insulate my home?

Though the concept of energy conservation through home insulation is theoretically a great idea, the use of urea formaldehyde as an insulant has caused deleterious effects on pregnant women's health. Until it was banned in 1982, urea formaldehyde foam had been the most commonly used preparation for home insulation, with an estimated 500,000 to 750,000 homes having been treated with this material. With time, formaldehyde gas may seep out of the foam, penetrate the walls, and pass into the room air, where it exerts its toxic effects.

The common symptoms of formaldehyde toxicity are tearing and itching of the eyes, headache, sneezing, frequent colds, flu-like symptoms, nasal infections, cough, shortness of breath, eczema-like skin rash, a general feeling of fatigue, sore throat, insomnia, and loss of appetite. The severity of reported symptoms have ranged from mild to incapacitating. Animal research and human experience suggest that maternal exposure during pregnancy will increase a child's risk of chromosomal damage, mutations, and birth defects, though more research is necessary before this can be stated with certainty.

In 1982, the Federal Consumer Product Safety Commission banned the sale of urea formaldehyde foam insulation. Prior to this move, Massachusetts had taken the most radical steps by not only banning the foam but ordering its removal from existing homes at the manufacturers' expense.

Paints and Solvents

What precautions should I take while preparing and painting my baby's room?

There is no danger associated with painting during pregnancy, provided that the room you're working in is well ventilated to dispel any fumes. It is healthier to leave a window open and feel uncomfortably cold than to inhale noncirculating air. In addition to paints, work with floor and furniture polishes is also associated with noxious fumes, and the same precautions must be followed. Avoid using all these agents in confined and windowless spaces.

Lead-base paints are dangerous and must never be used to paint a baby's room. If you are renovating an older house which was built before World War II, there is a good chance that the paint on the walls contains lead. In tearing down walls or scraping paint, a do-it-yourselfer may expose herself and her family to dangerously high concentrations of lead dust.

Extensive exposure to spray paint which contains M-butyl ketone, or MBK, may be associated with severe neurological abnormalities. Pregnant women should avoid working with this chemical. Use of turpentine and other liquid paint-stripping agents should also be considered hazardous during pregnancy. The main ingredient in most paint removers is methylene chloride, which rapidly metabolizes to carbon monoxide, a colorless, odorless, deadly gas. The amount of carbon monoxide formed in a person's body is directly related to the amount of methylene chloride absorbed during a paint-stripping project. Exposure for two or three hours can reduce oxygen levels in maternal and fetal blood to dangerously low levels. This effect is significantly exaggerated in heavy smokers, who already have high levels of carbon monoxide in their blood. Pregnant women with heart disease are extremely susceptible to even a slight decrease in oxygen concentrations. Such individuals should be advised not to use paint removers and varnishes that contain methylene chloride during pregnancy.

Toxic Crafts Materials

What hazards may be encountered if I work with arts and crafts materials during pregnancy?

There is a growing concern among artists, hobbyists, and craftswomen about the hazards of the materials with which they work. Sixty percent of the 80 million people engaged in arts and crafts in this country are women. Though there are no large-scale studies, scientists believe that most chemicals found in art materials have the capacity to cross the placental barrier. In addition, the amount necessary to damage the fetus is much smaller than that which can injure an adult. The most sensitive time for these chemicals to alter normal development is from the eighteenth to sixtieth day after conception.

Many artists, jewelers, and craftswomen who make ceramics and ceramic enamel may be exposed to arsenic, a chemical deadly to both a mother and her fetus. Other toxic agents which rapidly cross the placenta are found in glues, asbestos, metallic dust, lead, cadmium, plastics, resins, paint and varnish removers, dyes and pigments, turpentine, glazes, finishes, lacquers, paint thinners, adhesives, silica-containing dusts and clays, and vinyl chloride. Exposure to benzene, a constituent of some paint strippers, has been associated with chromosomal breaks and central nervous system defects in the fetus. Methylene chloride is a popular solvent found in paint strippers and other art materials which, when inhaled by the pregnant woman, reduces the amount of oxygen carried to the fetal bloodstream. Lithium, used by potters, may be responsible for cardiac and other fetal anomalies (see chapter 7).

Art chemicals, especially heavy metals and solvents, can be found in a woman's breast milk several hours after exposure. Animal studies actually show that nursing increases lead absorption from the intestine, leading ultimately to higher levels of lead in the breast milk. In one study, methylene chloride was shown to be present in women's milk up to seventeen hours after exposure had ended.

If you are an artist, or involved in crafts as a hobby, you must inform your obstetrician of all the materials that you use in your work. During pregnancy, try to substitute less hazardous materials whenever possible and store materials safely. Most importantly, be sure that you have proper ventilation in your working environment. In general, there are two basic types of ventilation: general or dilute ventilation and local exhaust ventilation. Local exhaust ventilation is better because it traps the toxic agents at their source and exhausts them before the air in the room becomes contaminated.

Other Environmental Pollutants

What other environmental pollutants should I try to avoid?

Benzene is a colorless liquid which evaporates rapidly to form harmful vapors. It is frequently used in photographic labs, as well as in the production of plastics, pharmaceuticals, rubber products, pesticides, and textiles. Drycleaning establishments also use abundant amounts of benzene. It has been estimated that more than 1 million American workers receive some exposure to benzene. Benzene increases a person's risk of leukemia and has been proven to cause chromosomal breaks in humans.

Exposure to benzene and other organic solvents during pregnancy has been reported to increase a woman's risk of bearing children with central nervous system defects. In addition to benzene, other chemicals inplicated were styrene, acetone, denatured alcohol, alkylphenol, dichlormethane, methanol, ether, toluene, xylene, methylethylketone, petrol, butanol, and ethylene oxide. Of this group, **ethylene oxide** has long been suspected of causing birth defects. This chemical is used in the production of antifreeze and as a fumigant for dried fruit and cereals.

Spray adhesives have a wide variety of uses in the home. In 1973, the Consumer Product Safety Commission suddenly banned all spray adhesives because of a report which claimed that they caused chromosomal and genetic damage among men and women using them. The ban was lifted several months later for lack of evidence to support these allegations. Sadly, before the ban was lifted, several women underwent abortion because of their fears following exposure to spray adhesives. At the present time, there is no proof that chromosomal damage results from their use.

Nitrosamines are widely distributed carcinogens and mutation-inducing chemicals which may enter the body by inhalation, ingestion, or absorption through the skin. They are formed when chemicals called nitrites combine with substances known as amines. Various nitrosamines have been found in foods, cosmetics, alcoholic beverages, cigarette smoke, and many industrial processes, including leather-tanning, rocket fuel, and rubber and tire manufacture. Vegetarian diets also contribute to the level of nitrosamine exposure. Naturally high amounts are found in beets, spinach, celery, lettuce, and turnip greens although the concentration in these foods varies according to the soil, fertilization, and harvesting conditions. Though there is no direct evidence that nitrosamines cause cancer in humans, a number of epidemiologic studies of the tire industry have reported a high incidence of cancer where nitrosamine levels are most likely to be high.

A study sponsored by the National Science Foundation reported the presence of a nitrosamine named N-nitrosodimethylamine (NDMA) in six of seven scotch whiskies and in eighteen brands of beer. Since the concentration of NDMA is higher in beer than in scotch, beer probably constitutes a hazard to the pregnant woman. A woman will often drink beer during pregnancy rather than "hard liquor" because of

Environmental and Occupational Health Hazards and Manifestations

Organ System (Primarily Affected)	Manifestations Acute and Chronic	Environments and Practices Conveying an Increased Risk of Developing Disease	Chemical and Physical Agents

From their extensive study of environmental and occupational health hazards, scientists have come to realize that toxins produce specific organ system manifestations and symptoms. Knowledge of these relationships will often help in the early diagnosis and rapid initiation of treatment. The Health Systems Agency of New York City has provided a valuable table for early identification of some of these environmentally related symptoms.

Organ System (Primarily Affected)	Manifestations Acute and Chronic	Environments and Practices Conveying an Increased Risk of Developing Disease	Chemical and Physical Agents
Skin	Dermatitis "Cola-colored" skin Skin cancer	Electroplating; photoengraving; metal cleaning; wood preserving; food preserving; contact with foods and cosmetics; use of household chemicals and soaps	Hydrocarbon solvents; beryllium; arsenic, zinc oxide, PCB, nickel, dioxane, soap, pentachlorophenol, bismuth, alcohol, drugs
Respiratory System	Acute pulmonary edema and pneumonitis Asthma Chronic lung disease Lung cancer	Construction and insulation; textile manufacturing; painting; arc-welding; meat wrapping; animal handling; in-flight airline services; radiological work; exposure to traffic exhausts, dust, and industrial air pollution; improper ventilation and heating	Arsenic, asbestos, chromium, iron oxide, ionizing radiation, beryllium, ozone, nitrogen oxides, textile dusts, nickel, carbonyl, aerosolized plastics (e.g., vinyl chloride, teflon), dusts, fumes, vapors, TMA
Cardiovascular System	Arrhythmias Angina Intermittent circulatory disease of the legs Arteriosclerosis	Exposure to traffic exhaust; diesel engine operation; sewage treatment; cellophane and plastic manufacturing; motor vehicle repairing; extreme hot/cold; contact with synthetic film and hazardous agents in art and hobby supplies; pest extermination	Carbon monoxide, hydrogen sulfide, barium, organophosphates, freon, glues and solvents, heat and cold
Gastrointestinal System	Abdominal pain, nausea Vomiting, diarrhea, bloody stools Hepatic necrosis Hepatic cancer Hepatic fibrosis	Jewelry making; dry cleaning; refrigerant manufacturing; food processing; chemical handling; printing; contact with lead-based paints and components of batteries and electrical equipment; consumption of improperly handled food.	Heavy metals (e.g., lead, cadmium), carbon tetrachloride, chlorinated hydrocarbons, phosphorus, beryllium, arsenic, nitrosamines, vinyl chloride, aflatoxin, bacterial toxin

Environmental and Occupational Health Hazards and Manifestations (*continued*)

Organ System (Primarily Affected)	Manifestations Acute and Chronic	Environments and Practices Conveying an Increased Risk of Developing Disease	Chemical and Physical Agents
Genitourinary System	Amino acid (protein) in the urine Chronic renal disease Bladder cancer	Plumbing; soldering; exterminating; textile manufacturing; contact with components of batteries	Cadmium, lead, mercury, organic dyes, halogenated hydrocarbons
Nervous System	Headache/convulsions/coma Extrapyramidal disorders Peripheral neuropathy	Wood working; painting; exposure to traffic exhausts; fireproofing; plumbing; soldering; manufacturing of textiles and petrochemicals; contact with pesticides and battery components; consumption of improperly prepared food	Mercury, manganese, lead, carbon monoxide, boron, fluoride, organophosphates, hexane, organic solvents, wood preservatives (pentachlorophenol)
Auditory System	Hearing loss (and stress reactions)	Subway operations; metal working; construction; activities involving loud music	Loud noise, high frequency noise
Ophthalmic System	Eye irritation Cataracts	Petroleum refining; chemical handling; paper production; laundering; contact with photographic films: glass blowing	Nitrogen oxides, acetic acid, formaldehyde, radiation
Reproductive System	Spontaneous abortions Birth defects Infertility	Operating room procedures; contact with pesticides and contact with battery components	Anesthetic gases, ionizing and nonionizing radiation, lead, chemicals (dioxane) pesticides (DBCP)
Hematological System	Dangerous decrease in the number of blood cells, leukemia, lymph node enlargement, and anemia	Dye manufacturing; dry cleaning; chemical handling; contact with hazardous agents in art and hobby supplies; contact with rodent excreta, rodent bites	Benzene, arsenic, organic dyes, arsine, nitrates, drugs, lead
Nasal Cavity and Sinuses	Inflammation Cancer	Welding; photoengraving; manufacturing of glass, pottery, linoleum, textile, wood and leather products; contact with battery components	Arsenic, selenium, chromium, nickelcarbonyl, wood

its lower alcoholic content. While such women may diminish their chances of giving birth to a baby with the fetal alcohol syndrome, they may be exposing their unborn infants to a new risk. For this reason, if you must have an alcoholic beverage during pregnancy, a glass of wine is probably your best bet.

When to Stop Working and Rights of Pregnant Workers

How long should I continue to work and what limitations, if any, should I observe?

Of the more than 40 million female workers in the United States, 70 percent of them in the reproductive age group between sixteen and forty-four, it is estimated that, by 1990, 2 out of 3 women will be working, compared to 1 out of 20 in 1890. Based on present fertility rates, well over 1 million pregnancies can be expected among working women every year.

In the past, if a woman was discovered to be pregnant, she was quickly discharged from her job or refused employment. Many misunderstandings and taboos about work during pregnancy still exist, but, in general, normal pregnancy is no longer treated as an illness. To the surprise of their obstetricians, women are often capable of working until late in pregnancy. However, there are many differences between individuals and pregnancies, and two healthy women working at identical jobs often show different capacities for activity and productivity at this time. For this reason, women and their obstetricians must work together to make intelligent decisions about working and stopping work during pregnancy. Often, decisions made about employment are extremely difficult and challenging and involve economic, physiologic, and social factors as well as obstetrical considerations.

Obviously, jobs that are dangerous or cause physical or mental exhaustion should be given up, if possible, and a temporary transfer to an easier job arranged to enable the pregnant woman to prolong her working career during pregnancy. The American College of Obstetricians and Gynecologists, in cooperation with the National Institute for Occupational Safety and Health (NIOSH), published "Guidelines on Pregnancy and Work" in 1977. In general, the college recommends that physical exertion at work be somewhat reduced because the greater blood volume of pregnancy increases oxygen consumption and places greater demands on the circulatory system. In addition, loss of balance and coordination, combined with relaxation of joints and musculature, increases the likelihood of experiencing muscle sprains and injuries if the pregnant woman's job requires heavy lifting or excessive physical exertion. While many women now work until the onset of labor, some evidence in the medical literature suggests that this trend may be ill advised. Several studies support the view that lack of rest during the last two to four weeks of pregnancy may have an unfavorable effect on the fetus. When European working women of poor socioeconomic levels were allowed rest in maternity homes for several days prior to delivery, a significant decrease in perinatal mortality was observed among those resting for longer than one week.

In a 1982 study from the Pennsylvania State University College of Medicine in Hershey, Pennsylvania, researchers analyzed the work activity of 7,722 women during pregnancy. They found that those who worked past their twenty-eighth week gave birth to infants weighing 150 to 400 grams less than women who did not work. They also noted a higher incidence of placental infarcts among some working women. A placental infarct is an area of dead tissue in the placenta caused by impairment of its blood supply from the uterus. Extensive infarcts can be responsible for growth retardation and even fetal death. The investigators found that large infarcts, having a diameter of 3 centimeters or more, occurred with a very high frequency of 250 per 1,000 births among women who did "stand-up work" after their thirty-seventh week. Included in this group were retail sales workers, private household workers, and laborers. Women who quit this type of work before their thirty-third week had only 47 infarcts per 1,000 births, while the incidence for those who quit between the thirty-third and thirty-seventh weeks was 96 per 1,000 births. Women who did "sitting work" throughout pregnancy, such as clerical workers and students, experienced large infarcts at a rate of 51 per 1,000, compared with 53 per 1,000 for women who remained at home. Despite these statistics, the researchers found no evidence to prove that working women were more likely to give birth to babies with long-term mental or physical impairment. However this report does suggest that if you have a "stand-up" job it might be advisable to curtail this activity during the last two months of your pregnancy.

Though there are many exceptions, here is a guide as to when you should leave your job and return to work following delivery, assuming you are in good health:

1. Stop working two to four weeks before your due date if your pregnancy is uncomplicated and six to twelve weeks early if your job places you in physically or emotionally demanding situations involving undue stress.
2. Stop working at least twelve weeks before your due date if you are expecting twins, have a previous history of premature rupture of the amniotic membranes, or have had premature labor during two or more previous pregnancies.
3. Return to work four to six weeks after a vaginal delivery and six to eight weeks after a cesarean section.
4. If you prefer to work until labor begins, you should be allowed to do so provided that you are examined and evaluated by your doctor at weekly intervals during the last six weeks of pregnancy.

Are there certain women who should definitely not work during pregnancy?

Yes. Most knowledgeable obstetricians would agree that certain women should not be allowed to work during pregnancy. This includes the following categories:

1. Those who have delivered two previous premature infants weighing less than 5 pounds.
2. Those with a history of an incompetent cervix, have had surgery for an incompetent cervix, or have had more than one spontaneous midtrimester abortion.
3. Those with uterine malformations, such as a septum (wall) in the uterus or a double uterus, who have lost a fetus in the past.

4. Those with heart disease who experience shortness of breath when doing less than a normal amount of activity.
5. Those with diseases classified as hemoglobinopathies, such as sickle-cell disease and thalassemia, and those with severe anemia regardless of its cause.
6. Those with significantly elevated blood pressure before or during pregnancy.
7. Those with moderately severe lung and kidney disease.
8. Those with third-trimester bleeding, premature rupture of the amniotic membranes, placenta previa, or abruptio placenta.
9. Those who are expecting a multiple birth.
10. Those with long-standing and severe forms of diabetes characterized by narrowing of the blood vessels carrying oxygen to the uterus. (Most diabetics, however, do not have this problem and are usually able to work until early in the third trimester.)

What should all pregnant woman know about their legal rights and medical benefits during pregnancy?

The most important legislation ever passed for the pregnant working woman was the 1978 amendment to Title VII of the 1964 Civil Rights Act. Simply stated, it prohibited job discrimination based on pregnancy, childbirth, or related medical conditions. While most employers are usually sympathetic and supportive of the pregnant worker, many others become unresponsive and even hostile to the point of demanding an immediate resignation. Remember, you cannot be forced to resign simply because you are pregnant! The most important factor to consider is your ability to do your job. If you can function as you did before pregnancy, the fact that you are pregnant should never determine how you are treated. Furthermore, even if you are partially disabled by pregnancy, you need not necessarily resign. If your employer regularly assigns light work to other partially disabled employees, he or she is obliged to do the same for you. If you are temporarily unable to work, your employer should give you the same rights as other employees who are temporarily disabled by accident or by illness, including the same medical insurance benefits provided to other workers. Finally, you should be permitted to return to the job just as other employees who have temporary disability conditions.

If you believe that you are being unfairly treated because you are pregnant, object to your personnel director or union shop steward. To determine exactly what your rights are and the legality of your claim, contact your state's human rights commissioner, a local chapter of the National Organization for Women, the American Civil Liberties Union, or the federal Equal Employment Opportunity Commission.

Maternal financial benefits vary significantly from one company to another. Ask about the exact coverage provided by your corporate and private health insurance plans. Many women assume because their employers' group health insurance plan provides some maternity benefits, every pregnancy-related bill will be covered. Unfortunately, this is often not the case. Be sure to determine if your policy includes items such as special tests, additional hospital stay, hospital nursery costs, and medications. Some policies also require that you pay the bills and then await reimbursement. This can often create an impossible financial burden for a young couple.

Disability payments cover the period of time from when you stop working to have your baby until you return to your job following delivery. Most employers treat pregnancy as any other disability and continue your salary and benefits while you are away from the office. Some companies allow you additional sick leave as part of your maternity leave. Others offer partial disability while continuing other benefits. Be sure that your employer is not among those miserly few who offer no disability payments. From a financial point of view, it is better that you continue working for as long as you can rather than to quit on a specific predetermined date prior to your due date. Delivery dates are usually unpredictable, and if you or your doctor have miscalculated and you are late, you could use up several weeks of maternity leave before your baby is born. In addition, by leaving voluntarily before it is medically necessary, you might disqualify yourself from your company's health insurance, disability, and sick pay provisions.

If your employer does not have a temporary disability plan, you may qualify for full or partial unemployment or temporary disability benefits from your state. However, not all states provide coverage, and payments may vary significantly.

To find out about the benefits to which you may be entitled, check with your local state employment office.

10.
The New Obstetrical Technology

Pregnant women of today are far more knowledgeable than their predecessors about their own bodies and about childbirth. Words such as amniocentesis, chromosomal analysis, and fetal monitoring are not foreign to them. But many women and men have reacted to this new technology with skepticism and antagonism. In the eyes of many expectant parents the new gadgetry has only helped to further depersonalize the birth experience and intensify the rift between parents and what they see as uncaring, scientifically oriented obstetricians. The recent surge in midwifery and home births in the United States is a direct result of women's widespread dissatisfaction with technically competent but emotionally deficient obstetricians and the hospitals in which they work.

Despite the significant drawbacks of our new technology, even the most skeptical person would have to agree that modern obstetrical discoveries have been an invaluable comfort to women. Just ask any forty-year-old who has recently carried a pregnancy to term, secure in the knowledge that her baby would not be born with a chromosomal abnormality. Similarly, many babies are alive today because laboratory studies determined the ideal time for delivery to occur without fear of respiratory complications.

The proper use of the new obstetrical methods is critical. Doctors who have not kept abreast of the latest advances may compensate by haphazardly ordering a wide variety of unnecessary and expensive tests. To have meaning, these studies must be done at specific times during pregnancy and in an orderly sequence. If not, the interpretation of results and subsequent proper treatment is impossible. Some procedures impose a risk to the fetus and mother as well; their use should provide benefits that clearly outweigh the potential dangers and expense.

Some doctors enjoy impressing their patients with their medical double-talk and the complicated names of various tests. In fact, there is no test so complex that its indications and interpretations cannot be accurately explained to the lay person. This chapter evaluates some of the newer obstetrical tests and procedures. It is not my purpose to convert all pregnant women to Board-certified obstetricians but rather to help you understand these procedures and decide if you need them.

Amniocentesis   **What is amniocentesis and how is it performed?**

Amniocentesis is the sampling of the amniotic fluid from the pregnancy sac, or bag of waters, which surrounds the fetus in order to evaluate the well-being of the fetus. By analyzing the amniotic fluid, it is now possible for doctors to detect fetal chromosomal abnormalities, the presence of a wide variety of hereditary diseases, the severity of Rh disease, and the maturity of the baby's lungs. Chromosomal analysis also reveals the sex of the baby, information which is invaluable for those unfortunate women who are carriers of so-called sex-linked diseases. A needle is passed through the anesthetized skin of the abdominal wall to obtain the amniotic fluid for testing. The test is usually not performed before the sixteenth week of pregnancy. This insures that an adequate quantity of amniotic fluid is present so that the procedure can be safely performed.

The safety to the fetus and the accuracy of the amniotic fluid tests depends upon obtaining clear rather than bloody fluid. It is, therefore, imperative that the doctor performing the amniocentesis be skilled in the technique. To minimize the risk of fetal injury or accidental puncture of the placenta, an ultrasound examination must be performed immediately before inserting the needle. It is also important that the pregnant woman urinate immediately before the needle is inserted in order to be certain that the needle does not perforate the distended urinary bladder which lies just in front of the uterus. On rare occasions, doctors have had the embarrassing experience of obtaining maternal urine rather than amniotic fluid for analysis.

The procedure is very simple. Wearing sterile gloves, the doctor cleans the skin overlying the needle site with an antiseptic solution. A local anesthetic, such as Novocain, is sometimes injected into the skin with a very fine needle. This is followed by the larger and longer amniocentesis needle, which may cause a moderate amount of pain as it enters the tissues below the skin. The pain will be minimized if the needle is inserted rapidly. Correct placement is confirmed by a free flow of clear amniotic fluid through the tip of the needle. Approximately 30 cubic centimeters, or a tenth of a cup, is all that is needed to perform the required prenatal studies. After the fluid is obtained, the needle is rapidly withdrawn and the heartbeat of the baby is checked to be certain that all is well. The entire procedure usually takes no more than five minutes, but the information obtained lasts a lifetime.

What are the risks of amniocentesis?

When the fetal position and placental site is determined by ultrasound immediately before amniocentesis, the incidence of complications will be extremely low. However, even in the best of hands, it is not a totally innocuous procedure. Trauma to the fetus, placental and umbilical cord hemorrhage, injury to maternal structures, inadvertent rupture of the amniotic membranes, uterine and amniotic fluid infections, premature labor, and spontaneous abortion have all been reported. The passage of fetal red blood cells into the maternal circulation following a midtrimester amniocentesis may be far more common than is currently believed; 8.4 percent in one study. This is especially significant for Rh-negative women, who may become sensitized by Rh-positive fetal cells.

Fortunately, severe complications are infrequent and several large studies have confirmed that fetal loss following amniocentesis will increase by no more than 0.5 percent.

Injury to the fetus, when it occurs, is more common if the volume of amniotic fluid is small or if it is thick and does not flow freely through the needle. Both conditions are more likely to be encountered in a pregnancy that extends beyond the expected delivery date. Performance of amniocentesis before the sixteenth week of pregnancy also increases the risk of fetal injury because of the smaller volume of amniotic fluid—actually 50 percent less at fourteen weeks than that at sixteen weeks. The location of the placenta is also very important; when the ultrasound examination reveals that the placenta is attached to the front (anterior) wall of the uterus, rather than the back (posterior) wall, the risk of placental injury and fetal bleeding is greater.

What vital information does amniocentesis provide about the X and Y sex chromosomes?

The sex of the fetus can easily be determined when amniocentesis is performed at, or after, the sixteenth week of pregnancy. Unlike other prenatal studies which require culturing of the amniotic fluid cells over a period of two or more weeks, rapid staining techniques often allow instant identification of the X and Y chromosomes. The accuracy of these rapid methods is approximately 97 percent. Complete accuracy can only be obtained if the cells are cultured.

The sex of the fertilized egg is determined by the type of sex chromosome present in the head of the sperm. The adult male has two sets of sex chromosomes in his body cells; they are called X and Y. The adult woman contains two X sex chromosomes in each of her body cells, but no Y's. Therefore, her egg always contributes an X to the future offspring. If a sperm cell carrying a Y chromosome fertilizes the X egg, the result is an XY male. However, if a sperm cell carrying an X gets there first, the result is an XX female (see top figure on opposite page).

Knowing the sex of the fetus is invaluable in offering genetic counseling to couples at risk of conceiving a child with a so-called X-linked or sex-linked disease. Such diseases are carried on one of a woman's two X chromosomes and only appear in the offspring when the affected chromosome is fertilized by a man's Y chromosome. Only male fetuses inheriting the disease-carrying X will be afflicted with the disease. Those males inheriting the nonaffected X chromosome will be normal. (The bottom figure on the opposite page illustrates the mechanism of transmitting X-linked diseases.) The odds, therefore, of a carrier mother transmitting the disease to her male offspring is 50 percent, but for female offspring it is zero. Each daughter has a 50 percent chance of being a carrier and transmitting the disease to one half of her sons. No male-to-male transmission of X-linked disorders can occur. That is, a father cannot pass the disorder on to his son.

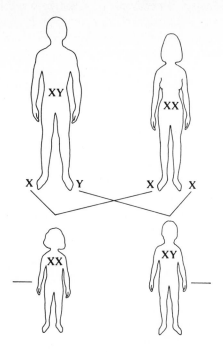

How sex is determined.

Carrier mother   Normal father

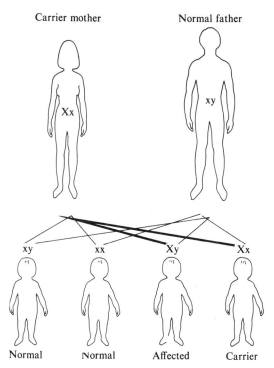

Normal   Normal   Affected   Carrier

How X-linked inheritance works.

In the most common form of X-linked inheritance, the female sex chromosome of an unaffected mother carries one faulty gene (X) and one normal one (x). The father has normal male x and y chromosome complement.

The odds for each *male* child are:
50 percent risk of inheriting the faulty **X** *and the disorder*
50 percent chance of inheriting normal x and y chromosomes

The odds for each *female* child are:
50 percent risk of inheriting one faulty **X** to be a *carrier* like mother
50 percent chance of inheriting no faulty gene

Though color blindness is an example of a benign condition passed on through the X chromosome, deadly diseases, such as a common form of muscular dystrophy known as Duchenne; classic hemophilia, or hemophilia A; hemophilia B; and rare diseases with names, such as Hunter syndrome, Lesch-Nyhan syndrome, Fabry's disease, and Menke's disease also fall into this category. At the present time geneticists are often quite limited in their ability to determine with certainty if a male fetus is affected. A couple is faced with the dilemma of a midtrimester abortion on all male fetuses, while allowing females to survive. Unfortunately, this will necessitate aborting healthy males 50 percent of the time, but it will also prevent the despair of caring for an infant afflicted with one of these terrible diseases.

Research in the prenatal diagnosis of muscular dystrophy has been quite frustrating. Although clinical symptoms of the disease do not become obvious until early in childhood, an enzyme in the blood named creatine phosphokinase, or CPK, is elevated at birth in individuals with Duchenne muscular dystrophy. Investigators are currently determining if CPK levels in utero can be used to diagnose Duchenne muscular dystrophy.

Far better success has been achieved with the in utero diagnosis of hemophilia A, or classic hemophilia. With the use of the fetoscope, a viewing instrument placed inside the amniotic sac, fetal blood samples can be collected and analyzed. Abnormally low levels of a blood clotting factor called factor VIII are found in the hemophilic male fetus. Diagnostic accuracy has approached 100 percent. Hemophilia B is characterized by a deficiency of factor IX clotting factor. The intrauterine diagnosis of this condition has also shown initial success.

Occasionally, a couple requests amniocentesis merely to know the sex of their child. Some have even requested a second-trimester abortion based solely on the fact that the fetus, though healthy, is not of the desired sex. Important ethical questions have been raised as to whether or not modern technology should be used to abort potentially healthy offspring simply because of a couple's sex preference for their child.

Abnormalities of the sex chromosomes make up approximately 20 percent of all chromosomal defects. Approximately 1 out of 950 females are born with the so-called triple X, or super female, chromosomal abnormality. These individuals have three X chromosomes, or a trisomy, rather than the normal female complement of two. Their total chromosomal count is forty-seven rather than the usual forty-six. While many triple X females have no symptoms and lead perfectly normal lives, others may experience infertility, premature menopause, congenital abnormalities, and mental retardation. At the opposite end of the spectrum are the 1 in 10,000 female infants who are born with only one X chromosome, or monosomy, rather than two, giving them a total of forty-five chromosomes. This condition, called ovarian dysgenesis, is characterized by short stature, small streaks of tissue instead of ovaries, infertility, infantile genitals, sparse pubic hair, undeveloped breasts, and a failure to menstruate. About a third of these young girls will also have multiple congenital deformities, such as webbing of the neck, abnormalities of the heart and its blood vessels, abnormal loss of bone minerals, bony abnormalities, and visual defects. This constellation of bizarre abnormalities is known as Turner's syndrome.

Klinefelter's syndrome is characterized by the presence of an XXY sex chromosome pattern. It occurs as frequently as 1 in 1,000 male births. In addition to having forty-seven chromosomes, these men often demonstrate abnormally small genitals, minimal if any sperm cell formation, and prominent breasts.

Men with an XYY chromosomal pattern, known as "supermales," also have forty-seven chromosomes. The incidence of this abnormality is equal to that of Klinefelter's syndrome. XYY men may be asymptomatic and lead normal lives. Others have been described as being tall, thin, acneed, and excessively aggressive, and violent individuals. There is some evidence that a higher percentage of XYY men are in penal institutions; lawyers for Richard Specks, the mass murderer from Chicago, claimed that his XYY genetic makeup was responsible for his violent deeds.

The most recently described sex chromosome abnormality is referred to as the "fragile X" chromosome. The presence of a small, delicate constricted spot at the end of the long arm of a man's X-chromosome has been found in as many as 20 percent of all mentally retarded men. In addition to mental retardation, these individuals have large gonads and abnormally large ears. It has been theorized that this condition may be related to a folic acid deficiency or a defect in folic acid metabolism. In families with a strong history of mental retardation, it may be helpful to perform amniocentesis in order to detect this condition.

Is there any other way to determine a baby's sex without performing amniocentesis?

Successful studies have been carried out in the People's Republic of China by sampling cells that are shed into the cervical canal from the placenta. The cells are obtained in a manner similar to a Pap smear, and the accuracy of sex prediction was originally reported to be 94 percent. Equally optimistic results were reported in 1977 by American doctors who suctioned cells from the inner cervix. Studies conducted in 1980 by doctors at the Center for Disease Control, using the identical technique, have not confirmed these early enthusiastic reports. Instead, it was found that specimens obtained from within the cervix were most likely to be maternal rather than fetal in origin.

During pregnancy male cells (XY), presumably of fetal origin, are present in the bloodstream in 80 percent of mothers with a male fetus. Based on this fact, researchers in Switzerland have successfully predicted the fetal sex 86 percent of the time. The greatest number of successful tests occurs between the fourteenth and eighteenth week of pregnancy. It was hoped that this method could be used as a simple blood test for screening all women, young or old, for chromosomal defects early in pregnancy, but fetal cells recovered from maternal blood did not respond to laboratory testing and culturing in the same way as those obtained from the amniotic fluid, so genetic studies are not yet possible with cells obtained in this fashion.

Amniocentesis and Genetic Disorders

Can Down's syndrome be diagnosed by amniocentesis?

Yes. It is estimated that 15,000 infants with chromosomal abnormalities are born each year in the United States. Practically all these genetic disorders can be diagnosed prenatally by studying the fetal cells and fluid obtained at the time of amniocentesis. By far, the most common reason for amniocentesis is to detect Down's syndrome, commonly known as mongolism.

Normally, a person has twenty-two pairs of body, or autosome, chromosomes and one pair of sex chromosomes in each body cell, for a total of forty-six chromosomes. Down's syndrome is also known as trisomy 21 because affected infants have three chromosomes rather than the normal two, on the chromosome named number 21. Consequently, these infants have a total count of forty-seven chromosomes in each of their body cells. Trisomy 21 occurs when the paired number 21 chromosomes fail to divide and separate at the time that either the sperm or egg cell is being formed. This inability of chromosomes to divide normally is called nondisjunction. When one of these cells with an extra chromosome is fertilized by a normal sperm or egg cell, a chromosome trisomy, or threesome, is inevitable. The chances of producing an infant with a trisomy increases with advancing maternal and paternal age (see below). Parents of these infants show a normal chromosome pattern when their blood cells are analyzed.

Three percent of all infants with Down's syndrome inherit their extra number 21 chromosome through a process called translocation. Though parents of children with this condition appear normal, they are genetically abnormal because they are born with a fragment of their 21 chromosome attached to another chromosome such as the eighteenth, thirteenth, fifteenth, or twenty-second. Carrier parents produce Down's syndrome infants at a frequency ranging from 2 to 100 percent, depending on where the 21 fragment is attached. Unlike Down's syndrome caused by nondisjunction, this form of the disease is not related to parental age and can be diagnosed by studying the chromosomes of the affected parents' blood cells. In the case of Down's syndrome, the extra amount of chromosomal material is responsible for significant fetal damage. It has been estimated that two-thirds of the fetuses with this abnormal chromosome configuration undergo spontaneous abortion, stillbirth, or neonatal death. The remaining one-third who survive present a striking clinical picture, which is easily recognized at birth. Characteristics are mental retardation, short stature, a thick and fissured tongue, low-set ears, slanting and closely set eyes, and abnormal hands and fingers. Many of these infants suffer from congenital heart disease and respiratory infections.

What are my chances of having a baby with Down's syndrome?

Women under thirty years of age have only 1 chance in 900 of giving birth to an infant with a trisomy 21 chromosomal abnormality. Although the incidence of Down's syndrome increases with each year during the twenties, as well as the thirties, after thirty the risk increases perceptibly with each advancing year (see table 10–1).

Amniocentesis should be performed for women over age thirty-five to detect Down's syndrome. The availability of midtrimester abortion to women carrying abnormal fetuses, combined with more efficient sterilization techniques, have resulted in relatively few such babies being born to mothers thirty-five and older when compared to earlier decades in this century. The incidence of older women having babies with Down's syndrome has not changed, but younger women are having a greater

Table 10–1. Risk of Giving Birth to a Down's Syndrome Infant for Each Maternal Year over the Age of 20

Maternal Age	Frequency of Down's Syndrome Births
20	1 in 1,923
21	1 in 1,695
22	1 in 1,538
23	1 in 1,408
24	1 in 1,299
25	1 in 1,205
26	1 in 1,124
27	1 in 1,053
28	1 in 990
29	1 in 935
30	1 in 885
31	1 in 826
32	1 in 725
33	1 in 592
34	1 in 465
35	1 in 365
36	1 in 287
37	1 in 225
38	1 in 176
39	1 in 139
40	1 in 109
41	1 in 85
42	1 in 67
43	1 in 53
44	1 in 41
45	1 in 32
46	1 in 25
47	1 in 20
48	1 in 16
49	1 in 12

proportion of the births, because younger women are not being screened. As a result, women over thirty-five are now having only 30 percent of the infants with Down's syndrome.

In about 20 to 30 percent of cases of Down's syndrome, the additional chromosome 21 comes from the father. Regardless of the mother's age, a father over the age of fifty-five doubles his wife's chances of giving birth to an affected child.

What other genetic diseases can be detected by studying amniotic fluid?

Autosomal recessive diseases are carried by healthy individuals who themselves show no symptoms of the disease. The disease appears in the offspring when those who are carriers of the same harmful gene mate. Under these circumstances, the theoretical risk of giving birth to an affected infant will be one out of four. Two out of four, or 50 percent, will be healthy carriers capable of transmitting the disease, while one out of four will be normal and unaffected. Actual experience, however, does not always follow this theoretical scheme, and many parents have had the misfortune of giving birth to two or more diseased infants in succession. The genetics of autosomal recessive inheritance is demonstrated in the figure below.

Sickle-cell anemia, cystic fibrosis, Tay-Sachs, and phenylketonuria are among the better known autosomal recessive diseases. However, there are about one hundred others—serious and rare disorders with names such as Gaucher's, Nieman-Pick, maple syrup urine disease, cystinosis, and Pompe's disease. Many of these disorders involve specific enzyme deficiencies which can only be detected by studying the amniotic fluid of a fetus believed to be at risk. Individuals afflicted with autosomal recessive diseases show no obvious abnormalities in the makeup of their chromosomes obtained at the time of amniocentesis. Unfortunately, the fact that both parents are carriers of one of these diseases is often not known until after the birth of an affected infant. Despite the availability of biochemical laboratory studies, there are still many autosomal recessive diseases in which no method has been found to screen for asymptomatic carriers before a woman becomes pregnant. One notable exception is Tay-Sachs disease (see page 310).

In utero detection of severe autosomal recessive blood disorders, such as sickle-cell disease and beta thalassemia, involves studying the fetal red blood cells rather

How recessive inheritance works.

Both parents, usually unaffected, carry a normal gene (N) that takes precedence over its faulty recessive counterpart (r).

The odds for each child are:
A 25 percent risk of inheriting a "double dose" of r genes, which may cause a serious birth defect.
A 25 percent chance of inheriting two N's, thus being unaffected.
A 50 percent chance of being a carrier, as both parents are.

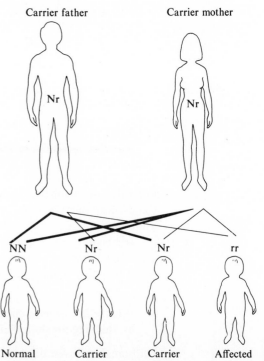

Carrier father   Carrier mother

Nr   Nr

NN   Nr   Nr   rr

Normal   Carrier   Carrier   Affected

than the amniotic fluid. Unbelievable success has been achieved in obtaining direct fetal blood samples through an instrument called a fetoscope. It is much easier and safer to perform amniocentesis rather than fetoscopy. Recently developed enzyme tests on the amniotic fluid may eventually lead to simpler methods for diagnosing these conditions. There are some autosomal recessive diseases in which the fetal appearance is markedly abnormal. Under these conditions, diagnosis is possible by visualization of the fetus through the fetoscope, combined with the use of ultrasound.

Unlike autosomal recessive diseases, there are usually no healthy carriers of autosomal dominant conditions and inheritance in autosomal dominant genetic diseases follows a different pattern. An afflicted person with the disease trait on one of a pair of genes shows symptoms of the disease and has a 50 percent chance of transmitting the condition to his or her offspring. The other 50 percent are normal, with no chance of passing on the disease. Children who inherit the abnormal gene have symptoms of the disease, regardless of the normal genetic makeup of the unaffected parent, because the dominant gene overwhelms the effect of the normal gene. This is demonstrated in the figure below.

Examples of some of the many autosomal dominant diseases are acute intermittent porphyria, Huntington's disease, achondroplastic dwarfism, the adult type of polycystic kidney disease, Marfan's syndrome, and neurofibromatosis.

There is convincing evidence that some autosomal genetic diseases may suddenly appear as a result of a gene change, or mutation, in the sperm or egg of an otherwise healthy parent. Statistically, two-thirds of these mutations occur in the

How dominant inheritance works.

One affected parent has a single faulty gene (D) that dominates its normal counterpart (n). Each child's chances of inheriting either the D or the n from the affected parent are 50 percent.

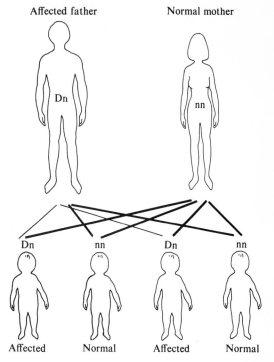

sperm and one-third affect the egg. Even when there is no previous family history of the disorder, once a mutation occurs, the disease is passed to subsequent generations by the afflicted person in the usual pattern of autosomal dominance.

Is Tay-Sachs disease inherited and can its presence be detected in carriers?

Yes. This autosomal recessive disease which is ninety-nine times more common in Jewish families than among non-Jews is always fatal. Specifically, it is the Jews of Central and Eastern European (Ashkenazi) ancestry who run the highest risk of carrying Tay-Sachs. Ninety percent of American Jews are of Ashkenazi origin, and of this group 1 out of every 30 men or women will be carriers of the disease. Statistically, this means that approximately 1 in 900 Jewish couples is at risk of having children with Tay-Sachs. As with other autosomal recessive diseases, there is a 1 in 4 chance in each pregnancy of two carrier parents having an affected child.

The cause of Tay-Sachs disease is the absence of a vital enzyme named hexosaminidase A. In normal individuals this enzyme helps to break down fatty chemicals, named glycolipids, in body cells. When absent in a Tay-Sachs child a glycolipid named GM_2-ganglioside accumulates, leading to the degeneration and eventual destruction of nerve cells in the brain and other body tissues. Tragically, affected children appear normal at birth. Symptoms of physical weakness and uncoordination first appear at six months of age. From this point, deterioration is rapid and is characterized by blindness, seizures, severe mental retardation, and death by the age of four. There is no cure or treatment for this disease.

Fortunately, scientists have discovered that healthy Tay-Sachs carriers can be identified by a simple blood test which measures hexosaminidase A levels. Carriers show a 50 percent reduction in the level of this enzyme. If it is determined that both parents are carriers, detection of hexosaminidase A levels in the amniotic fluid can be accurately determined during the sixteenth week of pregnancy. A woman found to be carrying a Tay-Sachs fetus can be offered the alternative of terminating the pregnancy. With repeat pregnancy attempts, the odds are that a carrier couple will eventually conceive an unaffected baby or a healthy carrier.

Routine blood screening is not as accurate when performed during pregnancy. If testing was not done before conceiving, the father should be tested immediately. If he proves not to be a carrier, no further testing is necessary during the pregnancy, because the birth of an affected baby would be an impossibility. However, if he is a carrier, the mother must undergo a somewhat more time-consuming and more specific blood test to determine her hexosaminidase A levels. If this test proves positive, amniocentesis is mandatory.

The routine blood test for Tay-Sachs carriers may be unreliable for some women. Included in this group are those using oral contraceptives and others with diabetes, hepatitis, heart disease, or other debilitating diseases.

Through the tireless efforts of the National Tay-Sachs Association and many state and local organizations, millions of Jews throughout the United States have undergone Tay-Sachs screening. It appears that this combination of scientific expertise and community participation will put an end to the birth of infants with this terrible disease.

Can analysis of amniotic fluid detect the presence of cystic fibrosis?

Despite intensive efforts by scientists to detect healthy carriers of cystic fibrosis, until recently results have been quite disappointing. Similarly, amniotic fluid analysis has failed to diagnose the disease in the fetus. Fortunately, some promising research suggests that this situation may soon change.

Cystic fibrosis is the most common lethal inherited disease of white Americans, afflicting approximately 1 in every 2,000 babies born in the United States. Like Tay-Sachs disease, it has an autosomal recessive inheritance pattern and is rare in racial groups other than whites. Children with this condition lack the normal body enzymes needed to clear thick mucous secretions from their respiratory tract. As a result, they become prone to respiratory complications and repeated infections and often die in their late teens or early twenties. The diagnosis of cystic fibrosis is made by measuring the high concentration of sodium chloride in the sweat and body secretions of affected children.

Doctors at Northwestern University have made encouraging strides in the in utero diagnosis of cystic fibrosis. A chemical named methylumbelliferyl-guanidinobenzoate, or MUGB for short, has the ability to measure the concentration of certain enzymes which are deficient in the saliva and plasma of patients with cystic fibrosis. When MUGB is mixed with a sample of amniotic fluid, it has been found that the enzyme levels are significantly lower among fetuses later proven to have cystic fibrosis. A control group of normal fetuses demonstrated normal enzyme concentrations. To date, doctors have reported almost 100 percent success rates in the intrauterine detection of cystic fibrosis, though the number of patients studied has been limited.

Who should undergo amniocentesis?

I would recommend amniocentesis to all women over the age of thirty-five and to those married to men who are older than fifty-five. In addition, any woman, regardless of her age, who has given birth to an infant with a chromosomal abnormality should also be encouraged to undergo diagnostic amniocentesis. A family in which one parent is a known carrier of a genetic disease is at especially high risk of conceiving an abnormal infant. Similarly, pregnancies among women who are known carriers of serious X-linked disorders must have the fetal sex verified with amniocentesis and appropriate measures taken if it is male. When both parents are discovered to be carriers of one of the few autosomal recessive diseases which may be diagnosed in utero, amniocentesis is mandatory. The same is true for autosomal dominant conditions. Unfortunately, fewer than 100 of the 1,200 autosomal dominant and autosomal recessive disorders can be diagnosed during pregnancy. Amniocentesis is also indicated when a woman's prenatal blood test or previous history strongly suggests that she may give birth to an infant with a neural tube defect such as anencephaly or spina bifida.

As mentioned in chapter 2, spontaneously aborted fetuses are significantly more likely to be chromosomally abnormal. It is believed that if a woman has experienced three or more spontaneous abortions prior to her present conception she will be at a much greater risk of giving birth to an infant with a genetic defect. Similarly, if her husband's previous wife experienced several miscarriages, the odds are slightly greater that he may be contributing chromosomally abnormal sperm to the present union. Many geneticists believe that couples with this type of history should be offered diagnostic amniocentesis.

Amniocentesis and Respiratory Distress Syndrome (RDS)

How is amniocentesis used in the last few weeks of pregnancy to determine the respiratory status of the fetus?

The leading cause of death among newborn infants, particularly premature infants, is respiratory distress syndrome, or RDS. Newborns suffering from RDS lack a substance named surfactant, which is produced by the cells lining the small air spaces (alveoli) within the lungs. Surfactant prevents the baby's lungs from collapsing with each expiration. As a result, newborns with sufficient amounts of surfactant rarely succumb to RDS. When adequate concentrations of surfactant are present in the fetal lungs, some is transported into the amniotic fluid. Its concentration in the amniotic fluid can then be measured if a sample is obtained through amniocentesis.

The components of surfactant are chemicals called phospholipids, which have names such as lecithin, phosphatidylglycerol, and phosphatidylinnositol. Lecithin is the most important of the surfactant phospholipids. Its relationship to another phospholipid in the lung, named sphingomyelin, has been the basis for one of the most important laboratory tests now available to obstetricians. During a normal pregnancy, lecithin and sphingomyelin are present in amniotic fluid in approximately equal amounts until the thirty-fourth week. At this point the concentration of lecithin relative to sphingomyelin begins to rise.

The relationship between the lecithin and sphingomyelin concentrations in the amniotic fluid is referred to as the L/S ratio. It has been convincingly proven that the risk of RDS in the newborn will be less than 3 percent whenever the concentration of lecithin is at least twice that of sphingomyelin, meaning that the L/S ratio is two or greater. When the L/S ratio is less than two, the prognosis for the newborn becomes significantly worse. An L/S ratio that predicts adequate functioning of the lungs can often be the deciding factor in favor of an immediate early delivery when the fetus' and/or mother's health is in doubt. When the L/S ratio is too low, amniocentesis can be repeated at weekly intervals until a higher ratio is obtained.

The L/S ratio may be misleading in the presence of maternal diabetes, and infants delivered with a normally mature ratio of two may still experience a significantly higher incidence of RDS. Similar results have also been noted among infants with erythroblastosis fetalis (see RhoGam, page 342). When these medical conditions complicate pregnancy, most obstetricians prefer to see L/S ratios of at least three before the baby is delivered. Meconium, or greenish-yellow fetal feces in the amniotic fluid, may also invalidate the L/S ratio.

Approximately 3 percent of all infants experience RDS despite an L/S ratio of two or more. This is thought to be due to a deficiency of a phospholipid named phosphatidylglycerol. Many laboratories now test for this phospholipid along with the L/S determination. Phosphatidylglycerol appears in the amniotic fluid at about the thirty-sixth week of pregnancy and increases in amount from that point on. In pregnancies complicated by mild diabetes, it may first be noted one to one and one-half weeks later than in normal pregnancies. Amazingly, RDS has never been observed whenever phosphatidylglycerol has been detected in the amniotic fluid. Another advantage of this measurement is that it, unlike the L/S ratio, is unaffected by contamination of amniotic fluid with blood, meconium, or vaginal secretions. In critical situations, where the L/S ratio is between 1.5 and 1.9, the phosphatidylglycerol determination enables doctors to decide which babies can be safely delivered and which ones are at high risk of RDS.

There is no longer any excuse for a newborn to develop RDS just because a doctor decided to induce labor for his or her convenience or for the convenience of a patient. Similarly, a prescheduled, nonemergency cesarean section should hardly ever result in the birth of a baby who develops RDS. Judicious use of ultrasound and amniocentesis before induction of labor or a scheduled nonemergency cesarean section, in which a woman's due date is not absolutely certain, should prevent this physician-induced complication from occurring.

What is the shake test?

The shake test, also known as the foam stability test, provides a rapid half-hour estimate of the presence of surfactant in the amniotic fluid. If surfactant is present in sufficient concentrations, a ring of bubbles and foam will form after alcohol is added to the amniotic fluid and the mixture is shaken vigorously. If the ring of foam persists for at least fifteen minutes after the mixture is shaken, the risk of respiratory distress will be very low.

The great advantage of the shake test is that it takes only half an hour to interpret the results, compared to several hours for the L/S ratio. This is vital in situations where decisions must be made within minutes. Most problems with the shake test have arisen with false negative results, meaning that the quantity of surfactant is adequate but the ring of foam does not persist for fifteen minutes. For this reason, shake test results that are negative for lung maturity should always be confirmed by an L/S ratio.

Other Uses of Amniotic Fluid Studies

How can the study of amniotic fluid be used to detect fetuses with neural tube defects?

So-called neural tube defects, such as anencephaly and hydrocephaly, occur with a frequency of approximately 2 out of every 1,000 births and afflict between 3,000 and 6,000 babies each year in the United States. Interestingly, black women have approximately one-half the chance white women have of bearing a child with a neural tube disorder. The frequency of occurrence of neural tube defects is unrelated to the age or sex of either parent, and chromosomal studies of the amniotic fluid are of no value in making the diagnosis. Once a woman has given birth to a baby with a neural tube defect, her odds of giving birth to a second affected infant will increase to 2 to 5 out of 100. After 2 such births, the chances of a thrid will be 6 to 10 out of 100.

While some neural tube defects may be mild, others are severe and the baby may die after the first few days. When the neural, or nerve, tissue is not covered by the scalp or skin it is called an open neural tube defect. Anencephaly is the most abnormal open defect. It is characterized by incomplete closure of the fetal skull and retarded development of the brain. Open spina bifida is caused by an incomplete closure of the lower spine with exposure of nerve tissue of the lower back. It is often associated with paralysis of the legs and blockage of the fluid which surrounds the brain and spinal cord. The result is hydrocephaly, or an abnormally large head caused by the accumulation of obstructed fluid.

Most open neural tube defects can be diagnosed before the twentieth week of pregnancy, by the measurement of a protein, named alpha-fetoprotein, or AFP, in the amniotic fluid and maternal bloodstream. Alpha-fetoprotein is produced by all fetuses. Under normal circumstances its concentrations in the amniotic fluid increases until the 15th week of pregnancy, and then drops precipitously. Traces of AFP also cross the placenta and enter the maternal circulation. Maternal blood levels, however, follow a different pattern, rising slowly during the second trimester and reaching a plateau during the third trimester. When a pregnancy is complicated by an open neural tube defect, AFP levels in the amniotic fluid and maternal bloodstream are extremely high between the fifteenth and twentieth week. A blood test, should be used as the initial screening for neural tube defects rather than amniocentesis, except when amniocentesis is being performed for other suspected abnormalities or the mother's advanced age. This blood test has its greatest accuracy when performed between the fifteenth and eighteenth week of pregnancy. Then, almost all cases of anencephaly and about 75 percent of open spina bifida defects can be detected. If this initial test is positive, it should be repeated immediately to be sure that it was not in error. If it is still positive, ultrasound examination of the fetal skull and spinal cord should be performed in order to demonstrate the presence of these abnormalities followed by sampling of amniotic fluid if the ultrasound examination does not pinpoint the exact cause of the elevated AFP levels in the maternal bloodstream. If the amniotic fluid AFP is normal, no further action is necessary. However, if it is elevated and this is confirmed with a second amniocentesis, a woman should be offered a midtrimester abortion, because a high percentage of these infants will prove to be abnormal. Statistically, of all women initially screened with the blood test, 50 out of every 1,000 will have elevated serum AFP levels. A second blood test reduces this number of suspect pregnancies to 30 per 1,000, while ultrasound further lowers this number to 15 per 1,000 who will require amniocentesis. Even at this stage, only about 8 to 12 percent of the tested babies prove to have anencephaly or an open spina bifida. It is still unclear why some women have elevated serum AFP values in the presence of normal amniotic fluid specimens. In some cases, this occurs when the baby is of low birth weight.

At the present time, there is a lack of agreement among obstetricians as to whether or not the AFP blood test should be routinely performed on all pregnant women. The strongest argument in favor of screening is that 95 percent of women at risk of bearing a child with a neural tube defect will have no previously affected child or family history of neural tube abnormalities. The blood tests are painless and easy to perform, and the high yield of 8 to 12 abnormal fetuses per 100 amniocenteses makes these tests extremely worthwhile.

What other medical and obstetrical conditions are capable of producing an abnormally high AFP blood test?

An elevated AFP blood test indicates one of several possibilities, the most likely of which is that the pregnancy is more advanced than previously suspected. A subsequent ultrasound exam will confirm this fact 35 percent of the time. Women with twins have higher than normal AFP levels, and this accounts for 10 to 15 percent of all abnormal blood tests. Maternal liver disease may also give a false positive test. If the fetus is severely compromised, has died, is suffering from a kidney ailment known as nephrosis, or is small-for-date, the maternal blood levels of AFP are elevated. Bleeding from the placental site, as noted with abruptio placenta and placenta previa, may result in passage of fetal blood cells into the maternal circulation. This so-called fetomaternal hemorrhage elevates maternal blood levels of AFP, and this could lead to the erroneous diagnosis of a neural tube defect in a normal fetus. Amniotic fluid specimens also show high concentrations of AFP in the presence of twins, oligohydramnios (reduction in the quantity of amniotic fluid), fetal death, and impending fetal death. Accidental fetal blood contamination of the amniotic fluid specimen, a congenital anomaly named osteogenesis, Turner's syndrome (see question on sex chromosomes, page 302), and defects of the fetal abdominal wall such as omphalocoele (large umbilical hernia) and gastroschisis (herniation of intestinal contents due to an absence of abdominal wall musculature) also significantly elevate the AFP concentrations in the amniotic fluid.

What else does study of amniotic fluid reveal about the maturity and well-being of the fetus?

Prior to the discovery of surfactant, doctors used a variety of other amniotic fluid tests to determine a baby's overall body maturity and health. These tests are still performed today in many laboratories as confirmation of the accuracy of the L/S ratio findings and in situations where the L/S ratio is questionable or borderline. Each of these tests requires only a small amount of amniotic fluid, can be performed within a few minutes, and provides the obstetrician with valuable information about the well-being of the baby.

One fascinating test involves examination of a sample of amniotic fluid after it is stained with Nile blue sulfate dye. The presence of unusual-looking orange cells, which clump together and do not have a nucleus, is often indicative of fetal maturity. These cells are believed to originate from the fetal sebaceous glands of the skin, and first begin to shed into the amniotic fluid in significant amounts after the thirty-fifth week of pregnancy. Scientists have determined that the fetus is likely to be more than thirty-six weeks of age when these cells make up more than 30 percent of the total number seen under the microscope.

Creatinine is a chemical which is easily measured in the serum and urine in order to determine a person's kidney function. The concentration of creatinine in the amniotic fluid increases significantly during the last four weeks of pregnancy. This is believed to be due to maturation of the fetal kidney and passage of creatinine-rich urine into the amniotic fluid. A level of at least 1.8 milligrams of creatinine per liter of amniotic fluid is indicative of fetal maturity in 85 percent of all cases. This test is not valid if the mother has kidney disease.

The breakdown, or hemolysis, of circulating red blood cells yields a yellow pigment named bilirubin. Exact measurements of bilirubin concentrations in the amniotic fluid are accomplished with a special light meter called a spectrophotometer. Bilirubin is found in the amniotic fluid during normal pregnancies. It decreases in amount during the second half of pregnancy, and eventually disappears during the last four weeks. Its absence from the amniotic fluid is of some assurance that a baby is mature, but it is not specific enough to be used as the sole test for determining if a jeopardized infant should be delivered early.

The greatest application of the amniotic fluid bilirubin measurement has been in determining the severity of fetal hemolytic disease, or erythroblastosis fetalis, caused by blood type incompatibility between an Rh-negative woman and her Rh-positive fetus. In this condition, an Rh-negative mother forms antibodies against the Rh-positive infant she is carrying. These antibodies then cross the placenta and hemolyze, or destroy, the fetal red blood cells. The most severely affected fetuses have the highest bilirubin concentrations recorded on the spectrophotometer. Infants most in jeopardy require immediate delivery or an intrauterine exchange transfusion of blood (see question on Rh disease, page 342). To this day, scientists are still unable to explain how bilirubin reaches the amniotic fluid from the fetal circulation since none is excreted in the fetal urine. The most likely routes are through the amniotic membrane or the fetal respiratory tract.

Amniography and Fetography

What are amniography and fetography and when are these procedures used by obstetricians?

Amniography is the injection of water-soluble radiopaque x-ray dyes into the amniotic fluid in order to identify abnormalities of the fetus and placenta. An x-ray taken following injection of the dye can determine the volume of the amniotic fluid, the location of the placenta, and the presence of a hydatidiform mole or tumor associated with pregnancy. When taking of the x-ray is delayed for several hours after the dye is injected the intestinal tract of the fetus can be seen because the fetus will swallow the dye from the amniotic fluid. If there is an abnormality, this fetal G.I. series actually outlines it. If the fetus does not swallow the dye this may mean a severely compromised infant, a fetal death, or a congenital defect.

Fetography is amniography performed with fat-soluble dyes. When injected into the amniotic sac, these dyes adhere to the fetal skin and outline the fetus with greater clarity than water-soluble agents.

One obvious disadvantage of amniography and fetography is that they expose the fetus to radiation (see chapter 9) and the potential complications of amniocentesis. In addition, the dangers of fetal ingestion of radiopaque materials have not been adequately studied. Both procedures are rarely used today because they have been replaced in most diagnostic situations by ultrasound. Occasionally, however, they may be helpful if it is necessary to clearly outline abnormalities, such as spina bifida, which may not be diagnosed with certainty following an ultrasound examination.

Amnioscopy and Hysteroscopy

What are amnioscopy and hysteroscopy, and how do they differ?

In amnioscopy the amniotic fluid is observed by placing a thin viewing instrument through the cervix. Though this has been endorsed by some European investigators as a means of detecting meconium in the amniotic fluid, it has not become popular in the United States. One reason for this lack of enthusiasm is that the amnioscope can't be inserted until late in pregnancy, when the cervix is partially dilated. In addition, the instrument may inadvertently rupture the amniotic membranes and introduce potentially harmful bacteria into the uterus from the vagina and cervix.

Hysteroscopy is similar to amnioscopy in that a viewing instrument is passed through the cervix and into the endometrial cavity. The hysteroscope, however, is not used during pregnancy. It has it greatest application in retrieving IUDs which are lost or embedded in the uterine cavity, and it is also helpful in evaluating and cutting out scar tissue or small tumors lining the endometrium.

Fetoscopy

What is fetoscopy and how is it used in obstetrics?

A fetoscope, or needlescope, is a viewing instrument which has a diameter that is slightly greater than a large needle. It is placed through the abdominal wall and into the amniotic cavity in much the same manner as in performing amniocentesis (see illustration on following page). The fetoscope contains a high-powered fiberoptic light source which allows a view of the fetal and placental surfaces, but due to the small diameter of the fetoscope, the area observed at any one moment is quite limited. The fetoscope is equipped with a biopsy forceps which can be used to obtain a small piece of the baby's skin for chromosomal and biochemical studies. The prenatal diagnosis of a variety of congenital skin diseases is also possible with this technique. By inserting a tiny needle into the placenta and umbilical cord, doctors have been able to obtain samples of fetal blood for analysis. To date, less than a handful of fetal liver biopsies have been performed successfully with fetoscopy.

The development of expertise in fetoscopy is very difficult, and at the present time its use is limited to a very few medical centers in the United States. The procedure must still be considered a research tool because of the increased risks to the fetus and mother compared to other methods of prenatal screening and diagnosis. Fetal hemorrhage, accidental rupture of the amniotic membranes, uterine infection, premature labor, and second-trimester abortion are all possible complications. Therefore, fetoscopy is only indicated when the risks of giving birth to a severely compromised infant clearly outweigh the dangers of the procedure.

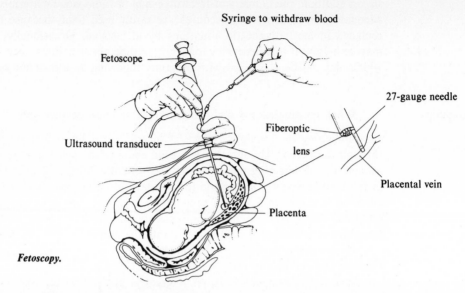

Fetoscopy.

Laparoscopy

What is laparoscopy, and how is it used in pregnancy?

A laparoscope is an instrument with a diameter slightly larger than a pencil. It contains a powerful light source which, when inserted through the naval, allows visualization of the upper abdominal and pelvic contents.

The injection of two or more liters of carbon dioxide or nitrous oxide gas into the abdomen moves the intestine out of the lower pelvis and makes viewing of the pelvic organs easier. Specially designed instruments can then be passed through the laparoscope to accomplish such procedures as tubal sterilization; biopsy of the ovary, liver, or intestinal wall; removal of misplaced IUDs; diagnosis of tubal pregnancies; and evaluation and treatment of infertility, pelvic pain, pelvic infection, and endometriosis. When the laparoscopic procedure is completed the carbon dioxide or nitrous oxide is removed from the abdomen, and the tiny incision in the navel is closed with one absorbable suture. The suture is then covered with a Band-Aid—hence the name "Band-Aid surgery." Another synonym for laparoscopy is "belly-button surgery." The procedure may be performed under general anesthesia or local anesthesia, though the former method is preferred by most doctors in this country.

One of the most important uses of laparoscopy is in the diagnosis of an ectopic pregnancy, one located outside its normal site within the uterine cavity. Ectopic pregnancies may on rare occasions be located in the ovary or the abdominal cavity, but the vast majority implant in one of the fallopian tubes. The early diagnosis of an ectopic pregnancy is vital because with time it can eventually burst through the tube and cause intraabdominal hemorrhage, shock, and even death. Vaginal bleeding and abdominal cramps early in pregnancy may indicate either a threatened abortion or an ectopic pregnancy. The correct diagnosis can be determined rapidly by combined use of diagnostic laparoscopic examination, modern sensitive pregnancy tests (see chapter 2), and ultrasound. If laparoscopy confirms the presence of an ectopic pregnancy, it must be surgically removed through a lower abdominal incision. Removal of a tubal pregnancy through the laparoscope was first described in the medical literature by this writer. Since then it has been successfully accomplished by many other doctors.

Diagnostic laparoscopic procedures performed beyond the sixteenth week of pregnancy are potentially dangerous because the enlarged uterus may be injured by the instrument as it is passed through the umbilicus.

In the days immediately following childbirth, laparoscopic tubal sterilization may be performed instead of the traditional tubal ligation. This is easily accomplished by coagulation, or burning, of the tubes. Despite the impressive statistics from several medical institutions, most doctors have never performed this operation postpartum and some have even claimed that it is hazardous. My experience with the technique on over 100 postpartum women at Norwalk Hospital in Connecticut has been excellent. There have been no complications, and all patients have experienced significantly less discomfort and a shorter hospitalization than those undergoing the abdominal procedure. There is also the added benefit of no visible scar. One great advantage of the procedure over the abdominal postpartum operation is that it may be performed on the second or third day following delivery rather than immediately after. This gives a woman more time to decide if she really wants the operation.

Hormonal Testing

How is the measurement of maternal estrogen used as a test of fetal well-being?

A woman's body produces three different estrogens: estradiol, estrone, and estriol. Estradiol is the principal hormone secreted by the ovaries of nonpregnant women, but during pregnancy, the placenta, fetal liver, and fetal adrenal glands all contribute to the production of abundant amounts of estriol. As pregnancy advances, progressively greater concentrations of estriol are found in the maternal bloodstream and urine. As a matter of fact, the amount of estriol produced in one day by a normal pregnant woman near her due date may actually exceed the total produced by a nonpregnant woman over a three-year period.

Doctors have used both urinary and plasma estriol measurements as a means of evaluating placental function and fetal well-being during the last two months of pregnancy. Though urinary estriol determinations are of some value in the management of certain high-risk pregnancies, they also have many drawbacks. One problem is that a woman must collect, save, and refrigerate all urine specimens over a twenty-four-hour period.

Another problem is that there is a wide range of normal estriol values, and the decline from a high to a low level from one day to the next is difficult if not impossible to interpret. For this reason, the test is only meaningful if at least three 24-hour urine specimens are collected each week. An estriol which is outside the normal range must be verified by at least one other twenty-four-hour specimen. Unfortunately, the finding of a low urinary estriol gives the doctor no information as to the site of the problem. A fetal adrenal gland insufficiency or liver disease, maternal kidney disease, or a poorly functioning placenta may all be responsible for the low laboratory reading. Some medications, such as aspirin, cortisone, and certain antibiotics, may also lower urinary estriols even though the fetus is in no distress. Falsely high estriol levels may be present in diabetic women and in Rh-negative women carrying a severely affected Rh-positive fetus. High rates of estriol excretion also occur in women with multiple fetuses.

The great advantage of plasma estriol determinations is that they can be carried out with a simple blood test. Plasma determinations are not affected by factors such as a woman's kidney disease or her diminished urinary output. Despite this, most laboratories in the United States still perform the more cumbersome twenty-four-hour assay.

Though estriol determinations are extremely disappointing as predictors of fetal well-being, at the present time they are still more accurate than any other hormonal determination during the last two months of pregnancy.

What other hormonal and chemical tests have doctors used to evaluate fetal well-being?

Human chorionic gonadotropin, or HCG, is known as the pregnancy hormone. This hormone is produced by the placenta and its assay is the basis of all pregnancy tests. Quantitative measurements of HCG are helpful early in pregnancy in making the diagnosis of threatened abortion and ectopic pregnancy.

The rate of excretion of HCG into the maternal serum and urine during pregnancy gradually increases following fertilization, reaching peak levels between the sixtieth and seventieth days of pregnancy. Its concentration declines between the 100th and 130th day and remains constant throughout the rest of the pregnancy. HCG concentrations will vary little between healthy and unhealthy pregnancies after the fourth month, so measurements beyond the fourth month are valueless in assessing placental function and fetal well-being.

Human placental lactogen, or HPL, is a hormone which is produced in abundance by the placenta. Also known as human chorionic somatomammotropin, or HCS, it can first be detected in the serum of pregnant women by the sixth week of pregnancy and rises gradually throughout the last trimester. The hormone prepares the breasts for later milk secretion which is sustained by prolactin, a pituitary gland hormone. When the measurement of HPL was first introduced, it was hailed as an excellent method of evaluating fetal health, especially in post-term pregnancies. Unfortunately, it has not fulfilled these early expectations, as shown by the fact that very few obstetrical services presently use this test.

Ultrasound

What is ultrasound, and how are the various ultrasound instruments used in obstetrics?

The medical use of high-frequency sound waves, or ultrasound, has revolutionized the practice of obstetrics and gynecology. This painless and safe technique has provided significantly more information about the status of a woman's pregnancy than had ever been achieved with the use of potentially harmful x-ray examinations. The intensity of diagnostic high-frequency sound waves is extremely low and well within the upper limits of safety.

An ultrasound machine generates sound waves when a current is applied to the probe or transducer of the machine. The transducer is moved gently over the skin of the abdomen during the examination. A pulse of sound waves passes through the tissues below the skin. As the sound waves are bounced back to the transducer from the tissues deep within the abdominal cavity, an image, displayed as a picture on a fluorescent screen, is created. Since tissues of different densities reflect sound differently, the trained ultrasonographer is usually able to identify abdominal and pelvic structures and interpret abnormalities which may be present. To diminish the loss of ultrasound waves at the point where the transducer meets the skin, a large amount of mineral oil or gel is first applied liberally to the skin surface.

Ultrasound machines perform the following techniques: A-scan, B-scan, and real-time. The A-scan is helpful in measuring the exact size of structures, such as the diameter of the fetal head, but is otherwise quite limited in the things that it can do. The B-scan, especially the type known as the gray scale, provides a detailed longitudinal and cross-sectional view of structures and gives their size, shape, and location. It is especially useful in the precise evaluation of placental structure and gynecological conditions such as ovarian cysts and uterine tumors. Though the real-time image gives a less detailed picture than that of the gray-scale B-scan, it is able to show fetal body movement and breathing and pulsations of the heart and its blood vessels, including those of the umbilical cord. Another advantage of the real-time machine is that it is portable, and in the case of an emergency it can be rushed to wherever it is needed. An entire real-time obstetrical study can be completed in five to ten minutes, compared to twenty to forty-five minutes with the B-scan. Finally, the cost of a real-time machine is significantly less than that of a B-scanner.

The small Doppler ultrasound devices used by many obstetricians to hear the fetal heartbeat in their offices also employ high-frequency sounds. However, they provide no other diagnostic information and lack the sophistication of the other devices. The ultrasound wave produced by the Doppler is emitted continuously while those of the real-time and B-scan are pulsed or intermittent. Though these procedures are considered harmless, you should realize that the innocuous-looking hand-held listening device that your doctor uses produces greater sound-wave exposure than the machines with the more imposing appearance. This bit of news may come as a surprise to the pregnant woman who joyfully listens to her baby's heartbeat with each office visit but resists a B-scan or real-time examination for fear of fetal injury or chromosomal damage.

What does ultrasound detect during the first trimester of pregnancy?

With the use of ultrasound it is possible to detect the presence of a fetal sac within the uterine cavity as early as the fifth week after conception. The fetal heartbeat can actually be observed with the real-time ultrasound at seven weeks of pregnancy, while limb movements are noticeable at the ninth week. As early as the eleventh week of pregnancy, movements of the fetal chest wall may be observed. The so-called crown-rump measurement is probably the most precise way to determine the fetal age during the first fourteen weeks of pregnancy. In the hands of an expert, this measurement gives the fetal age within one week in 95 percent of patients studied. However, crown-rump measurements are often difficult to obtain after the fourteenth week.

If a woman experiences vaginal bleeding, or if it appears that her uterus is not growing during the first trimester, an ultrasound examination usually reveals the cause of the problem. Defects and breakage of the pregnancy sac and displacement of the sac to an abnormally low position in the uterine cavity often signal that spontaneous abortion is inevitable. Similarly, failure to detect a fetal heartbeat after the seventh week is an ominous sign. When examination by a qualified ultrasonographer demonstrates unequivocally that an early pregnancy is lost, it should be terminated and the woman spared further anguish and delay. It is doubtful that a doctor's old-fashioned prescription of complete bed rest has ever prevented a first trimester abortion from taking place. It is inexcusable for an obstetrician not to order an ultrasound examination for a pregnant woman who is bleeding over a period of several days. When an abortion occurs spontaneously, ultrasound will help to determine if any residual pregnancy tissue is still in the uterine cavity. This knowledge often indicates if dilatation and curettage is necessary for removal of retained fragments of tissue.

As previously mentioned, a positive pregnancy test, vaginal bleeding, and abdominal cramps early in pregnancy may indicate either a threatened abortion or an ectopic pregnancy. When ultrasound examination shows an empty uterine cavity, further diagnostic measures must be taken immediately to be sure that an ectopic pregnancy is not present.

The identification of multiple fetuses may be easily made by using ultrasound during the first trimester. Formerly, this diagnosis was often delayed until confirmed by an x-ray examination during the second or third trimesters. As use of ultrasound has increased, doctors have discovered that significantly greater numbers of women carry twins early in pregnancy. In many cases, however, one of the twins never develops or is expelled from the uterus during an episode of bleeding.

Rare pregnancy tumors, called hydatidiform moles, produce human chorionic gonadotropin, or HCG, and therefore give a positive pregnancy test. The diagnosis of a mole, rather than a healthy pregnancy, can be made accurately with ultrasound during the first trimester.

For the woman with a healthy, intact pregnancy who experiences first-trimester bleeding, ultrasound confirmation that all is well can be tremendously reassuring. Similarly, a woman with presumably retarded fetal growth may in reality be carrying a healthy pregnancy that is not as far advanced as the menstrual history would suggest. Ultrasound is invaluable in clarifying these and other first-trimester questions.

What information can be gained by using ultrasound during the second and third trimesters of pregnancy?

The presence of fetal anomalies such as anencephaly, hydrocephaly, and spina bifida can be confirmed with ultrasonography during the second trimester. In the case of hydrocephaly, an abnormally large fluid-filled head, the diagnosis can usually be made during the second trimester before grossly abnormal changes have occurred. The diagnosis of other fetal anomalies, such as limb defects, kidney and urinary bladder abnormalities, abnormalities of the heart and great vessels, and microcephaly, or abnormally small head, is also possible during the second and third trimesters.

The distance between the outside edges of the two parietal bones of the fetal skull is known as the biparietal diameter. Normal fetuses, regardless of their eventual weight differences at birth, have similar biparietal diameters between the eighteenth and twenty-eighth weeks of pregnancy. Two biparietal measurements taken at four-week intervals at this stage of pregnancy may be plotted on a graph and should accurately determine the duration of pregnancy within five to eight days. This information is especially helpful if confusion exists as to a woman's last menstrual period and her estimated delivery date, if the pregnancy is complicated by medical diseases, such as hypertension and diabetes, if a repeat cesarean section is scheduled, or if early induction of labor is contemplated for obstetrical or medical reasons.

Biparietal diameters taken at the very end of pregnancy are less reliable than those obtained earlier in predicting fetal age. However, if this measurement is 9.3 centimeters or more, one can be reasonably certain that the pregnancy is at least thirty-eight weeks along, the fetus is mature, and probably more than 5½ pounds. Most likely, such infants would not suffer from RDS if delivered at this time, the one notable exception being a pregnancy complicated by diabetes. When biparietal measurements are inconclusive, many doctors are now measuring the length of the fetal femur, or thigh bone. This provides a good indication of the due date if performed during the second and third trimester.

When periodic measurements of the biparietal diameter during the second and third trimesters lag behind those expected for the normal fetus, it is a strong possibility that the infant may be suffering from intrauterine growth retardation, or IUGR. Such infants must be carefully and frequently evaluated. To more adequately assess the presence of IUGR, doctors are using ultrasound to calculate the total intrauterine volume. They correctly reason that amniotic fluid volume, placental weight, and fetal size are all diminished in the presence of IUGR, and their formula for determining the volume of all the uterine contents has more accurately pinpointed those infants that are lagging in growth.

The position of the fetus can easily be determined with an ultrasound examination, and an abnormal situation, such as a breech or transverse position, can be promptly diagnosed without exposure to x-rays. This information is especially important with a twin pregnancy, in which an abnormal position of one of the babies is more likely. The sex of the fetus can occasionally be detected when a thorough ultrasound examination of the genitals is performed during the second and third trimesters. However, one should never rely solely on these results in vital clinical situations, such as the diagnosis of a sex-linked disease. Under such circumstances, amniocentesis must be performed.

Movements of the fetal chest wall have been detected as early as the eleventh week of pregnancy, and actual breathing has been noted from the fourth month until birth. Changes in fetal breathing patterns on ultrasound examination have been associated with fetal distress. The evaluation of fetal body movements at different stages of pregnancy has also been studied with ultrasound. Both the absolute number of movements per day as well as the degree of change in the frequency of fetal movements may serve as indicators of fetal well-being.

It is helpful to follow the progress of a twin pregnancy with serial ultrasound examinations. Occasionally, identical twins share a common blood supply, with one twin receiving too much blood and the other too little. As a result, there is a great difference in the size of the twins. This is called the "twin transfusion syndrome." It places both fetuses in jeopardy; the larger twin from heart failure due to an over-abundance of blood in its circulatory system and the smaller one from IUGR. Repeated ultrasound examinations can follow the progress of such pregnancies and help doctors decide on the ideal time to deliver these distressed infants.

Conjoined or Siamese twins are a very rare phenomenon. They are most commonly attached at the chest, though they may also be joined at the head and back. This extremely rare abnormality may be detected with ultrasound.

The amount of amniotic fluid in comparison to the size of the fetus can be diagnosed with ultrasound examinations during the second and third trimesters. Hydramnios, or polyhydramnios, is the presence of excessive amounts of amniotic fluid. It may be associated with a wide variety of conditions such as diabetes, twins, under-developed fetal lungs, and fetal anomalies, such as anencephaly and hydrocephaly. Excessive amniotic fluid causes overdistention of the uterus, often to the point where it is impossible to palpate the fetal parts. In addition to causing severe discomfort, it may precipitate premature labor and a variety of other obstetrical complications.

Oligohydramnios, or too small a volume of amniotic fluid, can also be diagnosed with ultrasound. It is often associated with pregnancies that extend several weeks' duration beyond the expected delivery date but may also be noted with fetal anomalies involving obstruction of the urinary tract and underdevelopment of the kidneys and lungs. When oligohydramnios occurs early in pregnancy, adhesions of the amniotic sac may cause serious deformities and a peculiar fetal appearance characterized by dry, leathery, and wrinkled skin.

One of the most important uses of ultrasound is the evaluation of vaginal bleeding during the second and third trimesters of pregnancy. Premature separation of the placenta from the uterine wall (abruptio placenta) occurs when a blood clot forms behind the placenta and actually shears it off from its uterine wall attachment. In addition to uterine bleeding, maternal symptoms often include a tense, tender abdomen and shock due to blood loss. This potentially catastrophic situation for both mother and fetus can often be diagnosed in its early stages with ultrasound.

Less serious conditions, such as bleeding from a small sinus at the edge of the placenta, may be readily distinguished from the more severe abruptio. Structural abnormalities of the placenta, as well as variations in its size and its maturity, may also be diagnosed. An ultrasound scan will accurately demonstrate the placental location in relation to the cervix so that preparations for cesarean section may be made when indicated. A doctor should not perform a cesarean section, however, based on a second-trimester report of placenta previa (placenta situated over the cervix). Dr. Donald King, a pioneer in the use of ultrasound, was the first to observe that the placenta may actually migrate from a low to a normal position as pregnancy progresses. As a result, vaginal delivery is often possible even when an earlier ultrasound suggests a dangerously low placental position.

Since all obstetrical problems that may occur at the end of pregnancy can never be foreseen, some obstetricians have recommended that at least two ultrasound examinations be performed on all pregnant women between the eighteenth and twenty-eighth weeks of pregnancy. Though this idea has not gained universal acceptance, I would strongly endorse second-trimester ultrasonography whenever there is a possibility of a complicated pregnancy or if an elective cesarean section is to be scheduled.

While most ultrasonographers rely solely on the biparietal diameter to estimate fetal weight, this method may not always be accurate. Researchers at various medical centers have had a greater degree of success by combining several ultrasonic measurements and subjecting them to complex computer analysis. It is likely that within the next five years ultrasound machines will be manufactured which will give three-dimensional images of the fetus and placenta. These should permit very precise weight measurements of the fetus.

What are the potential dangers of ultrasound?

When ultrasound is used medically, the wave frequency is very high but the power of the sound wave is extremely low. Despite the exposure of thousands of women and their fetuses to both diagnostic ultrasound and ultrasonic monitoring of the fetal heart rate over a period of at least ten years, there is no evidence to show that these procedures are harmful. Follow-up studies of children exposed to ultrasound in utero have detected no physical or developmental difficulties when compared to a control group and more studies are being conducted.

The only reports of ultrasound damage have been to chromosomes in laboratory tissue cultures. Though I heartily endorse the use of ultrasound for a variety of obstetrical indications, until the final verdict on safety is in, I would not use it for such trivial reasons as parental amusement and attempts at determining fetal sex solely out of curiosity.

What is known about in utero fetal body movements, and how can this information be used as a test of fetal well-being?

Though pregnant women noted fetal movement long before the invention of obstetricians, it is only in recent years that we have used this observation as an indicator of fetal well-being. While most women first experience fluttering movements between the seventeenth and twentieth weeks of pregnancy, real-time ultrasound actually enables us to observe motion at the eleventh week. Obviously, the absence of fetal movement after this time would be an ominous sign of fetal death or severe distress.

If real-time ultrasonography is not readily available during the last trimester, fairly good determinations of fetal movement may be obtained by placing two external pressure-measuring devices, called tocodynometers, over the maternal abdomen.

This device is part of the electronic monitoring equipment that is routinely used in most delivery rooms for measuring the strength and frequency of uterine contractions. A woman's perception of fetal movements often is less sensitive than the actual number detected by the ultrasound machine. In a 1978 report, published in the *British Medical Journal*, doctors compared movements felt by forty women between the twenty-fifth and fortieth week of pregnancy with those measured ultrasonically. They found that the ultrasound recorded an average of sixty movements in forty-five minutes while the mothers sensed only thirty-one. Other investigators have shown that the accuracy of maternal perception is closer to 90 percent, rather than this finding of 50 percent.

Doctors at Hadassah-Hebrew University Hospital in Jerusalem have electronically studied fetal body movements during pregnancy and found that the "daily-fetal-movement recording," or DFMR for short, rises from an average of 200 in the twentieth week to approximately 500 in the thirty-second week. From this point, the number of daily movements gradually declines to an average of 282. One important observation was the wide range of normal DFMRs, from a low of 50 to a high of almost 1,000. The actual number, however, is of much less significance than a sudden change from active to inactive, since this may portend fetal distress.

It is unknown why fetal movements decrease in number toward the end of pregnancy. One theory routinely quoted in most obstetrical textbooks is that the relative decrease in the amount of amniotic fluid and uterine volume restricts fetal movement. If this is so, fetal motion following rupture of the amniotic membranes should be markedly decreased. Dr. William F. Rayborn, of Ohio State University has decisively disproved this theory. In his 1980 article published in the *American Journal of Obstetrics and Gynecology*, he noted that fetal movements occurred more than twice as frequently following rupture of the amniotic membranes. In addition, maternal perception of fetal motion following membrane rupture was as accurate as that of women with intact membranes.

Though fetal movement may decline slightly at the end of pregnancy, one must never believe the myth that complete cessation of movement at the end of pregnancy, for several hours at a time, is a healthy sign that labor is imminent. It is more likely to indicate that the baby is in severe distress and that the doctor should be notified immediately. He or she, in turn, would be well advised to instantly perform a nonstress test (NST). If, during the nonstress test, no fetal movements are detectable over a ten-minute period of time, immediate delivery should be strongly considered. Remember, a "quiet" fetus is more likely to be a sick fetus than one with a placid disposition.

A mother's perception of fetal activity is a rapid and reliable method of ascertaining the fetal condition. The results of a 1979 Swedish study in which mothers kept track of their own fetus's activity, indicated that fetuses are most active between 8:00 and 11:00 P.M. and that fetal activity diminished in high-risk pregnancies. Reduced fetal movements were, in most cases, associated with IUGR and often accompanied hypertension, toxemia, premature labor, hemorrhage, and postmaturity.

At the present time, there are no universal criteria for determining the number of perceived or recorded fetal movements indicative of fetal distress. The Hadassah University group regard less than three perceived movements per hour as abnormal. When this occurs, patients are asked to chart for six to twelve hours and those with no fetal movements after twelve hours are delivered immediately. Doctors at the University of Pennsylvania consider a fetus to be distressed when its mother perceives fewer than ten movements in twelve hours, while those at Ohio State University define "alarming fetal movement" as less than two movements recorded over an hourly period for two consecutive days. Also defined as "abnormal" is a drop of 50 percent or more in the number of fetal movements on two consecutive days. For example, a drop from seven movements on one day to three on the next would be a cause for concern. Other researchers have evaluated fetal activity over a period of two successive days, recording movements for a total time period of two hours per day. Less than ten fetal movements during this time period is considered abnormal. They also consider a progressive decline in fetal activity to be equally as important, even if the total number of movements is still within the normal range.

Though the use of fetal movement as a predictor of pregnancy outcome and as a guide to the management of high-risk pregnancies is still in its scientific infancy, the evidence strongly suggests that it will become an important method for studying the distressed fetus.

What can be learned by studying fetal breathing movements during pregnancy and labor?

Though a pregnant woman is unable to perceive fetal breathing movements (FBM), they can be readily detected with the use of a real-time ultrasound machine. Researchers are presently attempting to determine if the assessment of fetal breathing rates can be of value when incorporated with other tests of fetal well-being.

Though we eagerly await the newborn infant's first breath at birth, the patterns of breathing activity and use of the muscles of respiration actually begin in utero. Faint breathing movements may be seen as early as the eleventh week, with a periodic pattern appearing at about twenty-four weeks of pregnancy. The onset of regular breathing activity first becomes obvious at about the thirty-fourth week, and some investigators have claimed that this observation can be used to accurately assess fetal age. It is also interesting to note that there is a circadian variation in breathing movements in the human fetus, with maximum activity observed between the hours of 4:00 and 7:00 A.M. while a woman is asleep. The fetus seems to have spurts of either breathing or moving but rarely does both simultaneously. Data from several studies have demonstrated that healthy human fetuses normally make breathing movements about 30 to 35 percent of the time during the last ten weeks of pregnancy.

Apnea is defined as the absence of breathing movements, and it is not unusual to see this in the fetus for varying periods of time throughout pregnancy. Gasping motions, rather than breathing, are a more ominous indication of fetal distress than no breathing at all.

Dr. Kenneth Boddy and his associates at the University of Edinburgh have made some interesting and important observations of FBMs under a variety of conditions. For example, the second twin has a lower rate of FBMs and a longer period of apnea than the first-born twin, confirming the clinical impression that first-born twins have a higher survival rate. A reduction in breathing movements may also be associated with a mother's disturbed emotional state. Cigarette smoking reduces fetal breathing for as long as ninety minutes, while maternal alcohol consumption exerts a similar effect for up to one hour (see chapter 9). Active labor causes fetal breathing to diminish and occasionally cease even among healthy fetuses. Exercise initially reduces and later increases FBMs. Drugs may affect FBMs as well. When diazepam (Valium) is administered intravenously to women in labor, there is a marked reduction in FBMs during the next two hours, followed by a return to normal. Doctors at the University of Western Ontario in Canada observed FBMs following meals during the last trimester. They reported a significant increase during the two to three hours following meals. This pattern appeared to coincide with levels of maternal plasma glucose.

While some research groups hold the opinion that there is little or no correlation between FBMs and fetal outcome, others enthusiastically endorse the opposite view. Doctors at the University of Southern California Medical Center studied 136 fetuses in an attempt to correlate FBMs with a newborn's Apgar score at one and five minutes of age.

The Apgar score is a number which is arrived at by evaluation of the newborn's color, heart rate, respiratory rate, reflexes, and muscle tone. Each of these five factors is given a value of either 0, 1, or 2, with an Apgar of 10 being awarded to the healthiest babies. Apgar scores serve as an important indication of a newborn's condition immediately after birth. When investigators measured fetal breathing movements with real-time ultrasound during the thirty minutes prior to delivery, they found a strong correlation between the presence of fetal breathing and the one- and five-minute Apgar score.

Much remains to be learned about the significance of fetal breathing movements. At the present time they would appear to have their greatest use when combined with other indicators of fetal well-being.

Fetal Monitoring

What is fetal monitoring and how is it used to assess fetal well-being?

In recent years, electronic monitoring has become the most frequently employed method of assessing fetal health during the last trimester of pregnancy and throughout labor. Though great controversy has arisen between consumer groups and obstetricians over the use and possible abuse of this new electronic gadgetry, most experts agree that it has been invaluable in the management of high-risk pregnancies.

Many obstetricians and delivery-room nurses would like you to believe that the interpretation of fetal monitor recordings is beyond your limited comprehension, but actually it is surprisingly simple to understand.

There are two basic methods of electronic fetal monitoring: external (noninvasive) and internal (invasive). With the external technique, an ultrasonic transducer is strapped to the maternal abdomen over the area where the fetal heartbeat is most easily heard. The heartbeat is recorded on a strip of graph paper which runs through the monitoring machine. A second detector, known as a tocodynometer, is strapped to the upper abdomen at a point over the top of the uterus. This detector records the frequency and strength of the uterine contractions. Alterations in the fetal heartbeat, in relation to the uterine contractions, are of great importance in determining if the fetus is in jeopardy. The external fetal monitor is demonstrated in the figure below.

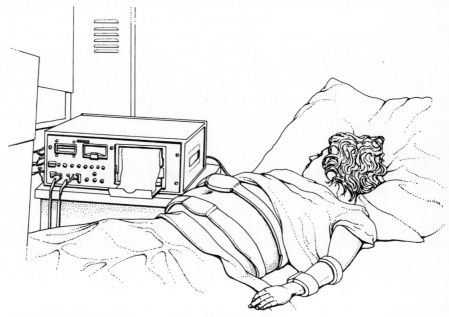

Fetal monitoring (external).

The upper detector strapped to the abdomen senses uterine contractions from the change in the curvature of the abdomen. The lower one detects fetal heart action using the Doppler principle and ultrasound.

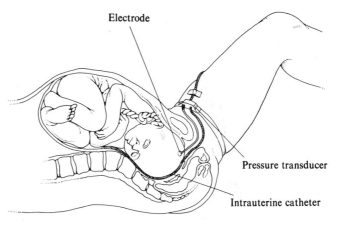

Fetal monitoring (internal).

Internal, or invasive, fetal monitoring involves the placement of monitoring devices into the uterus through the vagina (see illustration at bottom of preceding page). With this method, the fetal heartbeat is recorded from a tiny spiral electrode which is attached to the baby's scalp. A specially designed catheter, inserted through the cervix, monitors the uterine contractions from within.

Internal fetal monitoring usually gives a more accurate recording of fetal heart rate and uterine contractions than the external method. However, it can only be used during active labor when the amniotic membranes are ruptured and the cervix is sufficiently dilated to allow insertion of the spiral electrode and the uterine catheter. During labor, a doctor may elect to use only the external equipment, a combination of one external device and one internal method, or two internal monitors. The choice would depend on a variety of factors, such as the degree of cervical dilatation, the position of the baby, the location of the placenta, the doctor's familiarity and skill with the more difficult internal methods, the degree of potential distress, and the wishes of the woman being monitored.

How is external monitoring used to evaluate fetal status before labor begins?

The normal fetal heart rate usually ranges between 120 and 160 beats per minute, though a rate which is 20 beats above or below this standard does not necessarily mean fetal distress. Under normal conditions, the fetal heart rate fluctuates from one moment to the next. This fluctuation, called beat-to-beat variability, is a sign of a healthy infant who has a reactive and functioning nervous system. The fetal heartbeat that resembles a straight line on the electronic monitor is an ominous sign of diminished oxygen or central nervous system depression.

The nonstress test (NST), or fetal heart acceleration determination (FAD), is the most commonly used method of assessing the condition of the fetus during the last trimester. It is extremely simple to perform and to interpret. An ultrasonic transducer is placed over the maternal abdomen at the point where the fetal heartbeat is most easily detected. The heartbeat is recorded on the fetal monitor's paper strip. Each time the pregnant woman detects fetal movement, she immediately presses a button which she holds in her hand. This is recorded as an arrow on the same paper strip. The test is considered to be normal or reactive when two or more fetal movements over a period of 20 minutes are immediately followed by an increase of the fetal heartbeat by at least fifteen beats per minute, for a minimum of at least fifteen seconds. A reactive NST is shown in figure 10–1.

A reactive nonstress test implies that a fetus possesses reactive nervous and cardiovascular systems. Though there have been notable exceptions to this rule, a reactive test usually indicates that the fetus is healthy enough to survive for at least one more week in the uterus, and the obstetrician need not plan an immediate delivery. This assumption is incorrect—meaning that the fetus dies within a week of a negative NST—in less than 1 percent of all women tested. In managing a high-risk pregnancy, nonstress testing often begins as early as two months before the expected

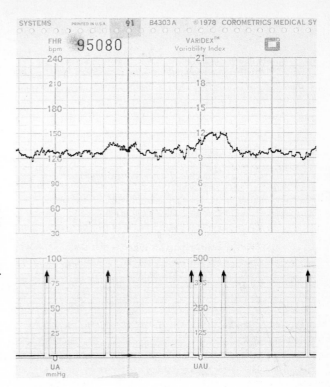

Fig. 10–1

***Example of a reactive nonstress
test (NST).***

Mother's perception of fetal
movement (arrow) is followed by
an immediate acceleration of the
fetal heart rate by at least 15
beats per minute for a minimum
of at least 15 seconds. This
suggests that the baby is healthy.

delivery date and continues each week until the baby is delivered. It is invaluable for
assessing most complicated pregnancies.

Occasionally, the nonstress test is unsatisfactory because the fetus does not
move during the time that the test is being performed. This situation can be remedied by gently shaking the mother's abdomen, thereby stimulating the fetus. Failure
of the fetus to move over a prolonged period of time, however, may indicate that a
problem exists.

When there is a lack of heart-rate acceleration in response to a perceived fetal
movement, it is called a nonreactive nonstress test. This is a potentially ominous sign
which requires another test, known as a contraction stress test, or CST. Of all NSTs
performed, less than 10 percent will be nonreactive and necessitate further testing. A
nonreactive stress test is illustrated in figure 10–2 on the following page.

What is a contraction stress test, or CST, and when is it used?

Though it is usually not performed as the initial screening test for evaluating fetal
well-being, the contraction stress test (CST), or oxytocin challenge test (OCT), is
invaluable in studying the fetus suspected of being in jeopardy. This is especially
true when the nonstress test is either nonreactive or inadequate for proper interpretation.

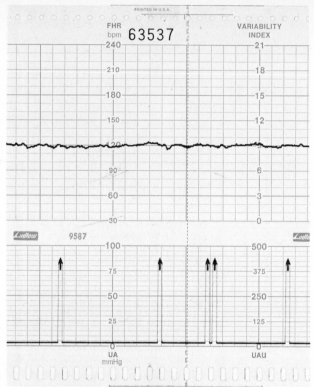

Fig. 10–2

Example of a nonreactive nonstress test (NST).

Mother's perception of fetal movement (arrow) is not followed by an acceleration of the fetal heart rate. This suggests that the baby may be experiencing distress.

To perform this test, the fetal heartbeat is recorded with an external monitoring device in a manner identical to that used for the NST. However, maternal perception of fetal movement is not recorded. Instead, uterine activity and contractions are monitored by placing a tocodynometer, secured by a belt, around the upper abdomen. The CST is only meaningful if three uterine contractions take place over a period of ten minutes and each contraction lasts approximately forty seconds. Some women have these contractions spontaneously during the third trimester without being in labor, but most require a dilute solution of intravenous oxytocin (trade name Pitocin) to stimulate the required number of contractions. You need not fear that this procedure will inadvertently induce labor prematurely, because only minimal amounts of oxytocin are used at a controlled rate of flow.

Under normal conditions, the fetal heart rate does not decrease following a uterine contraction. However, in the presence of a poorly functioning placenta and a severely distressed infant, the contractions of the uterus cause a decrease in oxygen flow to the baby. This in turn results in a drop in the fetal heart rate beginning as the contraction intensity peaks. The lowest level of the heart rate is usually recorded approximately thirty seconds after the contraction is most intense. When the fetal heart rate shows this characteristic decline in response to a uterine contraction, it is called a positive CST. Doctors have given this pattern of fetal heart change a variety of names, including late decelerations, late dips, and Type II dips. Regardless of the name, this pattern indicates that fetal distress may be present, and immediate delivery should be considered if the fetus is mature. This is especially true when a positive contraction stress test is preceded by a nonreactive NST.

A negative CST means that the fetal heart rate does not decelerate following the peak of the contraction. This is a reassuring indication that there is no fetal distress. A negative contraction stress test implies that a woman possesses sufficient placental function to maintain the fetus safely in utero for at least one more week. This is true even in the presence of a nonreactive nonstress test. The test must be repeated at weekly intervals as long as it remains negative. (For examples of negative and positive CSTs see figures 10–3 and 10–4).

The NST and CST complement each other as predictors of fetal well-being. When both the CST and the NST are in agreement that the fetus is distressed, there is a very high probability that this is so. In a 1981 study from the University of Chicago, doctors found that the joint occurrence of a nonreactive and a positive NST correctly predicted a distressed fetus 92 percent of the time. However, either test used without the other is associated with an unacceptably high incidence of tests which falsely show a healthy fetus to be distressed.

While a reactive NST in a high-risk pregnancy is very reassuring that the fetus will survive for at least one more week, the one disturbing exception to this rule appears to be the postterm pregnancy. Two different studies in 1981 have demon-

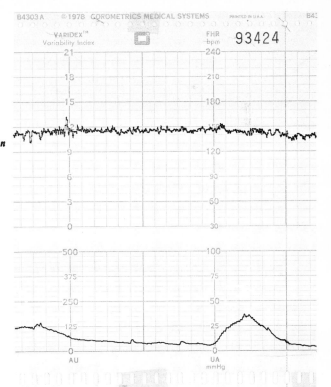

Fig. 10–3

Example of a negative contraction stress test (CST).

Uterine contraction (C) is not followed by a drop in the fetal heart rate. This indicates that there is probably good placental function and the baby is not in distress.

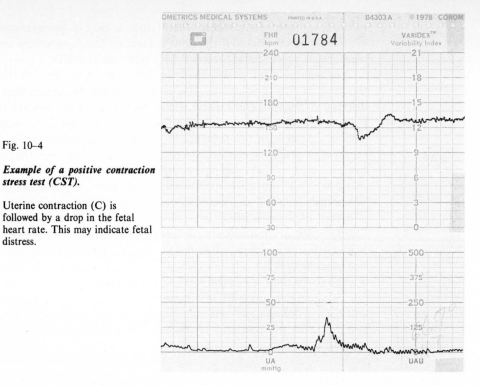

Fig. 10–4

Example of a positive contraction stress test (CST).

Uterine contraction (C) is followed by a drop in the fetal heart rate. This may indicate fetal distress.

strated that the CST may be the more appropriate initial test for detecting a postmature infant in distress.

To reproduce the results of a CST without the inconvenience of using intravenous pitocin, doctors have recently devised the nipple self-stimulation test. It has long been known that nipple stimulation results in release of oxytocin from the pituitary gland and subsequent uterine contractions (see chapter 4). By firmly massaging her nipples, the pregnant woman will note contractions almost immediately. This method has the advantage of taking less time than intravenous pitocin, is less expensive, and is more acceptable to most women. The contraindications to the nipple self-stimulation test are identical to those for the CST (see next question).

Are there any women who should not undergo a contraction stress test?

If a woman has a history of premature labor, or if examination reveals that she may start labor several weeks before her estimated delivery date, the use of oxytocin is not recommended because it may be just enough of a stimulus to trigger labor in her sensitive uterus. This advice also applies to women with premature rupture of the amniotic membranes, because contractions may induce premature labor or disperse bacteria which are capable of causing a uterine infection. In the presence of placenta previa, abruptio placenta, and undiagnosed uterine bleeding CST should not be performed.

Most cesarean sections are performed through an incision in the lower segment of the uterus. However, on rare occasions it is necessary to do the surgery through the muscles in the upper part of the uterus. This is called a classical cesarean section, and its scar is far more likely to weaken and rupture if the uterus is stimulated to contract. For this reason, if a previous classical cesarean section has been performed a CST is not recommended.

Finally, the presence of multiple fetuses and hydramnios may overly distend the uterus and make oxytocin stimulation more hazardous. If the CST is performed under these circumstances it must be done with great care, using the lowest possible dose of intravenous oxytocin.

What is the significance of fetal heart rate changes which occur during labor?

When labor contractions produce late fetal heart rate decelerations, or Type II dips, it is an indication that the baby may be in jeopardy. However, the heart rate can often be converted to normal by the pregnant woman's taking simple measures such as lying on her left side and breathing oxygen through a face mask or nasal catheter. If labor is being induced or stimulated, stopping the oxytocin often improves the heart rate within seconds. If all of these measures fail, prompt vaginal or abdominal delivery is often indicated.

Doctors have described two other classic fetal heart rate patterns which may appear frightening to the novice but are usually harmless. One is known as an early fetal heart rate deceleration, or Type I dip. This pattern can easily be identified. It begins with the onset of the contraction and returns to normal with or before the end of the contraction. Type I dips are believed to be caused by mild compression of the baby's head with each contraction, and they become more pronounced as labor progresses. Another type of deceleration is referred to as nonuniform, or variable. It derives its name from the fact that it occurs at no specific time in relation to the contractions and it differs from those which precede and follow. Most variable decelerations are caused by mild compression of the umbilical cord, which may occur if the cord is draped around the baby's neck or body or is knotted. While most variable decelerations are not a cause for concern, others which reach a level of sixty beats per minute or last at least sixty seconds at a time may indicate fetal distress. Variable decelerations can often be corrected by changing body position since this relieves compression of the umbilical cord. If, despite this measure, a woman still experiences variable decelerations, the doctor may want to test the pH of the fetal scalp blood. This is the only way to determine with certainty if variable decelerations are innocuous or harmful (see page 336).

It is not uncommon for couples to express fear at the slightest variation of the heart rate pattern on the fetal monitor. Be assured that fluctuations in the heart rate are a normal and healthy sign. In contrast, a fetal heart rate pattern that looks like a straight line often means that an infant is compromised. This type of pattern is more apt to be seen among premature infants and following administration of drugs during labor such as narcotics, tranquilizers, barbiturates, and atropine.

A fetal tachycardia, meaning a heart rate greater than the normal limit of 160 beats per minute may be an early indication of fetal distress caused by oxygen deprivation. A moderate tachycardia defined as a rate of 160 to 180 beats per minute, is not nearly as ominous as rates above 180 beats per minute. Maternal fever is probably one of the more common causes of a rapid fetal heart rate, but other conditions and certain drugs and medications may also produce this effect.

An abnormally slow fetal heart rate, or bradycardia, may be associated with fetal distress. The lower limit of the normal fetal heart rate is 120 beats per minute, but a range between 100 and 119 beats during labor is usually not a cause for concern.

The most recently described fetal heart rate abnormality is known as the sinusoidal heart rate pattern. This has a characteristic wave-like appearance occurring at a frequency of three to five oscillations per minute. Many authorities consider the sinusoidal pattern to be a certain sign of fetal distress, though not all obstetricians share this pessimistic view.

Fetal Scalp Blood Test

How is fetal scalp blood obtained and what is the significance of an abnormal test?

The pH measurement is a laboratory test which determines the relative acidity of the blood in the capillaries of the fetal scalp. The blood specimen obtained from the scalp usually reflects the degree of acidity present in the rest of the fetal bloodstream, and an abnormally low pH level, or acidosis, is often associated with a severe lack of oxygen and fetal distress.

The technique of obtaining a fetal scalp blood specimen is painless, safe, and easy to perform. An endoscope, or funnel-shaped viewing device with a light attached to its end is inserted through the cervix and placed firmly against the fetal scalp. For this to occur, your cervix must be at least two centimeters dilated and the amniotic membranes ruptured. After the scalp is prepared so as to minimize bleeding, one or two superficial scalp incisions are made with a small knife blade placed within the endoscope. The blood which forms is collected in a special tube and immediately analyzed for its pH. Pressure applied to the scalp with a cotton swab will stop the blood flow within seconds. The procedure can be repeated periodically throughout labor.

The major advantage of fetal scalp blood sampling is that it will often clarify the significance of a confusing or abnormal heart rate pattern noted on the electronic monitor. In one study, only 5 percent of infants with a normal scalp pH required a cesarean section for fetal distress. There is no doubt that judicious use of this technique has reduced the incidence of unnecessary cesareans for what falsely appears to be fetal distress on the electronic monitor.

Sound Stimulation

How can sound stimulation be used as a test of fetal well-being?

Doctors from Queen Charlotte's Maternity Hospital in London have recently studied the fetal heart rate response to sound stimulation. They applied ten-second bursts of sound intermittently over the maternal abdomen, in the region of the fetal head, for periods ranging from five to twenty minutes. Following sound stimulation, the healthy fetus exhibited a heartbeat acceleration of at least fifteen beats per minute which was maintained for at least two minutes. This response was significantly impaired in cases of distressed fetuses and those subsequently born with low birth weights. They tested 116 women, first with NST and then with sound stimulation and concluded that the latter was a far better predictor of fetal health. Though these test results appear encouraging, further research will be necessary to confirm the accuracy of the sound stimulation test. The safety to the fetus must also be evaluated before this test can be fully endorsed (see question on noise pollution, page 266).

Prevention of Premature Labor

What are some of the newer methods of preventing premature labor?

Premature labor is unquestionably the main problem confronting the modern obstetrician. Although less than 10 percent of infants are premature, they account for 80 percent of all reported deaths of newborns and a significant number of neurologically handicapped infants. Most of the deaths attributed to prematurity are the result of respiratory distress syndrome (RDS) caused by immaturity of the fetal lungs. In an attempt to rapidly mature the lungs prior to delivery, doctors have administered cortisone medications, such as betamethasone, dexamethasone, and hydrocortisone, to susceptible pregnant women. This controversial treatment, however, does not inhibit contractions or prevent premature labor and delivery.

Though a wide variety of medications have been endorsed as labor-inhibiting drugs, most have failed miserably. Scientists have theorized that labor begins when maternal progesterone levels fall and that large amounts of progesterone will block the onset of contractions. In actual practice, however, the use of progesterone and other chemically similar hormonal preparations for this purpose has been disappointing. At the present time, I doubt that many doctors are using this hormonal method of treatment.

Until recently, a 10 percent solution of intravenous alcohol was the most widely used method of preventing premature births in the United States. Alcohol is believed to inhibit labor by blocking the release of oxytocin, the pituitary gland hormone that stimulates the muscles of the uterus. Unfortunately, the dose needed to stop uterine contractions is quite high and may cause complications for the mother, such as nausea, vomiting, restlessness, intoxication, stupor, and even death. Danger to the fetus, especially the fetal alcohol syndrome, makes the use of alcohol unacceptable.

Magnesium sulfate is an excellent drug for treating preeclampsia and toxemia. In recent years it has been used with some success in stopping premature contractions by relaxing the muscles of the uterine wall. Though relatively free of annoying side effects for the mother, it is known to cause respiratory depression and poor muscle tone in the newborn.

Prostaglandins, found in many body tissues, including the lining of the uterus and the fetal membranes, cause severe uterine contractions and are often used for inducing second-trimester abortions. A sudden increase in prostaglandin levels is believed by scientists to be most responsible for initiating and maintaining uterine contractions during labor. Drugs which inhibit prostaglandin release are capable of preventing premature labor. Aspirin, for example, is a prostaglandin inhibitor. It can prolong the onset of labor if taken in relatively high doses during the last weeks of pregnancy, but other factors preclude its use in this fashion. Indomethacin (trade name Indocin) has been used in the past to inhibit labor. Its main drawback, however, is its ability to increase fetal pulmonary artery pressure, which in turn may lead to a very serious and permanent condition known as pulmonary hypertension. Animal experimentation and human experience suggest that indomethacin may interfere with the normal uterine and placental circulation, causing a decrease in the volume of amniotic fluid, or oligohydramnios, meconium staining of the amniotic fluid suggestive of fetal distress, and impaired fetal kidney function.

The most promising group of drugs for inhibiting premature labor are known as the beta-sympathomimetics. These agents stop contractions and relax the uterus by stimulating special receptors, known as beta receptors, located in the muscle wall. Members of this group include isoxsuprine (trade name Vasodilan), fenoterol, salbutamol, ritodrine (trade name Yutopar), terbutaline (trade name Brethine), orciprenaline (trade name Alupent), and hexoprenaline. Terbutaline, orciprenaline, and hexoprenaline are also used in the treatment of asthma, while isoxsuprine is an important medication in the management of vascular diseases. Of these preparations, only ritodrine is approved by the FDA as therapy for the inhibition of premature labor. However, terbutaline, fenoterol, and salbutamol are used extensively for this purpose in many other countries throughout the world.

What are the side effects and risks of using beta-sympathomimetics to treat premature labor?

As these drugs have become more popular in the treatment of premature labor, the number of side effects and complications associated with their use has also increased. These include palpitations, nervousness, maternal and fetal tachycardia (rapid heartbeat), and alterations in the maternal blood pressure which at times may affect the fetus. Sudden pulmonary edema, the accumulation of fluid in the lungs, has been observed among a small number of women treated with terbutaline and other beta-sympathomimetics combined with cortisone preparations which were administered at the same time for the purpose of hastening fetal lung maturation. Though women with mild pulmonary edema usually respond to diuretic and oxygen therapy, more advanced cases may result in severe respiratory problems, heart failure, and even maternal death. Whenever cortisone and beta-sympathomimetics are used together, women and their doctors should be alert to early symptoms of pulmonary edema, such as cough and shortness of breath, so that treatment can be started immediately.

In a 1979 report from Duke University published in the *Journal of Pediatrics,* doctors noted a higher incidence of respiratory distress syndrome, a serious intestinal infection common to premature infants (necrotizing enterocolitis), abnormally low calcium levels in the blood (hypocalcemia), abnormally low blood sugar levels (hypoglycemia), low blood pressure, and death among newborns whose mothers were given isoxsuprine to prevent premature delivery. If the drug was given seventy-two hours or more before delivery, the risk of complications was diminished. In another 1979 study from Harvard Medical School, doctors noted a high incidence of hypoglycemia following maternal treatment with fenoterol and terbutaline.

Ritodrine was approved for general use by the FDA in 1979 because of its ability to inhibit uterine contractions without causing the severe maternal side effects observed with other beta-sympathomimetics. The relative safety of ritodrine has been established from worldwide clinical experience involving over 500,000 women. Shortly after it is administered intravenously, practically all women experience an increase in their heart rate of approximately twenty to forty beats per minute. The fetal heart rate also increases by less than ten beats per minute. These changes are easily tolerated by most women and are of no cause for concern. A person's blood pressure is composed of two numbers: a systolic or higher reading and a diastolic or lower number. Ritodrine will usually raise the systolic blood pressure and lower the diastolic pressure. For example, if a woman's normal blood pressure is 110/70, ritodrine may convert it to 120/60. This, too, is of no consequence for the vast majority of women.

Approximately 10 to 15 percent of women receiving intravenous ritodrine experience either tremors, nausea, vomiting, headache, or flushing of the face and body. Palpitations are experienced by 33 percent, while 5 to 10 percent note either nervousness or restlessness. Chest pain and abnormal heart rhythms have been observed in 1 to 3 percent of ritodrine-treated women, while pulmonary edema has been reported in only 4 of the more than 500,000 women evaluated. The incidence and severity of all of these complications is directly related to the dose of ritodrine which is administered. Diabetic women should be aware of the fact that ritodrine can elevate the blood sugar.

Unlike the other beta-sympathomimetics, infants born to ritodrine-treated mothers have demonstrated no medical problems during the neonatal period. In addition, no growth or developmental defects have been observed when these infants were evaluated at two years of age.

Oral ritodrine causes a slight increase in the maternal heart rate but has little effect on the systolic and diastolic blood pressure or the fetal heart rate.

In 10 to 15 percent of women, oral ritodrine produces palpitations or tremors. Nausea, jitteriness, and a mild rash have been reported. An abnormal cardiac rhythm occurs in only 1 percent of women given oral ritodrine.

When should ritodrine be used to inhibit premature labor, and when not?

Ritodrine is not harmless, and its use requires a careful clinical decision by a woman and her doctor as to whether the gain for the mother and child is worth the risk. Inhibition of labor is clearly indicated when the fetus is estimated to weigh less than 5½ pounds, the pregnancy is between twenty and thirty-six weeks in length, the contractions are coming at frequent intervals, the cervix is 4 centimeters or less dilated, the cervix is thinning out or effacing, and the amniotic membranes are not ruptured. Under these ideal conditions, labor can be successfully delayed for at least ten days in 80 percent of all women treated. On the average, ritodrine prolongs the length of pregnancy by sixteen days. This may not sound like very much, but in the case of a premature baby, every day is vital.

Though use of ritodrine may be attempted when labor is significantly advanced beyond 4 centimeters of cervical dilatation, the possibility of successfully prolonging the pregnancy is less than 10 percent. It is debatable whether or not ritodrine should be given if the amniotic membranes are ruptured. If a woman and her doctor elect to pursue this course, they should be aware of the increased risk of fetal and uterine infection when labor is inhibited for periods of time greater than twenty-four hours. Ritodrine should absolutely not be used when there is intrauterine or fetal infection, since these conditions can only be successfully treated by accomplishing an immediate delivery. Nor should it be used when there is active vaginal bleeding or evidence of a major malformation of the fetus, making it unlikely that the fetus will survive. Ritodrine is not approved for use before the twentieth week of pregnancy because its effects on early fetal development are not known. Its use in the prevention of early spontaneous abortion may also have the undesirable effect of prolonging chromosomally abnormal pregnancies.

Certain diseases preclude ritodrine therapy. It should never be given to women with heart disease, hypertension, severe preeclampsia, or hyperthyroidism because of its effects on the blood pressure and pulse. Though well-controlled diabetics may be given ritodrine, its use must be carefully maintained because it can raise the blood sugar and increase a woman's insulin requirements.

How is ritodrine administered to prevent premature labor?

Intravenous ritodrine may be started as soon as the diagnosis of premature labor is made. The maximum dose is 350 micrograms, but if side effects are severe, the dosage is reduced to a tolerable level. A woman's vital signs are checked frequently, and the external fetal monitor is used to observe the changes in contraction strength and frequency, as well as the fetal heart rate. To decrease the risk of a maternal drop in blood pressure and fetal distress, a woman should lie on her left side throughout the entire time that the ritodrine is running. For maximum success in stopping labor, the intravenous is continued for twelve to twenty-four hours after uterine contractions have ceased. Ritodrine in the form of a 10-milligram pill is started thirty minutes before the intravenous is stopped and continued until the risk of a premature birth is no longer present. If contractions do not recur, a woman can usually resume normal activity after two days. Occasionally, however, labor recurs and the intravenous therapy is required again.

Is there any way to speed up fetal lung maturation if there is a threat of premature labor and RDS in the newborn?

Since the principal defect in infants who develop RDS (respiratory distress syndrome) is the limited amount of surfactant coating their lung tubules, a great deal of research has focused on finding a drug that will hasten lung maturation by increasing surfactant concentrations. The principal phospholipid component of surfactant is lecithin; when lecithin is abundant, RDS will not occur (see question on amniocentesis for fetal maturity). To date, maternal intramuscular administration of corticosteroids (cortisone-like drugs) have shown the greatest promise in raising fetal surfactant levels. Betamethasone, dexamethasone, hydrocortisone, and methylprednisolone have all been used with varying degrees of success. Usually two injections are given twenty-four hours apart, and babies born less than twenty-four hours after the initial dose are unlikely to be helped. It is interesting to note that infants born more than seven days after the last corticosteroid injection may again be at risk of developing RDS. Therefore, proponents of this form of therapy recommend reinjection if the risk of prematurity still persists.

Researchers have found that corticosteroid therapy offers the greatest advantage between the thirtieth and thirty-fourth week of pregnancy. In one study of 1,431 women, 607 were treated with a corticosteroid prior to their thirty-sixth week. Of this group, 6.5 percent of the babies died. In an untreated group of 824 patients, the infant death rate was 22 percent. The total incidence of RDS was found to be 11 percent in the treated group, compared with 30 percent among those who did not receive corticosteroids.

While several other investigative groups have confirmed the above findings, many others remain skeptical and have not endorsed this form of therapy. One totally contradictory report from Columbia-Presbyterian Medical Center, published in 1979, studied eighty-four premature infants whose mothers received betamethasone. When compared with a control group of eighty-four infants, not similarly treated, there was no difference in the incidence of RDS and infant survival.

The long-term effects of corticosteroids on the infants exposed in utero have not been fully established. While preliminary evidence in human beings is encouraging, the results of some animal experiments have been somewhat pessimistic. In a 1979 report, monkeys exposed to betamethasone had smaller head circumferences than those not exposed. Rats similarly treated were noted to have lower body weights and smaller brains, hearts, livers, kidneys, and adrenal glands.

Some doctors oppose the use of betamethasone and other cortisone preparations, such as dexamethasone and hydrocortisone, because of their potential maternal hazards. For example, these agents alter the metabolism of glucose, and a diabetic woman treated with corticosteroids will often require greater daily amounts of insulin. Corticosteroids may also elevate a person's blood pressure, and this may be especially hazardous in hypertensives and those with preeclampsia. Infection rates are increased and wound healing is impaired among individuals receiving these drugs. This is an important consideration in the event that a cesarean section is necessary. Corticosteroids may make the detection of maternal infection somewhat more difficult because they elevate the white blood cell count. Doctors often use this important indicator to determine if an infection is present, and corticosteroid use will obscure the value of the test. Women with gastric (stomach) and duodenal ulcers may also fare poorly with this form of therapy.

At the same time that doctors are using corticosteroids to mature the lungs of a premature infant, they commonly give drugs that prevent the uterus from contracting prematurely. These so-called beta-mimetics have gained popularity in the prevention of premature labor (see page 338). However, when used in combination with corticosteroids, these drugs can cause maternal pulmonary edema, or the accumulation of fluid in the lungs. This very serious condition requires immediate treatment.

Based on all of the above evidence, one would have to agree that this method of treating prematurity is certainly not innocuous. Corticosteroids may cause significant maternal side effects, and their ultimate long-term fetal effects still remain unknown. For this reason, a significant number of medical centers have decided not to use corticosteroids in this manner. Certainly, if they are used, it must be for very specific situations in which the infant is extremely premature and at significant risk of developing severe respiratory distress following birth. An L/S ratio of the amniotic fluid should be obtained, if at all possible, prior to treatment, since it would be foolhardy to treat a mother whose baby has full lung maturity. In addition, corticosteroids are best used in medical centers equipped to handle these delicate infants after birth.

Rh Babies

How are Rh babies diagnosed and treated?

One of the first fetal problems to be treated successfully in utero was Rh-incompatibility disease. An Rh-negative mother may form antibodies against the red blood cells of her Rh-positive fetus. These antibodies cross the placenta and enter the fetal circulation, where they destroy the red blood cells, causing severe fetal anemia and heart failure and often result in death. For maternal Rh antibodies to form, Rh-positive red blood cells must first enter the maternal bloodstream. This is most likely to happen during the last trimester and at delivery of a first pregnancy, but it may also occur to a lesser degree following a spontaneous or induced first- or second-trimester abortion and at the time of an ectopic pregnancy. When blood tests confirm that a pregnant woman has Rh antibodies, bilirubin levels in the amniotic fluid are measured to determine how seriously the fetus is affected. High concentrations of bilirubin means that many red blood cells are being destroyed. If the fetus is found to be severely affected, certain to die, but too immature for immediate delivery, it is possible to transfuse small amounts of fresh adult Rh-negative red blood cells directly into its abdominal cavity. From there, the blood cells are absorbed into the fetal bloodstream, replacing those that were destroyed by maternal antibodies. This procedure must be repeated at ten-day-to-two-week intervals until the fetus is sufficiently mature to survive outside the uterus.

It is an amazing accomplishment to be able to accurately place a needle into a baby's abdomen so that blood can be transfused. Ultrasound is used to guide the needle, replacing the older procedure which required a significant number of x-rays. Recently, doctors at King's College Hospital in London were able to give blood transfusions directly into the fetal blood vessels within the umbilical cord by viewing the cord through a fetoscope, but this technique is still considered experimental.

What is RhoGam?

Fortunately, Rh incompatibility is infrequently seen today because of the introduction of Rh-immune globulin in 1969. More commonly known by its trade name

RhoGam, this medication consists of Rh antibodies. When given intramuscularly to an Rh-negative woman within seventy-two hours after birth or after an abortion, it destroys the Rh-positive fetal cells that may have passed into her bloodstream. RhoGam prevents the Rh-negative woman from producing her own antibodies to the Rh-positive cells. Once formed, these natural antibodies persist throughout a person's life and present an extreme hazard to Rh-positive offspring of all subsequent pregnancies. If a woman becomes sensitized, meaning that she has already formed her own Rh antibodies, the injection of RhoGam becomes valueless. For this reason, RhoGam injections must be given to all nonsensitized Rh-negative women following birth of each Rh-positive infant. Since the blood type of an early abortus is not determined, RhoGam must be given to all Rh-negative women at the time of a spontaneous or induced abortion or an ectopic pregnancy. The one exception to this rule is when the father is known to be Rh-negative, since two Rh-negative parents cannot conceive an Rh-positive infant.

The number of fetal red blood cells which enter the maternal circulation are significantly less following an abortion than a full-term delivery, so less RhoGam is needed. For this reason, a smaller amount of immune globulin, known by the trade name MICRhoGAM, may be given following an ectopic pregnancy or a spontaneous or induced abortion of twelve weeks or less.

The volume of fetal blood which passes into the maternal circulation during childbirth varies from one individual to another and from one pregnancy to the next. Greater amounts are transfused following a cesarean section or maternal bleeding complications such as placenta previa and abruptio placenta. One ampule of Rho-Gam protects against a 15-milliliter feto-maternal bleed. If more than this amount enters the maternal circulation, the one ampule of RhoGam will be inadequate for destroying all the fetal red blood cells, and the Rh-negative woman may form antibodies even though she received an ampule of RhoGam. This occurs in 2 percent of Rh-negative women but can be prevented by a simple blood test to determine if more RhoGam is needed.

Researchers in other countries have administered prophylactic RhoGam injections to all Rh-negative women between the twenty-eighth and thirty-second weeks of pregnancy and again during the postpartum period to reduce the 2 percent risk of maternal antibody formation to zero. Though no ill effects have been noted among infants delivered of mothers who received RhoGam in this manner, it is not the usual routine practiced in the United States.

Feto-maternal bleeding is a very real threat following amniocentesis. Therefore, RhoGam should be administered to all Rh-negative women at the time that the procedure is performed during the second or third trimester.

Fetal Therapy

Besides the use of intrauterine blood transfusions, what other forms of fetal therapy have been devised?

Maternal treatment with medications, such as betamethasone, dexamethasone, and hydrocortisone, has been used to stimulate surfactant production in the lungs of premature infants. A more radical procedure for achieving this goal has been to inject thyroxine, the thyroid hormone, directly into the amniotic sac.

In recent years, a host of ingenious methods of fetal therapy have been devised. For example, doctors have diagnosed abnormally fast fetal heart rates and have then successfully controlled them by administering digitalis to the mother injecting it directly into the fetus through the maternal abdominal wall. At Yale University School of Medicine, doctors have removed dangerously large amounts of fluid accumulations from the chest and abdomen of the fetus. Equally as miraculous was the report from the University of Colorado in which excess fluid was drained from the head into the amniotic fluid of a fetus with hydrocephalus with a tube, or shunt, placed into its head under ultrasonic visualization. Doctors at Harvard Medical School have used a similar technique to save a fetus from probable death from hydrocephaly. Instead of a shunt, they inserted a needle periodically into the fetal head to withdraw excess fluid.

Specialists at several medical centers have successfully drained urine from the fetal bladder in cases of congenital blockage of the urethra, or tube which carries urine from the bladder.

Regulating the diet of the mother can save her baby from a metabolic defect. This was proven in a recent case in which doctors prevented the death of a baby with a rare genetic defect in its ability to metabolize vitamin B12. The child's older sister had died of this disease, called methylmalonic acidemia (MMA), shortly after birth. When the mother became pregnant again, the condition was diagnosed early in the prenatal course and she was treated with injections of vitamin B12, almost 5,000 times the normal adult dose, during the last trimester. The idea was to force the vitamin across the placenta to stimulate the unborn baby's tissues, thus preventing the possible prenatal damage. As a result, a healthy female was born. She has maintained her good health on a controlled B12-supplemented diet. Biotin is another B vitamin that doctors at the University of California have given in high doses to a woman with a rare inherited enzyme disorder known as carboxylase deficiency. As a result, she gave birth to a healthy newborn.

Phenylketonuria is an autosomal recessive disease (see page 307) in which an afflicted newborn is unable to metabolize the amino acid phenylalanine. If phenylketonuria is not detected at birth and remedied with a low phenylalanine diet throughout childhood, severe mental retardation will occur because of toxic accumulations of the amino acid in the baby's body. Mass screening for the early detection of phenylketonuria among newborns was initiated in the 1960s, and as a result many women with the disease have led normal and healthy lives. As adults, these women are able to eat regular diets without ill effects. However, if they become pregnant, the phenylalanine in their foods may be readily transferred across the placenta to the fetus and cause mental retardation and microcephaly prior to birth. To prevent this, a woman with phenylketonuria must return to her phenylalanine-free diet prior to conception and throughout her pregnancy.

As previously mentioned (see page 233), recent studies have indicated that maternal use of folic acid and other vitamin supplements immediately before and throughout pregnancy may significantly reduce the number of babies born with neural tube defects.

Though the study of fetal therapeutics is new, more exciting discoveries are evolving each day. It is hoped that in the future a wide variety of fetal metabolic and enzymatic deficiencies may be treated in utero by replacing the deficient substance or by removing the offending agent. We are, however, light-years away from achieving this goal.

What are some of the advances made in the diagnosis and treatment of sickle-cell disease during pregnancy?

Sickle-cell disease is a debilitating and often fatal disorder which afflicts approximately 1 out of every 400 blacks. In this disease the hemoglobin in the red blood cells is abnormal, making the red cells more fragile than unaffected normal cells. Some of the red blood cells actually have a sickle shape, and the number with this configuration increases as the condition worsens. As many as 10 percent of healthy blacks are carriers of the sickle-cell trait. When two carriers mate, an average of one out of four of their children will have the full-blown disease, since it is inherited as an autosomal recessive condition (see autosomal recessive diseases pages 307–311). Until recently, it was impossible to diagnose sickle-cell disease in the fetus, and a black couple sharing the trait could only hope that their children would not be among the unfortunate 25 percent with the disease.

While many infants with sickle-cell disease die before reaching adulthood, the females who do survive to childbearing age often encounter severe difficulties if they become pregnant. The prognosis for pregnant women with sickle-cell disease, is dismal. There is a higher incidence of sickle-cell crisis and other life-threatening maternal complications, and a greater incidence of spontaneous abortion, prematurity, and stillbirth. So severe are the complications which may be experienced by the pregnant woman with sickle-cell disease that many obstetricians have advised prophylactic sterilization for affected individuals.

Recently, great strides have been made in the management of pregnancies complicated by this condition. The birth of an affected infant is no longer a matter of chance. Thanks to the development of the fetoscope, a sample of pure fetal blood can usually be obtained from a blood vessel on the fetal side of the placenta, ideally between the eighteenth and twentieth week of pregnancy. The blood can then be analyzed for the presence of abnormal sickle-cell hemoglobin. If it is confirmed that the fetus is destined to have sickle-cell disease, the parents may be offered the option of undergoing a midtrimester abortion. Medical centers throughout the world report that adequate fetal samples are obtained for analysis in 95 percent of all cases. As doctors have gained experience with fetoscopy, fetal loss following a blood sample has declined to slightly less than 5 percent, and the incidence of premature labor is estimated to be only 7 percent. Since the condition for which these women are being screened is very severe, the risks of fetoscopy would appear to be acceptable.

In an attempt to find a safer method than fetoscopy to diagnose sickle-cell disease in utero, doctors have studied the fetal cells obtained through amniocentesis. Though amniocentesis has a far lower complication rate than fetoscopy, the accuracy of this method is presently too low to be considered totally reliable.

Although women with sickle-cell disease are at significantly greater risk of developing complications during pregnancy than women without this condition, these risks have declined tremendously in recent years because of more meticulous management and better understanding of the disease by doctors, combined with the liberal use of blood transfusions for severe anemia and sickle-cell crises. Some medical centers advocate prophylactic transfusions of normal red blood cells at various intervals for all women with the disease during pregnancy, combined with the removal of many of the abnormal sickle cells to decrease the maternal risk of anemia and severe sickling of the abnormal cells. Other researchers believe that transfusions should only be given when absolutely necessary, since some women experience few if any problems during pregnancy and never require the blood. These doctors rightfully argue that a blood transfusion is not harmless and may be associated with a risk of an allergic reaction or infectious hepatitis from contaminated blood.

Doctors at the University of South Carolina have advocated the use of a prophylactic exchange transfusion at the twenty-eighth week of pregnancy for women with sickle-cell disease. To achieve this, they have developed an automatic blood separator that can remove a patient's red blood cells and replace them with normal donor cells while keeping the total blood volume constant. Since normal red blood cells have a life span of 120 days, one transfusion performed at week twenty-eight of pregnancy is sufficient to keep these cells from being destroyed until after delivery occurs at forty weeks. To date, the record of success with this method has been excellent, but large numbers of women must be studied before it can be enthusiastically endorsed.

What advances have been made in the diagnosis of thalassemia?

Thalassemia, like sickle-cell disease, is an autosomal recessive inherited condition caused by an abnormal hemoglobin in the blood. Also known as Cooley's anemia, thalassemia major, and Mediterranean anemia, this debilitating disease is one of the world's most common inherited disorders, yet few people have ever heard of it. It is estimated that there are close to 250,000 healthy thalassemia carriers in the United States in addition to thousands of severely affected children. Many of these individuals trace their ancestry to the Mediterranean region, especially Italy and Greece. Among persons of Italian and Greek ancestry, 1 in 25 will be found to be healthy carriers of the thalassemia trait, and 1 in 2,500 will exhibit the severe form of the disease. In a high-risk area of the world, such as Sardinia, 13 percent of the population are carriers and 1 out of 250 newborns are diseased. Other than supportive measures, such as periodic blood transfusions, there is no cure for thalassemia, and most affected individuals die before the age of thirty.

Though a healthy thalassemia carrier usually suffers from nothing more than a very mild anemia, the mating of two carriers produces an affected infant one out of four times suffering from severe anemia, frequent infections, abnormal enlargement of the liver and spleen, and thin, brittle bones. The abnormal hemoglobin in the infant is readily diagnosed by a test called hemoglobin electrophoresis. The microscopic appearance of characteristic red blood cells, known as target cells, is also a diagnostic test of this disease.

Healthy carriers of this disease have a small percentage of abnormal thalassemia hemoglobin in their blood, identifiable with hemoglobin electrophoresis. Couples of Mediterranean extraction should be encouraged to undergo thalassemia screening prior to a contemplated pregnancy so that genetic counseling may be offered where indicated.

When pregnancy occurs following the mating of two thalassemia carriers, it is now possible to diagnose the disease in the fetus with the use of fetoscopic blood sampling and placental aspiration techniques. As with sickle-cell anemia, study of enzymes in the amniotic fluid obtained via amniocentesis should eventually replace the more dangerous fetoscopy sampling method.

Roll-over Test

What is the roll-over test and how accurate is it in assessing fetal and maternal well-being?

Since its introduction in 1974, the supine pressor, or roll-over test, has been enthusiastically endorsed by some obstetricians and deemed totally worthless by others. To perform the test, a woman lies on her left side while four or five blood pressure measurements are taken at five minute intervals. She is then repositioned on her back and the blood pressure is immediately redetermined. If the change in position causes an increase in the diastolic pressure, or the lower number of the blood pressure reading, of at least 20 millimeters of mercury or more, the woman is said to have a positive roll-over test. Conversely, if the change in diastolic blood pressure is less than 20 millimeters of mercury, it is considered a negative test. Supposedly, when performed between weeks twenty-eight and thirty-two of pregnancy, a positive roll-over test predicts blood pressure elevations and preeclampsia later in pregnancy. In my opinion, studies indicate extremely poor predictability and limited clinical value of this test in the screening for potentially hypertensive women.

It has been suggested that the roll-over test may also be used for detecting fetuses destined to develop IUGR, or intrauterine growth retardation, later in pregnancy. In a report published in *Obstetrics and Gynecology* in 1980, doctors at the State University of New York at Stony Brook performed the test on 130 pregnant women between weeks twenty-eight and thirty-four of pregnancy. The authors concluded that women with positive tests, a low prepregnancy weight, and a poor weight gain during pregnancy should be followed by periodic ultrasound examinations throughout pregnancy in order to detect early signs of intrauterine growth retardation.

Second-Trimester Abortions

If studies reveal an abnormal fetus and a woman requests a second-trimester abortion, how is it performed?

In the past, major surgery in the form of a hysterotomy, or a cesarean-like incision in the uterus, was required to terminate a pregnancy during the fourth and fifth months. In addition to maternal mortality rates estimated to range from 45 to 270 per 100,000 women aborted, the hysterotomy incision often weakened the uterine muscles so that future full-term pregnancies required cesarean section.

Fortunately, physicians today have several safer options available to them for terminating pregnancies between the sixteenth and twenty-fourth weeks. One of these is the injection of either hypertonic saline (salt solution) or chemicals named prostaglandins into the amniotic fluid, using a technique identical to that used for obtaining amniotic fluid for chromosomal and chemical analysis. Several hours following the injection, contractions usually begin, followed by labor and eventual expulsion of the fetus and placenta. The labor is often described as a "mini-labor," slightly more painful than severe menstrual cramps. Nothing could be further from the truth. Despite the small size of the fetus, the labor is often prolonged and very painful, usually requiring liberal amounts of analgesics.

Prostaglandins in the form of vaginal suppositories have gained great popularity in recent years. By inserting one suppository in the vagina at three- to five-hour intervals, intense labor followed by expulsion of the fetus will usually occur within nine hours.

A survey conducted in 1982 found that the majority of American doctors now favor D and E, or dilatation and evacuation, of the uterine contents as a method of abortion after the twelfth week of pregnancy. This is accomplished with a large suction device and a variety of other instruments. Statistically, women undergoing this procedure are less likely to experience serious complications than those having saline or prostaglandin abortions. However, great skill is needed to perform a D and E, especially when the uterine size approaches twenty weeks. Since dilatation of the cervix is performed with instruments that have a large diameter, many doctors are fearful that D and E will prove to be responsible for significantly greater numbers of women with cervical incompetence and subsequent pregnancy loss.

What problems may be encountered with the hypertonic saline injection technique?

Though hundreds of these abortions have been performed with minimal side effects, the fact remains that it is a far more dangerous procedure than first-trimester suction curettage. The total complication rate for saline abortion in various studies is estimated at 20 to 26 per 100 women aborted. The death rate varies between 12 and 18 per 100,000 abortions, which means it is at least four times as likely as a first-trimester abortion to cause death.

The first potentially serious complication experienced with hypertonic saline may occur while it is being injected. If the doctor injects the solution into a uterine blood vessel, rather than the amniotic fluid, increased levels of salt solution in the blood can cause instant death. It is estimated that this occurs in less than 0.4 percent of all women undergoing saline abortions. The amount of saline required to produce abortion is approximately 200 cubic centimeters, about ¾ cup. When such a large amount is being used, the chances of accidental venous injection are greater. Because of this, your doctor must constantly observe you for early signs of hypernatremia while the solution is being injected—headache, restlessness, numbness of the fingers, a sensation of increased body warmth, and excessive thirst—and stop immediately if any of these warning signs are noted. It is obvious that a woman must be fully awake and alert and never sedated before or during the saline injection.

If the needle is accidentally placed in the muscle of the uterus and saline is then injected, necrosis, or death of the muscle, may occur. This complication, though very rare, may require hysterectomy. Rarer still is the placement of the needle into a woman's abdominal cavity rather than her amniotic sac, causing immediate and severe pain. No harm results if the injection is stopped immediately.

Even during an accurately performed procedure some saline is absorbed into the bloodstream over a period of several hours. If a woman has medical problems, such as heart disease, the increased salt load and expansion of the blood volume may be quite dangerous.

A temperature greater than 38° C (100.4° C) may occur in from 2 to 16 percent of women undergoing saline abortions. Those temperature elevations are usually due to necrosis (death of tissue) but may also be a result of infection. When infection is the cause of a fever, it can become a potentially lethal complication and is the leading cause of saline abortion death.

The incidence of hemorrhage has been calculated at 2.6 percent, while 1 to 2 percent of all women who have saline abortions hemorrhage to the point of requiring a blood transfusion. An unexplained but very serious complication of saline abortion is a decrease of several blood coagulation factors. Without these factors, severe hemorrhage requiring several units of blood may occur in 1 of every 1,200 women receiving saline.

Finally, 10 to 16 percent of women who abort the fetus retain the placenta and do not pass it within one to two hours. The placenta must then be removed, either by hand or with a sharp curette and other instruments under anesthesia. All these complications, while rarely mentioned to patients by their doctors, are potentially very serious and serve to emphasize the dangers that may occur with hypertonic saline abortions.

What are the advantages of prostaglandins as compared with saline for midtrimester abortion?

Several studies confirm that there are five definite advantages of using prostaglandins over hypertonic saline.

1. Only 8 cubic centimeters (40 milligrams) of the prostaglandin preparation, known as PGF2α, is injected into the amniotic fluid in order to induce abortion, compared with 200 cubic centimeters of saline, so the chances of that small amount entering the bloodstream are significantly less.

2. The time interval between abortion and injection is less with prostaglandins than with saline. In one study, 69 percent of patients given prostaglandins aborted within twenty-four hours, and 93 percent within forty-eight hours, compared with 22 and 85 percent with saline. Practically speaking, you spend less time in the hospital and thus incur less expense when prostaglandins are used. It should be noted that this injection-abortion time interval may be lengthened if pain medication containing aspirin is given to relieve the discomfort of contractions, because aspirin may obliterate prostaglandin contractions. Therefore, never take commonly used pain

medications which contain aspirin, such as Darvon and Percodan, when undergoing prostaglandin abortion.

3. Prostaglandins do not cause significant changes in the blood volume or salt load and can therefore be given with greater safety to women who have cardiac or other coexisting medical problems.

4. Prostaglandins do not alter the blood coagulation factors.

5. There is no risk of death from hypernatremia or necrosis of the uterine muscle when prostaglandins are given incorrectly.

Are there any adverse reactions when prostaglandins are used for an abortion?

The most frequent reaction to injection of prostaglandins is vomiting, which has been reported for at least 50 percent and as many as 75 percent of all women. There is a 25 percent incidence of extreme nausea without vomiting. These symptoms do not usually occur until several hours following the initial injection, and use of a rectal suppository to alleviate them before they occur is sometimes helpful. Diarrhea has been a problem in 16 percent of women aborted.

A rise in temperature has been observed 6 percent of the time and is of no clinical significance. However, it is sometimes difficult to distinguish from a fever caused by a uterine infection.

The most frightening side effect for both patients and doctors occurs as often as 1 to 3 percent of the time: the immediate onset of an asthmalike shortness of breath, nausea, vomiting, restlessness, and even seizures, a drop in blood pressure, slowing of the pulse, and irregularities of the heartbeat. It is believed this occurs if the prostaglandins pass directly into the circulation. Fortunately, prostaglandins are metabolized rapidly by the body, and all symptoms disappear within twenty minutes. However, because of this possibility, it is recommended that prostaglandins not be used in aborting asthmatic women.

The uterine muscle contractions caused by prostaglandins are often so strong that they can cause lacerations, or tears, of the lower cervix in approximately 0.5 percent of all patients. For this reason, the cervix must be carefully inspected following prostaglandin abortion, and all lacerations sutured immediately. The complication is more likely to occur in young women who have never experienced childbirth.

In one study of 600 prostaglandin abortions, it was noted that 30 percent of the women did not go into labor within twenty-four hours and required reinjection with half the initial 40-milligram dose. In addition, 140 women retained placental tissue following passage of the fetus. Removal of this retained tissue, requires rehospitalization.

Prostaglandin suppositories have a distinct advantage over prostaglandins injected into the amniotic fluid because of their painless and safe method of administration, requiring no special skill on the part of the person inducing the abortion. They are also invaluable in inducing labor when the diagnosis of fetal death has been confirmed. Before prostaglandin suppositories were available, women carrying a dead fetus were forced to await the onset of spontaneous labor. The injection of saline or prostaglandins into the amniotic fluid in the presence of a fetal death may be extremely dangerous, because these substances can enter the maternal circulation through the site of the nonfunctioning placenta. Once in the bloodstream, they may cause severe and even fatal reactions.

Is there any way to decrease the risk of trauma to the cervix during second-trimester abortions?

Laminaria digitata, a dried seaweed, has been used, both legally and illegally, as a cervical dilator for over 100 years. When inserted into the cervix it absorbs secretions and increases the diameter of the cervix by three to five times over a period of six to eight hours. This slowly and painlessly dilates the cervix before either suction curettage or prostaglandin abortion. Though the incidence of cervical injury may be greatly reduced with laminaria, the rate of cervical and uterine infection may be slightly higher because opening the cervix before abortion may introduce potentially harmful bacteria.

11.
Childbirth and the
Postpartum Period

For most women the word "childbirth" is synonymous with a moment of unequaled joy, but for others it represents an unforgettably painful, negative, and unhappy experience. Childbirth education classes have helped to relieve anxiety and create positive attitudes among many expectant couples, but even the most enthusiastic and prepared woman will readily admit that giving birth held some unanticipated and unwelcome surprises.

Though it is impossible to anticipate every conceivable situation which may arise during childbirth, an astute woman should have a pretty good idea about her obstetrician's attitudes toward a variety of subjects long before labor begins. When we hear of a doctor who was wonderful, humorous, and kind during the prenatal visits, only to become a villain at the time of labor and delivery, it is not uncommon to discover that the prenatal office visits were social encounters in which obstetrical philosophy was never discussed. Under such circumstances, misunderstanding and lack of communication during labor and delivery is not surprising.

It is highly unlikely that a busy obstetrician will find the time to volunteer information or explanations about childbirth unless asked. Take the initiative and make maximum use of each prenatal visit by carefully preparing a list of questions and concerns. For example, does your doctor monitor all patients routinely? How does he or she manage common problems such as breech positions, premature rupture of the amniotic membranes, and prolonged pregnancies? Is episiotomy routinely performed, and, if so, which type does he or she prefer? Are fathers permitted to observe cesarean section births as well as vaginal deliveries? Is breast-feeding enthusiastically endorsed? If you ask these questions, you may be able to identify a potential Dr. Jekyll early in pregnancy. But if you lack the temerity to challenge your doctor, you will undoubtedly experience a greater number of unwelcome surprises during labor. The woman who suddenly finds herself strapped to a fetal monitor, without explanation or previous discussion, is as foolish as the doctor who failed to mention that this was his or her standard procedure for all patients in labor.

Following childbirth, too, many women leave the hospital with unanswered questions. The vague postpartum instruction to "take it easy for six weeks" is of little help to a woman who wants to know when to resume intercourse and what type of contraceptive to use. Some postpartum instructions which doctors have given routinely for generations are without factual basis and are in many cases overly restrictive.

This final chapter presents the most current information concerning the proper management of labor, delivery, and the postpartum period. I do not discuss and compare the relative merits of the different methods of prepared childbirth or offer detailed instruction on the proper technique of breast-feeding; both subjects are very important, but many other books deal with them adequately. Rather, I want to discuss those equally important obstetrical subjects which most doctors understand but never seem to discuss with their patients so that the pregnant woman can evaluate the obstetrical care she receives. This chapter is meant to serve as a reference for women anxious to carry on a more intelligent dialogue with their doctors. Only with this knowledge can greater participation in obstetrical decisions be achieved.

Body Positions Before and During Labor and Delivery

How can a woman's posture during her pregnancy affect the fetus?

While a great deal of research has been devoted to analyzing the effects on the fetus of various maternal positions during labor and delivery, there are practically no reports dealing with the consequences of a woman's posture during the months which precede the onset of labor.

When a woman lies flat on her back during the second half of pregnancy, her enlarged uterus flops backward and compresses the aorta and vena cava, the largest artery and vein in the body. This phenomenon, known as aortocaval compression, has the effect of reducing the volume of blood returned to the heart and the amount which is pumped to the uterus and placenta. Consequently, the fetus receives less oxygen. For this reason, I encourage my patients to lie on their left side when they rest or sleep during the second half of pregnancy. The left side is preferred over the right because the vena cava passes slightly to the right of the midline and is less apt to be compressed if the uterus is tilted to the left.

Fetal growth lags slightly during the last ten weeks prior to delivery. This finding has led to speculation that markedly reduced activity and greater periods of time spent off one's feet may improve fetal growth, particularly during the last few weeks of pregnancy. Support for this position comes from a 1982 report from the Pennsylvania State University College of Medicine in Hershey, Pennsylvania. They found that women who worked at "stand-up" jobs throughout pregnancy were at significantly greater risk of having placental infarcts (see page 297) and giving birth to smaller babies.

How can a woman's posture affect the position of the baby at birth and can exercises influence the fetal position?

There has been much theorizing, but little scientific proof, to show that a woman's posture during pregnancy and labor helps to determine the in utero position of her baby. The size and shape of the pelvis, the location of the placenta, the presence of maternal uterine and pelvic anomalies, the amount of amniotic fluid which is present, the laxity of a woman's pelvic supports, and the presence of fetal anomalies are

354   *The Pregnancy Book for Today's Woman*

all factors which have been thought to contribute to the position the fetus assumes in its mother's uterus. More often than not, the reason why a woman's baby assumes an abnormal position, such as breech or occiput posterior, remains a mystery. The usual fetal position at the time of delivery is known as the occiput anterior position: the back of the baby's head, or the occiput, is anterior, or forward, and the baby is facing the maternal spine. In this position, the baby's back is closest to the maternal abdominal wall. In the occiput posterior position, the baby is facing in the same direction as the mother and its spine is closest to the maternal spine. This position is also known as a "sunny-side-up" position because the baby's head is facing upward at the moment of birth. Responsible for back labor (low back pain with labor), this position is more difficult and painful than the anterior position because a greater diameter of the fetal head must pass through the pelvis. Most often, the fetal head rotates to an anterior position just before delivery.

Physical theories of gravity and buoyancy have been quoted in attempting to explain fetal positions during pregnancy and labor. These theories assume that the fetal back is the heaviest, densest part of the fetus other than the head and will rotate to an inferior position. It is believed a woman lying on her abdomen is more likely to promote an occiput anterior fetal position, while a woman lying on her back is likely to be carrying a fetus in an occiput posterior position. The scientific literature to support these theories is minimal at best. Despite this, many midwives and childbirth instructors have devised "posturing exercises" for women so that occiput posterior positions can be avoided and rotation of the head to the anterior position can occur without medical intervention. Included among these exercises have been variations of the knee-chest position and pelvic rock maneuvers. In my experience, the use of these maneuvers has been of no help in rotating the fetal head. Enthusiastic supporters of this technique may claim excellent results, but the large majority of occiput posterior positions revert spontaneously to the more favorable anterior position. I would agree that all of these exercises are safe and simple, but I believe that they are ineffectual.

What is the ideal maternal position during labor and delivery?

While the standing position may not be the ideal prescription for fetal growth during the last trimester, there is no doubt that it offers great benefits for the woman in labor. As a matter of fact, just about any position is preferred to lying on one's back. In at least 30 percent of women, the supine position has been found to cause uterine occlusion of the common iliac artery, a branch of the aorta, which supplies blood and oxygen to the placenta, resulting in fetal heart rate decelerations, oxygen deprivation, and fetal distress.

Though our sudden condemnation of the supine position may seem like a radical departure from established obstetrical ideas, it is well documented that until late in the eighteenth century, most women in the world used an upright position during labor. This included standing, sitting, kneeling, or squatting, but always with the trunk more vertical than horizontal. The recumbent bed position became widely accepted during the ninteenth and twentieth centuries because it was more convenient for obstetricians to carry out vaginal examinations, forceps applications, and various other manuevers. Though the return to the more natural vertical position has been attributed to the research of many doctors, none has been as influential as Dr. Roberto Caldeyro-Barcia of Montevideo, Uruguay, who concluded that a woman's contractions are stronger, more efficient, but less frequent when she labors on her side rather than her back and even more efficient when she stands. When mothers were asked to describe if it was more painful to lie down, sit, or stand during labor, they indicated that they were more comfortable when upright.

The benefits to a mother and her fetus of walking during labor have been supported by a 1978 British study. Of sixty-eight women in spontaneous labor, thirty-four were randomly assigned to an ambulatory group while the remainder labored in the supine position. Electronic monitoring of the fetal heartbeat and uterine contractions was performed on all patients. Though the number of women studied was small, there were significant differences between the two groups. The ambulatory women experienced much shorter labors, were less likely to require intravenous oxytocin to improve the strength of their contractions, requested less medication for pain relief, delivered babies with significantly higher one- and five-minute Apgar scores, and were less likely to experience fetal heart-rate abnormalities. The frequency of contractions among ambulatory women was lower, the strength of their contractions was significantly greater.

When dilatation of the cervix fails to progress during labor, use of intravenous oxytocin often remedies the situation by increasing the strength and frequency of uterine contractions. Since there are some hazards associated with oxytocin use, it would be nice to employ a natural method of augmenting weak labor contractions. In a preliminary report from the University of Southern California School of Medicine, published in the *American Journal of Obstetrics and Gynecology* in 1981, doctors studied fourteen women who failed to progress during labor because of inadequate contractions. Six were given intravenous oxytocin to improve contraction strength while eight others were asked to walk. Labor progress was slightly better in the ambulatory group, with almost immediate improvement in the uterine contraction strength and frequency. It took two hours for the intravenous oxytocin to achieve an effect equal to that achieved simply by walking. Despite the small number of patients studied, the authors concluded that ambulation was as effective as oxytocin for the enhancement of labor. Certainly, if labor augmentation is needed, walking would appear to be a simpler and safer initial technique to try instead of the use of intravenous oxytocin.

Why is the upright position more efficient than lying on one's back during labor, and are there any hazards associated with its use?

When a woman assumes a vertical position, the effect of gravity on the fetus works harmoniously with the uterine contractions. It has been accurately calculated that gravity adds an additional 35 millimeters of mercury to the pressure exerted by the fetal head on the cervix during the first stage of labor. In addition, the same amount of pressure is exerted on the vaginal tissues during the second stage of labor, when the cervix is fully dilated.

The angle formed by the baby's body and the mother's spine also has an effect on the progress of labor. This angle, referred to as the "drive angle," is greater when a woman is standing than when she is lying on her back, and labor is significantly more efficient when the angle is greater.

The increased pressure on the fetal head when a woman is in the vertical position during labor has prompted some doctors to question if it may be responsible for some harmful fetal effects. However, studies do not bear this out.

In a 1977 study, comparing 189 women laboring in the horizontal position with 126 in the vertical position, doctors studied the incidence of caput succedaneum, or swelling of the tissues over the fetal scalp caused by pressure during labor. When the amniotic membranes were intact, the incidence of swelling was surprisingly higher among those in the former group. In addition, disalignment of the cranial bones, or molding, in the newborn was found not to be related to a woman's position during labor.

Though labor in the vertical position appears to be safe when the amniotic membranes are intact, there are no large studies demonstrating that the added pressure on the fetal scalp does not cause harm if the membranes are ruptured. Many hospitals have enthusiastically endorsed the use of the birthing chair during the end of the first stage and throughout the second stage of labor. A high percentage of women at this point in labor have spontaneously ruptured their amniotic membranes. One wonders if this significant increase in pressure on the fetal scalp could in any way be responsible for a higher incidence of head and brain trauma. Such information would be valuable in the management of the more delicate premature infant.

What is a birthing chair?

A birthing chair is exactly what its name says it is: a chair in which a woman gives birth. They have been in existence since 1500, and possibly even earlier. All sorts of chairs, tables, and boards have been developed over the years to elevate a woman's upper body so that it is in a near-vertical position during labor. Clinical experience suggests that women are most comfortable when their backs are between 30 and 45 degrees from the horizontal position.

The Birth EZ Birthing Chair (see illustration) was first introduced in the United States in 1979. Since then it has been used in hundreds of hospitals. It has the appearance of a modern molded chair and is set high on a pedestal which houses a motor capable of elevating, lowering, and tilting the seat. The chair costs $5,000 and for this price one would expect to receive power steering, power brakes, and air conditioning.

My impression of the chair to date, though not supported by scientific data, is that most patients find it more comfortable than the labor bed or the standard delivery room table, although I have not noted shorter second-stage labors among patients who have used the chair. While most women fit comfortably into the chair,

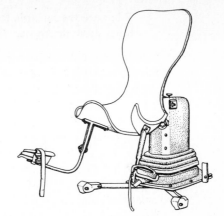

Birthing chair.

Drawing based on the Century Birthing Chair, Century Manufacturing Company, Industrial Park, Aurora, Nebraska.

those who are overweight or have large thighs have complained of uncomfortable pressure against the inner part of the leg and thigh supports. While repair of an episiotomy is easily done by tilting the chair backward, complicated suturing of vaginal wall lacerations is more difficult because of the limited amount of abduction, or turning out of the thighs, allowed by the chair. In the event of an emergency in which general anesthesia must be administered immediately, the chair is not properly equipped and a patient would have to be transferred to the standard delivery room table. Although the chair supposedly can be used with general anesthesia, in fact it is inadequate for this purpose. Until more extensive scientific data are available on the outcome of labor and the pressure effects of the added gravitational force on the fetal head, created by the sitting position, I withhold final judgment on the merits of the birthing chair.

Is there a preferred maternal position for a cesarean section?

A woman undergoing a cesarean section in the supine position is at the same risk of experiencing compression of the aorta and vena cava as one who labors in this position. This compression can markedly lower the maternal blood pressure, known as supine hypotension, as well as impair placental circulation and fetal oxygenation.

These effects may be intensified when epidural or spinal anesthesia is administered. To remedy this problem, most hospitals use operating room tables that tilt at least 15 degrees to the left while a cesarean section is performed. The tilt to the left allows the uterus and its contents to fall away from the vena cava thereby improving the return circulation from a woman's lower extremities to her heart. Hypotension is prevented, and normal placental blood flow returns.

Many hospitals use specially designed foam rubber wedges, positioned to the left of a mother's pelvis to hold her safely in position at the time of surgery. Some obstetricians have even devised methods of tilting the table to a full lateral or side position so that the cesarean section is performed with the doctor assuming a sitting position. This method, however, has not been endorsed by the majority of physicians.

What are the hazards to the fetus when the mother bears down during the second stage of labor?

It is not unusual to detect early fetal heart rate decelerations, or Type I dips, during the second stage of labor when a woman is bearing down. These decelerations are the result of fetal head compression and are practically always harmless. Prolonged bearing down efforts, however, may be dangerous to the fetus. Research by Dr. Caldeyro-Barcia of Uruguay suggests that best results are obtained when the bearing down or pushing effort lasts four to five seconds. Prolonging the attempt for longer than six to seven seconds at a time is ill advised and potentially very dangerous. When bearing down was encouraged for longer than fifteen seconds, Dr. Caldeyro-Barcia noted that the fetus was much more likely to experience hypoxia, or lack of oxygen, and a marked deceleration in heart rate. If bearing down efforts are spontaneously and voluntarily performed by a woman, the early fetal heart rate decelerations, or Type I dips, recover and return to normal after the last pushing effort of each contraction. However, if the pushing is extended and unnatural and each push is prolonged beyond six seconds, the fetal heart rate does not have time to recover between contractions.

The mechanism behind the development of fetal distress with prolonged pushing is easily explained. When a woman bears down she holds her breath. This closes the glottis at the opening of the trachea, or windpipe, increasing pressure within the thorax, or chest cavity, which in turn results in a drop in maternal blood pressure. The longer the bearing-down effort, the more marked the fall of a woman's blood pressure. As a result, there is a decline in the amount of blood reaching the placenta and the oxygen supplied to the fetus is reduced. These changes occur in all maternal positions, though they are intensified in the supine position.

Too often, obstetricians and nurses demand that their patients push as hard and as long as they can, and some women are criticized for not being "good pushers." Do not follow this advice. In labor bear down as you feel the need, without trying to produce very strong or prolonged efforts. Furthermore, push less if you are lying on your back. Though the second stage of labor may proceed more slowly when this advice is followed, the risks of cutting the supply of oxygen to the fetus will be reduced significantly.

Labor

Is there a particular time of the day or month when I am most likely to give birth?

Unfortunately for obstetricians, the maximum birth rate is between 6:00 and 8:00 A.M. In northern countries there is a significant increase in births in early spring, while in semitropical countries most births occur during the summer months. In the United States, far more births occur between Tuesday and Thursday than on the weekend, but this is probably because obstetricians perform more inductions or labor stimulations during the week.

Many obstetricians and midwives say childbirth is far more common at the time of a full moon, as did a study reported in the *American Journal of Obstetrics and Gynecology* in 1959. Further study of this lunar effect was reported in 1973, when researchers who studied 500,000 live births in New York City concluded that births are above average before a full moon and below average after a full moon.

Should a woman be routinely monitored electronically during labor even if she has no obstetrical or medical complications?

While few consumer advocates would deny that electronic monitoring, or EFM, has helped to improve fetal outcome in high-risk pregnancies, whether such monitoring is valuable for a woman with an uncomplicated pregnancy and labor is still unresolved. Those opposed to the routine use of fetal monitoring claim that attachment to the machine's wires and electrodes confines a woman to bed, is unnatural, detracts from the spontaneity of her birth experience and has been too frequently associated with a false diagnosis of fetal distress. This false diagnosis has helped to contribute to an incredibly high number of unnecessary cesarean sections. Though internal fetal monitoring has proven to be more accurate than the external technique (see fetal monitoring, page 328), it has also been accused of causing a greater incidence of maternal and fetal infection and hemorrhage, as well as a variety of other complications. Finally, those in opposition to monitoring point out the exorbitant costs of using it routinely on all women in labor.

In contrast to these negative views are the findings of some of the most highly respected obstetricians in the United States, who claim that routine monitoring of all women significantly reduces the incidence of fetal death during labor and permanent disability of the newborn infant. Support for their argument comes from statistics which show that 20 percent of apparently low-risk patients develop problems at some point during labor. According to recent estimates, events which occur during labor are currently believed to account for 20 percent of stillbirths, 20 to 40 percent of fetuses damaged by cerebral palsy, and 10 percent of children with severe mental retardation. It is estimated that 15,000 babies with cerebral palsy are born annually. In addition, approximately 126,000 children born each year will be diagnosed as retarded. Many of these tragedies could be prevented with widespread use of fetal monitoring. Although two highly publicized studies did not find any benefits of routine electronic monitoring, the vast majority of reports have concluded that widespread use of this technique can reduce the stillbirth and neonatal death rate by 1 to 5 babies per 1,000 births.

It is easy to understand the confusion that women experience when deciding whether or not to be routinely monitored. The main objection to EFM is that the technique is at variance with the concepts of family-centered childbirth and the return to a more natural homelike labor environment. Some have used words, such as "dehumanizing" and "humiliating," to describe EFM, despite the fact that the majority of objective evidence also shows that it helps to diagnose fetal distress caused by a lack of oxygen at an early stage. For the healthy woman whose pregnancy has been without incident, the ultimate decision on whether or not to be monitored is often extremely difficult. Certainly, the odds are well in her favor that her infant will encounter no problems if continuous electronic fetal monitoring is not used. However, in the unlikely event that the fetus suffers, she would have to bear some of the responsibility for not having taken advantage of this available technology. I firmly believe that EFM is compatible with family-centered care provided that it is accompanied by supportive and knowledgeable hospital personnel. A simple, unobtrusive monitor is not in itself dehumanizing and will not detract from the quality of the birth experience. However, the medical staff's attitudes and inflexibility of hospital regulations regarding birth may be.

The manner in which the option of routine fetal monitoring is understood by a woman also influences her decision. Question your obstetrician about the pros and cons of periodic listening with a stethoscope as opposed to continuous internal and external electronic monitoring during your prenatal visits rather than taking a "crash course" during labor. Some patients mistakenly believe that the hand-held Doppler device is as accurate as EFM in detecting fetal heart rate abnormalities. This is certainly untrue, though it is far better than the old-fashioned stethoscope.

Much of the negative reaction to internal monitoring is based on the fear that the scalp electrode can injure the baby. The truth is that the incidence of scalp infections is extremely rare, and when such infections do occur they are mild and superficial and do not represent any risk to the fetus. The chance of causing scalp hemorrhage, trauma, or lacerations with the scalp electrode is so rare as to be almost unheard of.

Many women are opposed to fetal monitoring because it hampers their movement during labor and confines them to bed. One way to avoid this restriction is to use the monitor intermittently. On admission to the labor room, an external fetal monitor can be applied for thirty minutes to be sure that no heart-rate abnormalities are present. The machine can then be unhooked and the woman allowed to walk about. Periodic five-minute tracings, taken at thirty-minute intervals during the first stage of labor, may be the ideal compromise for women who are opposed to continuous monitoring. This method of monitoring may be continued throughout labor as long as the fetal heart rate and cervical dilatation remain normal. Even with the application of the internal scalp electrode, monitoring may still be used intermittently simply by detaching the electrode from the wires leading to the machine. The electrode can then be taped to a woman's inner thigh when she leaves her bed to walk about. Some women are under the false impression that they have to lie perfectly still in bed in order to be monitored adequately. In fact, a change of position involves only a slight adjustment of the external transducer and no changes in the internal instruments. It is also possible to keep the monitor running while the mother is sitting in a chair or even standing near the machine. The view that fetal monitoring should be routinely employed is now shared by almost 80 percent of all practicing physicians. Though some may call EFM an intrusion in the natural birth process, if it can save at least 1 life per 1,000 births and decrease the incidence of children born with permanent brain damage, it is a worthwhile intrusion.

What constitutes normal progress during labor?

The historic work of Dr. Emmanuel A. Friedman enables us to understand and evaluate the normal course of labor. Dr. Friedman studied thousands of births and then derived a graph showing the approximate length of time that each phase of labor should last. Though these statistics represent averages, from which considerable deviation may occur, they allow for instant evaluation and detection of labor progress, as well as deviations from this normal pattern.

Normal labor is characterized by progressive cervical dilatation and descent of the fetal head in the pelvis. Descent is measured in terms of the relationship between the level of the lowest part of the fetal head and the maternal ischial spines. These two bony projections lie on either side of the pelvis, and a doctor can easily touch them during a vaginal or rectal examination. If the head is at the same level as the spines, the station, or point of descent in the pelvis, is said to be 0, and levels above and below the spines are referred to as minus (−) and plus (+) stations respectively. A station of −3 means that the leading part of the head is 3 centimeters above the maternal spines, while a +1 station signifies that it is 1 centimeter below. The station of the fetal head at any time during labor can be easily determined during a vaginal examination. Dr. Friedman was able to show that progress in labor could be followed by charting the results of periodic vaginal examinations on a labor graph. The results of each examination are plotted on the graph and then joined together to form a continuous line. By doing this, one can readily observe that during normal labor cervical dilatation will follow a characteristic S-shape curve. In contrast, the line measuring descent of the baby's head will follow a more angulated route. The classic configuration of the normal labor graph is demonstrated in figure 11–1. This method has become so successful that many hospitals throughout the world have now adopted the Friedman graph for following the progress of all women in labor.

The latent phase of labor (A–B on the curve) begins with the onset of regular uterine contractions and continues until the dilatation line begins to curve upward. In this phase the cervix softens for subsequent active dilatation. Most of the total time that a woman spends in labor is spent in this phase. The cervix during this phase may be as little as 1 centimeter and as much as 4 centimeters dilated. Under normal circumstances, the latent phase should not exceed twenty hours for a woman having her first baby (multipara or primigravida), or fourteen hours for someone who has previously given birth (multipara). Usually, however, the latent phase averages six and a half hours in primigravidas and slightly less than five hours in multiparas.

The active phase of labor (line B–D) is divided into three parts: the acceleration phase (B), in which cervical dilatation begins to increase; the phase of maximum slope (C), which is characterized by rapid cervical dilatation; and the deceleration phase (D), in which the rate of cervical dilatation slows just prior to full dilatation. During the phase of maximum slope, dilatation of the cervix should progress at a rate of no less than 1.2 centimeters per hour for primigravidas and 1.5 centimeters per hour for multiparas. All the phases of labor leading up to full dilatation of the cervix (A + E) make up the first stage of labor.

The second stage of labor (E) begins with full dilatation of the cervix and ends with delivery of the baby. Though there is a great deal of variability, the average length of the second stage of labor will be approximately fifty minutes for a primigravida and twenty minutes for a multiparous woman.

From the dotted line, which depicts fetal descent, it is readily apparent that the station of the baby's head rapidly moves downward during the active phase of cervical dilatation.

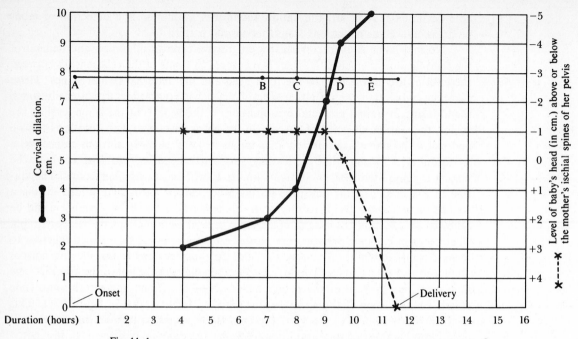

Fig. 11–1

Phases of labor.

Characteristic patterns of cervical dilatation and descent charted against elapsed time in labor, showing their component phases: A: latent phase; B-D: active phase; B: acceleration phase; C: phase of maximum slope; D: deceleration phase; E: second stage.

Couples taking childbirth education courses need not be confused trying to correlate this medical terminology with what they have learned. Most couples are taught that "active labor" is that period of time in which the cervix dilates from 3 to 7 centimeters. During this phase, the contractions are usually very strong and may occur as frequently as every two to three minutes, lasting one minute. This period of time corresponds to the acceleration and maximum slope components (B and C) of the active phase. The most difficult part of labor, from 8 to 10 centimeters of cervical dilatation, is commonly referred to by childbirth instructors as the transition stage. At this point, contractions are most intense, lasting as long as ninty seconds and coming as frequently as one minute apart. Fortunately, this stage usually lasts only twenty to forty-five minutes. The transition stage can be considered as being synonymous with Dr. Friedman's deceleration phase (D).

How do these objective measurements relate to what a woman actually experiences during labor?

Women have described these latent phase contractions, which are rhythmic and get stronger as time progresses, in a number of different ways, including pelvic pressure, backache, menstrual-like cramps, and a sensation of tightening in the area over the pubic bone. During this time, contractions are usually tolerated easily and most women feel quite sociable and are able to carry on a conversation between contractions. At this point in labor it is not necessary to time each contraction until the interval from the start of one to the start of another is approximately 5 minutes or less. Since the latent phase of labor may last for several hours, it is usually more comfortable to rest between contractions at home rather than rushing prematurely to the hospital.

During the "active labor" phase, with its more intense and more frequent contractions, most women do not feel like talking and usually become thoughtful, serious, and quiet, and totally preoccupied with their labor. Joking, loud noises, and conversations carried on during contractions are extremely distracting and annoying to a woman at this time, though companionship and sincere encouragement are invaluable and greatly appreciated. As dilatation approaches 7 centimeters, many women have some doubts about their ability to cope with the contractions that lie ahead. This is a normal reaction.

The most difficult part of labor, from 8 to 10 centimeters of cervical dilatation, is commonly referred to by childbirth instructors as the transition stage—Dr. Friedman's deceleration (D) phase. At this point, contractions are most intense, lasting as long as 90 seconds and coming as frequently as 1 minute apart. Fortunately, this stage usually lasts only 20 to 45 minutes. For many women, the contractions during this stage feel almost continuous, making it nearly impossible to relax. Restlessness, extreme irritability, expressions of discomfort, and request for help and medication are frequent during transition. Hiccups or belching , a feeling of nausea, and a desire to vomit are also frequently expressed as the cervix approaches full dilatation.

Contractions during the second active stage of labor (E) are often further apart than those of the transition stage, and they are accompanied by an irresistable urge to bear down and expel the baby. The feelings of insecurity and fear which characterize the transition stage are quickly substituted by a great sense of relief and confidence. A woman feels an almost unbelievable physical strength during this stage, knowing that each of her expulsive efforts is bringing her closer to the successful completion of labor. It is impossible for this male obstetrician to describe the incredible feeling of relief and joy which a woman experiences following the final herculean effort which results in the birth of her baby.

How can the doctor and patient diagnose and correct an abnormal pattern of cervical dilatation?

Dr. Friedman described four major types of abnormal cervical dilatation patterns: prolonged latent phase, protracted active-phase dilatation, secondary arrest of dilatation, and prolonged deceleration phase.

The latent phase is considered to be prolonged if it exceeds twenty hours in the primigravida or fourteen hours in the woman who has previously given birth. Excessive sedation at a point too early in labor is the most common factor associated with this problem. Similarly, administering a conduction anesthetic such as an epidural during the latent phase will also serve to prolong it. In addition, women who begin labor with a rigid, thick, and undilated cervix will be more likely to experience a long and difficult latent phase. Others, for unknown reasons, will have poorly synchronized uterine muscle contractions as the cause of their lack of cervical dilatation.

It is often very difficult for even the most experienced obstetricians to distinguish between false labor and a prolonged latent phase. The correct diagnosis can only be made after several hours of observation. Regardless of the cause of the prolonged latent phase, rest and sedation is the treatment. After fourteen or more hours of contractions, most women are exhausted and disheartened by their lack of progress. An intramuscular narcotic should be administered in a dosage which is sufficient to rest both the patient and her uterus for a period of six to eight hours. If, following this rest period, the contractions have stopped, the diagnosis of false labor can be made and the woman can be sent home.

Dr. Friedman found, however, that 85 percent of all women with a prolonged latent phase enter the active phase of labor following this period of therapeutic rest. Of this group, over 90 percent go on to normal active-phase dilatation of the cervix. Among the small number of women who continue to experience latent-phase labor following sedation, Dr. Friedman recommends initiation of intravenous oxytocin stimulation, provided there are no medical problems in the mother preventing its use. All too often, cesarean sections are performed for "failure to progress," when in reality one is dealing with a benign, though prolonged, latent phase. Nine times out of ten, surgery is unnecessary since these women spontaneously enter the phase of active cervical dilatation.

Protracted dilatation during the active phase is a rare type of abnormal labor in which cervical dilatation creeps along at a pace which is slower than the minimal normal amount of 1.2 centimeters per hour for primigravidas and 1.5 centimeters per hour for multiparas. It can be caused by excessive sedation, inappropriately early epidural anesthesia, or an abnormal position of the baby. However, in most cases, the cause remains unknown. Measures to speed up labor, such as artificial rupture of the amniotic membranes and intravenous oxytocin stimulation, only serve to complicate matters. Provided that some progress is being made, the best treatment is a hands-off policy. Two-thirds of all women with a protracted active phase eventually experience an uneventful vaginal delivery. However, one-third stop dilating at some point during labor and require a cesarean section because the baby's head size is too large to pass through the maternal pelvis. This condition is known as cephalopelvic, or feto-pelvic, disproportion.

The most ominous of cervical dilatation abnormalities is known as secondary arrest or cessation of dilatation during the active phase of labor. Approximately 40 percent of all women experiencing this problem ultimately require a cesarean section because of cephalopelvic disproportion. Other causes of secondary arrest of dilatation during the active phase of labor include sedation and improperly administered conduction anesthesia, such as an epidural. Among women who are believed to have adequate pelvic measurements, the use of intravenous oxytocin at this stage produces progressive dilatation of the cervix and subsequent vaginal delivery at least 80 percent of the time. X-ray pelvimetry can be avoided and oxytocin carefully administered if the pelvic measurements appear to be adequate, there are no significant heart-rate abnormalities on the fetal monitor, and there is no evidence of fetal distress. Failure of labor to progress following three to four hours of good oxytocin-induced contractions would warrant a cesarean section.

When arrest of dilatation is caused by analgesics or conduction anesthesia, rather than cephalopelvic disproportion, the effects of the drugs should be allowed to wear off. Progressive dilatation of the cervix and a successful vaginal delivery usually follow.

The final disorder of cervical dilatation, known as the prolonged deceleration phase, occurs just before full dilatation and is often associated with cephalopelvic disproportion. It can be recognized whenever dilatation of the cervix from approximately 8 or 9 centimeters to 10 centimeters (full dilatation) takes longer than three hours in the primigravida or more than one hour in the multipara. Management of this problem in a manner similar to that for arrest of labor in the active phase should bring a successful outcome, provided that your obstetrician does not attempt a difficult midforceps delivery after the cervix is fully dilated.

What happens when the baby's head does not descend in the normal way during labor?

The curve for descent of the fetal head during labor follows a flat line until the cervical dilatation curve reaches its maximum upward slope. It normally reaches its own maximum at the onset of the deceleration phase of cervical dilatation. During the second stage of labor, descent is usually progressive and at a rate of no less than 1 centimeter per hour in primigravidas and 2 centimeters in multiparas.

Dr. Friedman has described three abnormalities of fetal descent: failure of descent, protracted descent pattern, and arrest of descent. In a failure of descent situation the baby's head does not drop to a lower position in the pelvis at the time that the cervical deceleration phase begins. This failure is an ominous sign that cephalopelvic disproportion may be present. A protracted descent pattern is often related to a protracted active-phase cervical dilatation abnormality. The prognosis for vaginal delivery is generally good. Arrest, or cessation of descent for more than one hour after it has begun, is the third type of abnormal descent pattern described by Dr. Friedman.

Until recently, it was accepted obstetrical policy in many hospitals to attempt delivery following a maximum of two hours of full dilatation in women having their first baby and one hour in woman who have had a previous baby. Occasionally this rule was followed even if it involved a difficult midforceps operation. It was mistakenly believed that prolongation of the second stage of labor for periods longer than these limits adversely affects the fetus. Recent studies have shown, however, that this is not so. Labor can continue as long as descent is progressing and the fetus is monitored. Given enough time for their descent patterns to evolve, most women with labor abnormalities experience a normal vaginal delivery.

What happens when the bag of waters breaks prematurely?

The spontaneous breaking of the amniotic membranes, or bag of waters, at any time before the onset of labor is a common obstetrical problem in 6 to 12 percent of all pregnancies. This condition is sometimes called PROM (premature rupture of the membranes). For most women, labor usually follows rupture of the membranes within a few hours, but the time between the rupture of the membranes and the onset of labor tends to be longer for those women who are farthest from their estimated delivery date. Among all women with PROM, it is estimated that at least 80 percent will enter spontaneous labor and deliver within forty eight hours.

One must be sure that the amniotic membranes have actually ruptured. Quite often, pressure of the baby's head on a woman's urinary bladder produces urine which may be mistaken for leakage of amniotic fluid. Similarly, the passage of mucus from the cervix and an increase in vaginal secretions which are often noted at the end of pregnancy may confuse the diagnosis. Insertion of a sterile vaginal speculum resolves this question and allows visualization of the fluid as it passes from the cervix. Confirmation of the presence of amniotic fluid is easily accomplished by insertion of a thin strip of yellow nitrazine paper. Amniotic fluid is less acidic than vaginal secretions and turns the nitrazine paper from yellow to dark blue. Vaginal and cervical secretions and urine, however, are practically always acidic and therefore do not change the color of the nitrazine paper. When nitrazine paper test results are not clear a sample of the fluid may be studied under the microscope. Amniotic fluid assumes a characteristic appearance of a fern leaf due to its high concentrations of sodium chloride.

Statistically, 20 percent of all women with PROM give birth to a premature infant. Fetal immaturity is by far the most important cause of deaths of these infants. When a fetus is premature, the obstetrician must balance the risk of delivering it as soon as possible, to avoid the development of infection, against the dangers of not interrupting the pregnancy so that maturation of the fetus can occur in utero. Once the membranes have ruptured, the mortality rate at birth and the incidence of infection to the newborn is directly related to the length of the time between the rupture of the membranes and the onset of labor. A decision to deliver early exposes the infant to the risk of respiratory distress syndrome, or RDS, while prolonged observation increases the potential for fetal and maternal infection.

Though procedures vary from one medical center to the next, most experts recommend induction of labor when the fetus is believed to be at least thirty-three weeks mature or is judged to weigh at least 4½ pounds on ultrasound examination. Before thirty-three weeks, the risk of complications from fetal immaturity is greater than that of infection, and for this reason, watchful waiting is best. When the membranes rupture prior to the thirty-fourth week, it is possible that the fetus has major congenital anomalies since this is the condition in approximately 25 percent of such patients. For this reason, an ultrasound examination is very important in making the decision to wait or induce labor.

There is some evidence to suggest that the stress of the rupture accelerates fetal lung maturation, usually sixteen hours after the membranes rupture. For this reason, many obstetricians now delay labor induction for at least sixteen hours in order to reduce the incidence of RDS in low birth weight infants. Since the weight of the baby is not always correlated with lung maturity, an L/S ratio test (see page 312) may be performed on the amniotic fluid or abdominal amniocentesis may be used if leakage is not excessive, although this has been found to be successful only 50 percent of the time. To solve the problem of inaccuracies associated with measuring fetal lung maturity, doctors at Good Samaritan Hospital in Phoenix, Arizona, have used phosphatidylglycerol determinations from the vaginal secretions to assess fetal lung maturity. In their study RDS occurred in none of twenty-eight newborns in whom phosphatidylglycerol was present prior to delivery.

Many obstetricians believe that a conservative approach to PROM, rather than induction of labor, is both safe and beneficial even if a pregnancy is full term. In support of this position are statistics showing a three times greater cesarean section rate following induced rather than spontaneous labor. If an obstetrician elects to treat PROM conservatively, he or she must be constantly alerted to any early indications of fetal or maternal infection. A complete blood count should be performed at least every other day, since an elevation in the number of white blood cells will often indicate the presence of infection. Fever, abdominal tenderness, or foul-smelling vaginal discharge are all ominous signs. Although some obstetricians hospitalize women with ruptured membranes, I believe that this regimen is a bit too restrictive and expensive, but I do instruct my patients to take their temperatures at least twice daily and report any elevation above 37.5° C. (99.5° F.) immediately. Intercourse and the use of tampons should be strictly prohibited. There is no doubt that the chances of infection are significantly increased if even one digital vaginal examination is performed after the membranes rupture. Such an examination must be strictly avoided until labor has begun or the decision has been made to induce labor with intravenous oxytocin. Also, antibiotics taken at this time to decrease the risk of infection and improve the fetal prognosis are of no help and may even be harmful.

Whenever the diagnosis of infection is strongly suspected, the pregnancy must be terminated within eight hours, since the consequences of delay may be an overwhelming maternal infection and even death. Cesarean section is performed if it is determined that the baby will not be delivered within the approximate eight-hour time limit or if fetal distress warrants intervention. It is most important that pregnancies complicated by infection be treated at medical centers capable of handling all potential problems. Both mother and child will often require round-the-clock evaluation and treatment which these larger facilities are more capable of providing.

Induced Labor and Prolonged Pregnancy

Should labor be induced, and if so, how?

Labor induction may be classified as being either indicated or elective. Inducing labor is indicated when the medical benefits of delivery to the fetus or mother exceed those of continuing the pregnancy. IUGR, postmaturity syndrome, suspected fetal distress, abruptio placenta, fetal death, premature rupture of the membranes, amniotic membrane infections, preeclampsia, Rh disease, and maternal diseases such as diabetes, hypertension, and kidney disease are among the reasons for indicated induction of labor to benefit the fetus or mother.

Labor can be induced for convenience in an individual who is free of medical or obstetrical complications. Candidates for this elective induction are those with a history of a previous rapid labor or excessive travel time to the hospital. In the not too distant past, it was common practice among obstetricians to electively induce labor for a variety of nonmedical and nonobstetrical reasons, such as a planned vacation or a doctor's desire to avoid working at an inconvenient hour. Several large studies show this inadequate obstetrical care results in higher rates of fetal distress, ruptured uterus, maternal water intoxication due to too much oxytocin, cervical lacerations, birth injuries, postpartum hemorrhage, abruptio placenta, perinatal deaths, respiratory distress (RDS), and premature births due to miscalculation of the due date by an overanxious physician. The birth of a baby with RDS resulting from an elective induction of labor is inexcusable.

In response to the outcry of some prominent physicians, consumer groups, and the American Foundation for Maternal and Child Health, the FDA in 1978 issued restrictions on the use of oxytocin, the uterine stimulant, for the elective induction of labor. Even with use of modern monitoring techniques and delicately controlled intravenous infusion pumps, oxytocin use is still more likely than natural labor to be associated with a higher incidence of abnormally powerful, painful, and prolonged uterine contractions. During a natural labor, the rest time between uterine contractions allows a reservoir of oxygenated blood to accumulate in sufficient quantities to meet the needs of the fetus before the next contraction takes place. Since oxytocin-induced contractions are harder and faster than normal, there is less time for oxygen to accumulate between contractions, and fetal hypoxia and distress are more likely to result. This in turn leads to a higher incidence of emergency cesarean sections among women undergoing induction of labor. Some women who receive oxytocin experience greater tension of the uterine muscles which may persist even after the contraction has ended and further reduce the fetal oxygen supply. In one study, 94 percent of the women who were induced required pain relief, compared to only 60 percent of those who labored spontaneously. The excess amount of pain medication required can serve no helpful purpose for a compromised infant. It has been convincingly demonstrated that oxytocin crosses the placenta and enters the fetal circulation, where it produces distinct biochemical and physiological changes. Among these are hyponatremia, or a reduction in the sodium concentration of the newborn infant's blood, and jaundice during the first few days of life. Both these changes are temporary and are of little if any clinical significance. Despite an abundance of negative reports, however, there remains an unconvinced core of obstetricians in this country who continue to practice elective induction of labor.

Labor should not be induced with oxytoxin under certain medical and obstetrical conditions. Included among these are a weakened uterus due to a previous cesarean section or extensive uterine surgery, placenta previa, infections of the lower genital tract, such as herpes and gonorrhea, some abnormal positions of the baby, and marked disproportion between the large size of the baby and the small size of the pelvis. A woman who has had five previous viable pregnancies should not undergo oxytocin-induced labor since her uterus is more likely to rupture under the stimulus of potentially potent contractions. Overdistention of the uterus, as in the case of twins and hydramnios (excessive amount of amniotic fluid), are both conditions barring oxytocin stimulation.

In the past, oxytocin was commonly prescribed as tablets placed inside the cheek. Absorption into the bloodstream occurred unpredictably and dangerously when this method was used. Even more dangerous was the administration of oxytocin by intramuscular or subcutaneous injections. When oxytocin is medically indicated, it should only be given intravenously. Fortunately, the FDA has set limits on the initial dose of oxytocin used for induction at 1 to 2 milliunits per minute. This dose should be gradually and carefully increased in increments which do not exceed 1 to 2 milliunits per minute, until the contraction pattern is similar to that of a normal labor. Electronic fetal monitoring is mandatory whenever oxytocin stimulation is initiated. Oxytocin stimulation is not a procedure that can be delegated to a nurse while a doctor is seeing patients in the office; the obstetrician should be in attendance at the hospital, in the event that complications develop. In addition, the obstetrical unit should be prepared for an immediate cesarean section if indicated. Precautions of this type are vital if the incidence of poor pregnancy outcome following oxytocin induction is to be minimized.

The mere fact that a doctor intends to induce labor does not necessarily mean that success is assured. For a cervix to be favorable or "ripe" for induction, it must have a soft, yielding consistency, be more than half thinned out, and be sufficiently dilated to admit one examining finger with ease. Regardless of how much oxytocin is used, labor induction will most likely be unsuccessful if any of these conditions are not met. The many potential risks associated with the induction of labor may be minimized by proper selection of patients. The Bishop Scoring System, named after Dr. Edward Bishop, uses five objective criteria for determining if a woman can successfully undergo induction of labor: cervical dilatation, cervical effacement or thinning out, station of the fetal head, cervical consistency, and cervical position in relation to the vaginal axis.

Though many techniques and medications have been used by doctors over the years to "ripen" the cervix for induction of labor, to date all have failed. However, research at several hospitals throughout the world suggests that the use of very small doses of prostaglandin vaginal gels and suppositories are capable of markedly improving the Bishop score and initiating labor. In one study, 75 percent of the women who were considered unripe began labor within forty-eight hours after receiving prostaglandin gels.

When the cervix is truly ripe for labor, induction can often succeed simply by artificially rupturing the amniotic membranes. This technique, called amniotomy, is easily and painlessly performed by guiding a sterile clamp or stylet through the cervix in order to puncture the membranes. Amniotomy induces labor successfully, without oxytocin, in at least 90 percent of all women with a Bishop score of 4 or more. One distinct advantage of performing amniotomy is that it allows examination of the amniotic fluid for evidence of blood or meconium staining. In addition, it makes possible the placement of an intrauterine pressure catheter and a scalp fetal electrode and the taking of scalp pH blood samples in the high-risk patient. Amniotic membranes should never be ruptured if the baby's head is high in the pelvis, because the sudden release of fluid can cause a prolapse of the umbilical cord beneath the level of the head. This dire emergency requires immediate delivery, because the cord may then be compressed and fetal oxygenation impaired. The fetal heart tones should always be checked immediately before and after the membranes are ruptured in order to determine what effect the procedure may have on the fetus. Occasionally, a previously undetected low-lying umbilical cord may be compressed as the head descends. This can be detected promptly by the sudden bradycardia, or slowing of the fetal heart rate, and can be relieved by gently elevating the head with the fingers in the vagina, while emergency preparations for cesarean section are made. When amniotomy is performed during labor, it is best accomplished between contractions in order to avoid the potential risk of cord prolapse as the fluid gushes rapidly out of the uterus. Once the amniotic membranes have been artificially ruptured, delivery should be accomplished within twenty-four hours since the risk of an amniotic membrane infection increases significantly after this time. Though most obstetricians view amniotomy as a safe and simple procedure, some authorities, including Dr. Caldeyro-Barcia, condemn this common practice as being extremely dangerous. They claim that the fluid-filled membranes provide a liquid cushion that helps to protect the head of the fetus from damage caused by pressure against the pelvis during labor. It has been stated that artificial rupture of the membranes can produce massive tears in brain tissue due to misalignment of the unfused bones of the skull. To date, no studies support this assertion.

Obstetricians often claim that they are able to induce labor by manipulating the amniotic membrane. This technique, known as "stripping of the membranes," consists of inserting the examining finger into the cervix and then separating the amniotic membranes from their lower uterine wall attachment. One advantage of stripping, rather than rupturing the membranes, is that it can easily be performed in a doctor's office, and if it fails, nothing is lost because the membranes have not been ruptured and the risk of infection is practically nonexistent. Unfortunately, the efficacy of this method in inducing labor has never been proved, and it is too unreliable to use if labor must be induced.

When is a pregnancy considered prolonged?

A pregnancy is prolonged, or postdated, when it exceeds forty-two weeks, two weeks or more beyond the EDC. What makes labor begin remains unknown, and why it is delayed is also a mystery. For couples whose excitement has peaked in anticipation of labor, the delay is disappointing and frustrating. For the obstetrician it is nerve-wracking, because 10 to 15 percent of infants involved in prolonged pregnancies die or face serious illness. Since 85 to 90 percent of late pregnancies terminate in the delivery of a healthy infant, labor induction in the presence of an unripe or unready cervix is dangerous and foolhardy. Similarly, performance of cesarean section on all women who are late would result in unnecessary surgery 85 to 90 percent of the time.

What effect can a prolonged pregnancy have on the fetus?

Many pregnancies which are believed to be late are actually dated incorrectly. Problems are likely to arise by delivering a thirty-eight-week pregnancy erroneously believed to be forty-two weeks in length. Tests of fetal well-being should begin when, by the best estimate, forty-two weeks have elapsed since the last menstrual period.

Research has demonstrated that the placenta of an infant suffering from so-called fetal postmaturity syndrome undergoes degenerative changes which have the effect of decreasing the amount of oxygen and nutrients delivered to the fetus. Metabolic wastes also accumulate. Postmature infants are especially sensitive to the stress which labor produces and the degenerative changes described cause fetal death either before or during labor. It would be nice to have one accurate test which could distinguish between a healthy postdate fetus and one that is suffering from fetal postmaturity syndrome. Unfortunately, this is not the case. The determination of twenty-four-hour urinary estriols, three times a week, has proven to be notoriously inaccurate. The study of human placental lactogen, or HPL, once hailed as the most accurate test for evaluating postmaturity, has been abandoned by most medical centers.

The detection of meconium in the amniotic fluid through amnioscopy or amniocentesis, as a possible indicator of postmaturity, has many disadvantages. Furthermore, the significance of finding meconium in the amniotic fluid has been questioned. Formerly believed to be an indicator of fetal distress, it has been found that most babies with meconium are not compromised.

Most obstetricians use weekly electronic fetal monitoring. In a 1981 study, published in the *American Journal of Obstetrics and Gynecology* doctors found that the nonstress test (NST) was misleading and gave false reassurance of fetal well-being in 10 to 125 postterm patients. The CST, in contrast, accurately unmasked problem pregnancies. As a result of these studies, many doctors are now performing CSTs, rather than NSTs, as the initial test for evaluating the health of the postdate fetus. If the CST is negative, it should be repeated at five- to seven-day intervals, since the chance of fetal death occurring within a week of a normal test is usually less than 1 percent. If the CST becomes positive, immediate delivery is usually indicated. Ultrasound is rapidly becoming a valuable tool for evaluating the postdate pregnancy. Characteristic signs of placental aging, decreased amniotic fluid volume, and abnormal fetal movements can occasionally be identified by an expert ultrasonographer.

When it is firmly established that pregnancy is prolonged and the cervix is ripe, induction of labor should be carried out. It is imperative that electronic monitoring be used so that early evidence of distress may be detected. The condition of a severely compromised postmature infant will often worsen under the stress of labor. When the tests of fetal well-being indicate that immediate delivery is necessary but the cervix is unripe or unready for labor, cesarean section should be performed. Regardless of the route by which the baby is delivered, the obstetrician and pediatrician must be prepared to immediately suction the meconium from its mouth, nose, throat, and pharynx before it takes its first breath. Immediately following delivery, a tube should be placed into the trachea, or windpipe, of the postmature infant and as much meconium as possible should be removed by suction. If these precautions are not taken, the meconium may be aspirated into the lungs and cause pneumonia, respiratory distress, and even death. Postmature infants must also be carefully watched in the nursery for complications which may result from their low blood sugar and calcium levels.

**Forceps
Delivery**

What are obstetric forceps?

Obstetric forceps are paired metallic instruments designed for rotation and/or extraction of the baby's head after full dilatation of the cervix. The blades of the forceps, resembling the end of a shoehorn, are applied against the side of the head, and traction is exerted by pulling on the interlocked handles (see illustration).

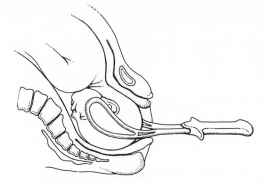

*Proper application of forceps
to the side of the baby's head.*

There are many types of obstetric forceps, most of them named after the doctors who invented them. Some are designed specifically for exerting traction, while others are used primarily for rotating or turning the baby's head into a more favorable position for delivery.

Forceps operations are classified according to the level and position of the head in the birth canal when the blades are applied and bear no relation to the type of instrument used. There are three classifications of forceps operations:

1. Low or outlet forceps. The scalp is visible at the vaginal opening, without having to separate the labia to see it. With low forceps, the head of the baby rests low on the pelvic floor, and its face is turned in the direction of the maternal spine. The baby's sagital suture, or the line formed in the middle of the top of its head by the joining of the two parietal bones, must be positioned front to back in relation to the maternal pelvis if the criteria of a low-forceps delivery are to be met. Some doctors differentiate outlet forceps from low forceps by the fact that the perineum is considerably more distended by the head. A low-forceps delivery is usually very easy to perform if carried out by a competent obstetrician.

2. Midforceps. In this more difficult operation, the forceps are applied after the head is engaged but before the conditions for low forceps have been met. The head is engaged if an imaginary line between the two parietal bones on the top of the baby's skull has descended to a level below the woman's bony pelvic inlet. Any forceps operation requiring rotation of the baby's head is a midforceps operation, regardless of how low in the pelvis the head has descended. Occasionally, a doctor may erroneously believe that the baby's head is engaged when it is not. This is especially likely to occur after a long, difficult labor, characterized by swelling and molding of the fetal head due to pressure against the cervix. In this situation the risk of trauma to the fetus and mother is greatly enhanced.

While some midforceps operations are extremely easy to perform, others are quite difficult and hazardous. Unfortunately, an obstetrician is not always able to predict the degree of difficulty until the midforceps delivery is attempted.

3. High forceps. In this operation, the baby's head is not engaged and may even be floating above the pelvic brim. High forceps has no place in modern obstetrics because it carries great risk for a mother and her baby.

Under what circumstances can an obstetrician justify the use of forceps?

Not too long ago, a large part of the "art" of obstetrics centered around the ability of an obstetrician to perform a difficult midforceps delivery soon after a woman's cervix was fully dilated. But, it was shown that the number of maternal complications, in the form of cervical and vaginal lacerations and hemorrhage, as well as the number of infant deaths, rose substantially following these difficult maneuvers. Though indications for attempting a forceps operation still remain, midforceps deliveries have been replaced by more cesarean sections. The tremendous popularity of prepared childbirth education has been a very important factor in reducing the number of women seeking anesthesia, forceps, or other forms of medical interference in the birth process.

Most forceps deliveries are termed "prophylactic" or "elective." Simply translated, this means that they are performed without clear-cut medical reasons. Included among these dubious indications are a desire to reduce a woman's effort and discomfort during the second stage of labor, to save her perineal tissues from overstretching, and to reduce the risk of fetal brain injury from prolonged pushing of the head against an unyielding perineum. In the presence of an uneventful pregnancy and labor, these alleged benefits would appear to be questionable at best. A more likely benefit of "prophylactic" forceps is that it shortens the doctor's stay in the hospital with his patient.

Forceps use is indicated if, for a variety of reasons, a woman is unable to push the baby's head out following a prolonged effort. Though there are no absolute and arbitrary rules, a second stage of labor exceeding two hours in a woman having her first child would be considered prolonged. For someone who has previously given birth, more than one hour of full dilatation with pushing would usually be considered to be abnormal. Arrest of progress during the second stage may be caused by fatigue, too much medication, poor uterine contractions, weak abdominal musculature, excessively resistant or inelastic perineal tissues, or a large baby. An abnormal position of the baby's head, such as the occiput posterior or transverse positions, may also be responsible for this problem.

One very important indication for the use of forceps is the diagnosis of fetal distress. Occasionally, an obstetrician must make a rapid decision and weigh the relative risks of an immediate forceps delivery against those of a cesarean section or further delay in hopes that the distress will correct itself. Often, valuable minutes may be lost while preparations are being made for a cesarean section.

Under certain medical conditions a forceps operation may be preferred to spontaneous vaginal delivery. For example, a woman with heart disease will fare better if she avoids bearing down efforts during the second stage. Similarly, a woman with a history of retinal detachment should not raise her intracranial pressure with excessive pushing. Obstetrical complications, such as severe abruptio placenta and a prolapsed umbilical cord, often demand instant delivery with forceps rather than a prolonged second stage of labor. Forceps are also valuable for delivery of very small babies because they are more prone to develop intracranial hemorrhage as a result of prolonged bearing down efforts.

Before a forceps operation is attempted, certain conditions must be fulfilled in order to minimize maternal and fetal hazards. These include the following:

1. The obstetrician must be skilled in the use of forceps.
2. The pelvis must be large enough to permit delivery of an undamaged baby.
3. The cervix must be completely dilated.
4. The woman's urinary bladder should be emptied with a catheter in order to prevent injuring it.
5. Adequate anesthesia must be given, and the anesthesiologist must remain in attendance throughout the delivery.
6. The fetal position must be precisely known.
7. The fetal head must be engaged in the pelvis.
8. The amniotic membranes must be ruptured so that the forceps can fit firmly against the baby's head.

Isn't a cesarean section safer for a baby than a forceps delivery?

Not always. There is no doubt that a low-forceps delivery is infinitely safer for both mother and child than a cesarean section. Fears of such a procedure are unfounded.

Many doctors believe that if an easy spontaneous or outlet forceps delivery is not possible, cesarean section should be performed so that the risk of fetal and maternal trauma may be reduced. The research of Dr. Emanuel Friedman noted 2 deaths per 1,000 spontaneous deliveries, compared with 11 deaths per 1,000 with midforceps, and 29 per 1,000 if the midforceps delivery followed a protracted labor. More importantly, Dr. Friedman found that the quality of life also suffers in newborns surviving midforceps deliveries. Speech and hearing disorders at the age of three were 6 per 1,000 following spontaneous vaginal delivery and 33 per 1,000 following arrested labors which were terminated by midforceps. Significantly lower IQ scores have also been noted at the age of four among babies delivered by midforceps. As a result, most obstetrical units in the United States are replacing the midforceps operative delivery with greater numbers of cesarean sections.

Vacuum Extraction

What is a vacuum extractor and how does its safety compare to that of forceps?

As a substitute for midforceps and low-forceps operations, the vacuum extractor has gained wide acceptance in Europe, but not in the United States. To use this instrument, a metal or plastic traction cup is first attached to the back of the baby's scalp. Negative pressure is then built up slowly over several minutes so that the cup adheres firmly to the area of the scalp on which it is attached. After adequate suction is obtained, an obstetrician exerts traction by pulling on a chain which passes through the suction tube.

Theoretically, the vacuum extractor has several advantages over the use of forceps. The overall severity of maternal and fetal injuries is less with this device. The procedure is easy to master. Unlike forceps, the vacuum extractor can be applied before the cervix is fully dilated, and anesthesia is not necessary for its use. In the case of fetal distress, in which a vaginal delivery is imperative, this can be a great advantage.

The vacuum extractor, however, is not harmless. In fact, it may be associated with trauma to the fetal scalp in the form of abrasions and lacerations. Hematomas, or blood clot formation under the skin of the scalp, are known to occur in 10 to 12 percent of infants delivered by vacuum extraction. Deaths following trauma, though extremely rare, have also been reported. Some studies have demonstrated a higher incidence of hemorrhage within the skull and the eyes among babies delivered with this device.

If your doctor is a vacuum extractor enthusiast, be sure that he or she adheres to the following criteria for use:

1. Your amniotic membranes must be ruptured.
2. Your pelvis must be of adequate size.
3. Your cervix must be sufficiently dilated to apply the vacuum cup. Advanced dilatation allows the use of larger cups and results in a safer and shorter labor.
4. The cup should be placed as close to the back of your baby's scalp as possible.
5. Negative-vacuum pressure should not exceed 0.7 to 0.8 kilograms per square centimeter.
6. The cup should not remain on the baby's scalp longer than a maximum of forty-five minutes. Short application times reduce the incidence of fetal scalp injury.
7. Your doctor should exert traction in synchrony with your uterine contractions and your voluntary bearing-down efforts.
8. The cup should not be allowed to "pop off," thereby causing sudden pressure changes in the scalp and increasing the risk of injury.
9. If progress is not evident after three or four pulls, your doctor should stop, reevaluate your situation, and consider the use of another method of delivery.

Breech Births

How frequent are breech births and what are the causes?

The breech, or buttocks-first, position of the baby occurs in 3 or 4 percent of all deliveries, with a much higher incidence noted among premature infants. Many theories have been proposed to explain why a baby assumes a breech position. Factors other than prematurity which appear related to this condition include uterine relaxation in a woman who has had several previous children, multiple births, excessive amounts of amniotic fluid (hydramnios), congenital abnormalities such as hydrocephaly and anencephaly, maternal uterine anomalies, and the location of the placenta. Women with placenta previa, an abnormally low-lying placenta, are more likely to carry a baby in the breech position. Similarly, a placental location in the cornua, or upper lateral part of the uterus, predisposes to a breech position. But the cause of a breech position remains unknown in the vast majority of cases. It also remains a mystery as to why a woman who gives birth to one breech will be more likely to do so again.

How is the breech position diagnosed?

The relationship between the legs and buttocks of a fetus in the breech position falls into one of three classifications: frank breech, complete breech, and incomplete breech (see illustration).

The frank breech position is the most common and is associated with the lowest number of complications (see below). As the cervix dilates during labor, one or both feet of an incomplete breech may drop down into the vagina through the dilated cervix. This is then known as a single and double footling breech, respectively, and both conditions are associated with a much higher complication rate (see below) than the frank breech and the complete breech.

Most experienced obstetricians can diagnose a breech position simply by palpating a woman's abdomen. Often, the patient suspects the diagnosis before her doctor because she detects the hardness of the fetal head in the upper abdomen, accompanied by a greater amount of lower abdominal kicking. If the findings on abdominal palpation are in doubt, a vaginal examination usually confirms the diagnosis. Occasionally, however, the buttocks of a frank breech can confuse an examiner into believing that he or she is palpating the head. Absolute confirmation of a breech can be made by ultrasound or abdominal x-ray examinations. The breech position is probably one of the few remaining valid indications for the use of x-ray pelvimetry. This x-ray examination has the great advantage of being able to demonstrate the relationship between the fetal breech and the bony structures of the maternal pelvis. Accurate assessment of the diameter and shape of the maternal pelvis is vital if vaginal delivery of a baby in the breech position is contemplated. This important information cannot be obtained with ultrasound. However, fetal anomalies, more

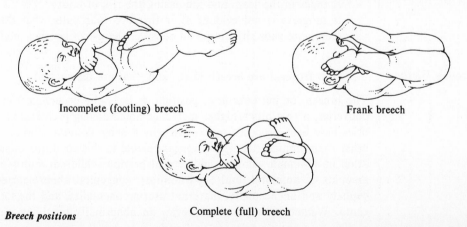

Incomplete (footling) breech   Frank breech

Breech positions   Complete (full) breech common among breech babies, are most readily identified with an ultrasound examination.

What problems may be encountered when a baby is in a breech position?

There is no doubt that the prognosis for a fetus in a breech position is considerably worse than that of a head-first position. This is true at every stage of pregnancy. In a report comparing the results of head-first deliveries with over 1,000 breech births, doctors at the University Hospitals in Cleveland noted a ten times greater overall mortality rate in the breech group. In addition, birth defects occurred in 6.3 percent of breech deliveries but only 2.4 percent of nonbreech births. When the same comparison is made between healthy babies weighing more than 5½ pounds, the results, though less striking, are still significant. In one study, conducted at Mount Sinai Hospital in New York City, the death rate was 3 percent among breech babies, compared to less than 1 percent for those in the head-first position.

While trauma to the baby may occur at any time during a vaginal breech delivery, problems are most commonly encountered when the obstetrician attempts to deliver the head. This is especially worrisome in the woman having her first baby. Unfortunately, x-ray pelvimetry demonstrating adequate maternal size is no guarantee that the head will be delivered easily. There is no obstetrical situation which is more frantic and desperately tragic than the inability to successfully and atraumatically deliver the head of a baby in the breech position. Time is crucial in these circumstances, since a delay of four or more minutes is likely to result in permanent brain damage due to a lack of oxygen received by the fetus. At this stage, the point of no return has been reached, because it is too late to perform an emergency cesarean section. Entrapment of the breech baby's head by a cervix which is not fully dilated is most likely to occur with a footling breech. In this situation, the legs easily pass through the cervix, but successively larger, less readily compressible parts must then be delivered. The largest structure, namely the head, may then be unable to pass. Head entrapment is also significantly more common when the baby weighs in excess of 8 pounds. While one would assume that a premature infant, weighing less than 5½ pounds, would be less apt to encounter this problem, the opposite is true. As previously mentioned, there is a disproportion between the large size of the head and the small buttocks of the premature infant. The incidence of head entrapment is greatest among those premature babies who are smallest.

Prolapse of the umbilical cord, an acute emergency requiring immediate delivery, is far more common among babies in the breech position. Even when prolapse is not present, delivery of the buttocks draws the umbilicus and attached cord into the pelvis and causes compression. Therefore, once the buttocks of the baby has passed the vaginal opening, the rest of its body must be delivered promptly.

Can anything be done to prevent the breech position from developing?

Whenever a breech position is recognized during the last trimester, some obstetricians attempt to turn the baby to the safer and more common head-first position by rotating it through palpation and manipulation over the maternal abdominal wall. This technique, known as external cephalic version, is accomplished by the obstetrician gently lifting the breech out of the pelvis with one hand while pushing the head downward with the other. External cephalic version is easier to accomplish if a woman has previously given birth because of the greater laxity of her abdominal wall musculature. Recently, doctors have claimed greater success with external cephalic version when it is immediately preceded by an intravenous injection of a uterine muscle relaxant such as ritodrine and terbutaline. However, the benefits of this form of therapy have not been fully evaluated.

Some doctors enthusiastically support external cephalic version, but this enthusiasm is not shared by most obstetricians, and the majority of residency programs in the United States devote little if any time to the mastery of this technique. Some doctors attribute complications, such as uterine hemorrhage, premature labor, fetal death, premature rupture of the amniotic membranes, and premature separation of the placenta, to attempts at external cephalic version. In one study in which 100 external cephalic versions were performed, a significant number of red blood cells were found to pass from the fetal to the maternal circulation. This co-called feto-maternal hemorrhage is especially significant among women who are Rh-negative. To prevent Rh sensitization, RhoGam should probably be administered whenever external cephalic version is attempted for these women.

This procedure should not be used if there is a marked disproportion between the size of the fetus and the maternal pelvis, the breech is too deep in the pelvis to safely lift it out, the abdominal wall or uterus is tense, the amniotic membranes are ruptured, and if there is only a minimal amount of amniotic fluid present (oligohydramnios). Anesthesia must never be administered when an external cephalic version is attempted because a woman's ability to detect pain is often the best indication that her doctor is exerting too much force.

Is there any way to predict which breech babies can be safely delivered vaginally and which ones will require cesarean section?

The Zatuchni-Andros Breech Scoring Index was developed by doctors of the same names in an effort to more accurately predict which infants would require cesarean section and which ones could safely deliver vaginally. Points are given for six determining factors: number of previous children, length of pregnancy in weeks, estimated fetal weight, delivery of a previous full-term breech, dilatation of the cervix at the initial vaginal examination in the hospital, and station or level of the breech in relation to the maternal ischial spines. The Breech Scoring Index is a helpful guide which has been used with success by many obstetricians, though it is certainly not infallible.

Whenever vaginal delivery of a breech is contemplated, an obstetrician must consider many different factors, the most important of which is the fetal size. The very large fetus is extremely likely to be traumatized when a vaginal breech delivery is attempted. Although estimates of fetal weight, based on the use of ultrasound, are an aid, these calculations are far from foolproof. If it is determined that the fetus weights 8 pounds or more, most experts would agree that a cesarean section should be performed. This advice applies even if the mother's pelvis appears to be of normal or above-normal size.

The adequacy and configuration of the maternal pelvis must be precisely determined before an attempted vaginal delivery of a full-term breech. Even if a minimal amount of pelvic contraction is detected on x-ray pelvimetry, cesarean section is necessary.

Marked extension of a fetal head may be detected by x-ray in 5 percent of all babies in the breech position. Cesarean section is indicated when the head is hyperextended to prevent injury to the baby's neck and spinal cord.

The use of x-ray and ultrasound in the evaluation of a baby in the breech position may help to determine the route of delivery if an abnormality is detected. The diagnosis of a severe defect, incompatible with survival, would be the deciding factor in opting for a vaginal, rather than a cesarean delivery.

While some doctors have advocated the use of oxytocin when needed to induce or improve labor in a woman with a breech, the majority of evidence suggests that this use is associated with lower Apgar scores and higher infant mortality rates. Cesarean section is undoubtedly the much wiser choice.

All infants in the single or double footling position are best delivered by cesarean section because of the possibility of cord prolapse and entrapment of the fetal head when vaginal delivery is attempted.

The extremely premature infant, or one weighing between 1 pound 2 ounces to 3 pounds 5 ounces, is best delivered by cesarean section because it is less traumatic and not associated with entrapment of the head by a cervix which is not fully dilated.

Many practicing obstetricians consider the vaginal delivery of a breech to be a relatively safe procedure if the following criteria are met:

1. The baby is in a frank breech position and there is no hyperextension of the head.
2. It is not the woman's first full-term delivery.
3. The fetus is estimated to weigh between 5½ and 8 pounds based on clinical impression and ultrasound examination.
4. The estimated gestational age is between thirty-six and forty-two weeks.
5. There is no evidence of fetal distress.
6. Progress in labor, as determined by dilatation of the cervix and descent of the buttocks in the pelvis is normal.
7. The obstetrician is skilled and experienced in the techniques of breech delivery.
8. Adequate anesthesia and nearby operating room facilities are readily available.

Unfortunately, even if all of these criteria are fulfilled, the infant may still not fare as well as when a cesarean section is performed. While it is true that a vaginal delivery is safer for the mother than a cesarean section, there is a far greater risk of permanent fetal damage, cerebral palsy, and perinatal mortality following a vaginal breech delivery.

If you are left with the impression that the vast number of babies in the breech position should be managed with a cesarean section, you are absolutely correct!

There is little question that fetal trauma, hypoxia, and perinatal deaths can only be reduced by liberalizing the use of cesarean section. In most medical centers, the cesarean section rate for breech births has risen from an average of 10 percent to approximately 75 percent over the past ten years. The breech position is now the fourth leading cause for the increase in the number of cesarean sections in the United States. Many obstetricians in teaching positions have expressed concern that young residents in training are not obtaining sufficient opportunities to deliver breeches vaginally. As a result, it is predicted that future specialists will lack this important skill. Perhaps this is a blessing in disguise. I am firmly convinced that the escalating cesarean section rate in the management of breech positions is a justifiable development in modern obstetrics.

Cesarean Section

What factors account for today's soaring cesarean section rates?

Over the past fifteen years, the cesarean section rate in the United States has increased from less than 5 percent to over 15 percent, with some medical centers reporting rates higher than 20 percent. Failure to progress in labor accounts for approximately 30 percent of the increase; previous cesarean section, 27 percent; fetal distress, 20 percent; and breech position, 16 percent (the remaining percentages being for a variety of reasons).

The obstetrical management of labor through most of the 1960s differed markedly from today's more sophisticated state of the art. Lacking objective methods of evaluating labor progress, obstetricians frequently made decisions based solely on their personal experience and clinical intuition. Patience was considered the hallmark of good obstetrical care, and labor often lasted for hours and even days, frequently culminating in a difficult midforceps delivery of a severely depressed infant. More often than most obstetricians would care to admit, these maneuvers were responsible for a significantly higher incidence of maternal trauma and permanent fetal damage.

Probably the most important obstetrical contribution of the late 1960s and the 1970s was that of Dr. Emanuel A. Friedman (see page 360). He was the first to objectively evaluate the labor patterns of thousands of women and establish guidelines for the assessment of normal and abnormal labor, making it possible for obstetricians to rapidly diagnose and remedy labor abnormalities without subjecting a woman to an endless labor. The failure to progress in labor has become the single most important factor for the rising cesarean section rate in the United States over the past ten years. It has also been one of the main reasons for the decline in fetal and maternal morbidity incurred with prolonged, nonprogressive labor. Through the research of Dr. Friedman and others, the use of difficult midforceps delivery has now been replaced by cesarean section when labor fails to progress following full dilatation of the cervix.

Changing ideas in the 1970s about maternal nutrition during pregnancy has resulted in the birth of larger babies. This has contributed to the higher cesarean section rates for disproportion between the size of the baby and that of the maternal pelvis.

Ten years ago, thirty-two weeks of pregnancy was considered as early as one could justify the risk of cesarean section, weighed against the benefits for the immature fetus. An obstetrician today is more apt to perform a cesarean section to save a small fetus if ultrasound and clinical history suggest that survival is likely. The following guide summarizes fetal prognosis:

Birth weight (grams)	Percent age survival
1,000 grams (2 lbs. 4 oz.)	80
1,500 grams (3 lbs. 5 oz.)	88
2,000 grams (4 lbs. 7 oz.) or more	99

Even in the absence of obvious fetal distress, some doctors have endorsed use of cesarean section for infants born before the thirty-fifth week and those weighing between 700 and 1,900 grams. The reason for this is that smaller babies are more likely to experience intracranial hemorrhage due to pressure on the head caused by uterine muscle contractions and the perineum.

The 20 percent increase in cesarean section rates for fetal distress over the past fifteen years can be attributed to the introduction of electronic fetal monitoring and other technology which allows for more rapid diagnosis of fetal distress.

The marked increase in cesarean section rates for babies in the breech position is a recent trend based on convincing clinical experience. It is now estimated that 75 percent of all breech births result in cesarean section, compared to 10 percent only ten years ago.

Since the incidence of cesarean section deliveries has increased dramatically in the last decade, it is not surprising to note a 27 percent rise in the number of repeat cesareans. However, the philosophy of "once a cesarean section, always a cesarean section" has been questioned in recent years.

With the development of newer and more potent antibiotics, modern blood bank facilities, more sophisticated anesthetic techniques, and improved postpartum care, cesarean section is no longer regarded as a significant risk to a woman. However, we tend to lose sight of the fact that it is still a major abdominal operation which is accompanied by a significantly higher incidence of maternal complications than a vaginal delivery. Occasionally a couple requests and even demands a cesarean section in preference to the pain and discomfort associated with childbirth. This apparently simple solution is not nearly as innocuous as one would imagine. Even under the most modern and ideal conditions, cesarean section is associated with a four- to fivefold increase in the maternal mortality rate. The most often quoted statistics are that there will be between 4 and 8 maternal deaths per 10,000 cesarean sections, compared to .3 per 10,000 following a vaginal birth. The incidence of postoperative pain, fever, hemorrhage, and other complications, combined with a longer, more expensive hospital stay and prolonged recovery period, makes a cesarean section a far less attractive option than a vaginal birth.

It has been claimed that physicians are using cesarean delivery as protection against malpractice suits. There is no doubt that in today's malpractice climate, many obstetricians are more comfortable performing a cesarean than attempting a simple and safe low-forceps delivery, particularly in view of the fact that many doctors have been sued for failure or delay in performing a cesarean. In fact, the second biggest malpractice charge related to cesarean section is failure of a doctor to perform an indicated cesarean which would have prevented injury or death. The most frequent complaint in cesarean-related litigation is failure to perform the procedure correctly. Of late, there has also been a rise in the number of malpractice cases alleging unnecessary surgery. Medicolegal experts agree that physicians who choose cesarean delivery for fear that a poor outcome with vaginal birth may result in a lawsuit must now fear legal action if a premature and unnecessary operation is performed.

I have heard it said that obstetricians are motivated to perform cesarean section because they can charge more than for a vaginal delivery. While a doctor does get a larger fee for doing a cesarean, I doubt that this is the prime consideration of most sane physicians. This is supported by statistics from the National Naval Medical Center in Bethesda, Maryland, which show that the cesarean section rate at naval hospitals is 15 percent. This rate closely parallels the national figures. Physicians at these hospitals are salaried and have no economic incentive to perform more cesarean deliveries. The contention that obstetricians perform significantly more cesarean sections on weekends for convenience and personal gain has been clearly refuted in a 1982 article published in the *Journal of the American Medical Association*. In this statistical study, it was shown that cesareans for both fetal distress and failure of labor progress were no more likely on any particular day of the week.

Despite the fact that obstetricians have been criticized for soaring cesarean section rates in the United States, the undeniable fact is that it has coincided with a significant drop in the infant death rates during the past decade. Although the significance of this association has been questioned by many researchers, in a 1977 report from California, investigators found that hospitals with higher cesarean section rates were more likely to use fetal monitoring, had more obstetrician-attended deliveries and provided better access to neonatal intensive care. In other words, those hospitals with the best technical facilities had the lowest infant death rate, as well as the highest number of cesarean sections. Indigent hospitals, lacking modern equipment and competent obstetrical personnel, also demonstrated lower cesarean section rates and subsequent higher numbers of perinatal deaths.

How can the number of cesarean sections in the United States be safely reduced?

Much has been written about the excessive number of cesarean sections performed in the United States, but few doctors or consumer advocates have offered rational suggestions for significantly reducing this amount below 15 percent. For example, many have voiced astonishment and rage at the rising number of operations performed for babies in the breech position, with some hospitals reporting rates as high as 75 percent or more. Professors of obstetrics tell us that the practicing physician should be able to safely deliver a breech if certain criteria are met despite the fact that 3 out of every 100 babies, even in their educated hands, will still incur significant injury at birth. The fact that a practicing obstetrician has elected to perform a vaginal breech delivery, based on criteria established by a group of professors, is no guarantee of a successful result or a malpractice-proof defense in the event of failure. In my opinion, the 75 percent cesarean section rate for breeches is probably too low, and I advise critics to look elsewhere in their efforts to reduce the number of unnecessary cesarean sections. There is no doubt in my mind that a well-performed cesarean section is infinitely safer for mother and child than a difficult breech birth. Part of the increase in the cesarean section rate for uterine dysfunction is due to the decrease in the use of difficult forceps operations to deal with poor progress in labor after full dilatation of the cervix. I hope this trend continues. We will all benefit from lower rates of infant death, fetal trauma, and tragic instances of cerebral palsy.

It may be possible to lower the number of cesarean section operations performed for fetal distress. Electronic fetal monitoring has enabled doctors to diagnose fetal distress both before and during labor. While this diagnosis is now the third leading reason for the increased number of cesarean sections, it can on occasion be less than totally accurate and reliable. Normal fetuses undergoing stress and those who are compromised and truly distressed may show the same abnormal patterns on the electronic fetal monitor. As a result, when cesarean sections are done solely because of abnormal patterns on the monitor, a significant proportion of healthy infants are delivered with good Apgar scores and no evidence of distress. When confronted with an abnormal fetal heart pattern, some obstetricians rush to deliver their patient by cesarean section. In most cases, conformation of fetal acidosis by scalp sampling techniques should be undertaken, and if fetal distress is not confirmed, close observation rather than surgery is usually indicated.

Surprisingly, less than half the obstetrical units in the United States employ scalp pH determinations because it is felt the technique is too cumbersome and time consuming. However, these reasons are unacceptable since scalp pH determinations significantly reduce the number of unnecessary cesarean sections. Even when a hospital has the facilities to perform scalp pHs, the technique is not always used. In one report, only 25 percent of patients with a diagnosis of intrapartum fetal distress were offered scalp pH blood sampling. Ask your doctor if the hospital in which you plan to have your baby has the equipment to perform scalp pH measurements, and if he or she makes use of these facilities when indicated.

The number of cesarean births may be significantly lowered by allowing more women with previous cesareans to attempt vaginal delivery (see page 384), reducing the need for a repeat operation by as much as 30 to 60 percent. Unfortunately, most obstetricians in the United States remain unconvinced of the many advantages of allowing labor among women with previous cesareans. Once again, only careful selection of your obstetrician and hospital will help to reduce your chances of an unnecessary repeat cesarean section.

A new, imprecisely defined, obstetrical term "failure to progress," has emerged, replacing the older term "dystocia." Whether it's called "failure to progress" or "dystocia," it is by far the largest contributor to the overall rise in the cesarean section rate in this country. It has been estimated that ineffectual contractions account for three-fourths of all cesareans performed for "failure to progress" and delivery of a fetus too large to pass through the maternal bony pelvis accounts for the remaining one-fourth. Ineffectual uterine contractions, in the absence of too large a fetus, can be made effective with intravenous oxytocin while carefully monitoring the fetus, thus improving labor efficiency and reducing the need for cesarean section. But not enough doctors use this obstetrically sound technique. In a 1980 study of 182 women with ineffectual labor contractions from Women and Infants Hospital of Rhode Island, doctors found that oxytocin was used in only 23 percent of women whose clinical indication for cesarean was uterine muscle dysfunction, or "failure to progress." Certainly more active physician intervention in the form of careful augmentation of uterine contractions with oxytocin will help reduce the number of operations performed for "failure to progress." When the cervix fails to dilate progressively during active labor, intravenous oxytocin usually brings progress within one to three hours. It is easier and less time consuming for a doctor to perform a cesarean than to carefully evaluate and monitor the strength of a woman's contractions or to sit with her while she is receiving intravenous oxytocin. There must be more valid reasons for cesarean section than that of doctor convenience.

Occasionally, the early or latent phase of labor is prolonged for more than twenty-four hours. Too often, the latent phase contractions prevent a woman from sleeping, and when the active phase of labor finally begins she is totally exhausted and unable to cope with the contractions. This problem is often intensified if an obstetrician restricts liquids during this phase of early labor and does not provide emotional support and a clear explanation of the prolonged latent phase to allay a woman's fears. A prolonged latent phase which can be managed successfully with rest, fluids, and sedation is too often mistakenly diagnosed as "failure to progress," and cesarean section is performed. In 1980, the National Institute of Health organized the Cesarean Birth Task Force to evaluate the reasons behind the rising cesarean section rates in the United States and to offer suggestions for safely improving these statistics. In addition to the above recommendations, they also endorsed peer review within hospitals to be sure that obstetricians were not too quick to perform "failure to progress" cesareans. I would heartily agree with this suggestion, in view of the fact that the task force found no infant survival advantage of cesarean over vaginal delivery when surgery was performed for this reason. Furthermore, in more than 90 percent of all cesarean deliveries performed for dystocia, the babies were of average size and were in the normal cephalic, or head-first, position.

Under what conditions can a woman attempt labor and vaginal delivery following a previous cesarean section?

"Once a cesarean section, always a cesarean section" was first proposed as a clinical dictum by Dr. Edwin B. Craigin in 1916. Until recently, American obstetricians have blindly followed this practice; 98 percent of women in this country who have had a cesarean section will undergo a repeat operation. Thanks to the objections of both consumer advocates and some leading obstetricians, this practice is now being questioned in many medical centers.

Evidence to date suggests that between 50 and 60 percent of women who have had cesarean sections should be able to subsequently deliver vaginally if allowed to try. While proponents of repeat cesarean section may argue that it is easier and safer than a vaginal delivery, statistics do not bear this out. Even under the most ideal conditions, cesarean section has a four- to fivefold higher maternal mortality than vaginal delivery. Though we have come to consider a cesarean section as a relatively minor procedure, in actual fact it is a major operation accompanied by a greater blood loss and anesthetic risk than vaginal delivery. Immediate postoperative problems such as infection, a greater degree of pain, and a longer and more expensive hospital stay cannot be denied. Later complications, such as abdominal and pelvic adhesions, may cause intestinal blockage in a small percentage of women years after the surgery has been performed. The newborn mortality rate and the incidence of respiratory distress syndrome (RDS) is higher among babies delivered by cesarean section. Though modern technology has decreased the incidence of RDS, the problem has not been eliminated and fetal and maternal complications have been known to occur following use of these techniques. Women undergoing cesarean section require significantly more pain medication during the postpartum period and greater amounts of these drugs pass into the breast milk and are ingested by the nursing infant.

Doctors are often too insensitive to the fact that vaginal delivery is far more emotionally satisfying for a woman than cesarean section. Many of my patients have expressed great disappointment and the feeling of having failed because they were unable to experience the physical and psychological "high" of delivering vaginally. The close maternal-infant contact and bonding so vital in the first few days of life is often never realized because the mother suffers from the pain and discomfort of surgery and is sleepy and nauseous from the potent analgesics used. Many women rightfully believe that they have been cheated from experiencing a very special event.

The main argument that proponents of repeat cesarean section have used for years is that rupture or tearing of the previous uterine scar, under the stress of labor contractions, will be accompanied by catastrophic hemorrhage and expulsion of the fetus into the abdominal cavity. This presumption, while possibly true in 1916, no longer applies today. In 1916, all cesarean sections were performed through a classical or vertical incision into the muscles of the upper uterine segment (see figure 11–5). Even after healing, the tissues of the scar from such an incision remain permanently weakened, and uterine expansion during a subsequent pregnancy or labor causes rupture 2 percent of the time. Of this 2 percent, one-half occurs during labor and the other half before its onset. The consequences of a classical incision rupture may be truly catastrophic since the entire uterine wall ruptures. The fetus and placenta extrudes into the abdominal cavity, through a complete uterine rupture, and the infant mortality rate is between 40 and 75 percent. The maternal mortality from hemorrhage has been estimated at less than 1 percent. Because of the dangers involved, a woman who has had a previous classical cesarean section should never be allowed to attempt labor and vaginal delivery. A repeat cesarean section is the much wiser option. Although still performed today, classical cesarean sections comprise less than 5 percent of the total number of cesareans. The operation is occasionally indicated for an unusual position of the baby, such as a transverse lie, or to minimize bleeding when the placenta is covering the usual incision site over the lower cervix, a condition known as placenta previa.

The so-called low cervical transverse cesarean section is performed through the tissues of the lower uterine segment and cervix. Today, practically all cesareans are of this type. Since connective tissue and only a thin layer of muscle is cut with this incision, it is far less likely to rupture than the classical operation. Another contributing factor is that most of the force of a uterine contraction comes from the upper segment, while the lower segment plays a more passive role. The reported rate of rupture of a low transverse scar is 0.25 to 0.5 percent. Even when it does occur, it hardly ever happens before the onset of labor and it is highly unlikely to be catastrophic. It may even go unrecognized because the rupture of a low transverse scar is usually incomplete. At least one tissue layer remains intact and consequently, the baby hardly ever is extruded into the abdominal cavity. Sometimes the uterine tissue layer is so thin that, at the time of a repeat cesarean section, the amniotic fluid and baby can actually be seen through the scar. This phenomenon, appropriately called a "window," is seen in 8 percent of all repeat low transverse cesarean sections. In the rare case where rupture is complete, the perinatal mortality rate is approximately 12 percent.

Several clinical studies support the claim that many women with a previous low cervical transverse cesarean section may safely labor and deliver vaginally during a subsequent pregnancy. A 1979 report from the University of Texas Health Science Center and Medical School at San Antonio, showed that of 526 women who were allowed to labor after a previous cesarean section, 313 successfully delivered and 213 required repeat cesarean sections. There were 3 instances of a ruptured uterus but no maternal or fetal mortalities. In a review of 110,000 deliveries and 4,000 cesarean sections at the Margaret Hague Maternity Hospital in New Jersey, between 1950 and 1962, there were no maternal deaths in patients whose uterus ruptured during labor after a previous cesarean section. Only 1 out of every 160 scars ruptured and no mothers lost their lives.

A small percentage of doctors perform low vertical, rather than transverse incisions (see figure 11–5). This technique, also known as a "semiclassical incision," is sometimes helpful for delivering small premature infants, babies in breech or transverse positions, and very large babies. However, this incision is associated with a 1.4 to 4 percent chance of sudden rupture and shock during a subsequent pregnancy or labor. Another type of incision, known as the "inverted T," usually occurs out of desperation when difficulty is encountered while trying to deliver a baby through a low cervical transverse incision. The base of the T is an ad-lib incision performed to allow more room for delivery. An inverted T heals into a significantly weaker scar, predisposed to rupture during a future pregnancy. For this reason, women with "semiclassical" and inverted T-type incisions should not be allowed to labor. The four types of incisions discussed are shown in the accompanying illustration.

Knowing the type of previous incision you had is crucial in determining whether or not you should be allowed to labor in a subsequent pregnancy. If you have moved or changed doctors and are contemplating an attempt at a vaginal delivery, it is vital

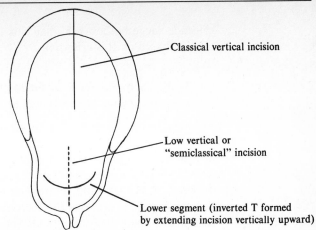

Types of cesarean section incisions.

Classical vertical incision

Low vertical or "semiclassical" incision

Lower segment (inverted T formed by extending incision vertically upward)

that you secure your previous doctor's operative notes. These are kept on file in the record room of the hospital in which you had your cesarean section. It is only in this way that you will know with certainty the type of incision you received. Many women confuse the scar on their abdominal skin with the type of uterine incision that they received. It is important to realize that a long, vertical scar on the skin is as likely to be associated with a low transverse cervical incision as is a "bikini," or horizontal hairline incision.

In addition to the type of previous uterine incision, doctors take several other factors into consideration when deciding if a woman should be allowed a trial of labor rather than a repeat cesarean section. Since this whole concept is relatively new, standards vary from one obstetrician to another and from one hospital to the next. For example, some obstetricians allow all women a trial of labor, regardless of the reason for the initial cesarean. Others exclude those whose first cesarean was for a "recurring" reason such as a small pelvis in relation to the size of the baby's head, although the diagnosis of cephalopelvic disproportion is often imprecise and based on unreliable data and doctors have observed the vaginal birth of many babies with greater birth weights than those previously delivered by cesarean section. Some doctors refuse to chance a vaginal delivery if a patient has had two or more previous cesareans because they believe that the scar may be weaker. There is no evidence to support or refute this claim. A woman who has had five or more previous full-term births may have a weakened uterus which can be accentuated if one or more of the births is by cesarean section. Under these conditions, I might agree that a repeat cesarean would be the most prudent option. Similarly, the presence of an overdistended uterus, caused by twins or an excessive amount of amniotic fluid, in a woman with a previous cesarean section, would make most obstetricians opt for a repeat operation. Some doctors foolishly insist that a woman have at least one vaginal delivery prior to the previous cesarean section before they will allow her to undergo labor again. Obviously, this would exclude too many women from attempting a vaginal birth and would disqualify all women not giving birth to three or more children. Other obstetricians believe that if a woman has experienced postoperative fever or infection with a previous cesarean section, she will be more likely to have a weakened uterine incision. They, therefore, prescribe a repeat cesarean section. Recent evidence suggests, however, that it is impossible to judge the future strength of an incision based on this criterion.

Is there any way for a doctor to predict if a transverse low cervical cesarean section scar will hold up when subjected to the stress of labor?

To evaluate the strength of a cesarean incision, doctors have taken special x-rays, called hysterograms, several weeks following surgery. With this procedure, radiopaque dye is injected into the uterine cavity through the cervix in order to detect defects which may be present in the scar. In a 1979 study from Holland, conducted by Dr. P. J. H. van Vugt, hysterograms were performed on sixty-eight women who had undergone a previous low cervical transverse cesarean section. He concluded that it was impossible to correlate the weakness of the scar with postpartum infection and fever in those studied. He noted more defects in the uterine scar in women who were sectioned after a long labor in which the lower uterine segment was well formed and thin than in those who underwent cesarean before labor began. Dr. van Vugt concluded that the thickness of the lower uterine segment at the time of cesarean section determines the eventual thickness of the scar. However, he cautioned that a thick uterine scar was not a guarantee against rupture and that a thin scar did not necessarily mean that it would be defective.

While it has been claimed that certain surgical techniques and the use of specific suture material at the time of cesarean section minimizes scar defects, most obstetricians now believe this is not true. Furthermore, the hysterogram appearance is a less than ideal predictor of the strength or weakness of the incision. In summary, the strength of the previous low cervical transverse incision is only known following a trial of labor during a subsequent pregnancy.

What precautions should be taken when caring for a laboring woman who has had a previous cesarean section?

Do not be surprised if you have difficulty finding a doctor who will agree to your request for a trial of labor following your previous cesarean section. An obstetrician who refuses to care for you is often more honorable than one who agrees but then does nothing to insure a successful pregnancy outcome.

Before labor begins, your doctor should be familiar with your previous obstetrical history and the operative description of your cesarean section in order to determine the type of incision which was performed and any complications which may have been encountered. It is vital that you and your doctor have a clear understanding as to how he or she is going to measure your progress in labor and at what point intervention, in the form of a repeat cesarean, would be necessary. Some doctors may promise you a trial of labor, but at the moment of truth will back down and claim that you need a repeat operation. The same criteria used to assess labor progress for all women should be applied to those undergoing a trial of labor, and you should object to a premature decision to perform a cesarean section. If labor fails to progress, cesarean section should be performed. The use of oxytocin to stimulate or augment the strength of your contractions is extremely dangerous and should be avoided.

You should be admitted to the hospital at the onset of your earliest contractions and preparations made for immediate cesarean delivery in the event that a uterine rupture is suspected. Adequate emergency preparations would include the availability of at least 2 units of blood for immediate transfusion, and intravenous infusion in a vein of your arm, twenty-four-hour availability of a fully equipped laboratory and blood bank, a readily available anesthesiologist stationed in the hospital, a nearby operating room ready for emergency surgery, and a sufficient number of experienced obstetrical nurses. Most importantly, your obstetrician should be actively managing your labor in the hospital and not from his or her office. During labor, fetal monitoring is imperative as is frequent maternal blood pressure and pulse readings, since, occasionally, a rapid pulse is the first sign of a uterine rupture and maternal hemorrhage. Early clues to uterine rupture include a "tearing" pain in the lower abdomen, tenderness on palpation over the previous scar, a bulge in the abdominal wall over the site of the previous surgery, and vaginal bleeding. If this diagnosis is even a remote possibility, it is best to immediately proceed with a cesarean section rather than wait for symptoms to worsen. Epidural anesthesia, a popular technique used to totally relieve pain during labor, is, in my opinion, not recommended for women undergoing a trial of labor after a previous cesarean section because by eliminating all pain, the early symptoms of uterine rupture may not be recognized.

Following delivery some doctors explore the inside of the uterus with their hand in order to determine if a defect is present along the previous cesarean section suture line. This practice is of little value and may even serve to further traumatize a weakened suture site.

Though the risk of uterine rupture and obstetrical complications is rare when a woman is allowed a trial of labor, if an emergency does arise it is best that it happen in a large, well-equipped medical center rather than in a small rural hospital. If you live in an area which lacks a hospital with a modern blood blank, adequate staffing, up-to-date obstetrical facilities, and full-time anesthesia coverage, it is probably best to undergo a repeat cesarean section instead of a trial of labor.

Anesthesia

How is local anesthesia used in obstetrics?

An anesthetic is defined as any substance that obliterates pain either through inducing unconsciousness or by interrupting the pathway of nerves which carry sensations of pain to the brain. Analgesics, on the other hand, are drugs, such as morphine and meperidine (trade name Demerol), which relieve or diminish the intensity of pain when given intravenously, intramuscularly, or subcutaneously (below the skin) during labor. (The effects of various analgesics are discussed in chapter 7.)

I am frequently asked which anesthetic is best, and my standard, but accurate, response is that the perfect anesthetic has not yet been invented. Even the safest of methods may occasionally be associated with undesirable side effects. For this reason, it is encouraging to note the growing number of couples enrolling in childbirth education classes. Regardless of whether one is a Lamaze, Grantly Dick-Read, or

Bradley enthusiast, women practicing these methods usually require or request less analgesia or anesthesia during labor and delivery.

The simplest and safest form of anesthesia is the injection of a medication, such as Novocain, just below the skin of the perineum at the site of the episiotomy (see page 400). This local anesthetic is administered just as the baby's head is crowning, as the emerging head is causing the perineum to bulge, and relieves pain only for the performance and repair of the episiotomy.

A **pudendal nerve block** anesthetizes the outer vagina, vulva, and perineum, or those areas containing branches of the two pudendal nerves. When performed correctly, this popular technique provides adequate perineal anesthesia for spontaneous delivery, as well as the performance and repair of the episiotomy. Though enthusiasts claim that a pudendal block provides adequate anesthesia for a low forceps delivery, most obstetricians would agree that it is less than adequate for this purpose. To anesthetize the left pudendal nerve, a doctor inserts the left index and middle finger deep into the left side of the vagina in order to locate the ischial spine. This bony landmark is important because it is in close proximity to the pudendal nerve. A long needle, housed in a protective sleeve or guide, is then inserted between the doctor's fingers and the vaginal wall and advanced to a point just below the spines. Though this needle is several inches long, only the last centimeter is inserted below the vaginal surface at this location. The anesthetic, most often lidocaine (trade name Xylocaine) in a 1 percent concentration, is then injected. The procedure is then repeated on the opposite side. Approximately 3 to 5 milliliters of a local anesthetic such as lidocaine (trade name Xylocaine) or mepivacaine (trade name Carbocaine) produces perineal anesthesia within five minutes, lasting at least one hour. Occasionally, one-half of the perineum will be completely anesthetized while the other side continues to elicit pain. When this occurs, the unanesthetized side should be reinjected.

The timing of the pudendal nerve block is very important. Ideally, it should be administered just after full dilatation of the cervix but before significant crowning has occurred. If the procedure is delayed until the last moment, it is much more difficult to perform and can be extremely uncomfortable if a woman is bearing down.

A **paracervical** (para=around) **block** is the injection of approximately 10 to 20 milliliters of a local anesthetic into the tissues surrounding the cervix. A properly placed paracervical block, in which 1 percent lidocaine or mepivacaine is used, can completely relieve the pain of cervical dilatation for one to two hours. Repeat injections may be given whenever the pain returns. A 2 percent chloroprocaine (trade name Nesacaine) solution may also be used for a paracervical block. This new anesthetic has the advantage of causing fewer adverse reactions but has the disadvantage of requiring reinjection as frequently as every forty to sixty minutes. Specially designed indwelling catheters, which pass out of the vagina and can be strapped to a woman's thigh or abdomen, make it possible to reinject additional amounts of anesthetic every forty-five minutes to one hour without having to reinsert the needle. Since a paracervical block provides no perineal, vaginal, or vulvar pain relief, another form of anesthesia is needed as the head begins to distend the vagina and perineum following full cervical dilatation.

A **spinal** or **subarachnoid block** is a frequently used anesthetic technique which provides complete pain relief for either a vaginal delivery or a cesarean section. To perform a spinal block, a long, fine needle is inserted between the bony processes of two adjacent vertebrae in the lower back. The needle is then advanced through the dura or outer membrane covering the spinal cord. When the dura has been punctured and the subarachnoid space entered clear spinal fluid flows through the end of the needle. The anesthetic is then injected through the needle, bringing almost instantaneous relief of pain, numbness over the lower half of the body, loss of voluntary movement of the legs, and an inability to use the abdominal muscles during bearing down efforts. Unlike other forms of anesthesia in which a catheter may be left in place for continuous injection of medication in a spinal block, the needle is removed immediately after the anesthetic is given.

A spinal block may be administered if a woman is sitting with her back arched outward or lying on her side with her head bent downward against her chest and her knees pulled tightly upward against her abdomen. By assuming these uncomfortable positions, the vertebrae of the lower back become more prominent, allowing the spinal block to be performed with greater ease. The choice of the sitting or lying position usually depends on the personal preference of the anesthesiologist, as well as the anesthetic effect sought. For example, a higher level of anesthesia is required for a cesarean section than for a vaginal delivery, and this is often best accomplished with a woman in the lateral position. If a woman is given a spinal block and then maintained in the sitting position for a minute or two after the anesthesia is administered, the medication settles to a lower level and only numbs her vagina, perineum, and inner thighs. This distribution of pain relief, with the exception of the vagina, covers most areas which would come in contact with a saddle if one were riding a horse. For this reason, a spinal block of this type is appropriately named a saddle block. A saddle block provides excellent anesthesia for a vaginal delivery and forceps operations, and also has the advantage of maintaining some voluntary bearing down efforts of the abdominal wall musculature.

Saddle block anesthesia should not be performed in a vaginal delivery until the cervix is completely dilated and the baby's head is deep in the pelvis, because the saddle block interferes with the normal descent of the head, possibly resulting in the need for a difficult midforceps delivery. Nearly all local anesthetic agents have been used for spinal block anesthesia. The two most popular are tetracaine (trade name Pontocaine) and lidocaine. However, chloroprocaine hydrochloride (trade name Nesacaine), a new rapidly acting anesthetic, should never be used for spinal block anesthesia because it has recently been associated with permanent neurological damage.

While an obstetrician is responsible for injecting a paracervical and pudendal nerve block, in most hospitals a spinal anesthetic is usually administered by a trained anesthesiologist. Though the technique of spinal block is extremely easy to learn and master, it may still be associated with serious complications. Patients receiving this form of anesthesia require careful monitoring of their vital signs and an anesthesiologist should be available throughout the delivery and for at least thirty minutes following its completion.

An **epidural** or **peridural block** is similar to a spinal anesthetic in that a woman assumes either a sitting or lying position and a needle is inserted into her lower back. The difference, however, is that the spinal needle passes through the dura and into the spinal fluid, while the epidural needle is more superficial and does not perforate the dura. Unlike a spinal block, an epidural may be given before the cervix is fully dilated and it provides excellent anesthesia during the active phase of labor, spontaneous vaginal delivery, forceps operations, or cesarean section. Though an epidural may dull a woman's bearing down reflex during the second stage of labor, it is less likely to do this than a spinal block.

Considerably more skill is required to perform an epidural than a spinal block. The quantity of anesthetic needed to provide an adequate epidural is considerably more than that used for a spinal block. Therefore, before the full amount is given, it is crucial that a very small test dose first be administered. Under normal circumstances, this minute amount will be too little to have any anesthetic effect. However, if the needle has inadvertently penetrated the dura, anesthesia in the form of numbness in the leg may be quite pronounced. When this occurs, it is best that the needle be withdrawn and the procedure abandoned since injection of the full dose may cause severe complications.

Depending on the obstetrical situation, an epidural block may be administered as a single injection or as a continuous anesthetic through a long plastic catheter. Whereas spinal block provides complete anesthesia within five minutes, it may take as long as ten to twenty minutes for an epidural to become effective. Several different local anesthetics have been used successfully for epidural block. As with spinal anesthesia, chloroprocaine hydrochloride should never be used for an epidural because of the possibility of causing permanent neurological impairment. Bupivacaine hydrochloride (trade name Marcaine) is a very long lasting anesthetic, effective for three to six hours. This is especially valuable if a single injection, rather than a continuous epidural is needed during labor. Bupivacaine hydrochloride is less likely to cause a drop in maternal blood pressure (hypotension), than other local anesthetics, and when used judiciously has no harmful effects on the fetus or newborn. Lidocaine usually provides excellent anesthesia for approximately two hours. However, several recent studies have shown that newborn infants of mothers receiving lidocaine and mepivacaine have a higher incidence of depression of muscle tone and reflexes than infants who are delivered with the use of other local anesthetics. When compared to other local anesthetics, lidocaine and mepivocaine were much more likely to reach higher concentrations in the fetal circulation.

In addition to an epidural block, peridural anesthesia may also be administered by inserting a needle into the lower end of the sacral bone at the base of the spine. This form of anesthesia is known as a **caudal** (meaning tail) **block.** Continuous caudal anesthesia is possible with a plastic catheter. The caudal block technique requires a great deal of skill and uses a far greater quantity of anesthesia than epidural in order to be effective. While caudal block was formerly a very popular method of childbirth anesthesia, it has been widely replaced by the simpler and safer epidural technique.

What complications may be encountered with the use of local anesthetics and how can these problems be minimized?

Whenever a local anesthetic is given, the danger always exists that some of the medication may be inadvertently injected into a blood vessel and then enter the general circulation. Symptoms of this potentially catastrophic situation include lightheadedness, dizziness, slurred speech, a metallic taste, numbness of the tongue and mouth, muscle twitching, loss of consciousness, convulsions, and even cardiac arrest and death. The severity of this reaction is likely to be less pronounced with chloroprocaine hydrochloride than with lidocaine hydrochloride or mepivacaine hydrochloride because it leaves the bloodstream rapidly. The injection of a local anesthetic into the bloodstream can be prevented if a doctor frequently draws back on the plunger of the syringe as the anesthetic is being injected. If blood appears in either the syringe or the needle, the anesthetic must not be injected. If symptoms of intravascular injection appear, an obstetrician and anesthesiologist must be prepared to immediately treat the convulsions, administer oxygen, and establish an airway with a tube into the trachea. As with most medical complications, it is easier to take the time beforehand to prevent the problem than it is to treat it.

Intravascular injection is the most serious complication of a pudendal nerve block. Of a less serious nature is the collection of blood that may result from needle perforation of a blood vessel lying near the pudendal nerve. On rare occasions, an infection may originate at the needle site.

It is only in recent years that doctors have noted fetal complications associated with paracervical block. Several studies have demonstrated that an abnormal slowing of the heart rate (bradycardia), may occur in as many as 25 percent of infants exposed to this type of anesthesia. This condition usually begins two to ten minutes after the block is performed and may last from three to thirty minutes. For the healthy infant, the bradycardia usually presents no problems. Complications including fetal death are far more likely to occur if the fetus is in difficulty before the administration of the anesthetic. The cause of this bradycardia remains unknown. Some investigators believe that the many blood vessels around the cervix allow more anesthetic to diffuse from the cervical tissues into the fetal circulation, where it slows the heart rate. Others claim that the bradycardia associated with paracervical block results from an increase in uterine muscle tone and constriction of uterine blood vessels, thereby decreasing the amount of oxygen carried to the placenta and fetus.

One of the most common complications of spinal block anesthesia is a drop in a woman's blood pressure (hypotension). This occurs because of a pronounced widening and loss of tone of the veins carrying blood to the heart. As a result, less blood is returned, and less oxygen-carrying blood is pumped to the uterus, placenta, and fetus. In addition, if a woman lies on her back following a spinal anesthetic the uterus can compress the veins carrying blood to the heart, further reducing the amount of oxygen delivered to her fetus and possibly resulting in severe distress.

To minimize the risk of maternal hypotension, an anesthesiologist should increase the blood volume by giving you an intravenous solution named Ringer's Lactate before administering a spinal block. In addition, the uterus should be displaced to the left side immediately after the spinal is given. If these measures fail, a valuable medication named ephedrine should be administered at the first sign of a fall in blood pressure. This drug immediately returns the blood pressure to normal or near-normal levels while maintaining uterine circulation and fetal oxygenation.

An uncommon, but frightening, complication of spinal anesthesia is known as total spinal blockade. In this situation, the anesthetic rises to a dangerously high level and causes respiratory paralysis and hypotension. Just prior to total blockade, a woman's final apprehensive exclamation will usually be "I can't breathe!" The subarachnoid space decreases in size during pregnancy and identical amounts of spinal anesthesia will produce a higher level when a woman is pregnant than when she is not pregnant. The spinal blockade calamity most often results when the dose of anesthetic given is more than the pregnant woman can tolerate. If spinal blockade does occur, it is vital that artificial ventilation of the lungs be continued until the effects of the anesthetic are out of the body. This may take several hours and will occasionally involve placing a tube in the trachea in order to maintain adequate breathing. Since a woman is aware of all that is happening during this harrowing experience, it is very important she understand that her condition will soon return to normal. As previously mentioned, permanent neurological impairment has recently been associated with the use of chloroprocaine as a spinal or epidural anesthetic.

Severe headaches following spinal block may occur in as many as 10 to 20 percent of all women receiving this form of anesthesia. These headaches, which are often incapacitating, usually begin as a pain in the back of the neck and head and then intensify during the second through the fourth postpartum day. Sitting or standing practically always intensifies the pain, and a woman with a spinal headache is most comfortable lying flat in bed. Improvement will usually occur rapidly after the fifth day. The cause of a spinal headache is believed to be the leakage of spinal fluid from the site of the needle puncture and the incidence of headache will be lowest if the anesthesiologist is skillful, using a small-gauge needle and avoiding multiple attempts at puncturing the dura. To prevent a headache from developing, most doctors recommend that a woman lie flat in bed for eight hours following a spinal block. Others suggest a high intake of liquids. In my experience, both of these measures have proven to be valueless. Once the headache is present, treatment usually consists of strong medications such as codeine and meperidine (trade name Demerol) for relief of pain, complete bed rest, the wearing of a tight abdominal binder, and reassurance to a woman that the condition is self-limited. For more severe headaches, the use of a so-called blood patch may prove to be very helpful. This is accomplished by drawing a small amount of blood from the woman's arm and injecting it into her epidural space at the site of the previous spinal. The blood has the effect of creating a seal over the leak. Some doctors have used saline solution, instead of blood, with equally good results.

Temporary urinary dysfunction and overdistention of the urinary bladder may follow spinal block anesthesia. It is important that the nursing staff be alerted to this potential problem when caring for a woman during the immediate postpartum period. If distention of the bladder with urine is suspected, catheterization is mandatory.

Epidural and caudal anesthesia may, like spinal, cause a drop in blood pressure and too high an anesthetic level. The latter is especially likely to occur if the dura has been accidentally punctured and an inadvertent spinal block has been given. Both complications are treated in the identical manner described for spinal anesthesia. A correctly performed epidural should never be complicated by a postprocedure headache.

One important difference between a spinal and epidural block is the amount of local anesthetic required. The large dose used in epidural anesthesia allows a significant amount to be picked up by the fetus, and this may produce neurobehavioral defects during the period immediately following birth. Since the dose of local anesthetic required for spinal anesthesia is extremely small by comparison, this problem almost never occurs. Of all local anesthetic techniques, caudal anesthesia requires the largest amount of anesthetic and for this reason imposes additional hazards to the fetus.

The amount of pain relief achieved with an epidural is far less predictable than that of a spinal. In one 1979 study, it was found that 12 percent of women receiving an epidural experienced only partial relief of pain while 3 percent continued to have severe pain. Often, your best assurance of the anesthetic "taking" will be your good fortune to have a skilled and experienced anesthesiologist. If you are scheduled to undergo a repeat cesarean section under epidural anesthesia, it is a good idea to ask your obstetrician to request an anesthesiologist who has a reputation for giving excellent epidurals. Even during labor, when there is less time to plan, there is no harm in requesting the doctor most skilled in this technique.

Epidural block may slow the progress of cervical dilatation during the first stage of labor or hinder the descent of the head during the second stage, possibly requiring a difficult and dangerous midforceps delivery. It is the wise obstetrician who, despite pressure from a patient, delays administering an epidural until the cervix is at least 6 centimeters dilated in a woman who has had previous babies and 8 centimeters dilated in a woman who has not.

What are some of the drawbacks of using general anesthetics for delivery?

The use of general anesthetics in obstetrics has declined dramatically in recent years. Several large studies show that any general anesthetic given to a mother rapidly crosses the placenta and enters the fetal circulation. Babies exposed to this form of anesthesia are more likely to be depressed at birth than those who are delivered under local, pudendal, spinal, or epidural block.

Childbirth education classes have emphasized the importance of viewing labor and delivery as a shared experience for a couple. A father will be deprived of seeing his baby being born because most hospitals will not allow him in the delivery room or the operating room when general anesthesia is being administered. In addition to preventing a woman from experiencing that unequaled moment of joy when her baby first cries, the drowsiness induced by general anesthesia also hinders early maternal-infant bonding and nursing during the immediate postpartum period.

One of the greatest disadvantages of general anesthesia is the ever-present threat that the contents of the stomach may be vomited and then aspirated into the lungs. The material from the stomach may contain undigested food which can cause airway obstruction and death. Even if a woman has fasted, and there is no food in her stomach, aspiration of the strongly acidic stomach secretions may be even more deadly. Chemical irritation and infection in the lungs, caused by acid stomach secretions, is known medically as Mendelson's syndrome. It has become the leading cause of anesthetic deaths in obstetrics and the fourth leading cause of all obstetrical deaths. The adverse fetal affects of general anesthetics administered early in pregnancy has been previously described (see chapter 10).

What types of general anesthesia are used in obstetrics?

In addition to eliminating painful sensations, general anesthesia also induces loss of consciousness, muscle movement, and reflex activity. Nitrous oxide, a gas administered through an anesthetic face mask, may be used to provide relief of pain during labor as well as delivery. Nitrous oxide should never be used for minor surgery or dental work during the first trimester because it may be associated with a higher incidence of birth defects. During the first stage of labor, a 50 percent concentration mixed with 50 percent oxygen can be inhaled as soon as each uterine contraction begins. It is then withdrawn as the contraction subsides. During the second stage of labor, a woman can take three or four deep breaths of gas, hold the last breath, and then bear down. Though nitrous oxide is classified as an anesthetic, it cannot provide total pain relief since concentrations required for complete relief provide too little oxygen for a woman and her fetus, and may even be fatal if administered over a period of several minutes. When combined with another anesthetic, it can usually provide adequate pain relief for episiotomy, delivery, and repair of the episiotomy.

Nitrous oxide may also be used effectively for cesarean section or difficult vaginal delivery if combined with an intravenous barbiturate named thiopental and a muscle paralyzing medication named succinylcholine. This so-called crash induction, or balanced inhalation anesthesia procedure begins with a small intravenous dose of a drug named D-tubocurarine to block muscle twitching, followed by a rapid intravenous injection of the thiopental to induce instant anesthesia and unconsciousness. Immediately after the thiopental is given, an intravenous injection of succinylcholine is administered in order to prevent movement and allow adequate muscle relaxation so that a plastic breathing tube may be placed in the trachea. The nitrous oxide gas is then given through the trachael tube in order to maintain an anesthetic that will not depress the infant. A cesarean section incision can usually be made immediately after the tube has been passed into the trachea. This technique provides adequate anesthesia for fifteen to twenty minutes, and the baby can almost always be delivered during this period of time. Additional anesthesia can then be added in order to prevent the mother from experiencing any discomfort for the remainder of the procedure. Any competent obstetrician can easily deliver a baby within three minutes after the skin incision is made. Rapid delivery in this fashion prevents these drugs from accumulating in the baby's body and causing respiratory depression at birth.

Recent studies from Harvard Medical School have confirmed that a slow-moving surgeon may adversely affect your baby's health. When cesarean sections were performed with thiopental, succinylcholine, and nitrous oxide, low Apgar scores and acidosis in the newborn were most likely to occur if the interval between the start of the anesthetic and the delivery of the baby exceeded eight minutes. Similar findings were noted when a doctor required more than three minutes to make the incision into the uterus and deliver the baby.

Ethylene is an anesthetic gas which is similar to nitrous oxide in its activity, but it has the distinct disadvantage of an unpleasant odor. It is also more likely to cause nausea and vomiting. As a result, it is rarely used in most obstetrical units.

Cyclopropane is a potent anesthetic gas which until recently was commonly used for both vaginal and cesarean section births. It is highly flammable and explosive, causes abnormal heart rhythms when administered with oxytocin or ergotrate, may induce an elevation of the blood pressure, and can cause severe maternal and fetal respiratory depression. This last complication may be intensified if cyclopropane is given following the use of narcotics or barbiturates earlier in labor. In addition to these drawbacks, cyclopropane is frequently associated with nausea and vomiting. One might logically ask, "Why on earth would anyone use this terrible anesthetic?" Though it is infrequently used in most hospitals today, in the past it was invaluable in inducing anesthesia rapidly during certain acute obstetrical emergencies.

The group of gasses classified as the volatile anesthetics include ether, chloroform, halothane (Fluorthane), methoxyflurane (Penthrane), and enflurane (Ethrane). Chloroform and ether will rarely if ever be found or used in a modern obstetrical suite because of unpleasant side effects and complications associated with their use.

Halothane, a potent, rapidly acting anesthetic gas, has the unique ability of totally relaxing the uterine muscles. For this reason, it is the anesthetic of choice for those rare situations which require complete uterine relaxation such as version or turning of a second twin or the emergency delivery of a baby in a difficult breech position. Halothane's major advantage, namely the relaxation which it provides, is also its main disadvantage because the uterine muscles may fail to contract following delivery. This may lead to severe postpartum hemorrhage. Attempts to remedy this situation with oxytocin and ergotrate are often unsuccessful. Other drawbacks of halothane anesthesia include maternal and newborn respiratory depression, abnormal lowering of the maternal blood pressure, and the rare but serious complication of liver toxicity.

Methoxyflurane, better known by the name of Penthrane, is a popular gas for both analgesia and light anesthesia at the time of delivery. It is pleasant to breathe and can be self-administered. A woman actually holds the inhaler in her hand and rapidly breathes the Penthrane throughout her contractions. During the second stage of labor, the anesthetic may be inhaled just before the bearing down begins. In proper analgesic concentrations, the gas will cause no harm to a mother or her fetus, but close nursing surveillance is necessary to be sure that too much Pentrane is not inhaled. Though somewhat helpful for relief of pain during a spontaneous vaginal delivery, self-administered Penthrane is totally inadequate if forceps are to be applied. In higher anesthetic concentrations, it may cause maternal and newborn respiratory depression, bradycardia, impairment of kidney and liver function, a drop in blood pressure, an abnormal amount of postpartum uterine relaxation, and a higher incidence of postpartum blood loss. Induction of full anesthesia with Penthrane often takes several minutes, and for this reason it is less than adequate when immediate delivery is indicated.

Enflurane is rarely used for complete obstetrical anesthesia because of its many side effects, its possible role in causing impaired kidney function, and its depressive effects on the heart. However, in low concentrations it can provide excellent pain relief when inhaled during contractions in the second stage of labor. In addition to providing rapid analgesia, enflurane is pleasant to breathe and does not cause respiratory depression in the baby.

Thiopental (trade name Pentothal) is a rapidly acting barbiturate which is given intravenously to induce sleep for a cesarean section. It is also given intravenously, though less frequently for a vaginal delivery combined with a general anesthetic. Ketamine hydrochloride (trade name Ketaject), a new nonbarbiturate anesthetic which can be administered intravenously or intramuscularly, has recently been gaining popularity because, unlike thiopental, it is unlikely to cause maternal or infant respiratory depression. Barbiturates may impair reflexes in the pharynx and larynx and cause choking, but ketamine in properly administered doses is less likely to do this. Instead, it produces an almost trancelike state in which the patient appears to be awake but experiences no pain, an effect termed "dissociative anesthesia" because it selectively interrupts pain pathways to the brain without altering other nervous reflexes. Ketamine has been used as the sole anesthetic for vaginal delivery, for short minor surgical procedures, and for inducing anesthesia prior to administering other agents. It is also combined with a low potency anesthetic, such as nitrous oxide, to enhance its efficacy.

No anesthetic is perfect, and ketamine is certainly not an exception. It can elevate the blood pressure, and women with heart disease and hypertension must be carefully monitored. One of the most serious and common problems associated with ketamine use is bizarre psychological behavior, a reaction reported to occur in as many as 12 percent of women who are anesthetized with this drug. Reactions may range from a pleasant dreamlike state to hallucinations and delirium. Though no known permanent psychological effects have been reported, the bizarre behavior pattern may last for a few hours and in some cases for as long as twenty-four hours. Experience with ketamine use for vaginal delivery and cesarean section is limited, but reports suggest that it is safe for both mother and fetus.

How can the complications associated with general anesthesia be decreased?

Given the choice between general anesthesia and one of the local anesthetic techniques, it is the wise woman who selects the second option. If general anesthesia is contemplated, the hazards associated with aspiration of stomach contents can be markedly reduced if food is withheld for at least eight hours before the onset of contractions. Unfortunately, one is never clairvoyant enough to predict when labor will begin, and the fullness of one's stomach is often a matter of chance. However, if your amniotic membranes rupture before the onset of contractions, do not eat any solid foods since it is a good bet that labor will begin within a few hours. Another important point to remember is that peristalsis, or the propulsion of food from the stomach into the intestine, often stops completely with the onset of labor. Even when labor is prolonged for twelve hours or more, food may still be in the stomach at the time of delivery, posing a severe risk of regurgitation and aspiration of food into the respiratory tract. It is, therefore, essential, that all women receiving general anesthesia for delivery have a tube inserted into the trachea immediately after sleep is induced. To neutralize the deadly chemical reaction in the lungs caused by aspiration of acidic gastric juices, most anesthesiologists now recommend that pregnant women ingest approximately 30 milliliters of an antacid, such as Maalox, milk of magnesia, or Gelusil, within one-half hour of the anesthetic induction. It has recently been suggested that an intramuscular injection of cimetidine (trade name Tagemet), a new drug which inhibits gastric acid secretions, be administered one hour before delivery. Studies to date have shown that cimetidine does not impair labor progress and is harmless to the fetus. It goes without saying that the important factor in reducing general anesthetic complications is an attentive, alert and skilled Board-certified anesthesiologist.

When is general anesthesia more appropriate than spinal, caudal, or epidural anesthesia?

Caudal, epidural, and spinal anesthesia can cause significant lowering of the blood pressure. When administered in the presence of obstetrical hemorrhage, they only intensify the problem and create difficulties in supplying blood and oxygen to a woman's vital organs and placenta. For this reason, a general anesthetic is a far better choice in the presence of abruptio placenta, placenta previa, and other conditions which cause heavy bleeding.

Women with severe hypertension and preeclampsia are far more likely to experience a drastic drop in blood pressure following caudal, epidural, and spinal block. Though this may sound like a good method of treating high blood pressure, it is extremely dangerous for the maternal and fetal circulation. Proponents of using caudal, epidural, or spinal block in the presence of hypertension maintain that severe complications caused by a drop in blood pressure are unlikely if a woman is carefully monitored and precautions are taken. The choice of anesthesia for the hypertensive woman is not always very simple especially since recent studies have shown that there may be a tremendous increase in blood pressure accompanying the induction of general anesthesia and insertion of an endotracheal tube.

The presence of a superficial skin infection at or near the intended puncture site as well as bony deformities of the spine, previous low back surgery, a blood clotting disorder, a history of a herniated disc, evidence of neurologic disease, and chronic low back pain of unknown cause, should serve as deterrents to the use of local anesthetic techniques.

When fetal distress is extreme and immediate delivery becomes urgent, epidural and caudal anesthesia are extremely poor anesthetic choices. Spinal is better because it takes effect at least twice as fast, but a rapid "crash induction" is probably the fastest method of delivering the infant.

If anesthesia is needed for a vaginal delivery of a baby in the breech position, general anesthesia is preferred to spinal or epidural because the head can be more easily manipulated and delivered without trauma. Other abnormal fetal positions requiring uterine relaxation and manipulation may be encountered in the delivery of a second twin. In these situations, no anesthetic compares to halothane. The various local anesthetic techniques are totally inadequate for this type of intrauterine manipulation.

Episiotomy

Should I allow my doctor to perform an episiotomy at the time of delivery?

Many women consider the episiotomy to be totally contrary to their desire for a natural childbirth experience. Many believe that midwives possess a unique and magical ability to avoid unnecessary episiotomies, while obstetricians hunger for a chance to perform the procedure, even when it isn't indicated. In addition, it has been said that if women were allowed to squat or sit during delivery, instead of being forced to lie down, episiotomy would be unnecessary because the laboring mother could then work with, and not against, the forces of gravity. Opposition to the episiotomy is growing.

Briefly stated, an episiotomy is a minor procedure in which an incision is made through the outer vagina and perineum, or the area between the vagina and the rectum. An episiotomy is most often performed as the baby's head is crowning, which means the emerging head is causing the perineum to bulge. If adequate amounts of local anesthesia are used, the performance of the episiotomy and its repair with sutures should both be painless. Childbirth instructors often speak of the natural anesthesia created by the pressure of the baby's head on the perineum during a contraction, stating that if an episiotomy is made during contraction, it will be painless. Don't believe it! Insist that anesthesia be given before the episiotomy is performed. Even if you are lucky enough to experience the natural anesthetic effect, the repair of the episiotomy following delivery is extremely painful in the absence of anesthesia. In addition, injection of a local anesthetic following delivery, when a woman is most sensitive, is often far more painful than if it is given when the baby's head is crowning.

An episiotomy prevents excessive stretching and ragged lacerations of the perineal muscles which may result from the pressure of the baby's head and shoulders at the moment of birth. Occasionally, the laceration may even extend into the lower portion of the rectum. The timing of the episiotomy is very important. If done too early, before crowning is evident, bleeding from the incision can be quite brisk. The crowning of the head puts firm pressure against the perineum and its muscles, and the episiotomy site bleeds far less if it is performed at this time. When the episiotomy is made too late, the perineal muscles may be stretching and tearing, thereby defeating the purpose of the procedure. For some women an episiotomy may shorten the final stage of labor. However, the claim that it prevents infant brain damage, by decreasing the amount of time that the baby's head pounds against the perineum, is grossly exaggerated and is highly unlikely. The two exceptions would be the birth of a premature infant and the rare situation in which the pushing stage was incorrectly managed and allowed to persist for several hours.

Myths abound about the effects of an episiotomy on a woman's future anatomical appearance and sex life. Proponents of episiotomy claim that prolonged bearing down causes prolapse, or droppage of the uterus, urinary bladder (cystocele) and rectum (rectocele). In actual fact, however, the presence of these conditions is more a matter of an inherited predisposition that some women have toward developing weakened pelvic support following childbirth. Some women have given birth to five or more children without benefit of episiotomy and still have far healthier vaginal and uterine tissues than other women who have had episiotomies with the delivery of their only child.

The main muscle cut at the time of an episiotomy is named the bulbocavernosus. When you consciously contract this muscle, you narrow the vaginal opening, and this can enhance your sexual enjoyment to some degree. Some obstetricians believe that episiotomy will prevent the tearing, stretching, and weakening of the bulbocavernosus muscle, thereby enhancing a woman's future sexuality. Opponents of episiotomy, take just the opposite view: that a woman's sexuality may be diminished because these important muscles, and the nerves which supply it, are permanently weakened when episiotomy is performed. No surveys or studies have ever been done to show if the performance or nonperformance of episiotomy ultimately enhances or detracts from a woman's sex life. All women, regardless of whether or not they have had an episiotomy, benefit from muscle setting or Kegel's exercises. They are very useful in overcoming mild or moderate amounts of bulbocavernosus weakening following childbirth and also strengthen other muscles which surround the vagina, bladder, and rectum following delivery. The simplest Kegel exercise is to tighten the muscles of the buttocks as though trying to prevent the escape of feces from the anus. The same group of muscles is also used in trying to stop the flow of urine in midstream. After learning Kegel's exercises, you must practice them at least 100 times per day for a minimum of 6 months. In addition, each time you pass your urine, voluntarily interrupt the flow several times. If you perform these exercises diligently, you will note improvement in your ability to tighten the muscles surrounding the vagina and perineum.

As soon as the baby's head distends the perineum, a doctor or midwife may place a towel over the woman's rectum and exert upward pressure on the baby's chin through the perineum. This technique, known as the Ritgen maneuver, allows a slow and careful delivery of the baby's head and also helps to prevent perineal lacerations. However, excessive pressure placed in this fashion can occasionally force the head upward and cause lacerations around the mother's urethra. Since these lacerations are often more painful and difficult to anesthetize and suture than perineal lacerations a Ritgen maneuver should be done with moderation and not in excess.

Another technique that has gained great popularity is referred to as "ironing out the perineum," in which the perineal muscles are gradually stretched by applying digital pressure against the vaginal wall during the final stages of labor. Some women tolerate this very well but others find it quite annoying and irritating. It is believed that this procedure decreases the necessity for episiotomy, but there is no proof that it does. Neither has use of various lotions for massaging the perineum been shown to increase its capacity to stretch and accommodate the birth of the baby.

Obstetricians generally believe that episiotomy should be performed for most women having their first baby. Naturally, there are many exceptions, and babies of smaller than normal size can usually be delivered without an episiotomy. Women with a greater degree of laxity of their perineal tissues can also avoid the procedure. However, avoidance of episiotomy when a woman demands none be done can sometimes create large and extensive perineal lacerations which require many sutures. The great majority of women who have previously given birth can avoid a repeat episiotomy. Then, if a laceration does occur, it usually follows the old incision line and it can easily be repaired as if an episiotomy had been performed. Many women bearing extremely large babies require episiotomies, regardless of their previous obstetrical history. Breech deliveries often present unique problems and complications and it is best to perform an episiotomy on all women undergoing a vaginal delivery of a baby in the breech position. The use of forceps will usually require an episiotomy. It takes sound judgment on the part of the person delivering the baby to decide if an episiotomy is absolutely indicated. Even in the hands of an expert, mistakes in judgment can take place.

An incision made exactly in the center is called a median episiotomy, while the mediolateral technique veers off to one side or the other (see illustration). The median episiotomy has many advantages over the mediolateral, which is extremely painful, is associated with a greater blood loss than the median technique, leaves a larger and more permanent scar, and may occasionally cause painful intercourse following healing. Proponents of this method claim that it allows more room for difficult deliveries and large babies. However, most experts, familiar with both techniques question this. Admittedly, the incidence of extension of the episiotomy into the rectum is greater with the median episiotomy, occurring in 2 to 5 percent of all cases in which this technique is used and is seen in only 1 percent of all mediolateral episiotomies. However, repair of an extension into the rectum is actually quite simple and is by no means a major catastrophe. Overall, the advantages of the median episiotomy far outweigh the mediolateral method and, if your doctor performs only mediolateral episiotomies, I strongly suggest that you find another obstetrician.

Natural Childbirth

What is your opinion of the different methods of natural childbirth?

From the above discussion of anesthesia, one can readily understand that the best method of anesthesia is none at all. By the same token, the best method of childbirth is "prepared childbirth"—a term used to describe a number of methods for preparing and educating both mother and father so that pregnancy, labor, and delivery are positive and beautiful experiences, resulting in the birth of a healthy infant.

The term "natural childbirth," often used synonymously with "prepared childbirth" had its origins in 1933 with the publication of a book with that same title,

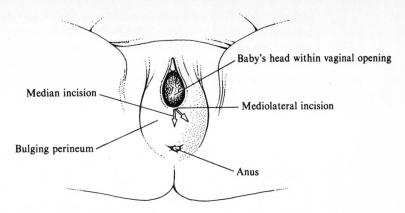

Median incision

Bulging perineum

Baby's head within vaginal opening

Mediolateral incision

Anus

The two types of episiotomy incisions.

written by the English physician Grantly Dick-Read. In this book and in another, *Childbirth Without Fear*, Dick-Read formulated his "fear-tension-pain" theory. Simply stated, he observed that those women who were most fearful experienced the most pain, while those who appeared calm had the easiest labors. The Grantly Dick-Read method, therefore, involved educating women so that they would be more knowledgeable about and less fearful of labor, thereby breaking the vicious cycle of fear, tension, and pain. Grantly Dick-Read further emphasized the importance of physical fitness, relaxation, and breathing exercises. Today, his method is widely practiced in Britain and Canada, though it is far less popular in the United States.

The Bradley method named after Robert Bradley, an American physician, has gained great popularity in the United States in recent years. Dr. Bradley adopted Grantly Dick-Read's principles and later added emphasis to "husband-coached" childbirth in which vital and active participation of the father becomes necessary for success. Bradley classes differ from most other types of childbirth education in many important ways. A special series of eight "early bird" meetings begin as soon as a woman's pregnancy is confirmed. Some of the early pregnancy topics include anatomy, nutrition, and physiology of pregnancy. Regular weekly sessions start at the sixth month of pregnancy to allow parents plenty of time to evaluate their needs and to find cooperative medical care. Other methods of childbirth usually begin during the last six weeks, and for some couples this is hardly enough time to prepare for labor. Unlike the more publicized Lamaze method, Bradley instructors deplore special breathing techniques which can, on rare occasions, lead to exhaustion, dizziness, and hyperventilation, as well as reduction in the oxygen supplied to the fetus. Instead, the Bradley method emphasizes that mothers continue to breathe normally throughout labor and birth. Bradley instructors teach relaxation training to the woman and her partner so that even under the stress of labor she can relax groups of muscles. Her partner's role is to instruct her and determine if she has indeed achieved this relaxed state. In childbirth classes and practice at home the couple feel and learn to detect the difference between tense and relaxed muscles and the immediate relaxation of tense muscles at the first sign of simulated contractions. The father-coach whispers encouragement and praise to the mother in labor. To date, I have seen only a handful of Bradley-coached couples, but I have been most impressed with the success they have achieved.

The most popular method of prepared childbirth in the United States is the Lamaze method or Psychoprophylaxis. Introduced in France in 1951 by the now-immortalized French obstetrician Fernand Lamaze, the method has made it possible for millions of women to experience controlled childbirth with a minimum of anesthesia. The Lamaze method was first popularized in this country by Marjorie Karmel in 1959 with the publication of her book, *Thank You, Dr. Lamaze.*

With the Lamaze method, a woman under the direction of her partner carries out a variety of controlled breathing exercises. The rate of breathing is determined by the strength and frequency of the contractions. By totally focusing on the breathing patterns and a "concentration point," which may be a picture on a nearby wall, a woman is able to block out the pain stimuli to that area of the brain which interprets them. Psychoprophylaxis enthusiasts do not deny the existence of pain in labor, but they distract themselves with their controlled breathing techniques so completely that many report painless labor.

Several large studies have documented the medical value of the Lamaze method. One at Northwestern University in 1978 noted that Lamaze-prepared women had only 25 percent the number of cesarean sections and 20 percent the incidence of fetal distress compared to a group of women who had not undergone childbirth preparation. Infant death was 25 percent lower in the Lamaze group, and maternal infection rates and perineal lacerations were also significantly lower. Other studies have concluded that women trained in the Lamaze method were more likely to have a shorter first stage of labor (the time from the onset of regular contractions to full dilatation of the cervix) and required significantly less narcotic medication than another group not using this method. These statistics would appear, at first glance, to be quite impressive. However, one deficiency common to all of these reports is that women in the Lamaze group are really quite different from those in the control group. Those who choose to participate in childbirth education courses are often better educated, enthusiastic, less fearful, and more knowledgeable about the birth process than women not requesting natural childbirth. Fear of childbirth (parturiphobia) intensifies the pain of labor and stimulates the release of chemical substances known as catecholamines, in turn, causing narrowing or constriction of blood vessels which carry oxygen to the fetus and placenta. This can result in a higher incidence of fetal distress among women in the control group. In addition, the fearful woman who has not participated in childbirth education classes is more likely to request pain medication during labor with its attendant complications.

Though much has been written about the potentially harmful effects of hyperventilation with Lamaze breathing, I believe that this danger has been grossly exaggerated. It is true that excessive rapid breathing can lead to exhaustion, dizziness, muscle spasms, and even a decrease in oxygen supplied to the baby. However, such instances are extremely rare. Furthermore, an attentive nurse or doctor can prevent or correct the problem simply by having a woman breathe into a bag. When the woman rebreathes her exhaled carbon dioxide gas, the symptoms associated with rapid breathing quickly disappear.

In summary, all methods of prepared childbirth are definitely worthwhile. A couple should never let a lack of enthusiasm by a friend, relative, or obstetrician deter them from learning one of these techniques.

Gentle Birth

What is meant by the term "gentle birth"?

Until recently, American obstetricians took great pride in bringing newborns into the world with a vigorous slap on the buttocks while hoisting the baby aloft by its ankles. The latter procedure, reported to cause orthopedic problems for some babies, has been abandoned by most doctors. Thanks to the influence of a French obstetrician named Frederick Leboyer, the slap on the buttocks is being replaced by the more humane and natural "gentle birth."

Leboyer's thesis, outlined in his book, *Birth Without Violence* (1974) is that birth is a violent experience for a baby and is made even more violent by insensitive treatment in the delivery room. Examples of this insensitivity are excessive amounts of noise, bright lights, early clamping of the umbilical cord, and excessive suctioning of the baby's mouth secretions. To correct this trauma, the Leboyer remedy is to darken the delivery room, keep it warm and quiet, and to place the newborn immediately on its mother's abdomen and enhance this skin-to-skin contact by gently massaging the baby at the same time. The umbilical cord is cut approximately five minutes later when it has stopped pulsating. Then the baby is placed in a tepid bath, which Dr. Leboyer claims is a soothing return to the weightlessness of existence in the amniotic fluid.

It was only natural that many caustic comments came from the medical establishment in response to Dr. Leboyer's unscientific book, but claims that the dim lights and lack of suctioning would endanger the baby have not been substantiated. Furthermore, Dr. Leboyer never advocated abandoning good sound medical practice when it proves necessary. The pundits may ridicule the simplicity of the Leboyer method, but the contentment noted on the face of a Leboyer baby is the best argument in its defense.

To date, the few published reports evaluating the Leboyer method have all attested to its safety. In 1980, doctors at Pennsylvania State University compared the outcome of pregnancy among eighty-seven mothers delivered by the Leboyer method with a control group using conventional techniques. Mothers and infants in both groups did equally well. Nurses caring for the newborns, when asked to make six subjective assessments of the infants, noted no significant differences between the Leboyer and control group in contentment, "smilability," sleep-wake cycle, sucking ability, reaction to circumcision, and reaction to eye care. Couples participating in Leboyer births are enthusiastic about the method, particularly praising the father's participation and the serene atmosphere of the delivery room.

Dr. David A. Kliot and Dr. Max I. Lilling of the Brookdale Hospital Medical Center, in New York City, who have attended hundreds of Leboyer births find this method to be as safe as traditional delivery styles and note medical benefits as well. The maternal abdomen proved to be as effective a heat source as the radiant warmers used in most delivery rooms. In addition, they found that by placing the baby in the prone position on the mother's abdomen and massaging its back the possibility of aspiration of secretions and mucus into the mouth, nose, throat, and lungs was decreased and the use of a suction apparatus to remove secretions was rarely needed. The postural drainage achieved in the face-down position effectively cleared the nasopharyngeal cavity.

While placing a baby on its mother's abdomen immediately after birth has several positive effects, it should be pointed out that it does have the disadvantage of depriving the newborn of all the blood that it should receive. Contrary to popular belief, the transfusion of blood from the placenta to the baby via the umbilical cord immediately after birth can only occur if the baby is held at a level below the placenta for 1 to 3 minutes. Since the blood in the cord cannot flow upward, the newborn placed on its mother's abdomen will receive no therapeutic benefits even if the clamping of the cord is delayed until all pulsations stop. It has been calculated that a baby held below the level of the placenta will receive an additional 40 to 60 milliliters of blood, equivalent to a 15 percent increase in its hematocrit or red blood mass. Most healthy full-term infants are unaffected by early clamping of the cord or their position on their mother's abdomen. However, a premature infant should be given the advantage of a placental transfusion by holding it below the level of the vaginal opening until there are no longer pulsations in the umbilical cord.

The reports in newspapers and popular women's magazines claiming that Leboyer children are socially and psychologically better adjusted than conventionally delivered infants are based on some very unscientific observations made by a French psychologist. To date, there are no large scientific studies to support these claims.

The natural extension of a "gentle birth" is the immediate nursing of the baby on the delivery room table and extensive close contact of a mother with her baby during the early hours and days of life. Both experimental animal studies and observations of human behavior emphasize the importance of early maternal-infant bonding, which is achieved by close physical and emotional contact immediately after birth. Eye-to-eye contact, tactile contact, caressing, and verbal contact all enhance this relationship. Routine eye care with silver nitrate is a hindrance to maternal-infant bonding and should be delayed for at least one hour following birth except when there has been a recent positive gonorrhea culture from the cervix or prolonged rupture of the membranes.

Home Birth and Family-Centered Facilities

What are the advantages and disadvantages of giving birth at home?

In recent years there has been an alarming increase in the number of women having their babies at home. Estimates are that they make up 2 to 3 percent of all deliveries in the United States and that mortality rates are higher than among babies born in a hospital environment. Dr. Warren H. Pearse of the American College of Obstetricians and Gynecologists refers to this trend as an example of "maternal trauma" and "child abuse." In a recent review of statistics from all over California, infant deaths were 20 per 1,000 in hospitals and 42.3 per 1,000 at home. The stillbirth rate was 9.9 per 1,000 in hospitals and 25 per 1,000 at home.

The dangers of home delivery to a baby are obvious when one considers that one-third of the infants admitted to newborn intensive care units are born of healthy mothers who develop complications during labor or who developed problems that were not anticipated. (The rate of complications arising in apparently normal pregnancies is estimated to be about 7.5 to 10 percent.) Furthermore, trying to transfer a sick infant from the home to the hospital shortly after birth heightens the danger to the baby. One doctor with many years of home-birth experience has recently estimated that, even among carefully screened women, 20 percent attempting birth at home will have to be taken to the hospital during delivery.

Some home-birth advocates acknowledge its hazards but assert that dangerous complications are almost always predictable. Nothing could be further from the truth! Obstetrical emergencies, such as premature separation of the placenta, ruptured uterus, cervical and vaginal lacerations, and postpartum hemorrhage due to failure of the uterine muscles to contract often happen suddenly and pose a great threat to a woman's life if they are not expertly managed in a hospital environment. Regardless of the skill and training of the nurses, midwife, or doctor attending a home delivery, the absence of a laboratory, blood bank, monitoring equipment, and special resuscitative procedures place both mother and child in unnecessary jeopardy.

If, despite all logic, you still intend to give birth at home, it is vital that you take certain precautions. Though a rare few uncertified or lay midwives have achieved a limited degree of competence following years of trial and error, most cannot evaluate an abnormal labor pattern. If you do opt for a home birth, please be sure to obtain the services of a certified Nurse-Midwife. Call the American College of Nurse-Midwives (1522 K Street NW, Washington, D.C. 20005; telephone 202-347-5445) to verify an individual's credentials. In addition, be certain that the midwife has adequate back-up coverage of a qualified obstetrician.

To support their claim that home births are safe, enthusiasts often refer to the fact that in Scandinavia, where practically everyone gives birth at home, infant death rates are lower than those in the United States. Unfortunately, one cannot compare the pregnancy outcome of this homogeneous population with that of countries having individuals of more diverse ethnic origins. For example, England has a home-birth program which has a significantly higher infant mortality than Canada, which does not.

Is there a happy medium between home delivery and hospital delivery?

Couples requesting childbirth at home are usually normal individuals who want to avoid the depersonalized environment of most hospital delivery rooms and the authoritative attitudes of the doctors and nurses who staff them. These couples reject the contention of some medical authorities that every labor must be monitored routinely with electronic equipment. They would rather chance the greater risks of home delivery than be placed in the typical hospital environment of increasing automation and mechanization. Advocates of home birth deeply believe that this experience confers unmatched psychological advantages on the parents, the newborn infant, and its siblings. They especially believe that the bonding between baby and mother can take place more easily at home, in a relaxed environment, supported by close friends.

To discourage this trend of childbirth at home, many hospitals throughout the United States are attempting to find a happy medium by creating a homelike atmosphere within the hospital. This concept, called family-centered maternity/newborn care, tries to include the entire family in the childbearing experience so that all members may benefit. There are childbirth preparation classes and a tour of the hospital's maternity and newborn units before delivery. Labor rooms are converted into bright attractively decorated rooms which resemble living rooms or bedrooms and some hospitals have provided family waiting rooms and early-labor lounges near the obstetrical unit where patients in early labor can walk and visit with friends and family members. A vital member of the obstetrical team in many family-centered units is the nurse-midwife. In addition to participating in delivery of the baby, this individual is skilled at providing prolonged emotional support which, though needed, is often not provided by the obstetrician.

A recent addition to many obstetrical suites has been the "birthing room" which is equipped with a labor-delivery bed. This unique bed is quite comfortable during labor, and it can have stirrups added to it easily when delivery is imminent. This allows a woman the opportunity to give birth in the same bed in which she labors, avoiding transfer to a separate delivery room at a time when she is most uncomfortable. "Birthing rooms" are also equipped with a cribette and warmer for the newborn, as well as emergency resuscitation apparatus if needed.

I have found that a father's clamping and cutting of the umbilical cord and his bathing of the baby following delivery adds immeasurably to his joy and sense of participation in the birth process. If the delivery is uncomplicated, his guiding of the baby out of the birth canal with coparticipation and supervision of the obstetrician is perfectly safe and will be remembered as probably the greatest moment of a young father's life. Assisting in the delivery of a baby under the watchful eye of a doctor is not nearly as dangerous as some obstetricians would have you believe. After all, even the busiest obstetrician once delivered his or her first baby under the supervision of another doctor.

Family-centered care permits fathers to have extended visiting hours after the birth and gives them the opportunity to assist in the care and feeding of the baby. Other children in the family are allowed special hours for visiting with their mother and father in a special family room. Flexible "rooming-in" allows mothers and newborns to remain together in the same room rather than to have the newborn separated in a nursery. It also encourages breast-feeding immediately after delivery in a quiet environment free of all distractions.

"Rooming-in" varies from one hospital to another and runs the gamut from a mother having twenty-four hour access to the baby in the room to visits only at the time of nursing, followed by the return of the baby to a central nursery. To avoid disappointment, be sure to get a complete explanation of a hospital's definition of "rooming-in" before your expected date of delivery. The extent of family-centered facilities differ tremendously from one hospital to another and couples should compare obstetrical units from this point of view. For more complete details about family-centered care, order a copy of *Family-centered Maternity/Newborn Care in Hospitals,* from the American College of Obstetricians and Gynecologists, 600 Maryland Avenue SW, Washington, D.C. 20024.

Family-centered alternative birth centers, or ABCs, have recently gained great popularity. An ABC may be either hospital-based or located in a converted residence within minutes of a fully-equipped obstetrical unit. Patients are carefully screened for medical or obstetrical complications before they are allowed to deliver in an ABC. These facilities are usually furnished with comfortable sofas and rocking chairs, carpeting, cheerful wallpaper, quilt-covered beds, stereos, television, coffee machines, and other items which make the room as cozy and homelike as possible. Equipment is minimized, often discreetly concealed behind curtains. In this one room, a mother labors, delivers, and recovers with her husband and often their other children, until she leaves the hospital. Many women and their babies are discharged within six hours following birth.

The obvious advantage of a hospital-based facility is that it can offer both a homelike environment and the security of stand-by medical expertise and equipment. This would appear to be the most satisfactory compromise for women who are rejecting hospitals for home births.

How can I make my admission and discharge from the hospital as easy as possible?

Often, the greatest obstacles encountered by a couple electing to have their child in a hospital arise at the time of arrival to the admitting office. Entering an unfamiliar environment for the first time can be unnerving, and under such circumstances it is often difficult to be assertive when dealing with unyielding and narrow-minded hospital employees. Be assertive! Your efforts will be rewarded. Tour and inspect the hospital earlier in your pregnancy so that admission to the delivery room will be less foreboding. You should find out ahead of time which entrance to use, what the admission procedures are, and what financial arrangements are necessary. Many hospitals have preadmission procedures which enable you to complete much of the paperwork during the last two months of pregnancy. Remember, it's much easier to attend to these matters before the need is urgent. At the time of admission if you are faced with a new admissions clerk asking unnecessary and irrelevant questions, the best advice is to insist on seeing the nursing supervisor immediately. Don't let the hospital or obstetrical staff intimidate you.

After being admitted to the hospital, you will be taken to the labor and delivery area. Most hospitals have a variety of labor and birthing rooms, with some being more attractive and comfortable than others. If you did not make note of this during your previous hospital tour, you should ask to look at the rooms which are available. After you are in the room which you have selected, you will be given a hospital gown to wear and a nurse or resident physician will ask some brief questions about your previous medical and obstetrical history, allergies, medications which you may be taking, the time you last ate, and the exact contents of the meal. This last question is very important since the onset of labor stops the normal digestive processes. If it is necessary to use general anesthesia for delivery, solid food eaten several hours earlier can be regurgitated and cause a catastrophic emergency. Don't be surprised if an insensitive nurse or doctor pursues the questioning during your contractions. If this occurs, just wait and reply between contractions. After the brief history is taken, the nurse will ask you for a urine sample and record your pulse, blood pressure, temperature, respiratory rate, and listen to your baby's heart rate. You will probably be given an identification bracelet that lists your name, the date of admission, your doctor's name, and your hospital number. Later, your baby will be given a bracelet in the delivery room with the identical hospital number as yours. You must carefully check this number whenever your baby is brought to you from the nursery.

Vehemently resist any attempt to separate you from your prepared childbirth partner. Equally protest attempts at shaving your entire perineum, the starting of a routine intravenous solution, the total restriction of clear fluids or ice chips, or confinement to bed during the early stages of labor. Shaving of the pubic hair is especially dehumanizing and it does not decrease your chances of contracting an infection as was previously believed. If anything, it may increase your risk of a hair follicle infection during the uncomfortable period of time when the hair is growing back. Clipping the few hairs between the vagina and rectum will provide your doctor with more than adequate exposure for performance of an episiotomy. All of your special requests should be discussed with your doctor prior to labor and noted on your obstetrical record which he or she forwards to the delivery room during the last month of pregnancy.

An initial pelvic examination by a resident physician, obstetrical nurse, or nurse-midwife may be acceptable and indicated on admission, but if the doctor whose fee you are paying does not arrive within a reasonable amount of time, demand his or her presence in the delivery room. Too many doctors follow the progress of their patients by telephone, and arrive in a blaze of glory only at the very last minute before delivery.

Some physicians believe that an enema should be given in labor because women are often constipated late in pregnancy, and expulsion of feces during the bearing down stages may contaminate the episiotomy site. It has also been stated that the passage of the baby through the birth canal may be easier if the colon and rectum are empty. I know of no scientific studies to support this claim. However, it is true that an enema given early in labor may occasionally bring on more effective uterine contractions. Some women prefer to take an enema because they fear embarrassment caused by the expulsion of feces. For this reason, I allow my patients to decide for themselves if they want an enema. Another option is take a mild Fleet's enema at home just at the onset of labor, but I do not recommend this for women with a history of very rapid labors. When you are in the hospital, you should avoid an enema if your labor is advanced to a cervical dilatation of 7 centimeters or more since it will only intensify your discomfort and increase the risk of a delivery which is too rapid and uncontrolled.

While some women thoroughly enjoy the days spent in the hospital following delivery, others are anxious to return as quickly as possible to their more familiar home surroundings. To accommodate the latter group, many hospitals and birthing centers offer an almost immediate release from the hospital following delivery. On rare occasions, I have discharged a healthy mother and her baby as early as three hours following delivery, without apparent ill effects. An early release from the hospital should only take place after the baby has been carefully examined by a qualified pediatrician. Provisions must also be made for careful follow-up of the baby on an almost daily basis during the first few days of life and for proper rest and care for the mother at home.

How do you feel about the presence of siblings in the delivery room?

Though I was initially enthusiastic about the idea of having other children present during childbirth, I have become less than enamored with this idea. Older children are especially disturbed by the pain which their mother is experiencing and younger children are often totally unable to comprehend the intensity of the birth experience. Until such time that children can be given extensive indoctrination and undergo careful evaluation by trained personnel before labor, I do not endorse sibling presence in the delivery room.

Midwifery

Can you evaluate the competency of the nurse-midwife?

Modern midwivery is a far cry from the stereotype of the early 1900s in which babies were delivered at home by "grannies" and an assortment of untrained persons. The incompetence of these individuals was reflected in the incredibly high number of maternal and infant deaths. Today's nurse-midwives are well-educated, highly qualified, dedicated professionals who have contributed immeasurably to the practice of modern obstetrics in the United States.

To become a nurse-midwife, one must first graduate from a three-year or four-year nursing school and become a registered nurse. Following this, one must get a year's experience in obstetrical nursing and then take a course in nurse-midwifery in one of approximately twenty medical centers offering training programs which are recognized by the American College of Nurse-Midwives. The course of instruction usually lasts for twenty-four months and includes subjects such as anatomy, physiology, embryology, neonatology, and genetics. Students are required to assist in as many as forty or fifty deliveries and manage at least twenty by themselves, under supervision. After graduation, one must take a national certification examination given by the American College of Nurse-Midwives. Passing this test is indicated by the initials C. N. M., or Certified Nurse-Midwife after the nurse-midwife's name. Unfortunately, many unqualified individuals calling themselves nurse-midwives have capitalized on the public's enthusiasm for home births. If you have elected to deliver your baby at home carefully check the midwife's credentials.

Nurse-midwives attend only normal, uncomplicated deliveries, and they always work under the supervision of an obstetrician who must be available for immediate consultation. This applies for deliveries which take place in a hospital, alternative birth center, or at home. Midwives can give local anesthesia for vaginal delivery, perform episiotomies, and suture vaginal and perineal lacerations. They do not perform complicated deliveries or prescribe medications. Following delivery, midwives are trained to provide full postpartum care.

Since the midwife's expertise is limited to uncomplicated births, one might ask, "Why not use an obstetrician who can treat all complications?" The answer is that a midwife offers invaluable minute-by-minute emotional support, enthusiasm, and family-centered care which most busy obstetricians seem incapable of giving. Doctors have been trained to treat diseases with objectivity and detachment, and this can be a great barrier to providing meaningful emotional support to a woman in labor. The overwhelming majority of midwives are women, and patients in labor often remark that they are most comfortable and secure in a first-name relationship with a woman whom they consider to be a friend, rather than an authoritative figure. There are also taboos against the physician, especially if he is a male, giving the intense physical support that the woman in labor often needs. The touching, stroking, and applications of pressure performed by the nurse-midwife can often relieve the stress of labor without use of excessive amounts of analgesics.

Despite official endorsement of certified nurse-midwives by the American College of Obstetricians and Gynecologists, some of the greatest antagonism and scorn of nurse-midwifery has come from Board-certified obstetricians who remain highly suspicious of the nurse-midwife's ability and simply cannot understand how some women could prefer an individual less qualified than themselves to deliver their baby. Hopefully, as doctors learn more about the midwife's skills and sense of commitment, some of these negative attitudes will change. As a member of the obstetric team, the special skills of the nurse-midwife can complement those of the physician in meeting the needs of the patient.

Circumcision

What are the advantages and disadvantages of newborn circumcision?

Circumcision is the most commonly performed operation in the United States, with almost one and a half million procedures recorded each year. Yet, most who give permission for circumcision of their newborn sons have practically no knowledge of the procedure or its attendant risks.

In most hospitals, circumcision is performed on the second day after birth. In some hospitals, the pediatricians do the surgery, while in others it is the job of the obstetrician. The Jewish ritual circumcision is performed on the eighth day of life by a trained religious leader, or mohel. Since few women will remain in the hospital for eight postpartum days, this joyous occasion, for everyone but the baby, is usually celebrated at home.

The operation itself is simple. The prepuce, or fold of skin covering the glans, is removed by applying a specially designed clamp. The clamp crushes any blood vessels as the skin is being removed. The result of the operation is that the glans of the circumcised male is permanently exposed. In contrast, the uncircumcised male must retract his foreskin in order to expose his glans.

Phimosis is the name given to the condition in which the prepuce adheres to the glans. Occasionally, the prepuce will retract but then can't be repositioned. This causes a painful constriction at the base of the glans and is known as paraphimosis. The supposed advantage of circumcision is that it prevents the accumulation of smegma, or penile secretions, and dirt from accumulating under the prepuce, which may cause infection and phimosis. However, daily bathing and retraction and cleaning of the glans with soap and water, can prevent practically all cases. It is estimated that only 6 percent of all males medically require circumcision. Use of circumcision solely for the purpose of avoiding the chore of teaching your son proper penile hygiene would appear unwarranted.

In the opinion of many doctors, the only currently valid indications for circumcision are religious preference and the psychological concerns of parents who want their infant to have a penile appearance resembling that of a father or older sibling. Previous claims of a higher incidence of cervical cancer among wives of uncircumcised men are unfounded. Similarly, uncircumcised males are not less likely to contract gonorrhea, syphilis, or herpes. Although it is believed that the absence of the prepuce may slightly reduce the incidence of penile cancer, the protective benefits are minimal because the disease is extremely rare even in uncircumcised men.

Circumcision is certainly not painless, and individuals observing the procedure for the first time are often appalled at the amount of pain that some infants appear to experience. Though short-lived, the experience certainly is not in keeping with attempts to provide a peaceful and serene environment for all newborns. If anything, this practice recalls a more primitive era of medicine. Studies conducted on newborns suggest that circumcision does affect behavior. In one report, changes in the infants' sleep patterns, characterized by wakefulness, agitation, and crying, were noted following the procedure. The endocrine response of newborns to this procedure supports the behavioral evidence that the operation is stressful.

Physical complications from circumcision occur no more often than 1 in 500 cases, and most of these are very mild. Complications include excessive bleeding, postoperative infections, injuries to the glans, penile shaft, and damage to the urinary opening or meatus. There are several cases in which too much foreskin had been removed. The need to perform a second circumcision on as many as 10 percent of babies occurs because inadequate removal of tissue has been followed by phimosis. The rare deaths following circumcision, estimated at 2 out of every 1 million operations, can be attributed to extremely poor surgical technique or to a blood clotting deficiency of the affected infants.

Parents should think twice about their decision to circumcise their newborn if it is not being performed solely for religious purposes.

Lactation Suppression

If a woman prefers not to nurse her baby, what can she do to relieve breast engorgement and lactation?

Breast engorgement can usually be relieved with simple measures such as use of a breast binder or good maternity brassiere, ice packs, and analgesics. Contrary to popular belief, restricting fluid intake does not decrease breast engorgement. Discomfort is most pronounced between the second and fourth postpartum day. All signs and symptoms usually disappear by the end of the first postpartum week, provided that the breasts are not stimulated by pumping.

One of the most exciting pharmacological discoveries in recent years has been the synthesis of bromocriptine mesylate (trade name Parlodel). This nonhormonal drug has been used effectively to inhibit postpartum lactation and lactation associated with a variety of endocrine disorders.

To prevent postpartum lactation, a 2.5 milligram Parlodel tablet is ingested twice daily with meals for fourteen days. If necessary, it may be prescribed for an additional seven days. Since an abnormal drop in blood pressure has been reported in as many as 28 percent of postpartum women receiving Parlodel, the first tablet should be taken no earlier than four hours following delivery, and only after it is certain that a woman's postdelivery vital signs are stable. While estrogen preparations (see below) must be taken immediately after delivery if they are to be effective, an advantage of bromocriptine is that it remains effective even when taken days, weeks, or months following childbirth. In addition to these benefits, bromocriptine, unlike estrogens, is not associated with an increase in blood clotting factors or an abnormal increase in uterine bleeding patterns.

To date, hundreds of postpartum women have been treated with Parlodel with excellent results. Bromocriptine, however, is not free of adverse reactions. In addition to the previously mentioned 28 percent incidence of drop in blood pressure, it may cause headaches (10 percent), dizziness (8 percent), nausea (7 percent), vomiting (3 percent), fatigue (1 percent), fainting (0.7 percent), diarrhea (0.4 percent), and abdominal cramps (0.4 percent). Lactation and mild breast engorgement may return after the bromocriptine is stopped.

When a woman takes bromocriptine to inhibit puerperal lactation, her ovulatory function and ability to conceive returns earlier than is normal. It is, therefore, imperative that she use adequate contraception even if intercourse is resumed as early as the second or third postpartum week.

Metergoline is a drug which has shown great promise in preventing and treating postpartum lactation. It is also effective in relieving breast pain and congestion. When taken orally for five to ten days, metergoline has achieved success rates of 95 to 100 percent. Unlike Parlodel, metergoline use does not appear to be associated with unpleasant side effects. Further studies related to its safety and efficacy are being anxiously awaited.

There is some evidence to suggest that vitamin B6, or pyridoxine, may inhibit prolactin release and reduce breast milk secretion. A minority of scientists have gone as far to urge nursing women to avoid the long-term use of multivitamins which contain pyridoxine. Further research on this subject is required before definite conclusions can be reached, but it is certain that the use of pyridoxine as a lactation suppressant is far from becoming a reality.

How safe or effective are estrogens or other hormonal preparations in inhibiting lactation?

Though hormonal preparations have been widely used to inhibit postpartum breast engorement and lactation, they are less than adequate for this purpose. Estrogens remain the most popular medication prescribed, even though they prevent breast engorgement in only 25 percent of all nonnursing women and do not prevent lactation. Of all preparations, the best results are probably achieved with an intramuscular injection of a lactation suppressant containing a long-acting estrogen named estradiol valerate combined with the male hormone testosterone enanthate (trade name Deladumone). For maximum results, it is best taken immediately after delivery. Other natural and synthetic estrogens, including the popular chlorotrianisene (trade name Tace) and the infamous DES (see chapter 1), have also been used to suppress lactation. All of these preparations, however, may increase a woman's risk of abnormal blood coagulation and the formation of blood clots or thrombi in the veins of the legs and pelvis. On very rare occasions, dislodged clots called emboli may travel to vital organs, such as the lungs, and cause death. It has been estimated that postpartum estrogens may increase the maternal death rate by 1 to 2 deaths per 100,000 women. Though this may not sound like very much, I believe that even 1 preventable death should be enough to discourage doctors from prescribing these hormones for lactation suppression.

Federal law now requires that all women first read a patient information paper before receiving postpartum estrogens. Although I would agree with the information in this paper regarding blood clotting factors, I do take exception to the way in which other risks are evaluated. For example, it is known that cancer of the endometrium of the uterus and diseases of the gallbladder may be associated with long-term and continuous estrogen use. However, it has never been proven that these complications can result from a single postpartum exposure. In my opinion, the patient information paper falsely implies such a relationship.

Breast-Feeding

What are some of the myths related to breast-feeding?

Not every woman wishes to nurse her infant, and this decision must be respected. Unfortunately, this negative feeling is often based on misinformation, fears, and anxieties which are without basis. For example, many women believe that breast-feeding causes sagging of the breasts and excessive weight gain. Both beliefs are untrue. In fact, it has been proven that women who nurse lose most of their stored pregnancy fat faster than those who do not nurse.

The quantity of breast milk is dependent upon good nutrition and adequate caloric intake. Ideally, a balanced food intake providing approximately 500 extra calories a day allows the production of enough breast milk to meet the needs of an average growing baby. There is a common misconception that at least 1,000 extra calories must be consumed each day to achieve this end. The quality of breast milk varies from one woman to another, but it is of interest to note that the quality remains fairly consistent for each individual even when the quantity changes.

For the first few days following childbirth, colostrum is secreted from a woman's breasts. This differs significantly from the later milk in that it is deep yellow in color and is not as sweet. Nevertheless, it is rich in antibodies for fighting infection, contains proteins and salts, and has a laxative effect on the baby. The frequent bowel movements help to remove the bilirubin pigment from the body and reduce a baby's likelihood of jaundice during the first few days of life. Colostrum usually disappears from the milk in four to five days and is replaced by the more nutritious breast milk.

It is a common misconception that nursing women should drink excessive amounts of water in order to maintain adequate milk production. In fact, excessive fluid intake may actually diminish milk supply due to stimulation of a complex pituitary gland mechanism. One quart of milk daily is also not necessary. A woman who doesn't like milk can get the calcium her body needs from other dairy products (see chapter 8).

Although nursing mothers are often instructed to allow their infants to feed for at least ten minutes on each breast, a 1979 study from England has demonstrated that 80 to 90 percent of the nutritive value of milk is obtained during the first four minutes. Within the first two minutes, over 50 percent of the total nutritional content has usually been ingested. This statistic should in no way encourage women to rapidly nurse their infants since the untold emotional benefits of prolonged nursing will never be adequately studied by scientists.

Some women decline to nurse because they fear their breasts are too small to produce a sufficient milk supply. Larger breasts are large because they contain more fat, not more milk ducts. It is the glandular tissue which produces the milk, and this functions just as well in the "flat-chested" woman as in the more abundantly endowed individual.

There are very few medical situations which would preclude successful nursing. Preparation of the breasts is best accomplished during pregnancy. For women with special problems such as inverted nipples, breast shields and other aids are usually helpful. Literature and details about breast care, prenatal nipple conditioning, and specific problems related to nursing can be obtained from your local chapter of the La Leche League or from national headquarters (9616 Minneapolis Avenue, Franklin Park, Illinois 60131).

What advice do you have for a working woman who wants to nurse her baby?

A lack of time is frequently cited as a reason why many working mothers decline to nurse. However, even the most demanding job schedule should not deter the ambitious woman from successfully breast-feeding. Many working women actually state that the moments spent nursing their babies are the most restful and enjoyable part of every day. For those who are fortunate enough to work close to home, it is often possible to nurse during the lunch break, while part-time jobs with flexible hours provide greater latitude in planning a nursing schedule. For those who cannot return home during the day, a baby can be nursed just before you leave for work and immediately after you return. With this schedule probably only one supplemental bottle will be required in the middle of the day, but it is important that such mothers take an occasional break to express milk from their breasts so that their breasts do not become overly full. Painful breast engorgement and embarrassing leakage can be avoided in this way, and the mothers can maintain continuous milk production and lessen their risk of blockage and infection of the milk ducts. While expression by hand is probably the simplest method, a small hand pump can be used. Many women prefer to collect their breast milk in sterile containers so that their babysitter can serve it the next day as a supplemental feeding. If you are considering this, do not hesitate to request a quiet and private area in your work environment so that you can take a few minutes during the day to express your breast milk in an unhurried manner without unpleasant interruptions. And remember that expressed milk must be kept refrigerated at all times.

In addition to the emotional benefits derived from nursing, what are the medical advantages?

As a result of new research showing that a mother may transmit temporary but effective immunity to her nursing infant, the American Academy of Pediatrics has enthusiastically endorsed the value of breast-feeding. Though this same idea was presented several years ago and rejected, it was rekindled by the findings of a 1977 study which compared episodes of significant illness between 164 breast-fed infants and 162 who were receiving a formula. Among the former group, episodes of significant illness were uncommon and there were no life-threatening diseases. In contrast, 5 formula-fed babies developed pneumonia, 1 contracted meningitis, and 1 died of sudden infant death syndrome or SIDS. Other studies, including the most recent in 1979, have confirmed a higher incidence of SIDS among bottle-fed infants. Infant botulism, a deadly disease caused by a bacterial organism named Clostridium botulinum, is also more likely if an infant does not nurse. It is interesting to note that the onset of the disease is at a younger age in bottle-fed infants and is likely to be of greater severity if iron supplements are added to the milk formula.

Infants who nurse extensively are also less likely to experience common complaints such as colic, skin rashes, ear infections and upper respiratory infections, when compared to those receiving formula. In a 1979 study, published in the *Journal of Pediatrics,* it was reported that middle ear infections and episodes of severe diarrhea and vomiting were approximately twice as frequent in the bottle-fed group studied than in the breast-fed group. Lower respiratory tract infections were five times more likely to occur and hospital admissions and total episodes of illness were reported to be three times more frequent among the artificially fed infants.

There are a host of disease-fighting antibodies contained in breast milk. Three antibody types, known as immunoglobulins G, A, and M, are especially important. They offer protection against a wide variety of infectious diseases until the newborn is capable of producing its own immunoglobulins at three months of age. Polio, mumps, influenza, whooping cough, diphtheria, and salmonella are but a few of these diseases. It has recently been shown that some antibodies are ingested in the breast milk and then reside in the intestine where they protect the newborn's susceptible gastrointestinal tract against a variety of bacterial infections. This finding supports earlier studies showing that breast-fed infants had gastrointestinal infections at a rate of 0.2 per 1,000 compared to 8 per 1,000 among those fed cow's milk. In addition to antibodies, breast milk is now known to contain macrophages, living cells capable of preventing infection by killing harmful bacteria and viruses. Living white blood cells named lymphocytes when found in mother's milk were once considered to be a sign of recent infection. New studies, however, show that their presence may be essential to a baby's ability to resist infections.

Breast milk contains a substance known as "bifidus factor" which encourages the growth of the beneficial bacterium *Lactobacillus bifidus,* and helps to explain the greater resistance of breast-fed infants to intestinal infections. Breast milk also contains other bacterial-fighting agents with names such as lysozyme, lactoperoxidase, lactoferrin, and complement factors C3 and C4. The protective effect of breast milk is especially vital for the premature infant.

Breast-feeding also offers protection against childhood food allergies, asthma, and allergic skin rashes. This is especially true when the period of nursing lasts for at least six months. Cow's milk is loaded with foreign proteins, or allergens, which may incite allergic reactions in children. One such protein, named beta lactoglobulin, is probably the chief culprit. Lactalbumin is the main protein of human milk, and since it is not a foreign substance, it is well tolerated.

A 1979 study from the Children's Hospital, University of Helsinki, Finland showed that compared with formula feeding, prolonged breast-feeding for longer than six months was associated with a significant decline in the incidence and severity of allergic reactions during this period of time. In babies who were solely breast-fed for at least six months, food allergy was suppressed for up to one year of age, and eczema for as long as three years. This was particularly significant among families with an allergic disease history, leading the authors to endorse prolonged breast-feeding for these susceptible individuals. They also recommended the avoidance of common allergenic foods, such as fish, citrus fruits, chocolate, eggs, peanuts, honey, and tomato, for at least the first year of life.

The nutritional content of breast milk makes it ideal for meeting the specific needs of the newborn infant. On the average, human milk contains 8 percent protein, 55 percent fat, and 37 percent carbohydrate. This ratio is constant and is not affected by the mother's diet. Human milk has one-third as much protein as cow's milk, but this is all a baby needs to ensure normal growth. Excretion of excess protein only adds stress to a newborn's immature kidneys. Counterbalancing the decreased quantity of protein available in human milk is its higher quality. The main protein in human milk is lactalbumin, while cow's milk contains an abundance of casein protein. The latter often forms large and hard curds in a baby's stomach, making it far more difficult to digest.

Lactose, the carbohydrate in breast milk, is helpful in stimulating the growth of bacteria in the baby's intestine, an aid in the protection against intestinal diseases. Lactose also provides energy, aids in the production of certain vitamins, and helps in the absorption of minerals from the intestinal tract.

Breast milk has less sodium and phosphorus than cow's milk, and a better phosphorus-calcium ratio. This balance prevents an overload on the baby's kidneys and reduces the baby's need for fluids other than breast milk. The low sodium or salt content may be beneficial since high salt intake in infancy may be related to high blood pressure in later life.

Though human milk consists of an abundance of fats, it also contains enzymes called lipases which aid in their digestion and absorption. In contrast, the saturated fat content of cow's milk is difficult for a baby's body to absorb. Breast milk contains more cholesterol than cow's milk or infant formulas. Many nutritionists believe that an infant needs this higher level of cholesterol in early life in order to stimulate enzyme systems that will metabolize cholesterol throughout life. Based on this observation, some doctors have theorized that adults who have been breast-fed as children may show a lower incidence of coronary artery disease than milk- or formula-fed individuals. Though this theory has not been supported by any large-scale studies, researchers at Harvard School of Public Health have studied cholesterol levels of adult men and women who were exclusively breast-fed for more than two months as infants. Amazingly, these individuals had lower cholesterol values than those who were not breast-fed.

The vitamin and mineral content of breast milk reflects the amount of these nutrients that a woman consumes in her daily diet. In table 11–1, I have compared the relative amounts of these vitamins in human and cow's milk. However, some doctors recommend vitamin supplements for nursing infants (see below for a full discussion).

Mothers of low birth weight babies should be encouraged to breast-feed. Preterm breast milk has higher sodium and nitrogen content than term breast milk and is better suited to the nutritional needs of the preterm infant. Nitrogen availability in the form of protein, urea, and amino acids provides the rapidly growing premature infant with higher amounts of compounds necessary for building tissue protein. Early milk produced by preterm women contains about 30 percent more fat than that of full-term mothers. This higher energy content makes the premature infant better able to use the protein and other nutrients of breast milk for growth.

In addition to this impressive list of breast-feeding benefits, one must not forget that nursing immediately following delivery will help to release oxytocin. This will help to contract uterine muscles and reduce the incidence of postpartum hemorrhage. Nursing also helps to restore the mother's uterus to its prepregnancy size at a faster rate than occurs among women who do not nurse. The limited benefits of nursing as a method of birth control have been previously discussed.

Are there any potentially harmful aspects to breast-feeding?

Not all pediatricians agree that mother's milk is the nutritionally perfect food. Some doctors have reported deficiencies of vitamin D, vitamin K, iron, and fluoride among healthy infants who are nourished with unsupplemented human milk over an extended period of several months. In a 1978 report, published in the *New England Journal of Medicine*, doctors recommended supplements of iron, vitamin K, and vitamin D for all nursing infants.

In addition, they cautioned that the breast-fed child of a strict vegetarian may suffer from a severe vitamin B12 deficiency. Since a vitamin B12 deficiency may prove fatal, it is best to add this supplement to the diet of those babies. Nursing babies of vegetarian mothers should also receive iron, vitamin K, and vitamin D.

Calcium, phosphorus, and iron levels are especially low in human milk, and this

Table 11–1. Comparison of Vitamin Content in Breast Milk and Fresh Cow's Milk

	*Mature Breast Milk**	*Cow's Milk**
Vitamin A	150 USP units	100 USP units
Carotenoids	27 μg	38 μg
B vitamins		
Thiamine	16 μg	42 μg
Riboflavin	43 μg	157 μg
Nicotinic acid	172 μg	85 μg
Pyridoxine	11 μg	48 μg
Pantothenic acid	196 μg	350 μg
Folic acid	0.18 μg	0.23 μg
Choline	9 mg	13 mg
Inositol	39 mg	13 mg
Biotin	0.4 μg	3.5 μg
B$_{12}$	0.04 μg	0.41 μg
Vitamin C	4.3 mg	1.8 mg
Vitamin D	0.4–10.0 USP units	0.3–4.0 USP units
Vitamin K	26 Dam-Glavind units	100 Dam-Glavind units

* Vitamin content in 100 ml.

may pose serious problems to low birth weight infants who are nursing. For this reason, many pediatricians recommend supplements of these elements for premature infants. The lack of sodium in human milk may be particularly dangerous for premature infants since they may experience an abnormally low sodium concentration in their blood (*hyponatremia*). Premature infants who are nursing should have their serum sodium levels closely monitored and sodium added if there is a deficiency.

When jaundice, a yellow pigmentation of the skin and eyes, occurs in a healthy newborn for a short period of time it is termed physiologic jaundice. It is hardly ever severe and usually disappears by the seventh day of life. A breast-fed infant will, on rare occasions, develop deeper and more prolonged jaundice than normal. This is believed to be due to the interaction between a metabolite of progesterone hormone in the breast milk and an enzyme in the baby. If the jaundice seems severe enough to cause concern, breast-feeding is interrupted for three or four days to rapidly reduce the jaundice and allow time for the baby's liver to deal with the pigment more efficiently.

Practically all medications given to a mother pass into her breast milk in various concentrations. Some drugs even cause serious problems for the nursing infant (see chapter 7). To minimize the concentration of medication, even if it is safe, take the medication fifteen minutes after the baby has nursed or three to four hours before the next feeding to allow enough time for reduction in the amount of medication in the blood and consequently in the breast milk. Alcohol, harmful drugs, certain viruses, and environmental contaminants may all be passed on to the nursing infant through breast milk. The effects of this are discussed more fully in earlier chapters. Despite these drawbacks, however, there is no doubt that the benefits of breast-feeding far outweigh the risks for the vast majority of healthy women.

Are there any medications that can be used to increase the quantity of a woman's breast milk?

If prolactin was available as a pill or injection, it would probably be helpful in stimulating milk production among women who want to nurse but lack an adequate supply of milk. Though this medication does not exist, there are lactation-inducing agents including antidepressants and tranquilizers, such as chlorpromazine (trade name Thorazine) and thioridazine (trade name Mellaril) (see chapter 7). It is not unusual for nonpregnant women to experience lactation following long-term use of these drugs.

The antidepressant sulpiride has been studied by doctors at Osaka University Medical School in Japan. In their 1979 and 1982 reports they noted significant increases in yield of milk among the sulpiride-treated women as early as the second postpartum day. Though the results are encouraging, two important questions remain unanswered. One concern is that antidepressants, such as sulpiride, are transmitted to the breast milk, and it is not yet known what effect this has on the nursing infant. In addition, it has not yet been demonstrated that sulpiride can maintain the increase in milk quantity for prolonged periods of time. Whether sulpiride or a chemically related drug finds a place in obstetrical practice will only be determined after extensive clinical experience. Maternal side effects of tranquilizers, such as fatigue and drowsiness, may also serve as a deterrent to their use.

In addition to its effects on uterine muscle contractions, oxytocin also stimulates cells in the breast, known as myoepithelial cells, to contract. This causes milk "let-down" or ejection from the nipple and helps to initiate the nursing process. Oxytocin in the form of a nasal spray or tablet placed below the tongue has been used extensively to aid milk ejection. Contrary to popular belief, it will not increase the total yield of milk and should not be used for this purpose.

Postpartum

What emotional feelings may be experienced during the postpartum period?

For the majority of women, the euphoria which they experience at the moment of birth continues throughout the postpartum period. However, for as many as 40 percent, the emotional "high" of childbirth is often followed by varying degrees of postpartum depression, or "blues," usually manifested by one or two crying episodes without apparent cause during the first three to seven postpartum days, followed by a rapid recovery with no further difficulties. For other less fortunate individuals, the depression may become deeper, last longer than two weeks, and cause serious psychological impairment requiring professional help. The risk of recurrence of postpartum depression in subsequent pregnancies is believed to be between 25 and 33 percent.

Despite extensive study, the cause of postpartum depression remains a mystery. Some psychiatrists attribute this condition to the many sudden physical, social, and psychological changes which occur immediately following the birth of a child. Other doctors believe it is caused by the dramatic decline in concentration of circulating female hormones, combined with a reduction in a woman's blood volume following childbirth. These factors, in addition to a variety of physical discomforts, such as episiotomy and hemorrhoid pain, "afterbirth" pains caused by contractions of the postpartum uterus, breast engorgement, and lack of sleep, all contribute to the problem. Women who, for a variety of medical reasons, are separated from their infant during the first two days of life are believed to be more susceptible to postpartum depression because they have lost the opportunity to bond with their infant during this critical time.

Interviews with women suffering from postpartum depression reveal a wide range of concerns. The most commonly reported problem is arguments with their husbands or partners. For some the reality of caring for a demanding and irritable baby twenty-four hours a day is far more difficult than they had anticipated, while for others the concern is the change that their bodies have undergone. Some women express feelings of isolation because the baby has suddenly become the focus of everyone's attention.

Women who have had a cesarean section are also more likely to experience depression. Such women often express a feeling of inadequacy and a sense of having deprived their spouse of the birth experience. A great aid for such women has been the emergence of cesarean section support groups. Too often, hospitals isolate babies born by cesarean section in a special nursery. If a baby is healthy and a woman is awake during the cesarean section, holding her baby as soon as possible after the operation is completed should be allowed.

While postpartum "blues" usually start when a woman is in the hospital, they may intensify when she arrives home and is confronted with the added burden of household chores, unannounced visitors, a demanding mate, and too little sleep. Of all these factors, a lack of sleep is probably the greatest underlying reason for postpartum depression. For this reason it is vital that you sleep whenever your baby sleeps and nap during the day when your baby does not demand attention.

Interestingly, a significant number of fathers suffer from postpartum "blues." In one study as many as 62 percent of new fathers experienced some form of this feeling. Among those men who have been interviewed, many seemed frustrated in their inability to help cope with the new baby. Others expressed helplessness in caring for the babies themselves, while some of the men who experienced prolonged depression described themselves as "overwhelmed" by the problems that their spouses were having in caring for the infants. A small number of fathers expressed frustration because the amount of time allotted to them with their baby was limited.

Though postpartum "blues" can't be prevented, their intensity and duration can be dramatically reduced. The most important thing you can do is to get help with the housework, shopping, and cooking so that you are free to concentrate on the care of your baby during the first two to three weeks at home. Don't be afraid to ask for help—there is nothing to be gained by suffering silently. A professional baby nurse, though expensive, is a luxury which is well worth it. By caring for your baby, a nurse allows you the opportunity to catch up on your sleep and enjoy leisure time away from the house. A quiet evening out to a favorite restaurant is great therapy for postpartum depression, though you should not expect it to be an instant cure. Discuss your feelings openly with your mate and let him ventilate as well. It is through this process of communication that the problems and depression of the early postpartum days can be corrected.

When friends, relatives, nurses, and other helpers have all departed after the first few weeks, you can continue to enjoy your leisure time if you join or form a babysitting co-op with other new mothers. One of the great cures for postpartum depression is a mothers' support group. Such groups are usually made up of a handful of women from the same neighborhood whose children are roughly the same age. Frequently local Y's or community centers sponsor such groups. During weekly meetings, a wide range of topics dealing with the physical and emotional concerns of motherhood can be discussed. This will often help you to realize that your problems are not unlike those of other young mothers. While you may have prided yourself on being the perfect cook, homemaker, and lover prior to the birth of your baby, you must accept the fact that the limited number of hours in the day will prevent you from achieving unrealistic and unnecessary goals. Furthermore, make it clear to your partner that he should not demand more than you are capable of giving and that he must actively participate in the management of the household. Assertiveness is the key to preventing and curing postpartum depression.

How do most women feel about sex during the postpartum period?

Needless to say, women demonstrate a variety of sexual responses during the postpartum period. While a minority experience an early return to erotic interest within four weeks, do not be surprised if it takes as long as six to twelve weeks before your libido returns to its prepregnancy levels (see chapter 4). One hindrance to complete sexual enjoyment during the early postpartum weeks is a woman's fear that her episiotomy is not completely healed. In addition, pain with intercourse during the first three months is more likely to occur among women who nurse because their vaginal tissues are thin and fragile because of a lack of estrogen. While some doctors prescribe estrogen cream vaginally twice a week to correct this problem, it is a form of therapy which I don't endorse because significant amounts of the hormone may be absorbed through the vaginal walls and enter the bloodstream and breast milk. Instead, a lubricant such as K-Y may be used. Though this is not as effective as estrogen cream, it is in my opinion much safer.

In addition to the physical and hormonal changes which occur during the postpartum period, a woman's libido may be dampened by a variety of other factors such as fatigue, anxiety, lack of sleep, a crying baby, and financial concerns. Patience, love, understanding, communication, and elixir of time will cure an overwhelming number of postpartum sexual problems.

When can intercourse be resumed after childbirth?

Contrary to what most doctors recommend, there is no scientific evidence to show that a couple must wait the standard six weeks before resuming intercourse. Following an uncomplicated vaginal delivery, in which there are no lacerations and no episiotomy is performed, intercourse should be perfectly safe at two weeks postpartum. The stitches of an episiotomy or a sutured laceration usually completely dissolve three weeks later. At that time, intercourse can be attempted gingerly, and if there is no discomfort there is no need to abstain. Following a cesarean section, the abdominal incision usually takes two weeks to heal, and barring unusual medical complications, intercourse should be safe at this time.

Noncoital lovemaking techniques should be undertaken gingerly. The mouth contains a wide variety of potentially harmful bacteria which, when introduced into a vaginal, urethral, or vulvar laceration may be capable of causing an infection. If you are contemplating oral-genital sex prior to three weeks postpartum, I advise that you carefully inspect your vulva and vagina with a hand mirror for evidence of a laceration that has not healed. If you are unable to do this, consult your obstetrician. While some doctors believe that bacteria from a man's mouth may be introduced into the nipple of a nursing mother during lovemaking, there is no scientific evidence to show that this would cause mastitis or breast inflammation.

Is contraception necessary prior to the six-week postpartum examination?

I must confess that I have never seen a woman who has conceived prior to her six-week postpartum visit, and many studies have confirmed that ovulation rarely occurs before the fifth postpartum week. However, there is scientific evidence which clearly documents ovulation in a nonnursing woman as early as twenty-eight days following a full-term delivery. Though you may have a period prior to your six-week visit, it will most likely be anovulatory, meaning that it will not be preceded by ovulation and the risk of pregnancy. It has been estimated, on the basis of available statistics that 5 percent of nursing women and 15 percent of nonnursing women ovulate by the sixth postpartum week. By the twelfth postpartum week, the percentages increase to 25 to 40 percent respectively. At the twenty-fourth postpartum week, the theoretical risk of conception jumps to 65 percent if you nurse and 75 percent if you don't. In actual practice, however, the number of women who conceive is much lower than the above figures since most couples use some type of contraceptive technique during this time. When this is taken into account, only 1 percent of nursing mothers and 3 percent of nonnursing mothers conceive within three months of delivery. At six months, actual conception rates increase to 5 percent and 15 percent respectively.

Some recent studies from Europe suggest that enthusiastic breast-feeding with more than five feedings in twenty-four hours, including one at night, may inhibit ovulation for a year or more. This form of birth control, referred to as "push-button contraception," requires further evaluation among many nursing women before it can be enthusiastically endorsed. Until that time, I will continue to encourage my patients to use more traditional methods of contraception if they resume intercourse prior to their six-week postpartum examination.

What form of contraception can I use before the six-week postpartum check-up?

Since the risk of pregnancy is minimal during the first six postpartum weeks, the use of condoms and vaginal spermicides in the form of nonprescription aerosal foams, jellies, tablets, creams, and suppositories provides adequate and easy-to-use contraception. When choosing a condom, be sure that it is lubricated so that the sensitive vaginal tissues are not irritated.

All spermicidal agents must be inserted high into the vagina, as close to the cervix as possible, if they are to be effective. It is best to do this within thirty minutes before intercourse and repeated acts of coitus should be preceded by insertion of additional spermicide. Contraceptive aerosol foam is probably the best of the vaginal spermicides because it is more rapidly distributed throughout the vagina and quickly forms a barrier over the cervix so that intercourse and ejaculation can immediately follow its insertion. Allow creams or jellies slightly more time for them to adjust to your body temperature and melt and allow suppositories and tablets at least ten minutes to completely liquefy. Since intravaginal distribution of jelly, tablets, and suppositories is partially dependent on penile thrusting, a greater chance of pregnancy exists if a man ejaculates quickly after penetration. Foam is also not nearly as messy as the other vaginal spermicides. It is less likely to drain out of the vagina after use, and is also less likely to leak out of the vagina during intercourse.

Can a diaphragm be used during this early postpartum period?

No. Don't try to use your old diaphragm prior to your six-week postpartum visit because, as a result of your changing anatomy and greater sensitivity of your vaginal tissues, it will be difficult to insert and may not adequately cover your cervix. Ask your doctor to recheck your diaphragm size at your six-week visit since it is quite possible that you will require a larger size than you previously used. If you have intentions of losing additional weight, be sure to have your diaphragm size rechecked after each fifteen pounds of weight loss.

If you have never used a diaphragm, your doctor can measure or fit you for the correct size at the time of your postpartum visit. The prescription for the specific type and size and the spermicidal cream or jelly used with it is then filled by a pharmacist. The actual measuring of the diaphragm takes only a few minutes, but once the size is determined, it is the obligation of your doctor to take the time to explain the simple anatomy involved, as well as the proper insertion technique. You should take the time to practice inserting the diaphragm without assistance, and your doctor should then check the proper position by doing a vaginal examination. Regardless of how many failures are encountered, don't leave the office until you are satisfied and you fully understand the insertion technique. Occasionally, when a woman has become discouraged at several unsuccessful insertion attempts, I tell her to practice in the privacy of her home and then return to the office on another day wearing the diaphragm so that we can be sure that it is now inserted correctly. But remember that other contraception should be used during this learning period. Once the insertion technique is learned, it becomes extremely simple and is never forgotten.

What is a cervical cap, and how effective is it as a postpartum contraceptive?

A cervical cap looks like a small diaphragm but fits securely over the cervix rather than against the vaginal walls. Though women have shown a tremendous amount of interest in cervical caps, they are not approved for use by the FDA and they are fitted by very few doctors. Since the size of the cervix continues to decrease during the first two postpartum months, it would be foolish to be fitted for a cervical cap during this time. While some reports have noted cervical cap pregnancy rates equal to the diaphragm, others have found higher rates caused by slippage during intercourse and difficulty in using it correctly.

What problems may be encountered if I use birth control pills during the postpartum period?

Aside from permanent sterilization, no other method of birth control approaches the efficacy of oral contraceptives. If you are not nursing and your doctor finds no medical reasons for not prescribing the Pill, it can be started at the time of your six-week postpartum visit. Practically all birth control pills contain estrogen combined with a synthetic progesterone-like chemical known as a progestin. Minipills such as Ovrette, Micronor, and Nor-Q.D. contain only a progestin. The estrogen contained in the combination birth control pills is capable of reducing the quantity of a woman's breast milk. In addition, a small amount of the estrogen may enter the breast milk and on rare occasions cause breast enlargement of a nursing infant. The progestin-only minipill, on the other hand, does not appear to adversely affect the quantity of milk produced. As a result, many obstetricians prescribe the minipill as contraception for nursing women. Other doctors are reluctant to do this because no large-scale studies have been conducted to prove that small amounts of progestins ingested in the milk over a prolonged period of time are harmless to a nursing infant. Progestins are chemically similar to the male hormone testosterone and it has been theorized that their passage into the breast milk may be associated with masculinization of a breast-fed female infant. While minipills do not appear to decrease milk quantity, there are statistics available which show that they do alter the basic composition of breast milk, including a decrease in total protein content, milk fats, lactose, phosphorus, calcium, magnesium, and zinc. It is for these reasons that minipills should not be your first choice of contraception if you are nursing.

What is your opinion of the intrauterine device as a method of postpartum contraception?

An intrauterine device, or IUD, is a device inserted into the endometrial cavity and left there for various periods of time for the purpose of contraception. Although the

Copper-7 (Cu-7) is by far the most popular brand in this country, the Lippes Loop, Saf-T-Coil, and Copper-T (Cu-7) are also frequently used. While a vocal minority of obstetricians have advocated the insertion of IUDs immediately following childbirth, this technique has not gained popularity because it may be associated with a number of complications, such as perforation of the enlarged and soft uterus, infection, postpartum bleeding, and expulsion of the device. Until recently, the consensus among doctors was that IUDs should not be inserted prior to the eighth postpartum week because of the greater likelihood of these problems. However, a 1982 study from the University of Southern California School of Medicine clearly demonstrated that complication rates were no higher among women who had a Cu-7 inserted between the fourth and eighth postpartum weeks when compared to those who waited until after the eighth for their IUD insertion. The authors of this report confirmed my opinion that the IUD can be safely inserted at the time of your six-week postpartum visit.

The obvious advantages of an IUD are its extremely low pregnancy rate of 2 women per 100 who use the device and the convenience of not having to take elaborate precautions in preparation for each coital act. However, before you receive an IUD be sure to carefully read and understand the accompanying booklet which describes the unlikely but serious complications which you may encounter. For example, the risk of infection is less than 3 percent, but if it occurs it may be quite serious. Symptoms that should alert you to the possibility of an early pelvic infection are vague lower abdominal pain, any temperature above 37.5°C (99.5°F), a foul-smelling yellowish discharge, chills, and pain with intercourse. Unfortunately, sometimes these infections become far advanced before a woman experiences any symptoms at all. Vague symptoms such as fatigue and flulike aches and pains should also be cause for alarm. If you are in doubt, consult your doctor immediately.

What advice do you have for couples seeking permanent sterilization?

Emotionally, a woman may believe that she wants a tubal ligation, or tying of her tubes, immediately following a difficult nine months of pregnancy and a painful labor. However, studies show that she may later regret this decision. In one report, a significant number of women who requested postpartum sterilization but had surgery delayed for various reasons, declined to undergo the operation when given the opportunity at a later date. For this reason, it is best not to have the surgery if there is even the slightest doubt. Nothing is lost by waiting.

An abdominal tubal ligation during the immediate postpartum period is extremely easy to perform. Under either general or local anesthesia, an incision of an inch or less is made just under the navel and a small segment of each tube is then tied and cut. When a tubal ligation is performed immediately after delivery or on the following day, a woman can return home three to five days later. This lengthens her total postpartum hospitalization time an average of only two days.

Instead of the traditional abdominal tubal ligation, many doctors now perform postpartum tubal sterilization through a viewing instrument called a laparoscope which is inserted through the umbilicus. Using this instrument, a doctor can block the tubes by burning them or by applying special bands or clips. In my experience with this technique, I have found that patients have experienced significantly less discomfort and a shorter hospitalization than those undergoing the traditional abdominal procedure. There is also the added benefit of no visible scar. One great advantage of laparoscopy over abdominal postpartum tubal ligation is that it may be performed on the second or third day following delivery rather than immediately after. This gives a woman more time to decide if she really wants the operation. Furthermore, if the newborn appears healthy at birth but develops serious complications after the first twenty-four hours, a hasty and tragic decision can be averted. With abdominal tubal ligation, both you and your doctor are rushed to have the surgery performed immediately following delivery in order to shorten the total time spent in the hospital.

Vasectomy means cutting of the vas deferens, the two tubes which carry sperm from each testicle in the male. Though vasectomy is a minor surgical procedure, it is the simplest, surest, and safest surgical or medical method known to prevent unwanted pregnancy. Unlike tubal sterilization, vasectomy may be performed easily in a doctor's office under local anesthesia. There is no doubt that the incidence of complications associated with tubal sterilization far exceed those related to vasectomy.

All too often, vasectomy is still looked upon with skepticism and fear, and misinformation about the operation is widespread. Many individuals mistakenly believe that vasectomy causes such ill effects as the inability to ejaculate, loss of fertility, inability to achieve orgasm, hair loss, premature aging, and a change in voice pitch. Vasectomy has even been accused of causing skin disease, kidney, lung, and liver diseases, narcolepsy (inability to stay awake), and multiple sclerosis. Sadly, such misinformation has been responsible for many men's avoidance of this simple and relatively harmless procedure.

What exercises do you recommend for improving physical fitness during the postpartum period?

There is no scientific indication that exercise during pregnancy and the postpartum period is responsible for sagging breasts or prolapse of the urinary bladder or uterus. Factors such as obesity and lack of good muscle tone probably contribute more to these conditions than any form of exercise. However, since activity levels of most women decline dramatically during the last trimester of pregnancy, the prudent course is to resume all forms of previous exercise gradually and carefully until you reach your prepregnancy levels of stamina and conditioning.

If you continue your prenatal exercises after you give birth (see chapter 3), you will increase your muscle tone and strength. Exercise can begin on the first day after you give birth and can build in frequency and intensity with each subsequent day. If your pregnancy and delivery was complicated or you required a cesarean section, you should consult with your obstetrician before resuming physical conditioning.

Afterword

In Chapter 11 I have discussed the newer concepts of family-centered obstetrical care that are gaining popularity in hospitals throughout the United States. Sadly, consumer advocates rather than obstetricians have been most responsible for this renaissance. Instead of initiating change, many doctors have resisted it and have refused to vary their old established attitudes and concepts of patient care. This is unfortunate, because today's women are seeking and demanding more humanistic medical care and are rejecting the detached and impersonal attitudes that prevail in many doctors' offices and hospitals. The home birth movement in America should not be viewed as an aberration but as a failure of the medical establishment that must be corrected. Instead of condemning the concept of home delivery, obstetricians would be well advised to spend their time in finding out what there is about home birth that appeals to so many couples.

The main cause of the growing negativism and skepticism among women is the failure of their doctors to communicate with them. Obstetricians have been too unwilling to get off their pedestals and share their knowledge with their patients. A doctor who listens attentively, explains carefully, encourages questions, corrects misconceptions, and involves the patient and her family in the decisions that affect their welfare will reap great benefits. Those who reject this new spirit of candor will never fully appreciate the degree of satisfaction that it can bring.

Selected Bibliography

Chapter 1
When Contraception Fails

Nora, J. J., and Nora, A. H. "Birth Defects and Oral Contraceptives." *Lancet* 1(1973): 941–42.

Nora, J. J., et al. "Exogenous Progestrogen and Estrogen Implicated in Birth Defects." *Journal of the American Medical Association* 240 (1978): 837–43.

Janerich, D. D.; Piper, J. M.; and Glebatis, D. M. "Oral Contraceptives and Congenital Limb-Reduction Defects." *New England Journal of Medicine* 291(1974): 697.

Janerich, D. T., et al. "Congenital Heart Disease and Prenatal Exposure to Exogenous Sex Hormones." *British Medical Journal* 1(1977): 1058.

Heinonen, O. P., et al. "Cardiovascular Birth Defects and Antenatal Exposure to Female Sex Hormones." *New England Journal of Medicine* 296(1977): 67–70.

Shapiro, H. I. "The Birth Control Book." New York: Avon, 1978, pp. 46–47, 48–49.

Rice-wray, E., et al. "Pregnancy and Progeny After Hormonal Contraceptives—Genetic Studies." *Journal of Reproductive Medicine* 6 (1971): 90–93.

Klinger, H. P.; Glasser, M.; and Kava, H. W. "Contraceptives and the Conceptus." *Obstetrics and Gynecology* 48(1976): 40–48.

Harlap, S., and Eldor, J. "Births Following Oral Contraceptives." *Obstetrics and Gynecology* 55 (1980): 447–51.

Harlap, S. "Multiple Births in Former Contraceptive Users." *British Journal of Obstetrics and Gynecology* 86(1979): 557–62.

Savolainen, E.; Saksela, E.; and Saxen, L. "Teratogenic Hazards of Oral Contraceptives Analyzed in a National Malformation Register." *American Journal of Obstetrics and Gynecology* 140 (1981): 521–24.

"Personality Difference in Children Tied to Prenatal Hormone Therapy." *Female Patient,* April 1978, p. 87.

Beral V. "Reproductive Mortality." *British Medical Journal* 2(1979): 632–34.

Bracken, M. B. "Oral Contraception and Twinning: An Epidemiologic Study." *American Journal of Obstetrics and Gynecology* 133(1979): 432–34.

Rothman, J. K., and Liess, J. "Gender of Offspring of Oral Contraceptive Use." *New England Journal of Medicine* 295(1976): 859.

Rothman, K. J. "Fetal Loss, Twinning and Birth Weight After Oral Contraceptive Use." *New England Journal of Medicine* 297(1977): 468–71.

Wilson, J. G., and Brent, R. L. "Are Female Sex Hormones Teratogenic?" *American Journal of Obstetrics and Gynecology* 141(1981): 567–80.

Rosenfield, A. "Oral and Intrauterine Contraception: A 1978 Risk Assessment." *American Journal of Obstetrics and Gynecology* 132(1978): 92–106.

Vessey, M., et al. "Outcome of Pregnancy in Women Using Different Methods of Contraception." *British Journal of Obstetrics and Gynecology* 86(1979): 548–56.

"Does Pill Affect IQ of Offspring?" *Medical World News,* Oct. 4, 1974, pp. 55–56.

Fuertes-De La Haba, A.; Santiago, G.; and Bangdiwala, I. S. "Measured Intelligence in Offspring of Oral and Nonoral Contraceptive Users." *American Journal of Obstetrics and Gynecology* 130(1976): 980–82.

Wertliak, L. F., et al. "Decreased Serum B_{12} Levels with Oral Contraceptive Use." *Journal of the American Medical Association* 221(1972): 1371–74.

Massey, L. K., and Davison, M. A. "Effects of Oral Contraceptives on Nutrition Status." *AFP* 19(1979): 119–24.

Martinez, O., and Roe, D. A. "Effect of Oral Contraceptives on Blood Folate Levels in Pregnancy." *American Journal of Obstetrics and Gynecology* 128(1977): 255–61.

Kent, D. R., et al. "Effect of Pregnancy on Liver Tumor Associated with Oral Contraceptives."

Obstetrics and Gynecology 51(1978): 148–51.

Klein, T. A., and Mishell, D. R. "Absence of Circulating Gonadotropin in Wearers of Intrauterine Contraceptive Devices." *American Journal of Obstetrics and Gynecology* 129 (1977): 626–28.

Beling, C. G.; Cederqvist, L. L.; and Fuchs, F. "Demonstration of Gonadotropin During the Second Half of the Cycle in Women Using Intrauterine Contraception." *American Journal of Obstetrics and Gynecology* 125(1976): 855–58.

Landesman, R.; Coutinho, E. M.; and Saxena, B. B. "Detection of Human Chorionic Gonadotropin in Blood of Regularly Bleeding Women Using Copper Intrauterine Contraceptive Devices." *Fertility and Sterility* 27(1976): 1062.

Ylikorkala, O., et al. "Trophoblastic Markers in Women Using Intrauterine Contraception." *Obstetrics and Gynecology* 55(1980): 329–31.

McArdle, C. R. "Ultrasonic Localization of Missing Intrauterine of Contraceptive Devices." *Obstetrics and Gynecology* 51(1978): 330.

Millen, A.; Austin, F.; and Bernstein, G. S. "Analysis of 100 Cases of Missing IUD Strings." *Contraception* 18(1978): 485.

Shapiro, H. I. *The Birth Control Book*. New York: Avon, 1978, pp. 72–74.

Vessey, M., et al. "Outcome of Pregnancy in Women Using Different Methods of Contraception." *British Journal of Obstetrics and Gynecology* 86(1979): 548.

Propper, N. S., and Moore, J. H. "Association of E. Coli Sepsis in Pregnancy with a CU-7 Intrauterine Device in Place." *Obstetrics and Gynecology* 48(1976): 76s–77s.

Eisinger, S. H. "Second-Trimester Spontaneous Abortion, the IUD, and Infection." *American Journal of Obstetrics and Gynecology* 4(1976): 393–97.

Osser, S.; Liedholm, P.; and Sjoberg, N. O. "Risk of Pelvic Inflammatory Disease Among Users of Intrauterine Devices, Irrespective of Previous Pregnancy." *American Journal of Obstetrics and Gynecology* 138(1980): 864–67.

Burkman, R. T. "Association Between Intrauterine Device and Pelvic Inflammatory Disease." *Obstetrics and Gynecology* 57(1981): 269–75.

Osser, S., et al. "Risk of Pelvic Inflammatory Disease Among Intrauterine Device Users Irrespective of Previous Pregnancy." *Lancet* 1(1980): 386.

Kaufman, D. W., et al. "Intrauterine Contraceptive Device Use and Pelvic Inflammatory Disease." *American Journal of Obstetrics and Gynecology* 136(1980): 159–62.

Gibbs, R. S. "The IUD and PID: Is the Contraceptive the Culprit?" *Contemporary OB/GYN* 11(1978): 163–67.

Kaye, B. M. "Patients' Concerns About IUD's." *Medical Aspects of Human Sexuality.* June

1978, pp. 63–64.

Westrom, L.; Bengtsson, L. P.; and Mardh, P. "The Risk of Pelvic Inflammatory Disease in Women Using Intrauterine Contraceptive Devices as Compared to Non-users." *Lancet* 2 (1976): 221.

Jain, A. K., and Moots, B. "Fecundability Following the Discontinuation of IUD Use Among Taiwanese Women." *Journal of Biosocial Science* 9 (1976): 137–51.

"Several Investigators Voice Caution over Use of IUDs." *Ob. Gyn. News,* Dec. 1, 1976, p. 2.

Evans, M. I.; Angerman, N. S.; and Moravec, W. D. "The Intrauterine Device and Ovarian Pregnancy." *Fertility and Sterility* 32(1979): 31–35.

Vessey, M. P.; Yeates, D.; and Flavel, R. "Risk of Ectopic Pregnancy and Duration of Use of an Intrauterine Device." *Lancet* 2(1979): 501–2.

Ory, H. W., and the Women's Health Study. "Ectopic Pregnancy and Intrauterine Contraceptive Devices: New Perspectives." *Obstetrics and Gynecology* 57(1981): 137–44.

Hallatt, J. G. "Ectopic Pregnancy Associated with the Intrauterine Device: A Study of Seventy Cases." *American Journal of Obstetrics and Gynecology* 125(1976): 754–56.

"Higher Ectopic Pregnancy Incidence with Progestasert IUDs." *Drug Therapy,* February 1979, p. 40.

"Data on Ectopia Risks with Progestasert IUD Ordered." *Ob. Gyn. News* 13(1978): 3.

"Progestasert Reappraisal Requested." *Medical World News,* Feb. 6, 1978, p. 63.

"Ectopic Pregnancy One of Main Complications with IUD." *Ob. Gyn. News,* June 1, 1979, p. 8.

Tatum, H. J., and Schmidt, F. H. "Contraceptive and Sterilization Practices and Extrauterine Pregnancy: A Realistic Perspective." *Fertility and Sterility* 28(1977): 407–21.

Tatum, H. J.; Schmidt, F. H.; and Jain, A. K. "Management and Outcome of Pregnancy Associated with the Copper T Intrauterine Contraceptive Device." *American Journal of Obstetrics and Gynecology* 126(1976): 869–74.

Barrie, H. "Congenital Malformation Associated with Intrauterine Contraceptive Device." *British Medical Journal* 1(1976): 488–90.

Layde, P. M., et al. "Failed IUD Contraception and Limb Reduction Deformities: A Case-Control Study." *Fertility and Sterility* 31(1979): 18–20.

Jick, H., et al. "Vaginal Spermicides and Congenital Disorders." *Journal of the American Medical Association* 245(1981): 1329–32.

Herbst, A. L. "Intrauterine Exposure to Diethylstilbestrol in the Human." *Proceedings of "Symposium on DES,"* 1977.

Robboy, S. J., et al. *Prenatal Diethylstilbestrol Exposure: Recommendations of the DESAD Project for the Identification and Management of Exposed Individuals.* United States Department of Health and Human Services, National Institutes of Health, March 1981.

Herbst, A. L., and Scully, R. E. "Update on DES Daughters." *Contemporary OB/GYN* 17(1981): 55–66.

O'Brien, et al. "Vaginal Epithelial Changes in Young Women Enrolled in the National Cooperative Diethylstilbestrol Adenosis (DESAD) Project." *Obstetrics and Gynecology* 53(1979): 300–308.

Spangler, S.; Bibro, M. C.; and Schwartz, P. E. "Diagnostic Evaluation of Patients with DES Exposure In-Utero." *Connecticut Medicine* 45 (1981): 215–19.

U.S. Department of Health, Education and Welfare. *Health Effects of the Pregnancy Use of Diethylstilbestrol,* Physician Advisory, Oct. 4, 1978, pp. 1–6.

Goldstein, D. P. "Incompetent Cervix in Offspring Exposed to Diethylstilbestrol In-Utero." *Obstetrics and Gynecology* 52(1978): 73–75.

Berger, M. J., and Goldstein, D. P. "Impaired Reproductive Performance in DES-Exposed Women." *Obstetrics and Gynecology* 55(1980) 25–27.

Kaufman, R. H., et al. "Upper Genital Tract Changes Associated with Exposure In-Utero to Diethylstilbestrol." *American Journal of Obstetrics and Gynecology* 128(1977): 51–56.

Kaufman, R. H., et al. "Upper Genital Tract Changes and Pregnancy Outcome in Offspring Exposed In-Utero to Diethylstilbestrol." *American Journal of Obstetrics and Gynecology* 137 (1980): 299–308.

Cousins, L., et al. "Reproductive Outcome of Women Exposed to Diethylstilbestrol In-Utero." *Obstetrics and Gynecology* 56(1980): 70–76.

Barnes, A. B., et al. "Fertility and Outcome of Pregnancy in Women Exposed In-Utero to Diethylstilbestrol." *New England Journal of Medicine* 302(1980): 609–13.

Sandberg, E. C., et al. "Pregnancy Outcome in Women Exposed to Diethylstilbestrol In-Utero." *American Journal of Obstetrics and Gynecology* 140(1981): 194–205.

Herbst, A. L., et al. "A Comparison of Pregnancy Experience in DES-Exposed and DES-Unexposed Daughters." *Journal of Reproductive Medicine* 24(1980): 62–69.

Schmidt, G., et al. "Reproductive History of Women Exposed to Diethylstilbestrol In-Utero." *Fertility and Sterility* 33(1980): 21–24.

Pillsbury, S. G. "Reproductive Significance of Changes in the Endometrial Cavity Associated with Exposure In-Utero to Diethylstilbestrol." *American Journal of Obstetrics and Gynecology* 137(1980): 178–82.

Veridiano, N. P., et al. "Reproductive Performance of DES-Exposed Female Progeny." *Obstetrics and Gynecology* 58(1981): 58–61.

Bibbo, M., et al. A Twenty-five-Year Follow-up Study of Women Exposed to Diethylstilbestrol During Pregnancy." *New England Journal of Medicine* 298(1978): 763.

Iffy, L. "Ectopic Pregnancy After Postcoital Diethylstilbestrol." *American Journal of Obstetrics and Gynecology* 125(1976): 876.

Henderson, B. E., et al. "Urogenital Tract Abnormalities in Sons of Women Treated with Diethylstilbestrol." *Pediatrics* 58(1976): 505.

" 'Morning After' Pill with Fewer Side Effects Reported." *NICHD: Research Highlights and Topics of Interest,* August 1978.

Haspels, A. A. "Interception: Postcoital Estrogens in 3016 Women." *Contraception* 14(1976): 375.

Proudfit, C. M. "Postcoital Contraception: How Effective and What Fetal Risk, if Ineffective? *Journal of the American Medical Association* 238(1977): 2728–29.

"Progress on a 'Morning After' Pill." *Medical World News,* July 25, 1977, p. 37.

Notelovitz, M., and Bard, D. S. "Conjugated Estrogen as a Post-ovulatory Interceptive." *Contraception* 17(1978): 443.

Dixon, G. W., et al. "Ethinyl Estradiol and Conjugated Estrogens as Postcoital Contraceptives." *Journal of the American Medical Association* 244(1980): 1336.

Gill, W. B., et al. "Association of Diethylstilbestrol Exposure In-Utero with Cryptorchidism, Testicular Hypoplasia and Semen Abnormalities." *Journal of Urology* 122(1979): 36–39.

Stenchever, M. A., et al. "Possible Relationships Between In-Utero Diethylstilbestrol Exposure and Male Fertility." *American Journal of Obstetrics and Gynecology* 140(1981): 186–91.

Iffy, L., and Wingate, M. B. "Risks of Rhythm Method of Birth Control." *Journal of Reproductive Medicine* 5(1970): 11–15.

James, W. H. "Down's Syndrome and Parental Coital Rate." *Lancet* 2(1978): 895.

Moscati, I. M., and Becak, W. "Down's Syndrome and Frequency of Intercourse." *Lancet* 2(1978): 629–30.

Liu, D. T. Y., et al. "Dilatation of the Parous Non-pregnant Cervix." *British Journal of Obstetrics and Gynecology* 82(1975): 246.

Cates, Jr., W. "Late Effects of Induced Abortion." *Journal of Reproductive Medicine* 22(1979): 207–12.

Slater, P. E.; Davies, A. M.; and Harlap, S. "The Effect of Abortion Method on the Outcome of Subsequent Pregnancy." *Journal of Reproductive Medicine* 26(1981): 123–28.

Harlap, S., et al. "A Prospective Study of Spontaneous Fetal Losses After Induced Abortions." *New England Journal of Medicine* 301(1979): 677–81.

Levin, A. A., et al. "Association of Induced Abortion with Subsequent Pregnancy Loss." *Journal of the American Medical Association* 243 (1980): 2495–99.

Shoenbaum, S. C., et al. "Outcome of the Delivery Following an Induced or Spontaneous Abortion." *American Journal of Obstetrics and Gynecology* 136(1980):. 19–24.

Madore, C., et al. "A Study on the Effects of Induced Abortion on Subsequent Pregnancy Outcomes." *American Journal of Obstetrics and Gynecology* 139(1981): 516–21.

Levin, A. A., et al. "Association of Induced Abortion with Subsequent Pregnancy Loss." *Journal of thè American Medical Association* 243 (1980): 2495–99.

Fleury, F. "Recognizing and Treating the Cervical Fistula." *Contemporary OB/GYN* 10(1977): 25–27.

Grimes, D. A., and Cates, Jr., W. "Gestational Age Limits of Twelve Weeks for Abortion by Curettage." *American Journal of Obstetrics and Gynecology* 132(1978): 207–10.

Cates, Jr., W. "D and E After 12 Weeks: Safe or Hazardous?" *Contemporary OB/GYN* 13 (1979): 23–29.

Grimes, B. A., and Cates, Jr., W. "Complications from Legally Induced Abortion: A Review." *Obstetrical and Gynecological Survey* 34(1979): 177–89.

Hodari, A. A., et al. "Dilatation and Curettage for Second Trimester Abortions." *American Journal of Obstetrics and Gynecology* 127(1977): 850–54.

Cadesky, K. I.; Ravinsky, E.; and Lyons, E. R. "Dilatation and Evacuation: A Preferred Method of Midtrimester Abortion." *American Journal of Obstetrics and Gynecology* 139(1981): 329–32.

Cates, Jr., W., and Grimes, D. A. "Deaths from Second Trimester Abortion by Dilatation and Evacuation: Causes, Prevention, Facilities." *Obstetrics and Gynecology* 58(1981): 401–7.

Phillips, J., et al. "Laparoscopic Procedures: The American Association of Gynecologic Laparoscopists' Membership Survey for 1975." *Journal of Reproductive Medicine* 18(1977): 227–32.

Gomel, V. "Tubal Reanastomosis by Microsurgery." *Fertility and Sterility* 28(1977): 59.

Siegler, A. M. "Microsurgery for Tubal Reconstruction." *JCAE Ob/Gyn,* September 1977, pp. 19–30.

Wolf, G. C., and Thompson, N. J. "Female Sterilization and Subsequent Ectopic Pregnancy." *Obstetrics and Gynecology* 55(1980): 17–19.

Mahnoodian, S. "Advances of Minilaparotomy Sterilization." *Female Patient* 6(1981): 18–21.

Gommel, V. "Microsurgical Reversal of Female Sterilization: A Reappraisal." *Fertility and Sterility* 33(1980): 587.

Brenner, W. E. "Evaluation of Contemporary Female Sterilization Methods." *Journal of Reproductive Medicine* 26(1981): 439–53.

Riedel, H. H.; Ahrens, H.; and Semm, K. "Late Complications of Sterilization According to Method." *Journal of Reproductive Medicine* 26(1981): 353–58.

Mumford, S. D.; Bhiwandiwala, P. P.; and Chi, I-C. "Laparoscopic and Minilaparotomy Female Sterilization Compared in 15,167 Cases." *Lancet* 2(1980): 1066.

Phillips, J. M., et al. "1979 AAGL Membership Survey." *Journal of Reproductive Medicine* 26 (1981): 529–33.

U.S. Department of Health and Human Services, Centers for Disease Control. Surgical Sterilization Surveillance. Public Health Service, Summary: 1976–1978, March 1981.

"Extraordinary Birth." *MD,* August 1979, p. 43.

Chapter 2
Conception and Early Pregnancy

Hutchins, C. J. "A Sensitive Hemagglutination Assay of Human Chorionic Gonadotropin in the Diagnosis of Ectopic Pregnancy." *Obstetrics and Gynecology* 52(1978): 499–502.

Lipman, A. G. "Drug Interferences with Urinary Pregnancy Tests." *Modern Medicine,* January 1980, pp. 103–4.

Regester, R. F., and Painter, P. "False-Positive Radioimmunoassay Pregnancy Tests in Nephrotic Syndrome." *Journal of the American Medical Association* 246(1981): 1337–38.

Poma, P. A. "Early Pregnancy Testing." *Female Patient* 5(1980): 49–51.

Braunstein, G. D., et al. "First-Trimester Chorionic Gonadotropin Measurements as an Aid in the Diagnosis of Early Pregnancy Disorders." *American Journal of Obstetrics and Gynecology* 131 (1978): 25–32.

Lundstrom, V., et al. "Serum Beta-Human Chorionic Gonadotropin Levels in the Early Diagnosis of Ectopic Pregnancy." *Acta Obstetrics and Gynecology of Scandinavia* 58(1979): 231.

Kadar, N.; DeVore, G.; and Romero, R. "Discriminatory HCG Zone: Its Use in the Sonographic Evaluation for Ectopic Pregnancy." *Obstetrics and Gynecology* 58(1981): 156–61.

Pelosi, M. A.; Apuzzio, J.; and Harrigan, J. T. "What to Expect from the New Generation of Pregnancy Tests." *Contemporary OB/GYN* 17 (1981): 233–46.

Rao, C. V. "Pregnancy Tests for Office and Home." *Contemporary OB/GYN* 16(1980): 107–12.

Morris, J. W. S. "RRA Versus RIA Methodology." *Obstetrics and Gynecology* 53(1979): 669.

Berry, C. M.; Thompson, J. D.; and Hatcher, R. "The Radioreceptor Assay for HCG in Ectopic Pregnancy." *Obstetrics and Gynecology* 54

(1979): 43–46.

Lorenz, R. P.; Work, B. A., and Menon, K. M. J. "A Radioreceptorassay for Human Chorionic Gonadotropin in Normal and Abnormal Pregnancies: A Clinical Evaluation." *American Journal of Obstetrics and Gynecology* 134(1979): 471–75.

Saxena, B. B., and Landesman, R. "Diagnosis and Management of Pregnancy by the Radioreceptorassay of Human Chorionic Gonadotropin." *American Journal of Obstetrics and Gynecology* 131(1978): 97–107.

Boyko, W. L., and Russell, H. T. "Evaluation and Clinical Application of the Quantitative Radioreceptorassay for Serum HCG." *Obstetrics and Gynecology* 54(1979): 737–45.

Corson, S. L.; Batzer, F. R.; and Schlaff, S. "A Comparison of Serial Quantitative Serum and Urine Tests in Early Pregnancy." *Journal of Reproductive Medicine* 26(1981): 611–14.

Rorvik, D. M., and Shettles, L. B. "You Can Choose Your Baby's Sex." *Look,* Apr. 21, 1970, pp. 87–98.

Glass, R. H. "Sex Preselection: Is It a Possibility?" *Contemporary OB/GYN,* 9(1977): 99–102.

Guerrero, R. "Type and Time of Insemination Within the Menstrual Cycle and the Human Sex Ratio at Birth." *Studies of Family Planning* 6(1975): 367–71.

Guerrero, R., and Rojas, O. I. "Spontaneous Abortion and Aging of Human Ova and Spermatozoa." *New England Journal of Medicine* 293 (1975): 573–75.

Harlap, S. "Gender of Infants Conceived on Different Days of the Menstrual Cycle." *New England Journal of Medicine* 300(1979): 1445–48.

Simpson, J. L. "More Than We Ever Wanted to Know About Sex—Should We Be Afraid to Ask?" *New England Journal of Medicine* 300 (1979): 1483–84.

Stolkowski, J., and Lorrain, J. "Preconceptional Selection of Fetal Sex." *International Journal of Gynecology and Obstetrics* 18(1980): 440–43.

Amankwah, K. S., and Bond, E. C. "Unreliability of Prenatal Determination of Fetal Sex with the Use of Y-Body Fluorescence in Midcervical Smears." *American Journal of Obstetrics and Gynecology* 130(1978): 300–301.

Glass, A. R., and Klein, T. "Changes in Maternal Serum Total and Free Androgen Levels in Early Pregnancy: Lack of Correlation with Fetal Sex." *American Journal of Obstetrics and Gynecology* 140(1981): 656–60.

Park, G. L. "The Duration of Pregnancy." *Lancet* 2(1968): 1388.

Eastman, N. J., and Hellman, L. M. *Williams Obstetrics,* 13th ed. New York: Appleton, 1961, pp. 218–20.

O'Sullivan, M. J. "Calculating Fetal Age." *Female Patient,* March 1976, pp. 26–28.

Adams, M. M.; Oakley, G. P.; and Marks, J. S.

"Maternal Age and Births in the 1980s." *Journal of the American Medical Association* 247 1982: 493–94.

Barclay, W. R. "Forecasting Motherhood." *Journal of the American Medical Association* 247 (1982): 497.

Kushner, D. H. "Fertility in Women After Age Forty-five." *International Journal of Fertility* 24(1979): 289.

Henahan, J. "80% of Preemies in Follow-up Essentially Normal by Age 2." *Medical Tribune,* Sept. 19, 1979, pp. 1, 20.

"Less Than 15 Oz. at Birth, This Little Lady Is Making It." *Medical World News,* Oct. 15, 1979, p. 43.

Tho, P. T.; Byrd, R.; and McDonough, P. G. "Etiology and Subsequent Reproductive Performance of 100 Couples with Recurrent Abortion." *Fertility and Sterility* 32(1979): 389.

Miller, J. F., et al. "Fetal Loss After Implantation: A Prospective Study." *Lancet* 2(1980): 554.

"Habitual Abortion: Etiology and Treatment." *Fertility Review* 6(1981): 1–4.

Evans, D. R. "Neural-Tube Defects: Importance of a History of Abortion in Aetiology." *British Medical Journal* 1(1979): 975–76.

"Spina Bifida Rate Linked to Abortion History." *Contemporary OB/GYN* 14(1979): 13–16.

Anderson, S. G. "Management of Threatened Abortion with Real-Time Sonography." *Obstetrics and Gynecology* 55(1980): 259–62.

DeCherney, A. H.; Minkin, M. J.; and Spangler, S. "Contemporary Management of Ectopic Pregnancy." *Journal of Reproductive Medicine* 26 (1981): 519–23.

Bergman, S.; Howards, S.; and Sanger, W. "Practical Aspects of Banking Patient's Semen for Future Artificial Insemination." *Urology* 13 (1979): 408–11.

Rothman, C. M. "The Usefulness of Sperm Banking." *CA* 30(1980): 186–88.

Frankel, M. S. "Human Semen Banking: Implications for Medicine and Society." *Connecticut Medicine* 39(1975): 313–17.

"Does Frozen Sperm Prevent Birth Defects?" *Modern Medicine,* Apr. 15, 1979, p. 24.

Jewelewicz, R. "Management of Infertility Resulting from Anovulation." *American Journal of Obstetrics and Gynecology* 122(1975): 909–19.

McCormack, S., and Clark, J. H. "Clomid Administration to Pregnant Rats Causes Abnormalities of the Reproductive Tract in Offspring and Mothers." *Science* 204(1979): 629.

Chapter 3
Sports and Physical Fitness

Carlson, K. M. "Fact vs. Fiction: Women and Sports." *Female Patient* 5(1980): 48–54.

Wilmore, J. H. "Inferiority of the Female Athlete:

Myth or Reality?" *Rx Sports and Travel* March–April 1975, pp. 19–22.

Wood, P. S. "Sex Differences in Sports." *New York Times Magazine,* May 18, 1980, pp. 30, 102.

Rebar, R. W., and Cumming, D. C. "Reproductive Function in Women Athletes." *Journal of the American Medical Association* 246(1981): 1590.

Fort, A. T., and Harlin, R. S. "Pregnancy Outcome After Noncatastrophic Maternal Trauma During Pregnancy." *Obstetrics and Gynecology* 35(1970): 912–15.

Gunby, P. "Increasing Numbers of Physical Changes Found in Nation's Runners." *Journal of the American Medical Association* 245 (1981): 547–48.

Haycock, C. E., and Gillette, J. V. "Susceptibility of Women Athletes to Injury." *Journal of the American Medical Association* 236(1976): 163–65.

Nicholas, J. A. "Are Sports More Dangerous for Women?" *Female Patient,* February 1976, pp. 16–20.

Orselli, R. C. "Possible Teratogenic Hyperthermia and Marathon Running." *Journal of the American Medical Association* 243(1980): 332.

Fraser, F. C., and Skelton, J. "Possible Teratogenicity of Maternal Fever." *Lancet* 1(1978): 634.

Miller, P.; Smith, D. W.; and Shepard, T. H. "Maternal Hyperthermia as a Possible Cause of Anencephaly." *Lancet* 1(1978): 519–20.

Halperin, L. R., and Wilroy, Jr., R. S. "Maternal Hyperthermia and Neural-Tube Defects." *Lancet* 2(1978): 212–13.

Schaefer, C. F. "Possible Teratogenic Hyperthermia and Marathon Running." *Journal of the American Medical Association* 241(1979): 1892.

"Infant Defects, Maternal Hyperthermia Tied." *Ob. Gyn. News* 15(1980): pp. 1, 24.

Siegel, A. J. "Exercise-Related Hematuria." *Journal of the American Medical Association* 242 (1979): 1610.

"Sports During Pregnancy, Other Questions Explored." Discussion. *Physician and Sportsmedicine,* March 1976, pp. 82–85.

"Pregnancy and Sports." Symposium. *Physician and Sportsmedicine,* May 1974, pp. 35–41.

Speroff, L. "Can Exercise Cause Problems in Pregnancy and Menstruation?" *Contemporary OB/GYN* 16(1980): 57–70.

Shrock, P. "Exercise and Physical Activity During Pregnancy." *Clinical Obstetrics* 2(1977): 1–11.

Pomerance, J. J.; Gluck, L.; and Lynch, V. A. "Physical Fitness in Pregnancy: Its Effect on Pregnancy Outcome." *Obstetrics and Gynecology* 119(1974): 867–76.

Korcok, M. "Pregnant Jogger: What a Record!" *Journal of the American Medical Association* 246(1981): 201.

Hobbins, J. C. "Sports During Pregnancy." *Contemporary OB/GYN* 3(1976): 36–38.

Hale, R. W. "Women and Sports: Keeping Up with Female Athletes' Needs." *Contemporary OB/GYN* 13(1979): 85–95.

Wallace, J. P. "Exercise in Pregnancy and Postpartum." *Female Patient,* 1979, pp. 78–83.

Dressendorser, R. H. "Physical Training During Pregnancy and Lactation." *Physician and Sportsmedicine,* February 1978, pp. 74–80.

Clapp, J. F. "Acute Exercise Stress in the Pregnant Ewe." *American Journal of Obstetrics and Gynecology* 136(1980): 489–93.

Newton, R. W., et al. "Psychosocial Stress in Pregnancy and Its Relation to the Onset of Premature Labor." *British Medical Journal* 2 (1979): 411.

Massey, E. W. "Carpal Tunnel Syndrome in Pregnancy." *Obstetrical and Gynecological Survey* 33(1978): 145–48.

Nicholas, J. A. "Exercises to Prevent Sports Injuries." *Female Patient,* March 1976, pp. 45–47.

"Scuba Diving During Pregnancy—How Safe Is It? *Diving Medicine and Physiology,* News Letter, May 1, 1979.

Newhall, Jr., J. F. "Scuba Diving During Pregnancy: A Brief Review." *American Journal of Obstetrics and Gynecology* 140(1981): 893–94.

Bolten, M. E. "Scuba Diving and Fetal Wellbeing: A Survey of 208 Women." *Undersea Biomedical Research* 7(1980).

Baum, J. L. "Kinetics: The Quiet Exercise." *American Baby,* July 1979, pp. 41–43.

Shoenfeld, Y., et al. "Walking: A Method for Rapid Improvement of Physical Fitness." *Journal of the American Medical Association* 243(1980): 2062–63.

Brody, J. E. "Walking Can Promote Physical Fitness Wihout the Risks and Bother of Jogging." *New York Times,* May 28, 1980, p. C10.

Ellenbogen, R. "Selection of Bras." *Medical Aspects of Human Sexuality*, September 1979, pp. 159–60.

Haycock, C. E. "Supportive Bras for Jogging." *Medical Aspects of Human Sexuality,* July 1980, p. 6.

Hauth, J. C.; Gilstrap, L. C.; and Widmer, K. "Fetal Heart Rate Reactivity Before and After Maternal Jogging During the Third Trimester." *American Journal of Obstetrics and Gynecology* 142(1982): 545–47.

Chapter 4
Sexuality During Pregnancy

Masters, W. H., and Johnson, Z. E. *Human Sexual Response.* Boston: Little, Brown, 1966.

Debrovner, C. H. "Vaginal Lubrication." *Medical Aspects of Human Sexuality,* November 1975, pp. 32–42.

Wagner, N. N., and Solberg, D. A. "Pregnancy

and Sexuality." *Medical Aspects of Human Sexuality,* March 1974, pp. 44–66.

Zalk, S. R. "Sexual Patterns During Pregnancy." *Medical Aspects of Human Sexuality,* October 1979, pp. 126–27.

Naeye, R. L. "Coitus Late in Pregnancy Linked to Antepartum Bleeds." *British Journal of Obstetrics and Gynecology* 88(1981): 765–70.

Falicove, C. J. "Sexual Adjustment During First Pregnancy and Postpartum." *American Journal of Obstetrics and Gynecology* 117(1973): 991–1000.

Perkins, R. P. "Sexuality in Pregnancy: What Determines Behavior?" *Obstetrics and Gynecology* 59(1982): 189–98.

Wales, E. "The Impact of Childbirth on Sexual Functioning." *Female Patient,* September 1979, pp. 44–51.

Schneider, R. A. "The Sense of Smell and Human Sexuality." *Medical Aspects of Human Sexuality,* May 1971, pp. 157–68.

Berle, B. B., and Javert, C. T. "Stress and Habitual Abortion: Their Relationship and the Effect of Therapy." *Obstetrics and Gynecology* 3(1954): 298.

Javert, C. T. "Repeated Abortion: Results of Treatment in 100 Patients." *Obstetrics and Gynecology* 3(1954): 420.

Goodlin, R. C.; Keller, D. W.; and Raffin, M. "Orgasm During Late Pregnancy." *Obstetrics and Gynecology* 38(1971): 916–20.

Wagner, N. N.; Butler, J. C.; and Sanders, J. P. "Prematurity and Orgasmic Coitus During Pregnancy: Data on a Small Sample." *Fertility and Sterility* 27(1976): 911–15.

Goodlin, R. C. "Orgasm and Premature Labor." *Lancet* 2(1969): 646.

Rayburn, W. F., and Wilson, E. A. "Coital Activity and Premature Delivery." *American Journal of Obstetrics and Gynecology* 137(1980): 972–74.

Perkins, R. P. "Sexual Behavior and Response in Relation to Complications of Pregnancy." *American Journal of Obstetrics and Gynecology* 134(1979): 498–505.

Goodlin, R. C.; Schmidt, W.; and Creedy, D. C. "Uterine Tension and Fetal Heart Rate During Maternal Orgasm." *Obstetrics and Gynecology* 39(1972): 125–27.

Grudzinskas, J. G.; Watson, C.; and Chard, T. "Does Sexual Intercourse Cause Fetal Distress?" *Lancet* 2(1979): 692–93.

Naeye, R. L. "Coitus and Associated Amniotic-Fluid Infections." *New England Journal of Medicine* 301(1979): 1198–1200.

Herbst, A. L. "Coitus and the Fetus." *New England Journal of Medicine* 301(1979): 1235–36.

"What Do You Advise Patients Concerning the Safety of Sexual Relations During Pregnancy?" Discussion. *Medical Aspects of Human Sexuality* 15(1981): 91–98.

Jensen, G. D. "Anal Coitus by Married Couples." *Medical Aspects of Human Sexuality,* July 1975, p. 115.

Bolling, Jr., D. R. "Prevalence, Goals and Complications of Heterosexual Anal Intercourse in a Gynecologic Population." *Journal of Reproductive Medicine* 19(1977): 120–24.

Swerdlow, H. "Significance of Relaxed Anal Sphincter During Rectal Examination." *Medical Aspects of Human Sexuality,* April 1977.

Semmens, J. P. "Orgasm via Anal Sex." *Medical Aspects of Human Sexuality,* January 1980, p. 121.

Aronson, M. E. "Fatal Air Embolism Caused by Bizarre Sexual Behavior During Pregnancy." *Medical Aspects of Human Sexuality,* December 1969, pp. 33–39.

DeCherney, W. A., and DeCherney, A. H. "Hazardous vs. Safe Douching," *Medical Aspects of Human Sexuality,* September 1977, pp. 77–78.

Davis, B. A. "Salivary Vulvitis." *Medical Aspects of Human Sexuality,* July 1974, pp. 104–25.

Bernstein, I. L., et. al. "Localized and Systemic Hypersensitivity Reactions to Human Seminal Fluid." *Annals of Internal Medicine* 94(1981): 459.

Jhirad, A., and Vago, T. "Induction of Labor by Breast Stimulation." *Journal of Obstetrics and Gynecology* 41(1973): 347–50.

Westheimer, O. "Facts About Postpartum Sex." *Mothers' Manual,* February 1980, pp. 21–24.

"Most U.S. Sex Clinics Bilk the Public!" *Medical World News,* May 10, 1974, p. 17.

Addictive Drugs and Pregnancy. ACOG Technical Bulletin no. 21, April 1973.

DuPont, R. L. "Problems of Using Cocaine as an Aphrodisiac." *Medical Aspects of Human Sexuality* 16(1982): 14.

Allport, S. "Epidemic of Cocaine Smoking Seen." *Medical Tribune,* Jan. 16, 1980, p. 12.

Herring, M. "Study Disputes Brain Defect from Chronic Marijuana Use." *Medical Tribune,* Mar. 17, 1976, p. 3.

"THC in Marijuana Impairs Reproduction in Primates." *Ob/Gyn News,* Oct. 1, 1979, p. 24.

Rosett, D. "Marijuana Linked to Menstrual Disorders, Anomalies in Sperm." *Medical Tribune,* Aug. 22, 1979, pp. 3, 16.

Rand, A. "Tie 'Pot' in Pregnancy to Jittery Neonates." *Medical Tribune,* May 13, 1981, pp. 1, 20.

Nahas, G. G. "Marijuana, Pregnancy, and Breast-feeding." *Journal of the American Medical Association* 242(1979): 1299.

Greaves, G. B. "Sexual Disturbances in Amphetamine Abusers." *Medical Aspects of Human Sexuality* 15(1981): 83–84.

Cohen, F. "Amphetamine Abuse." *Journal of the American Medical Association* 231(1975): 414–15.

McAllister, C. B. "Placental Transfer and Neonatal Effects of Diazepam When Administered to Women Just Before Delivery." *British Journal of Anaesthesiology* 52(1980): 423.

Williamson, R. A., and Stenchever, M. A. "The Effect of Diazepam on Rates of Fertilization in the CF/1 Mouse." *American Journal of Obstetrics and Gynecology* 139(1981): 178–81.

Dorrance, D. L.; Janiger, O.; and Teplitz, R. L. "Effect of Peyote on Human Chromosomes." *Journal of the American Medical Association* 234(1975): 299–302.

Bloom, A. D. "Peyote (Mescaline) and Human Chromosomes." *Journal of the American Medical Association* 234(1975): 313.

Golden, N. L.; Sokol, R. J., and Rubin, I. L. "Angel Dust: Possible Effects on the Fetus," *Pediatrics* 55(1980): 18.

Franek, B., and Franek, M. "Alcoholism and Sexual Performance." *Medical Aspects of Human Sexuality* 16(1982): 20–21.

Hanson, J. W. "Preventing the Fetal Alcohol Syndrome." *Female Patient,* October 1979, pp. 38–42.

Green, H. G. "Infants of Alcoholic Mothers." *American Journal of Obstetrics and Gynecology* 118(1974): 713–16.

Jones, K. L., and Smith, D. W. "The Fetal Alcohol Syndrome." *Teratology* 12(1975): 1.

Clarren, S. K. "Recognition of Fetal Alcohol Syndrome." *Journal of the American Medical Association* 245(1981): 2436–39.

Tennes, K., and Blackard, C. "Maternal Alcohol Consumption, Birth Weight and Minor Physical Anomalies." *American Journal of Obstetrics and Gynecology* 138(1980): 774–80.

Veghelyi, P. D., and Osztovics, M. "Fetal-Alcohol Syndrome in Child Whose Parents Had Stopped Drinking." *Lancet* 2(1979): 35–36.

Fox, H. E.; Steinbrecher, M., and Pessel, D. "Maternal Ethanol Ingestion and the Occurrence of Human Fetal Breathing Movement." *American Journal of Obstetrics and Gynecology* 132 (1978): 354–58.

Amarose, A. P., and Norusis, M. J. "Cytogenetics of Methadone-Managed and Heroin-Addicted Pregnant Women and Their Newborn Infant." *American Journal of Obstetrics and Gynecology* 124(1976): 635–40.

"Female Ejaculation Documented." *Sexual Medicine Today,* February 1982, pp. 14–15.

Mills, J. L.; Harlap, S.; and Harley, E. E. "Should Coitus Late in Pregnancy Be Discouraged?" *Lancet* 2(1981): 136–38.

FDA Drug Bulletin, vol. 11, no. 2 (July 1981).

Harlap, S., and Shiono, P. H. "Alcohol, Smoking, and Incidence of Spontaneous Abortions in the First and Second Trimester." *Lancet* 2(1980): 173–75.

Kline, J., et al. "Drinking During Pregnancy and Spontaneous Abortion." *Lancet* 2(1980): 176–80.

Rosett, H. L.; Weiner, L.; and Edelin, K. C. "Strategies for Prevention of Fetal Alcohol Effects." *Obstetrics and Gynecology* 57(1981): 1–7.

Greenland, S., et al. "The Effects of Marijuana Use During Pregnancy." *American Journal of Obstetrics and Gynecology* 143(1982): 408–13.

Chapter 5
Sexually Transmitted Diseases

Breen, J. L., and Smith, C. I. "Sexuality Transmitted Diseases." *Female Patient* 6(1981): 12–18.

Stamm, W. E. "Annual Update on Managing Sexually Transmitted Diseases." *Modern Medicine* Oct. 15–Oct. 30, 1979, pp. 95–108.

Krespo, J. H., and Rytel, M. W. "Venereal Diseases." *AFP* 18(1978): 90–101.

Thurnau, G. R.; Keith, L.; and Berger, G. S. "Syphilis." *Female Patient* 6(1981): 14–17.

Jones, J. E., and Harris, R. E. "Diagnostic Evaluation of Syphilis During Pregnancy." *Obstetrics and Gynecology* 54(1979): 611–13.

Fiumara, N. J. "When a Pregnant Woman Has Syphilis." *Contemporary OB/GYN* 17(1981): 75–99.

Morrissy, J. R. "Gonorrhea: Guidelines for Diagnosis." *Female Patient* 6(1981): 39–42.

Garagusi, V. F. "Gonorrhea in Genital and Nongenital Sites." *Female Patient,* March 1978, pp. 14–17.

Riccardi, N. B., and Felman, Y. M. "Laboratory Diagnosis in the Problem of Suspected Gonococcal Infection." *Journal of the American Medical Association* 242(1979): 2703–5.

Amstey, M. S. "Asymptomatic Gonorrhea in Pregnancy." *Human Sexuality* 15(1981): 52a–52e.

Felman, Y. M., and Nickitas, J. A. "Nongonococcal Urethritis." *Journal of the American Medical Association* 245(1981): 381–86.

Johannisson, G.; Lowhagen, G.; and Lycke, E. "Genital Chlamydia Trachomatis Infection in Women." *Obstetrics and Gynecology* 56(1980): 671–75.

Schachter, J. "Chlamydial Infections of the Genital Tract." *Female Patient* 5(1980): 10–11.

Duby, M. "Genital Chlamydia and Viral Infections." *Female Patient,* October 1979, pp. 62–65.

Bowie, W. R., et. al. "Efficacy of Treatment Regimens for Lower Urogenital Chlamydia Trachomatis Infection in Women." *American Journal of Obstetrics and Gynecology* 142(1982): 125–29.

Richmond, S. J., and Oriel, J. D. "Recognition and Management of Chlamydial Infection." *British Medical Journal* 2(1978): 480–83.

Eschenbach, D. A. "Recognizing Chlamydial Infections." *Contemporary OB/GYN* 16(1980): 15–28.

Sweet, R. L. "Approaches to Preventing Neonatal Chlamydial Infections." *Contemporary OB/GYN* 15(1980): 98–99.

Frommell, G. T., et. al. "Chlamydial Infection of Mothers and Their Infants." *Journal of Pediatrics* 95(1979): 28–32.

Martin, D. H., et. al. "Prematurity and Perinatal Mortality in Pregnancies Complicated by Maternal Chlamydia Trachomatis Infections." *Journal of the American Medical Association* 247(1982): 1585–88.

Alexander, E. R. "Chlamydia: The Organism and Neonatal Infection." *Hospital Practice,* July 1979, pp. 63–69.

Hammerschlag, M. R., et. al. "Erythromycin Ointment for Ocular Prophylaxis of Neonatal Chlamydial Infection." *Journal of the American Medical Association* 244(1980): 2291–94.

Graber, C. D., et al. "T-Mycoplasma in Human Reproductive Failure." *Obstetrics and Gynecology* 54(1979): 558–61.

Harrison, R. F.; Hurley, R.; and DeLouvois, J. "Genital Mycoplasmas and Birth Weight in Offspring of Primigravida Women." *American Journal of Obstetrics and Gynecology* 133 (1979): 201–3.

Adam, E., et al. "Persistence of Virus Shedding in Asymptomatic Women After Recovering from Herpes Genitalis." *Journal of Obstetrics and Gynecology* 54(1979): 171–73.

Aurelian, L. "Genital Herpes Update." *Female Patient,* November 1979, pp. 19–25.

Gardner, H. L. "Herpes Genitalis: Our Most Important Venereal Disease." *American Journal of Obstetrics and Gynecology* 135(1979): 553–54.

Wilbanks, G. D., and Chez, R. A. "How to Diagnose and Treat Genital Herpes." *Contemporary OB/GYN* 16(1980): 81–85.

Amstey, M. S. "Managing Herpes in Pregnant Patients." *Contemporary OB/GYN* 16(1980): 87–92.

Kibrick, S. "Herpes Simplex Infection at Term." *Journal of the American Medical Association* 643(1980): 157.

Grossman, J. H.; Wallen, W. C.; and Sever, J. L. "Management of Genital Herpes Simplex Virus Infection During Pregnancy." *Journal of Obstetrics and Gynecology* 58(1981): 1–4.

Boehm, F. H., et al. "Management of Genital Herpes Simplex Virus Infection Occurring During Pregnancy." *American Journal of Obstetrics and Gynecology* 141(1981): 735–40.

Whitley, R. J.; Nahmias, A. J.; and Visintine, A. M. "The Natural History of Herpes Simplex Virus Infection of Mother and Newborn." *Pediatrics* 66(1980): 489–94.

Baker, D. A. "Prospects for Treating Herpes." *Contemporary OB/GYN* 19(1982): 179–87.

Saral, R., et al. "Acyclovir Prophylaxis of Herpes-Simplex-Virus Infections." *New England Journal of Medicine* 305(1981): 63–67.

Sebastian, J. A.; Leeb, B. O.; and See, R. "Cancer of the Cervix—A Sexually Transmitted Disease." *American Journal of Obstetrics and Gynecology* 131(1978): 620–23.

Kessler, I. I. "Venereal Factors in Human Cervical Cancer." *Cancer* 39(1977): 1912–19.

Lurain, J. R., and Gallup, D. G. "Management of Abnormal Papanicolaou Smears in Pregnancy." *Journal of Obstetrics and Gynecology* 53 (1979): 484–88.

Kiguchi, K., et al. "Dysplasia During Pregnancy." *Journal of Reproductive Medicine* 26(1981): 66–72.

Townsend, D. E. "Colposcopy in Pregnancy." *Contemporary OB/GYN* 14(1979): 100–103.

Kohan, S., et al. "The Role of Colposcopy in the Management of Cervical Intraepithelial Neoplasia During Pregnancy and Postpartum." *Journal of Reproductive Medicine* 25(1980): 279–84.

Sever, J. J. "When the Mother Has Cytomegalovirus Infection." *Contemporary OB/GYN* 19 (1982): 40–41.

Stagno, S., et al. "Breast Milk and the Risk of Cytomegalovirus Infection." *New England Journal of Medicine* 302(1980): 1073–76.

Bobbitt, J. R. "Group B Streptococcal Neonatal Infection." *Contemporary OB/GYN* 15(1980): 119–25.

Yow, M. D., et al. "The Natural History of Group B Streptococcal Colonization in the Pregnant Woman and Her Offspring." *American Journal of Obstetrics and Gynecology* 137(1980): 34–41.

Allardice, J. G., et al. "Perinatal Group B Streptococcal Colonization and Infection." *American Journal of Obstetrics and Gynecology* 139 (1982): 617–20.

Merenstein, G. B., et al. "Group B B-Hemolytic Streptococcus: Randomized Controlled Treatment Study at Term." *Journal of Obstetrics and Gynecology* 55(1980): 315–18.

Lewin, E. B., and Amstey, M. S. "Natural History of Group B Streptococcus Colonization and Its Therapy During Pregnancy." *American Journal of Obstetrics and Gynecology* 139(1981): 512–14.

Faro, S. "Group B Beta-Hemolytic Streptococci and Puerperal Infections." *American Journal of Obstetrics and Gynecology* 139(1981): 686–89.

Anthony, B. F., et al. "Genital and Intestinal Carriage of Group B Streptococci During Pregnancy." *Journal of Infectious Diseases* 143(1981): 761.

Charles, D. "Listeriosis: Not Rare, but Rarely Diagnosed." *Contemporary OB/GYN* 15(1980): 111–15.

Anderson, G. D. "Listeria Monocytogenes Septicemia in Pregnancy." *Journal of Obstetrics and Gynecology* 46(1975): 102–4.

Kaufman, S. A. "Vulvovaginitis: A Digest of Diagnostic and Treatment Methods." *Female Patient* 5(1980): 16–19.

Young, A. W. "Candidiasis." *Female Patient,* July

1978, pp. 78–79.

McNellis, D., et al. "Treatment of Vulvovaginal Candidiasis in Pregnancy." *Journal of Obstetrics and Gynecology* 50(1977): 674–78.

Gardner, H. L. "Haemophilus Vaginalis Vaginitis After Twenty-five Years." *American Journal of Obstetrics and Gynecology* 137(1980): 385–91.

Malouf, M., et al. "Treatment of Hemophilus Vaginalis Vaginitis." *Journal of Obstetrics and Gynecology* 57(1981): 711–13.

Fleury, F. J. "Gardnerella." *Female Patient* 6 (1981): 44–47.

Vorherr, H., et al. "Vaginal Absorption of Providone-Iodine." *Journal of the American Medical Association* 244(1980): 2628–29.

Moore, G. E.; Norton, L. W.; and Meiselbaugh, D. M. "Condyloma." *Archives of Surgery* 113 (1978): 630–31.

Malfetano, J. H.; Marin, A. C.; and Malfetano, J. H. "Laser Treatment of Condylomata Acuminata in Pregnancy." *Journal of Reproductive Medicine* 26(1981): 574–76.

"Papilloma Virus and Cervical Dysplasia." *Journal of the American Medical Association* 245 (1981): 2483.

Tang, C.; Shermeta, D. W.; and Wood, C. "Congenital Condylomata Acuminata." *American Journal of Obstetrics and Gynecology* 131 (1978): 912–13.

Krugman, S., et al. "Viral Hepatitis, Type B." *New England Journal of Medicine* 300(1979): 101–6.

Parker, H. W., et al. "Venereal Transmission of Hepatitis B Virus." *Journal of Obstetrics and Gynecology* 48(1976): 410–12.

Valdiserri, R. O. "Venereal Transmission of Hepatitis B Virus." *Journal of the American Medical Association* 241(1979): 2379.

Hussey, H. H. "The Hepatitis B Saga." *Journal of the American Medical Association* 245(1981): 1317–18.

Wong, V. C. W.; Lee, A. K. Y.; and Ip, H. M. H. "Transmission of Hepatitis B Antigen from Symptom Free Carrier Mothers to the Fetus and the Infant." *British Journal of Obstetrics and Gynecology* 87(1980): 958.

Krugman, S. "The Newly Licensed Hepatitis B Vaccine." *Journal of the American Medical Association* 247(1982): 2012–15.

Alter, H. J. "The Evolution, Implications, and Applications of the Hepatitis B Vaccine." *Journal of the American Medical Association* 247 (1982): 2272–75.

Elster, A. B., et al. "Relationship Between Frequency of Sexual Intercourse and Urinary Tract Infections in Young Women." *Southern Medical Journal* 74(1981): 704–8.

Zinner, S. H. "Bacteriuria and Babies Revisited." *New England Journal of Medicine* 300(1979): 853–55.

Harris, R. E. "The Significance of Eradication of Bacteriuria During Pregnancy." *Journal of Obstetrics and Gynecology* 53(1979): 71–73.

Spellacy, W. N. "Detecting and Managing Urinary Tract Infections in Pregnant Women." *Contemporary OB/GYN* 18(1981): 119–28.

Chapter 6
Travel

Lichtendorf, S. S. "Travel for the Pregnant: When, Where—and Whether." *New York Times,* Oct. 24, 1976, section 10, p. 1.

Crosby, W. M. "Trauma During Pregnancy: Maternal and Fetal Injury." *Obstetrical and Gynecological Survey* 29(1974): 683–98.

Stuart, G. C.; Harding, P. G.; and Davies, E. M. "Blunt Abdominal Trauma in Pregnancy." *Canadian Medical Association Journal* 122 (1980): 901–5.

Pepperell, R. J.; Rubinstein, E.; and MacIsaac "Motor-car Accidents During Pregnancy." *Medical Journal of Australia* 1(1977): 203.

Fort, A. T., and Harlin, R. S. "Pregnancy Outcome After Noncatastrophic Maternal Trauma During Pregnancy." *Journal of Obstetrics and Gynecology* 35(1970): 912–15.

Crosby, W. M.; King, A. I.; and Stout, L. C. "Fetal Survival Following Impact: Improvement with Shoulder Harness Restraint." *American Journal of Obstetrics and Gynecology* 112 (1972): 1101–6.

Howe, H. F. *Physician's Guide to Medical Advice for Overseas Travelers.* American Medical Association, 1973.

Howard, R. G. "Viral Infections in Pregnancy." *Female Patient* 7(1982): 28–37.

Sabin, A. B. "Immunization." *Journal of the American Medical Association* 246(1981): 236–41.

"Immunization for Foreign Travel." *Medical Opinion,* 1976, pp. 63–69.

Mufson, M. A. "The New Vaccines." *Drug Therapy,* October 1980, pp. 39–48.

Tyler, C. W. Personal communication, Aug. 12, 1980.

Amstey, M. S., and Schwarz, R. H. "Immunization During Pregnancy." *Contemporary OB/GYN* 18(1981): 121–23.

Bernard, K. W., et al. "Human Diploid Cell Rabies Vaccine." *Journal of the American Medical Association* 247(1982): 1138–42.

Anderson, L. J.; Winkler, E. G.; and Hafkin, B. "Clinical Experience with a Human Diploid Cell Rabies Vaccine." *Journal of the American Medical Association* 244(1980): 781–84.

Stiehm, E. R. "Standard and Special Human Immune Serum Globulins as Therapeutic Agents." *Pediatrics* 63(1979): 301–19.

Richman, A. "Infectious Hepatitis." *Hospital*

Medicine, March 1978, pp. 72–86.

Hieber, J. P., et al. "Hepatitis and Pregnancy." *Journal of Pediatrics* 91(1977): 545.

Monif, G. R. G. "Do You Vaccinate for Influenza During Pregnancy?" *Contemporary OB/GYN* 16 (1980): 21–24.

Deinard, A. S., and Ogburn, Jr., P. "A/NJ/8/76 Influenza Vaccination Program: Effects on Maternal Health and Pregnancy Outcome." *American Journal of Obstetrics and Gynecology* 140 (1981): 240–45.

Polk, I. J. "Influenza Vaccine." *Journal of the American Medical Association* 247(1982): 1191.

"World Traveler's Immunization Guide." *Drug Therapy,* July 1979, pp. 119–25.

Bryant, G. "Malaria Is Ignored." *Toronto Star,* Jan. 26, 1980.

How to Protect Yourself Against Malaria. International Association for Medical Assistance to Travelers (IAMAT), New York.

Schmeck, Jr., H. M. "Malaria Still a Widespread Scourge, but Hope Grows for Vaccine to Defeat It." *New York Times,* Apr. 13. 1982, C1.

"Folk Cure for the Seasick." *New York Times,* Apr. 13, 1982, C2.

Holder, L. E. "X-ray Machines for Airport Security." *Journal of the American Medical Association* 233(1975): 1393–94.

"Pregnancy and Flying." *Travel Rounds* 1(1979): 2.

Kidera, G. J. "Preparing Patients for Plane Trips." *Consultant,* June 1979, pp. 21–27.

"Ozone Complaints Climbing." *Medicine Around the World* 2(1980): 2.

"Cloudy Issue." *Travel Rounds* 1(1979): 5–6.

Fried, F. A. "Sickle Cell Anemia and Plane Travel." *Consultant,* November 1979, p. 16.

McCullough, R. E.; Reeves, J. T.; and Liljegren, R. L. "Fetal Growth Retardation and Increased Infant Mortality at High Altitude." *Archives of Environmental Health* 32(1977): 36–39.

Cotton, E. K., et al. "Re-evaluation of Birth at High Altitude." *American Journal of Obstetrics and Gynecology* 138(1980): 220–22.

Sobrevilla, L. A.; Romero, I.; and Kruger, F. "Estriol Levels of Cord Blood, Maternal Venous Blood, and Amniotic Fluid at Delivery at High Altitude." *American Journal of Obstetrics and Gynecology* 110(1973): 596–98.

"Medical Plans." *New York Times,* Oct. 12, 1980, travel section, p. 9.

"For the Compleate Traveler—Be Your Own Dentist." *Medicine Around the World* 2(1980): 5.

Levine, N. "Sun Worship: Reducing the Ritual's Danger and Damage." *Modern Medicine,* June 15–June 30, 1980, pp. 37–47.

"Sunscreens: Playing the Numbers." *Parents,* August 1980, p. 10.

"Traveler's Black Bag." *M.D. Magazine,* November 1979, p. 60.

Kaplan, J. M. "Infectious Diarrhea: Knowing the New Causes and Picking the Right Rx. *Modern Medicine,* February 1982, pp. 119–33.

"Giardiasis." *American Family Physician* 23 (1981): 137–40.

Kreutner, A. K.; Del Vene, D. E.; and Amstey, M. S. "Giardiasis in Pregnancy." *American Journal of Obstetrics and Gynecology* 140(1981): 895–901.

Caruso, C. "Amebiasis, Giardiasis American Style." *Medical Tribune,* Mar. 10, 1982, p. 30.

Stevens, D. P. "Giardiasis." *Practical Gastroenterology* 4(1980): 23–28.

Barrett-Connor, E. "Traveler's Diarrhea: 1980 Update on Prevention and Rx." *Modern Medicine,* June 15–June 30, 1980, pp. 54–60.

Sack, D. A. "Arming Your Patients Against Traveler's Diarrhea." *Drug Therapy,* June 1981, pp. 46–55.

DuPont, H. L., et al. "Prevention of Traveler's Diarrhea: Prophylactic Administration of Subsalicylate Bismuth." *Journal of the American Medical Association* 243(1980): 237–41.

Kruesi, M. "Bismuth Preparations for Diarrhea." *Journal of the American Medical Association* 244(1980): 1435.

Chapter 7
Medications

Bracken, M. B., and Holford, T. R. "Exposure to Prescribed Drugs in Pregnancy and Association with Congenital Malformations." *Obstetrics and Gynecology* 58(1981): 336–44.

Howard, F. M., and Hill, J. M. "Drugs in Pregnancy." *Obstetrical and Gynecological Survey* 34(1979): 643–53.

Physicians' Desk Reference. 36th ed. New York: Medical Economics Company, 1982.

Compendium of Drug Therapy, 1981/1982. New York: Biomedical Information Corporation, 1982.

Obstetrics and Gynecology vol. 58, no. 5 (supplement), November 1981.

Bodendorfer, T. W.; Briggs, G. G.; and Gunning, J. E. "Obtaining Drug Exposure Histories During Pregnancy." *American Journal of Obstetrics and Gynecology* 135(1979): 490–94.

Jick, H., et al. "First-Trimester Drug Use and Genital Disorders." *Journal of the American Medical Association* 246(1981): 343–46.

Stirrat, G. M. "Prescribing Problems in the Second Half of Pregnancy and During Lactation." *Obstetrical and Gynecological Survey* 31 (1976): 1–7.

Brackvill, Y., et al. "Obstetric Premedication and Infant Outcome." *American Journal of Obstetrics and Gynecology* 118(1974): 377–84.

Soller, R. W., and Stander, H. "Maternal Drug Exposure and Perinatal Intracranial Hemorrhage." *Obstetrics and Gynecology* 58(1981): 735–40.

Borherr, H. "Drug Excretion in Breast Milk." *Postgraduate Medicine* 56(1974): 97–104.

Lipman, A. G. "Analgesics and Anti-inflammatories in Breast Milk." *Modern Medicine,* Nov. 15–Nov. 30, 1978, pp. 101–2.

Erickson, S. H.; Oppenheim, G. L.; and Smith, G. H. "Metronidazole in Breast Milk." *Obstetrics and Gynecology* 57(1981): 48–50.

Bartlett, J. G. "Metronidazole." *Johns Hopkins Medical Journal* 149(1981): 89–92.

Segal, S. "Primary-Infection Tuberculosis During Pregnancy." *Journal of the American Medical Association* 246(1981): 389.

Good, Jr., J. T., et al. "Tuberculosis in Association with Pregnancy. *American Journal of Obstetrics and Gynecology* 140(1981): 492–98.

Lynd, P. A.; Andreasen, A. C.; and Wyatt, R. J. "Intrauterine Salicylate Intoxication in a Newborn." *Clinical Pediatrics* 15(1976): 912–13.

Rumack, C. M., et al. "Neonatal Intracranial Hemorrhage and Maternal Use of Aspirin." *Obstetrics and Gynecology* 58 (suppl) (1981): 52S–56S.

Rudolph, A. M. "Effects of Aspirin and Acetaminophen in Pregnancy and the Newborn." *Archives of Internal Medicine* 141(1981): 358.

"New Warning on Propoxyphene." *FDA Drug Bulletin* 9(1979): 22–23.

Klein, K. L., et al. "Indomethacin: Placental Transfer, Cytotoxicity, and Teratology in the Rat." *American Journal of Obstetrics and Gynecology* 141(1981): 448–52.

Morrison, J. C., et al. "Meperidine Metabolism in the Parturient." *Obstetrics and Gynecology* 59 (1982): 359–64.

Pittman, K. A., et al. "Human Perinatal Distribution of Butorphanol." *American Journal of Obstetrics and Gynecology* 138(1980): 797–800.

Hodgkinson, R., et al. "Double-Blind Comparison of Maternal Analgesia and Neonatal Neurobehaviour Following Intravenous Butorphanol and Meperidine." *Journal of International Medical Research* 7(1979): 224–30.

Maduska, A. L., and Hajghassemali, M. "A Double-Blind Comparison of Butorphanol and Meperidine in Labour: Maternal Pain Relief and Effects on the Newborn." *Canadian Anesthesiology Society Journal* 25(1978): 398–404.

Lewis, J. R. "Evaluation of New Analgesics: Butorphanol and Malbuphine." *Journal of the American Medical Association* 243(1980): 1465–67.

Weis, O. F., and Weintraub, M. "New Developments in the Treatment of Nausea and Vomiting." *Drug Therapy,* January 1982, pp. 53–56.

Cordero, J. F., et al. "Is Bendectin a Teratogen?" *Journal of the American Medical Association* 245(1981): 2307–14.

Morelock, S., et al. "Bendectin and Fetal Development." *American Journal of Obstetrics and Gynecology* 142(1982): 209, 213.

Greenberger, P., and Patterson, R. "Safety of Therapy for Allergic Symptoms During Pregnancy." *Annals of Internal Medicine* 89(1978): 234–37.

Schwarz, R. H. "Use of Drugs in Pregnant Asthmatics." *Drug Therapy,* April 1982, p. 82.

Weinstein, A. M., et al. "Asthma and Pregnancy." *Journal of the American Medical Association* 241(1979): 1161–65.

Labovitz, E., and Spector, S. "Placental Theophylline Transfer in Pregnant Asthmatics." *Journal of the American Medical Association* 247 (1982): 786–88.

Liggins, G. C. "Report on Children Exposed to Steroids in Utero." *Contemporary OB/GYN* 19 (1982): 205–6.

Johnson, J. W. C., et al. "Long-term Effects of Betamethasone on Fetal Development." *American Journal of Obstetrics and Gynecology* 141 (1981): 1053–64.

Milkovich, L., and Vandenberg, B. J. "Effects of Prenatal Meprobamate and Chlordiazepoxide Hydrochloride on Human Embryonic and Fetal Development." *New England Journal of Medicine* 291(1974): 1268–71.

Hartz, S. C., et al. "Antenatal Exposure to Meprobamate and Chlordiazepoxide in Relation to Malformations, Mental Development, and Childhood Mortality." *New England Journal of Medicine* 292(1975): 762–68.

Safra, M. J., and Oakley, Jr., G. P. "Association Between Cleft Lip with or Without Cleft Palate and Prenatal Exposure to Diazepam." *Lancet* 1 (1975): 478–79.

"Teratogenicity of Minor Tranquilizers." *FDA Drug Bulletin* 5(1975).

Fieghner, J. "Pharmacology: New Antidepressants." *Psychiatric Annals* 10(1980): 35–41.

Sulser, F. "Pharmacology: Current Antidepressants." *Psychiatric Annals* 10(1980): 28–33.

Rosenbaum, A. H. "Manic-Depressive Illness in Pregnancy." *Journal of the American Medical Association* 243(1980): 1089.

Anticonvulsants and Pregnancy. Prepared by the AAP Committee on Drugs in Collaboration with the ACOG Committee on Obstetrics: Maternal and Fetal Medicine, January 1979.

Srinivasan, G., et al. "Maternal Anticonvulsant Therapy and Hemorrhagic Disease of the Newborn." *Obstetrics and Gynecology* 59(1982): 250–51.

Watson, J. D., and Spellacy, W. N. "Neonatal Effects of Maternal Treatment with the Anticonvulsant Drug Diphenylhydantoin." *Obstetrics and Gynecology* 37(1970): 881–84.

Swaiman, K. F. "Antiepileptic Drugs, the Developing Nervous System, and the Pregnant Woman with Epilepsy." *Journal of the American Medical Association,* 244(1980): 1477.

Stevenson, R. E., et al. "Hazards of All Anticoagulants During Pregnancy." *Journal of the American Medical Association* 243(1980): 1549.

Pauli, R. M., and Hall, J. G. "Warfarin Embryopathy." *Lancet* 1(1979): 144.

Dardick, K. R. "Warfarin During Lactation." *Connecticut Medicine* 44(1980): 693.

Berkowitz, R. L. "Anti-hypertensive Drugs in the Pregnant Patient." *Obstetrical and Gynecological Survey* 35(1980): 191–203.

Rubin, P. C. "Beta-Blockers in Pregnancy." *New England Journal of Medicine* 305(1981): 1323–25.

Milsap, R. L., and Auld, P. A. M. "Neonatal Hyperglycemia Following Diazoxide Administration." *Journal of the American Medical Association* 243(1980): 144–45.

Whitelaw, A. "Maternal Methyldopa Treatment and Neonatal Blood Pressure." *British Medical Journal* 283(1981): 471.

Witter, F. R.; King, T. M.; and Blake, D. A. "Adverse Effects of Cardiovascular Drug Therapy on the Fetus and Neonate." *Obstetrics and Gynecology* 58 (suppl) (1981): 100S–105S.

Bauman, D. J. "Are Antiarrhythmatic Drugs Contraindicated During Pregnancy?" *Journal of the American Medical Association* 245(1981): 2105–6.

Kampmann, J. P., et al. "Propylthiouracil in Human Milk: Revision of a Dogma." *Lancet* 1 (1980): 736.

Matsunaga, E., and Shiota, K. "Threatened Abortion, Hormone Therapy and Malformed Embryos." *Teratology* 20(1979): 469.

Peress, M. R., et al. "Female Pseudohermaphroditism with Somatic Chromosomal Anomaly in Association with In Utero Exposure to Danazol." *American Journal of Obstetrics and Gynecology* 142(1982): 708–9.

Chapter 8
Nutrition

Food, Pregnancy, and Family Health. ACOG Patient Information Booklet, American College of Obstetricians and Gynecologists, Chicago, February 1976.

Naeye, R. L. "Weight Gain and the Outcome of Pregnancy." *American Journal of Obstetrics and Gynecology* 135(1979): 3–9.

Harrison, G. G.; Udall, J. N.; and Morrow, G. "Maternal Obesity, Weight Gain in Pregnancy, and Infant Birth Weight." *American Journal of Obstetrics and Gynecology* 136(1980): 411–12.

Winick, M. "Preventing Growth-Retarded Children." *Current Prescribing,* July 1976, pp. 43–47.

Pitkin, R. M. "Is She Eating for Two?" *Contemporary OB/GYN* 19(1982): 130–40.

Brown, J. E., et al. "Influence of Pregnancy Weight Gain on the Size of Infants Born to Underweight Women." *Obstetrics and Gynecology* 57(1981): 13–17.

Gormican, A.; Valentine, J.; and Satter, E. "Relationships of Maternal Weight Gain, Prepregnancy Weight, and Infant Birthweight." *Journal of the American Diet Association* 77(1980): 662–67.

Edwards, L. E., et al. "Pregnancy in the Underweight Woman." *American Journal of Obstetrics and Gynecology* 135(1979): 297–302.

Grieve, J. F. K. "A Comment on the Relation Between Protein and Weight Gain in Pregnancy." *Journal of Reproductive Medicine* 14(1975): 55.

Swales, J. D. "Dietary Salt and Hypertension." *Lancet* 1(1980): 1177–79.

Atkinson, Jr., S. M. "Salt, Water, and Rest as a Preventative for Toxemia of Pregnancy." *Journal of Reproductive Medicine* 9(1972): 223–28.

Lindheimer, M. D. "Current Concepts of Sodium Metabolism and Use of Diuretics in Pregnancy." *Contemporary OB/GYN* 15(1980): 207–16.

Rosenberg, L., et al. "Selected Birth Defects in Relation to Caffeine-Containing Beverages." *Jouranl of the American Medical Association* 247(1982): 1429–32.

Weathersbee, P. S.; Olsen, L. K.; and Lodge, J. R. "Caffeine and Pregnancy." *Postgraduate Medicine* 62(1977): 64–70.

"Caffeine: What It Does." *Consumer Reports,* October 1981, pp. 595, 599.

Tyrala, E. E., and Dodson, W. E. "Caffeine Secretion into Breast Milk." *Archives of Disease in Childhood* 54(1979): 787–800.

Banner, Jr., W., and Czajka, P. A. "Acute Caffeine Overdose in the Neonate." *American Journal of Diseases in Children* 134(1980): 495–98.

U.S. Department of Health and Human Services, *Caffeine and Pregnancy.* Public Health Service Bulletin, 1981.

Webb, J. L. "Nutritional Effects of Oral Contraceptive Use." *Journal of Reproductive Medicine* 25(1980): 150–56.

Baker, H., et al. "Role of Placenta in Maternal-Fetal Vitamin Transfer in Humans." *American Journal of Obstetrics and Gynecology* 141 (1981): 792–96.

Moghissi, K. S. "Risks and Benefits of Nutritional Supplements During Pregnancy." *Obstetrics and Gynecology* 58(1981): 68S–78S.

Chez, R. A., and Pitkin, R. M. "Nutritional Supplements During Pregnancy." *Contemporary OB/GYN* 19(1982): 199–201.

Pitkin, R. M., et al. *Nutrition in Maternal Health Care.* Bulletin, Committee on Nutrition, American College of Obstetricians and Gynecologists, 1974.

Nutrition Labeling: How It Can Work for You. National Nutrition Consortium, Bethesda, Md., 1975.

Kitay, D. Z. "Folic Acid Deficiency in Pregnancy." *Modern Medicine,* June 15, 1970, pp. 77–84.

Smithells, R. W., et al. "Possible Prevention of Neural-Tube Defects by Periconceptional Vitamin Supplementation." *Lacet* 1(1980): 339–40.

Laurence, K. M., et al. "Double-Blind Randomised Controlled Trial of Folate Treatment Before Conception to Prevent Recurrence of Neural-Tube Defects." *British Medical Journal* 282 (1981): 1509.

McIntosh, E. N. "Treatment of Women with the Galactorrhea-Amenorrhea Syndrome with Pyridoxine (Vitamin B6)." *Journal of Clinical Endocrinology and Metabolism* 42(1976): 1192.

Lippe, B., et al. "Chronic Vitamin A Intoxication: A Multisystem Disease That First Reached Epidemic Proportions." *American Journal of Diseases in Childhood* 135(1981): 634–36.

Zucker, M. "Childbirth Made Easier with Vitamin C!" *Let's Live,* October 1979, pp. 22–30.

Roberts, H. J. "Perspective on Vitamin E as Therapy." *Journal of the American Medical Association* 246(1981): 129–30.

Archer, J. Vitamin E. Journal of the American Medical Association, 247:29, 1982.

Disler, P. D., et al. "The Effect of Tea on Iron Absorption." *Gut* 16(1975): 193–200.

Pitkin, R. M. "Calcium Metabolism in Pregnancy: A Review." *American Journal of Obstetrics and Gynecology* 121(1975): 724–34.

Brodey, J. E. "Enzyme Deficiency Is the Reason Many Can't Digest Milk." *New York Times,* May 5, 1982, C1–10.

Dilts, Jr., P. V., and Ahokus, R. A. "Effects of Dietary Lead and Zinc on Fetal Organ Growth." *American Journal of Obstetrics and Gynecology* 136(1980): 899.

Krieger, L. M. "Obs Look Cautiously at Report on Use of Prenatal Sodium Fluoride." *Ob.Gyn. News* 14(1979): 1–33.

Margolis, F. J., et al. "Fluoide Supplements for Children: A Survey of Physicians' Prescription Practices." *American Journal of Diseases in Childhood* 134(1980): 865–68.

"Caution Advised in Planning Vegetarian Diets for Gravidas Infants." *Ob.Gyn. News* 15(1980): 5.

Crosby, W. H. "Can a Vegetarian Be Well Nourished?" *Journal of the American Medical Association* 233(1975): 898.

Partners in Growth. Pamphlet. Rosemont, Ill.: National Dairy Council, 1977.

Assessment of Maternal Nutrition. Pamphlet, Task Force on Nutrition, American College of Obstetricians and Gynecologists, American Dietetic Association, 1978.

Kresina, M. "Are Fast Foods Nutritious for Adolescents?" *JCAM,* February 1980, pp. 26–28.

Metzger, B. E., et al. "'Accelerated Starvation' and the Skipped Breakfast in Late Normal Pregnancy." *Lancet* 1(1982): 588–92.

Chapter 9
Environmental and Occupational Hazards

Machol, L. "Environmental Hazards: What They'll Mean to Your Patients in the 1980s." *Contemporary OB/GYN* 15(1980): 22–43.

Duhring, J. L. "The Teratogenic Environment." *Female Patient* 7(1982): 36–44.

Longo, L. D. "Environmental Pollution and Pregnancy: Risks and Uncertainties for the Fetus and Infant." *American Journal of Obstetrics and Gynecology* 137(1980): 162–73.

Hale, M. "Preventing Toxic Insult to Fetus and Newborn." *Contemporary OB/GYN* 15(1980): 143–61.

Knuppel, R. A. "Recognizing Teratogenic Effects of Drugs and Radiation." *Contemporary OB/GYN* 15(1980): 171–83.

Guidelines On Pregnancy and Work. Booklet, American College of Obstetricians and Gynecologists, September 1977.

U.S. Department of Health, Education, and Welfare, Public Health Service. *Smoking and Pregnancy.* Reprinted from *The Health Consequences of Smoking: A Report of the Surgeon General,* 1971.

Evans, D. R.; Newcombe, R. G.; and Campbell, H. "Maternal Smoking Habits and Congenital Malformations: A Population Study." *British Medical Journal* 2(1979): 171–73.

Rush, D. "Smoking, Weight Gain, and Nutrition During Pregnancy." *American Journal of Obstetrics and Gynecology* 139(1981): 233–34.

Thaler, I.; Goodman, J. D. S.; and Dawes, G. S. "Effects of Maternal Cigarette Smoking on Fetal Breathing and Fetal Movements." *American Journal of Obstetrics and Gynecology* 138(1980): 282–87.

Manning, F. A., and Platt, L. D. "Maternal Hypoxemia and Fetal Breathing Movements." *Obstetrics and Gynecology* 53(1979): 758–60.

Phelan, J. P. "Diminished Fetal Reactivity with Smoking." *American Journal of Obstetrics and Gynecology* 136(1980): 230–33.

Cigarette Smoking and Pregnancy. ACOG Technical Bulletin, September 1979.

Quigley, M. E., et al. "Effects of Maternal Smoking on Circulating Catecholamine Levels and Fetal Heart Rate." *American Journal of Obstetrics and Gynecology* 133(1979): 685–90.

Mallov, J. S. "MBK Neuropathy Among Spray Painters." *Journal of the American Medical Association* 235(1976): 1455–57.

Stewart, R. D., and Hake, C. L. "Paint-Remover

Hazard." *Journal of the American Medical Association* 235(1976): 398–401.

"CNS Birth Defects Linked to Organic Solvent Exposure." *Contemporary OB/GYN* 15(1980): 11.

McCann, M. "The Impact of Hazards in Art on Female Workers." *Preventive Medicine* 7(1978): 338–48.

Jimenez, M. H., and Newton, N. "Activity and Work During Pregnancy and the Postpartum Period: A Cross-Cultural Study of 202 Societies." *American Journal of Obstetrics and Gynecology* 135(1979): 171–76.

"Working in Pregnancy: How Long? How Hard? What's Your Role?" Symposium. *Contemporary OB/GYN* 16(1980): 154–68.

Kuntz, W. D. "Pregnant Working Women: What Advice Should You Give Them?" *Contemporary OB/GYN* 15(1980): 69–79.

Pregnancy, Work, and Disability. ACOG Technical Bulletin no. 58, May 1980.

Briend, A. "Maternal Work During Pregnancy in Traditional Societies." *American Journal of Obstetrics and Gynecology* 137(1979): 630.

Naeye, R. L., and Peters, E. C. "Working During Pregnancy: Effects on the Fetus." *Pediatrics* 69(1982): 724–27.

Davies, J. M., et al. "Effects of Stopping Smoking for 48 Hours on Oxygen Availability from the Blood: A Study on Pregnant Women." *British Medical Journal* 2(1979): 355–56.

Hirayama, T. "Non-smoker Wives of Heavy Smokers Have a Higher Incidence of Lung Cancer: A Study from Japan." *British Medical Journal* 282(1981): 183–85.

Yerushalmy, J. "Mother's Cigarette Smoking and Survival of Infant," *American Journal of Obstetrics and Gynecology* 88 (1964): 505–18.

Yerushalmy, J. "Infants with Low Birth Weight Born Before Their Mothers Started to Smoke Cigarettes." *American Journal of Obstetrics and Gynecology* 112(1972): 277–84.

Brown, W. A.; Grodin, J.; and Manning, T. "Prenatal Psychological State and the Use of Drugs in Labor." *American Journal of Obstetrics and Gynecology* 113(1972): 598–601.

Rosa, F. W. "Birth Weight in Fiji and Western Samoa: A Pacific Prescription for Pregnancy?" *American Journal of Obstetrics and Gynecology* 119(1974): 1121–24.

Trudinger, B. J., and Boylin, P. "Antepartum Fetal Heart Rate Monitoring: Value of Sound Stimulation." *Obstetrics and Gynecology* 55(1980): 365–67.

Ames, B. N.; Kammen, H. O.; and Yamasaki, E. "Hair Dyes Are Mutagenic: Identitication of a Variety of Mutagenic Ingredients." *Proceedings of the National Academy of Science* 72(1975): 2423–37.

Kirkland, D. J.; Lawler, S. D.; and Venitt, S.

"Chromosomal Damage and Hair Dyes." *Lancet* 2(1978): 124–27.

"Are Hair Dyes Safe?" *Consumer Reports,* August 1979, pp. 456–60.

Kuhnert, P. M.; Kuhnert, B. R.; and Erhard, P. "Comparison of Mercury Levels in Maternal Blood, Fetal Cord Blood, and Placental Tissues." *American Journal of Obstetrics and Gynecology* 139(1981): 209–13.

Popescu, H. I.; Negru, L.; and Lancranjan, I. "Chromosome Aberrations Induced by Occupational Exposure to Mercury." *Archives of Environmental Health* 34(1979): 461–63.

Cohen, E. N., et al. "Occupational Disease Among Operating Room Personnel: A National Study." *Anesthesiology* 41(1974): 321.

Cohen, E. N., et al. "A Survey of Anesthetic Health Hazards Among Dentists." *Journal of the American Dental Association* 90(1975): 1291.

Tomlin, P. J. "Health Problems of Anaesthetists and Their Families in the West Midlands." *British Medical Journal* 1(1979): 779.

Wilson, C. B., et al. "Development of Adverse Sequelae in Children Born with Subclinical Congenital Toxoplasma Infection." *Pediatrics* 66(1980): 767.

Frenkel, J. K. "Congenital Toxoplasmosis: Prevention or Palliation?" *American Journal of Obstetrics and Gynecology* 141(1981): 359–61.

Wilson, C. B., and Remington, J. S. "What Can Be Done to Prevent Congenital Toxoplasmosis?" *American Journal of Obstetrics and Gynecology* 138(1980): 357–63.

Evans, M. E., et al. "Tularemia and the Tomcat." *Journal of the American Medical Association* 246(1981): 1343.

Cohen, M. L., et al. "Turtle-Associated Salmonellosis in the United States." *Journal of the American Medical Association* 243(1980): 1247–49.

Kaminester, L. H. "Suntanning Centers." *Journal of the American Medical Association* 244(1980): 1258–59.

Swartz, H. M., and Reichling, B. A. "Hazards of Radiation Exposure for Pregnant Women." *Journal of the American Medical Association* 239(1978): 1907–10.

Bross, I. D. J., and Nataragan, N. "Genetic Damage from Diagnostic Radiation." *Journal of the American Medical Association* 237(1977): 2399–2401.

Oppenheim, B. E. "Genetic Damage from Diagnostic Radiation?" *Journal of the American Medical Association* 242(1979); 1390–93.

National Council on Radiation Protection and Measurements. *Basic Radiation Protection Criteria.* NCRP Report no. 39, Washington, D. C., Jan. 15, 1971.

American College of Obstetricians and Gynecologists. *Guidelines for Diagnostic X-ray Examination of Fertile Women.* ACOG Statement of Policy, May 1977.

Shiono, P. H.; Chung, C. S.; and Myrianthopoulos, N. C. "Preconception Radiation, Intrauterine Diagnostic Radiation, and Childhood Neoplasia." *Journal of the National Cancer Institute* 65(1980); 681–86.

Philippe, J. V. "Fertility and Irradiation: A Preconceptional Investigation in Teratology." *American Journal of Obstetrics and Gynecology* 123(1975): 714–18.

Laube, D. W.; Varnar, M. W.; and Cruikshank, D. P. "A Prospective Evaluation of X-ray Pelvimetry." *Journal of the American Medical Association* 246(1981): 2187–88.

Barton, J. J., and Garbaciak, J. A. "Is X-ray Pelvimetry Necessary?" *Contemporary OB/GYN* 13(1979): 27–30.

Jukes, T. H. "Mercury in Fish." *Journal of the American Medical Association* 233(1975): 1001–2.

Wheaten, R. H. "Chemical Toxicants in Breast Milk." *Journal of the American Medical Association* 246(1981): 285.

Kreiss, K., et al. "Cross-sectional Study of a Community with Exceptional Exposure to DDT." *Journal of the American Medical Association* 245(1981): 1926–30.

Roberts, D. W. "Tissue Burdens of Toxic Pollutants." *Journal of the American Medical Association* 247(1982): 2142.

Harris, J. C.; Rumack, B. H.; and Aldrich, F. D. "Toxicology of Urea Formaldehyde and Polyurethane Foam Insulation. *Journal of the American Medical Association* 245(1981): 243–46.

Yodaiken, R. E. "The Uncertain Consequences of Formaldehyde Toxicity." *Journal of the American Medical Association* 246(1981): 1677–78.

Chapter 10
The New Obstetrical Technology

Chemke, J., and Schulman, J. D. "Pitfalls and Dilemmas of Prenatal Diagnosis." *Contemporary OB/GYN* 17(1981): 84–85.

Wilner, J. P., and Godmilow, L. "Prenatal Diagnosis of High-Risk Pregnancy." *Female Patient* 6 (1981): 25–29.

Galle, P. C., and Meis, P. J. "Complications of Amniocentesis." *Journal of Reproductive Medicine* 27(1982): 149–55.

Mennuti, M. T., et al. "Fetal-Maternal Bleeding Associated with Genetic Amniocentesis." *Obstetrics and Gynecology* 55(1980): 48–53.

Crandall, B. F., et al. "Follow-up of 2,000 Second-Trimester Amniocenteses." *Obstetrics and Gynecology* 56(1980): 625–28.

King, C. R. "Genetic Disease and Pregnancy." *Ob-

stetrical and Gynecological Survey* 37(1982): 151–57.

Henry, G. "Prenatal Diagnosis of Genetic Disorders." *Journal of Reproductive Medicine* 23 (1979): 185–93.

Simpson, J. L., et al. "Genetic Counseling and Genetic Services in Obstetrics and Gynecology: Implications for Educational Goals and Clinical Practice." *American Journal of Obstetrics and Gynecology* 140(1981): 70–80.

Simpson, J. L. "What Causes Chromosomal Abnormalities and Gene Mutations?" *Contemporary OB/GYN* 17(1981): 99–114.

Hook, E. B. "Rates of Chromosome Abnormalities at Different Maternal Ages." *Obstetrics and Gynecology* 58(1981): 282–85.

Adams, M. M., et al. "Down's Syndrome." *Journal of the American Medical Association* 246 (1981): 758–60.

"Paternal Age May Be Linked to Down's Syndrome." *Ob.Gyn. News,* Sept. 15, 1979, p. 46.

Fost, N. "Prenatal Diagnosis of Down's Syndrome." *Journal of the American Medical Association* 242(1979): 2326.

"Prevention of Tay-Sachs disease: Carrier Identification and Genetic Counceling." ACOG Technical Bulletin no. 34, January 1976.

Nadler, H. L., et al. "Prenatal Detection of Cystic Fibrosis." *American Journal of Obstetrics and Gynecology* 141(1981): 885–89.

Simon, N. V., et al. "Prediction of Fetal Lung Maturity by Amniotic Fluid Fluorescence Polarization, L.S. Ratio and Phosphatidyl Glycerol." *Obstetrics and Gynecology* 57(1981): 295–99.

O'Brien, W. F., and Cefalo, R. C. "Clinical Applicability of Amniotic Fluid Tests for Fetal Pulmonic Maturity." *American Journal of Obstetrics and Gynecology* 136(1980): 135–44.

Milunsky, A. "Prenatal Detection of Neural Tube Defects." *Journal of the American Medical Association* 244(1980): 2731–35.

Habib, Z. "Genetics and Genetic Counseling in Neonatal Hydrocephalus." *Obstetrical and Gynecological Survey* 36(1981): 529–33.

Weiss, R. R. "Maternal Serum Alpha-Fetoprotein Screening." *Obstetrics and Gynecology* 56 (1980): 669–70.

Macri, J. "Neural Tube Defects." *Female Patient* 6(1981): 75–79.

"Fetoscopy Shows Deformities Missed Previously." *Ob.Gyn. News,* 16(1981): 37.

MacKenzie, I. Z., and Maclean, D. A. "Pure Fetal Blood from the Umbilical Cord Obtained at Fetoscopy: Experience with 125 Consecutive Cases." *American Journal of Obstetrics and Gynecology* 138(1980): 1214–18.

Wenk, R. E., et al. "A Prospective Evaluation of Placental Lactogen as a Test for Neonatal Risk." *American Journal of Clinical Pathology* 71(1979): 72.

Diagnostic Ultrasound in Obstetrics and Gynecology. ACOG Technical Bulletin no. 63, October 1981.

"The Role of Ultrasound in High-Risk Obstetrics." Symposium. *Contemporary OB/GYN* 18 (1981): 44–80.

Shawker, T. H., et al. "Early Fetal Movement: A Real-Time Ultrasound Study." *Obstetrics and Gynecology* 55(1980): 194–97.

Hobbins, J. C. "Ultrasound Can Diagnose Fetal Malformations." *Contemporary OB/GYN* 19 (1982): 99–104.

Dunne, M. G., and Johnson, M. L. "The Ultrasonic Demonstration of Fetal Abnormalities in Utero." *Journal of Reproductive Medicine* 23 (1979): 195–206.

Sampson, M. D., et al. Prediction of Intrauterine Fetal Weight Using Real-Time Ultrasound. *American Journal of Obstetrics and Gynecology* 142(1982): 554–56.

O'Brien, G. D., and Queenan, J. T. "Growth of the Ultrasound Fetal Femur Length During Normal Pregnancy." *American Journal of Obstetrics and Gynecology* 141:833–37, 1981.

Hobbins, J. C.; Berkowitz, R. L.; and Grannum, P. A. P. "Diagnosis and Antepartum Management of Intrauterine Growth Retardation." *Journal of Reproductive Medicine* 21(1978): 319–24.

Mulhern, Jr., C. B.; Arger, P. H.; and Coleman, B. G. "Ultrasonic Diagnosis of Placental Abnormalities in Situ." *Journal of the American Medical Association* 244(1980): 2339–41.

Hobbins, J. C.; Berkowitz, R. L.; and Hohler, C. W. "How Safe Is Ultrasound in Obstetrics?" *Contemporary OB/GYN* 14(1979): 63–74.

"Question of Risk Still Hovers over Routine Prenatal Use of Ultrasound." *Journal of the American Medical Association* 247(1982): 2195–97.

Casano, K. "Little Concern on Ultrasound DNA Studies." *Ob.Gyn. News* 14(1979): 3–32.

Adamson, G. D.; Cousin, A. J.; and Gare, D. J. "Rhythmic Fetal Movements." *American Journal of Obstetrics and Gynecology* 136(1980): 239–42.

Sadovsky, E. "The Scoring System Using Fetal Movements." *Contemporary OB/GYN* 19 (1982): 142–44.

Patrick, J., et al. "Patterns of Gross Fetal Body Movements over 24-Hour Observation Intervals During the Last 10 Weeks of Pregnancy." *American Journal of Obstetrics and Gynecology* 142(1982) 363–71.

Hertogs, K., et al. "Maternal Perception of Fetal Motor Activity." *British Medical Journal* 2 (1979): 1183.

Rayburn, W. F., and McKean, H. E. "Maternal Preception of Fetal Movement and Perinatal Outcome." *Obstetrics and Gynecology* 56 (1980): 161–64.

Rayburn, W. F. "Clinical Significance of Percepti-

ble Fetal Motion." *American Journal of Obstetrics and Gynecology* 138(1980): 210–12.

Roberts, A. B., et al. "Fetal Activity in 100 Normal Third-Trimester Pregnancies." *British Journal of Obstetrics and Gynecology* 87 (1980): 480.

Ritchie, J. W. K. "Fetal Breathing and Generalized Fetal Movements in Normal Antenatal Patients." *British Journal of Obstetrics and Gynaecology* 86(1979): 612.

Harper, R. G., et al. "Fetal Movement, Biochemical and Biophysical Parameters, and the Outcome of Pregnancy." *American Journal of Obstetrics and Gynecology* 141(1981): 39–42.

Richardson, B., et al. "Effects of External Physical Stimulation on Fetuses Near Term." *American Journal of Obstetrics and Gynecology* 139 (1981): 344–52.

Trudinger, B. J., et al. "Fetal Breathing Movements and Other Tests of Fetal Well-being: A Comparative Evaluation." *Brisith Medical Journal* 2(1979): 577–79.

Trudinger, B. J., and Knight, P. C. "Fetal Age and Patterns of Human Fetal Breathing Movements." *American Journal of Obstetrics and Gynecology* 137(1980): 724–28.

Boddy, K. "Fetal Breathing: Its Physiologic and Clinical Implications." *Hospital Practice,* February 1979, pp. 89–96.

Boylin, P., and Lewis, P. J. "Fetal Breathing in Labor." *Obstetrics and Gynecology* 56(1980): 35–38.

Devoe, L. D. "Clinical Implications of Prospective Antepartum Fetal Heart Rate Patterns." *American Journal of Obstetrics and Gynecology* 137 (1980): 983–90.

Council on Scientific Affairs. "Electronic Fetal Monitoring." *Journal of the American Medical Association* 246(1981): 2370–73.

Schifrin, B. F. "The Rationale for Antepartum Fetal Heart Rate Monitoring." *Journal of Reproductive Medicine* 23(1979): 213–20.

Weingold, A. D.; Yonekura, M. L.; and O'Kieffe, J. "Nonstress Testing." *American Journal of Obstetrics and Gynecology* 138(1980): 195–202.

Rayburn, W.; Greene, Jr., J.; and Donaldson, M. "Nonstress Testing and Perinatal Outcome." *Journal of Reproductive Medicine* 24(1980): 191–96.

Gandhi, J., and Gugliucci, C. L. "Nonstress Test Prediction of Fetal Status." *Journal of Reproductive Medicine* 27(1982): 80–88.

Pratt, D., et al. "Fetal Stress and Nonstress Tests: An Analysis and Comparison of Their Ability to Identify Fetal Outcome." *Obstetrics and Gynecology* 54(1979): 419–23.

Druzin, M. L.; Paul, R. H.; and Gratacos, J. "Current Status of the Traction Stress Test." *Journal of Reproductive Medicine* 23(1979): 222–26.

Lin, C., et al. "Oxytocin Challenge Test and Intrauterine Growth Retardation." *American Journal of Obstetrics and Gynecology* 140(1981): 282–88.

Slomka, C., and Phelan, J. P. "Pregnancy Outcome in the Woman with a Nonreactive Nonstress Test and a Positive Contraction Stress Test." *American Journal of Obstetrics and Gynecology* 139(1981): 11–15.

Crane, J., et al. "Subsequent Physical and Mental Development in Infants with Positive Contraction Stress Tests." *Journal of Reproductive Medicine* 26(1981): 113–18.

Boehm, F. H.; Davidson, K. K.; and Barrett, J. M. "The Effect of Electronic Fetal Monitoring on the Incidence of Cesarean Section." *American Journal of Obstetrics and Gynecology* 140 (1981): 295.

Intrapartum Fetal Monitoring. ACOG Technical Bulletin no. 44, January 1977.

Krebs, H. B., et al. "Intrapartum Fetal Heart Rate Monitoring." *American Journal of Obstetrics and Gynecology* 137(1980): 936–43.

Gaziano, E. P.; Freeman, D. W.; and Endel, R. P. "FHR Variability and Other Heart Rate Observations During Second Stage Labor." *Obstetrics and Gynecology* 56(1980): 42–47.

Sacks, D. A., et al. "Sinusoidal Fetal Heart Rate Pattern with Intrapartum Fetal Death." *Journal of Reproductive Medicine* 24(1980): 171–73.

Petrie, R. H. "How Intrapartum Drugs Affect FHR." *Contemporary OB/GYN* 16(1980): 61–75.

Monheit, A., and Cousins, L. "When Do You Measure Scalp Blood pH? *Contemporary OB/GYN* 18(1981): 107–21.

Fetal Blood Sampling. ACOG Technical Bulletin no. 42, October 1976.

Young, D. C., et al. "Fetal Scalp Blood pH Sampling: Its Value in an Active Obstetric Unit." *American Journal of Obstetrics and Gynecology* 136(1980): 276–81.

Trudinger, B. J., and Boylan, P. "Antepartum Fetal Heart Rate Monitoring: Value of Sound Stimulation." *Obstetrics and Gynecology* 55 (1980): 265–67.

Ritchie, K., and McClure, G. "Prematurity." *Lancet* 2(1979): 1227–29.

Barden, T. P.; Peter, J. B.; and Merkatz, I. R. "Ritodrine Hydrochloride: A Betamimetic Agent for Use in Preterm Labor." *Obstetrics and Gynecology* 56(1980): 1–5.

Brazy, J. E., and Pupkin, M. J. "Effects of Maternal Isoxsuprine Administration on Preterm Infants." *Journal of Pediatrics* 94(1979): 444.

Schenken, R. S., et al. "Treatment of Premature Labor with Beta Sympathomimetics: Results with Isoxsuprine." *American Journal of Obstetrics and Gynecology* 137(1980): 773–79.

Tocolytic Agents. Proceedings of a symposium on tocolytic therapy. Society of Perinatal Obstetricians, New Orleans, May 2, 1980.

Obladen, M.; Merritt, T. A.; and Gluck, L. "Acceleration of Pulmonary Surfactant Maturation in Stressed Pregnancies: A Study of Neonatal Lung Effluent." *American Journal of Obstetrics and Gynecology* 135(1979): 1079–85.

Kaspi, E., et al. "Dexamethasome for Prevention of Respiratory Distress Syndrome: Multiple Perinatal Factors." *Obstetrics and Gynecology* 57(1981): 41–46.

The Selective Use of Rho(D) Immune Globulin (RhIG). ACOG Technical Bulletin no. 61, March 1981.

Harrison, M. R., et al. "Management of the Fetus with a Urinary Tract Malformation." *Journal of the American Medical Association* 246(1981): 635–39.

Fletcher, J. C. "The Fetus as a Patient: Ethical Issues." *Journal of the American Medical Association* 246(1981): 772–73.

Golbus, M. S., et al. "In Utero Treatment of Urinary Tract Obstruction." *American Journal of Obstetrics and Gynecology* 142(1982): 383–88.

Neonatal Metabolic Diseases. ACOG Technical Bulletin no. 60, January 1981.

Henig, R. M. "Saving Babies Before Birth." *New York Times Magazine,* Feb. 28, 1982, pp. 18, 48.

Lenke, R. R., and Levy, H. L. "Maternal Phenylketonuria: Results of Dietary Therapy." *American Journal of Obstetrics and Gynecology* 142(1982): 548–52.

Alter, B. P. "Prenatal Diagnosis of Hemoglobinopathies and Other Hematologic Diseases." *Journal of Pediatrics* 95(1979): 501–13.

Fletcher, J. C. "Prenatal Diagnosis of the Hemoglobinopathies: Ethical Issues." *American Journal of Obstetrics and Gynecology* 135(1979): 53–56.

Morrison, J. C.; Ruvinsky, E. D.; and Nicholls, E. T. "Sickling and Pregnancy: A Worrisome Combination" *Contemporary OB/GYN* 18(1981): 125–31.

Verma, U. L., et al. "Screening for FGR by the Roll-over Test." *Obstetrics and Gynecology* 56(1980): 591–94.

Kuntz, W. D. "Supine Pressor (Roll-over) Test: An Evaluation." *American Journal of Obstetrics and Gynecology* 137(1980): 764–68.

Chapter 11
Childbirth and the Postpartum Period

Briend, A. "Fetal Malnutrition: The Price of Upright Posture?" *British Medical Journal* 2(1979): 317–19.

Flynn, A. M., et al. "Ambulation in Labour." *British Medical Journal* 2(1978): 591–93.

Read, J. A.; Miller, F. C.; and Paul, R. H. "Randomized Trial of Ambulation Versus Oxytocin for Labor Enhancement: A Preliminary Report." *American Journal of Obstetrics and Gynecology* 139(1981): 669–72.

"Squatting Position for Childbirth?" *Female Patient* 7(1982): 36.

Haukeland, I. "An Alternative Delivery Position: New Delivery Chair Developed and Tested at Kongsberg Hospital." *American Journal of Obstetrics and Gynecology* 141(1981): 115–17.

Caldeyro-Barcia, R. "The Influence of Maternal Position During the Second Stage of Labor." In P. Simkin and C. Reinke, eds., *Kaleidoscope of Childbearing.* Seattle: Pennypress, 1978.

Brock-Utne, J. G., et al. "Advantages of Left Over Right Lateral Tilt for Caesarean Section." *South African Medical Journal* 54(1978): 489.

Bassell, G. M.; Humayun, S. G.; and Marx, G. F. "Maternal Bearing Down Efforts—Another Fetal Risk?" *Obstetrics and Gynecology* 56 (1980): 39–41.

Goodlin, R. C. "Maternal Bearing-Down Efforts." *American Journal of Obstetrics and Gynecology* 57(1981): 679–80.

Friedman, E. A. "An Objective Method of Evaluating Labor." *Hospital Practice,* July 1970, pp. 82–87.

Kappy, K. A., et al. "Premature Rupture of the Membranes at Term: A Comparison of Induced and Spontaneous Labor." *Journal of Reproductive Medicine* 27(1982): 29–33.

Varner, M. W., and Jalask, R. P. "Conservative Management of Premature Rupture of the Membranes." *American Journal of Obstetrics and Gynecology* 140(1981): 39–45.

Stedman, C. M., et al. "Management of Premature Rupture of the Membranes: Assessing Amniotic Fluid in the Vagina for Phosphatidylglycerol." *American Journal of Obstetrics and Gynecology* 140(1981): 34–38.

Induction of Labor. ACOG Technical Bulletin no. 49, May 1978.

Rindfuss, R. R.; Gortmaker, S. L.; and Ladinsky, J. L. "Elective Induction and Stimulation of Labor and the Health of the Infant." *American Journal of Public Health* 68(1978): 872.

"New Restrictions on Oxytocin Use." *FDA Drug Bulletin* 8(1978): 30.

Nichols, E. E. "Guidelines for Induction of Labor." *Journal of the American Medical Association* 245(1981): 777–78.

Brinsden, P. R., and Clark, A. D. "Postpartum Haemorrhage After Induced and Spontaneous Labour." *British Medical Journal* 2(1978): 855–56.

Ulmsten, U., et al. "Intracervical Application of Prostaglandin Gel for Induction of Term Labor." *Obstetrics and Gynecology* 59(1982): 336–39.

Homburg, R.; Ludomirski, A.; and Insler, B. "Detection of Fetal Risk in Postmaturity." *British Journal of Obstetrics and Gynecology* 86

(1979): 759.

Rayburn, W. F., and Chang, F. E. "Management of the Uncomplicated Postdate Pregnancy." *Journal of Reproductive Medicine* 26(1981): 93–95.

Miyazaki, F. S., and Miyazaki, B. A. "False Reactive Nonstress Tests in Postterm Pregnancy." *American Journal of Obstetrics and Gynecology* 140(1981): 269–76.

McBride, W. G., et al. "Method of Delivery and Developmental Outcome at Five Years of Age." *Medical Journal of Australia* 1(1979): 301.

O'Briscoll, K., et al. "Traumatic Intracranial Haemorrhage in Firstborn Infants and Delivery with Obstetric Forceps." *British Journal of Obstetrics and Gynecology* 88(1981): 577.

Leijon, I. "Neurology and Behavior of Newborn Infants Delivered by Vacuum Extraction on Maternal Indication." *Acta Pediatrics of Scandinavia* 69(1980): 625.

Fianu, S., and Vaclavinkova, V. "The Site of Placental Attachment as a Factor in the Aetiology of Breech Presentation." *Acta Obstetrics and Gynecology of Scandinavia* 57(1978): 371.

Collea, J. V.; Chein, C.; and Quilligan, E. J. "The Randomized Management of Term Frank Breech Presentation: A Study of 208 Cases." *American Journal of Obstetrics and Gynecology* 137(1980): 235.

Bowes, Jr., W. A., et al. "Breech Delivery: Evaluation of the Method of Delivery on Perinatal Results and Maternal Morbidity." *American Journal of Obstetrics and Gynecology* 135(1979): 965–73.

Mann, L. I., and Gallant, J. M. "Modern Management of the Breech Delivery." *American Journal of Obstetrics and Gynecology* 134(1979): 611.

Duenholter, J. H., et al. "A Paired Controlled Study of Vaginal and Abdominal Delivery of the Low Birth Weight Breech Fetus." *Obstetrics and Gynecology* 54(1979): 310.

Haberkern, T. M.; Smith, D. W.; and Jones, K. L. "The 'Breech Head' and Its Relevance." *American Journal of Diseases in Childhood* 133 (1979): 154.

Gimovsky, M. L.; Petrie, R. H.; and Todd, W. D. "Neonatal Performance of the Selected Term Vaginal Breech Delivery." *Obstetrics and Gynecology* 56(1980): 687.

Van Dorsten, J.; Schifrin, B. S.; and Wallace, R. L. "Randomized Controlled Trial of External Cephalic Version with Tocolysis in Late Pregnancy." *American Journal of Obstetrics and Gynecology* 141(1981): 417–24.

The Cesarean Birth Task Force. "National Institutes of Health Consensus Development Statement on Cesarean Childbirth." *Obstetrics and Gynecology* 57(1981): 537–44.

Amirikia, H.; Zarewych, B.; and Evans, T. N. "Cesarean Section: A 15-Year Review of

Changing Incidence, Indications, and Risks." *American Journal of Obstetrics and Gynecology* 140(1981): 81–86.

Leppert, P. C.; and Petrie, R. H. "Delivering the Preterm by Cesarean." *Contemporary OB/GYN* 19(1982): 116–25.

Evrard, J. R.; Gold, E. M.; and Cahill, T. F. "Cesarean Section: A Contemporary Assessment." *Journal of Reproductive Medicine* 24(1980): 147–52.

Boehm, F. H.; Davidson, J. J.; and Barrett, J. M. "The Effect of Electronic Fetal Monitoring on the Incidence of Cesarean Section." *American Journal of Obstetrics and Gynecology* 140 (1981): 295–98.

Neutra, R. R.; Greenland, S.; and Friedman, E. A. "Effect of Fetal Monitoring on Cesarean Section Rates." *Obstetrics and Gynecology* 55 (1980): 175–79.

Zalar, Jr., R. W., and Quilligan, E. J. "The Influence of Scalp Sampling on the Cesarean Section Rate for Fetal Distress." *American Journal of Obstetrics and Gynecology* 135(1979): 239–46.

Wilson, R. W., and Schifrin, B. S. "Is Any Pregnancy Low Risk?" *Obstetrics and Gynecology* 55(1980): 653–55.

Bottoms, S. F.; Rosen, M. G.; and Sokol, R. J. "The Increase in the Cesarean Birth Rate." *New England Journal of Medicine* 302(1980): 559–63.

Horowitz, B. J.; Edelstein, S. W.; and Lippman, L. "Once a Cesarean, Always a Cesarean." *Obstetrical and Gynecological Survey* 36(1981): 592–97.

Lavin, J. P., et al. "Vaginal Delivery in Patients with a Prior Cesarean Section." *Obstetrics and Gynecology* 59(1982): 135–47.

Vemianczuk, N. N.; Hunter, D. J. S.; and Taylor, D. W. "Trial of Labor After Previous Cesarean Section: Prognostic Indicators of Outcome." *American Journal of Obstetrics and Gynecology* 142(1982): 640–42.

Obstetric Anesthesia and Analgesia, ACOG Technical Bulletin no. 57, January 1980.

Fishburne, J. J. "Systemic Obstetric Analgesia." *Ob/Gyn Digest* 21(1979): 13–33.

Kim, W. Y.; Pomerance, J. J.; and Miller, A. A. "Lidocaine Intoxication in a Newborn Following Local Anesthesia for Episiotomy." *Pediatrics* 64 (1979): 643–45.

Van Dorsten, K. P.; Miller, F. C.; and Yeh, S. "Spacing the Injection Interval with Paracervical Block: A Randomized Study." *Obstetrics and Gynecology* 58(1981): 696–701.

James, F. M., et al. "Chloroprocaine vs. Bupivacaine for Lumbar Epidural Analgesia for Elective Cesarean Section." *Anesthesiology* 52 (1980): 488.

Endler, G. C. "Conduction Anesthesia in Obstetrics and Its Effects upon Fetus and Newborn." *Journal of Reproductive Medicine* 24(1980): 83–91.

Moore, D. C., et al. "Chloroprocaine Neurotoxicity: Four Additional Cases." *Anesthesia and Analgesia* 61(1982): 155–59.

Datta, S., et al. "Neonatal Effect of Prolonged Anesthetic Induction for Cesarean Section." *Obstetrics and Gynecology* 58(1981): 331–35.

Abboud, T. K., et al. "Enflurane Analgesia in Obstetrics." *Anesthesia and Analgesia* 60(1981): 133.

Pickering, B. G.; Palahniuk, R. J.; and Cumming, M. "Cimetidine Premedication in Elective Cesarean Section." *Canadian Anaesthesiology Society Journal* 27(1980): 33.

Oats, J. N.; Vasey, D. P.; and Waldron, V. A. "Effects of Ketamine on the Pregnant Uterus." *British Journal of Anaesthesiology* 51(1979): 1163.

Zax, M.; Sameroff, A. J.; and Farnum, J. E. "Childbirth Education, Maternal Attitudes, and Delivery." *American Journal of Obstetrics and Gynecology* 123(1975): 185–90.

Friedman, D. "Parturiphobia." *American Journal of Obstetrics and Gynecology* 118(1974): 130–35.

Samko, M. R., and Schoenfeld, L. S. "Hypnotic Susceptibility and the Lamaze Childbirth Experience." *American Journal of Obstetrics and Gynecology* 121(1975): 631–36.

Shapiro, H. I., and Schmidt, L. G. "Evaluation of the Psychoprophylactic Method of Childbirth in the Primigravida." *American Medicine* 37 (1973): 341–43.

Herrera, A. J. "Prepared Natural Childbirth vs. Regular Labor and Delivery: Differences in the Outcome." *Connecticut Medicine* 43(1979): 643.

Brewer, G. S. "Natural Childbirth: A Different Method." *Mother's Manual,* October 1980, pp. 38–41.

Crystle, C. D., et al. "The Leboyer Method of Delivery." *Journal of Reproductive Medicine* 25 (1980): 267–71.

Nelson, N. M., et al. "A Randomized Clinical Trial of the Leboyer Approach to Childbirth." *New England Journal of Medicine* 302(1980): 655–60.

Grover, J. W. "An Obstetrician Comments on Nonviolent Birth." *Female Patient,* July 1979, pp. 62–66.

Englund, S. "Birth Without Violence." *New York Times Magazine,* Dec. 8, 1974, pp. 113–24.

Mahan, C. S. "Ways to Strengthen a Mother-Infant Bond." *Contemporary OB/GYN* 17 (1981): 177–87.

Burnett, C. A., et al. "Home Delivery and Neonatal Mortality in North Carolina." *Journal of the American Medical Association* 244(1980): 2741–45.

Adamson, G. D., and Gare, D. J. "Home or Hospital Births?" *Journal of the American Medical*

Association 243(1980): 1732–36.

DeJong, Jr., R. N.; Shy, K. K.; and Carr, K. C. "An Out-of-Hospital Birth Center Using University Referral." *Obstetrics and Gynecology* 58(1981): 703–7.

Dobbs, K. B., and Shy, K. K. "Alternative Birth Rooms and Birth Options." *Obstetrics and Gynecology* 58(1981): 626–30.

Annexton, M. "Parent-Infant Bonding Sought in 'Birthing' Centers." *Journal of the American Medical Association* 240(1978): 823–26.

Goodlin, R. C. "Low-Risk Obstetric Care for Low-Risk Mothers." *Lancet* 1(1980): 1017–19.

Interprofessional Task Force on Health Care of Women and Children. *Family-Centered Maternity/Newborn Care in Hospitals.* June 1978.

Collins, N. "Birthing Rooms: The Happy Compromise." *Mothers' Manual,* May–June 1981, pp. 27–31.

Steinmann, M. "Now the Nurse-Midwife." *New York Times Magazine,* Nov. 23, 1975, pp. 34–36.

Mann, R. J. "San Francisco General Hospital Nurse-Midwifery Practice: The First Thousand Births." *American Journal of Obstetrics and Gynecology* 140(1981): 676–82.

Scott, W. C. "Lay Midwives: Some Solutions for a Serious Problem." *Contemporary OB/GYN* 16 (1980): 37–53.

Shannon, F. T.; Horwood, L. J.; and Fergusson, D. M. "Infant Circumcision." *New Zealand Medical Journal* 90(1979): 283.

Grimes, D. A. "Routine Circumcision Reconsidered." *American Journal of Nursing,* January 1980, pp. 108–9.

Dewhurst, C. J.; Harrison, R. F.; and Biswas, S. "Inhibition of Puerperal Lactation: A Double-blind Study of Bromocriptine and Placebo." *Acta Obstetrics and Gynecology of Scandinavia* 56(1977): 327.

Cavallero, A., et al. "Metergoline as a Lactation Inhibitor." *Journal of Reproductive Medicine* 27(1982): 202–6.

Greentree, L. B. "Inhibition of Prolactin by Pyridoxine." *American Journal of Obstetrics and Gynecology* 135(1979): 280.

Waterlow, J. C., and Thomson, A. M. "Observations on the Adequacy of Breast-Feeding." *Lancet* 2(1979): 238–41.

Weinstein, L. "Breast Milk: A Natural Resource." *American Journal of Obstetrics and Gynecology* 136(1980): 973–75.

The Womanly Art of Breastfeeding. La Leche League International, Franklin Park, Ill., 1981.

Saarinen, U. M., et al. "Prolonged Breast-Feeding as Prophylaxis for Atopic Disease." *Lancet,* 2 (1979): 163–66.

Welsh, J. K., and May, J. T. "Anti-infective Properties of Breast Milk." *Journal of Pediatrics* 94 (1979): 1–9.

Fallott, M. E.; Boyd, J. L.; and Oski, F. A. "Breast-Feeding Reduces Incidence of Hospital Admissions for Infection in Infants." *Pediatrics* 65(1980): 1121–24.

Cunningham, M. D.; Gesai, N. S.; and Charlet, S. S. "Human Milk for the Premature Infant." *Female Patient,* 1979, pp. 29–33.

Pitt, J. "Breast Milk and the High-Risk Baby: Potential Benefits and Hazards." *Hospital Practice,* May 1979, pp. 81–86.

Bolton-Maggs, P. H. "Breast or Bottle." *British Medical Journal* 2(1979): 371–72.

Cunningham, A. S. "Morbidity in Breast-Fed and Artifically Fed Infants." *Journal of Pediatrics* 95(1979): 685–89.

Aono, T., et al. "Augmentation of Puerperal Lactation by Oral Administration of Sulpiride." *Journal of Clinical Endocrinology and Metabolism* 48(1979): 478.

Robson, K. M.; Brant, H. A.; and Kumar, R. "Maternal Sexuality During First Pregnancy and After Childbirth." *British Journal of Obstetrics and Gynaecology* 88(1981): 882.

Keith, L., et al. *Postpartum and Postabortal Contraception.* Pittsburgh: Synapse, 1979.

Vorherr, H. "Contraception After Abortion and Postpartum." *American Journal of Obstetrics and Gynecology* 117(1973): 1002–22.

Campodonico, I.; Guerrero, B.; and Landa, L. "Effect of a Low-Dose Oral Contraceptive on Lactation." *Clinical Therapeutics* 1(1978): 454–59.

Breastfeeding and Oral Contraceptives. Franklin Park, Ill.: La Leche League International, 1975.

Mishell, Jr., D. R., and Roy, S. "Copper Intrauterine Contraceptive Device Event Rates Following Insertion Four to Eight Weeks Postpartum." *American Journal of Obstetrics and Gynecology* 143(1982): 29–35.

Haycock, C. E. "Jogging After Childbirth." *Journal of the American Medical Association* 246 (1981): 2500.

Brewer, G. S. "Fitting in Fitness." *Mothers' Manual,* September–October 1979, pp. 48–50.

Wallace, J. P. "Exercise in Pregnancy and Postpartum." *Female Patient* 1979, pp. 78–83.

Dressendorfer, R. H. "Physical Training During Pregnancy and Lactation." *Physician and Sportsmedicine,* February 1978, pp. 74–80.

Menaker, W., and Menaker, A. "Lunar Periodicity in Human Reproduction: A Likely Unit of Biological Time." *American Journal of Obstetrics and Gynecology* 77(1959): 905–14.

Osley, M.; Summerville, D.; and Borst, L. B. "Natality and the Moon." *American Journal of Obstetrics and Gynecology* 117(1973): 413–15.

Phillips, R. N.; Thornton, J.; and Gleicher, N. "Physician Bias in Cesarean Sections." *Journal of the American Medical Association* 248 (1982): 1082–84.

Index

Permissions
Acknowledgments

Grateful acknowledgment is made for the following:

Some of the material in Chapter 1 is based on *The Birth Control Book,* by Howard Shapiro. Reprinted by permission of St. Martin's Press, Incorporated.

Drawing on page 357: Century Mfg. Co., Industrial Park, Aurora, Nebraska 68818.

Table 2–2 List courtesy of Idant Corporation, 645 Madison Avenue, New York, New York.

Figures 3–1 through 3–9, exercises from the Pre-Natal Exercise Program developed by Ms. Ann Ljone of Norwalk, Connecticut, and Mrs. Aud Marcussen of Fairfield, Connecticut, certified aquatic instructors, are included by permission.

Table 5–1 from *Cutis* 28(1981) 124. Reprinted by permission of Yehudi M. Felman, M.D., Nikitas and Cutis.

Table 6–2 from ACOG Technical Bulletin *Immunization During Pregnancy,* no. 64, May 1982. Reprinted by permission of the American College of Obstetricians and Gynecologists.

Table 8–1 Copyright 1981 by Consumers Union of United States, Inc., Mount Vernon, New York 10550. Reprinted by permission from *Consumer Reports,* October 1981.

Table 8–2 from the Food and Drug Administration, U.S. Department of Health and Human Services Publication No. (FDA) 81-1081.

Table 8–3 from "Update: Nutritional Analysis of Fast Foods," by E. A. Young, E. H. Brennan, and G. L. Irving, *Public Health Currents,* Ross Timesaver, vol. 21-1103, May–June 1981. Reprinted by permission of E. A. Young and Ross Laboratories.

Table 9–1 reprinted by permission of Carl J. Collica, M.S. Chief, Section of Radiological Physics, Norwalk Hospital.

Table 9–2 from *Women's Occupations, Smoking, and Other Diseases* reprinted by permission of the College of Physicians & Surgeons of Columbia University.

The boxed material on pages 294–295 from *Environmental and Occupational Health Hazards: Primary Care Guide,* published by the Health Systems Agency of New York City. Reproduced by permission.

Table 10–1 from *Birth Defects* (13) (3A) : 123, 1977..Reprinted by permission of the Birth Defects Institute, New York State Department of Health.

Figures 10–2, 10–3, and 10–4 based on illustrations from *Genetic Counseling,* a publication of the March of Dimes Birth Defects Foundation. Reproduced by permission.

Figures 10–5 from "Prenatal Diagnosis of Inborn Defects: A Status Report." Reproduced by permission of Henry L. Nadler, M.D., Dean, School of Medicine, Wayne State University.

Figure 11–2 from *Female Patient,* May 1978. Reproduced by permission of Emanuel A. Friedman, M.D., Harvard Medical School and Beth Israel Hospital.